CONTENTS

CW01506684

PSYCHOLOGY
FOR MEDICINE
& HEALTHCARE

RICHARD DE VISSER & SUSAN AYERS

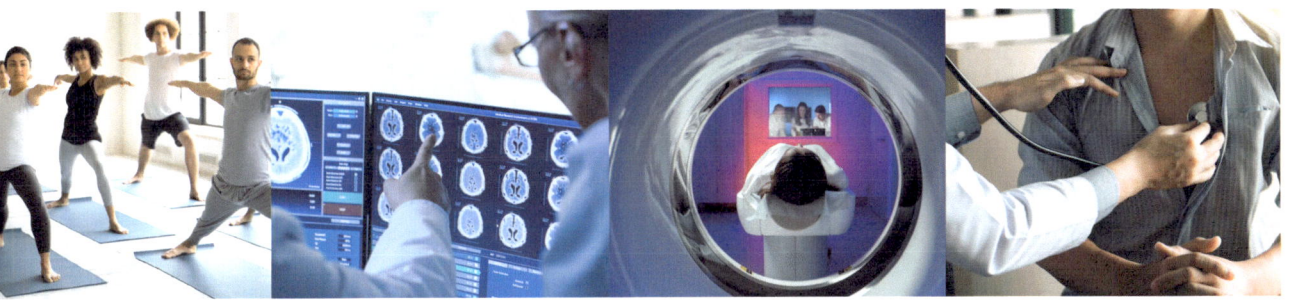

PSYCHOLOGY FOR MEDICINE & HEALTHCARE

FOURTH EDITION

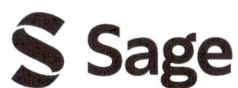

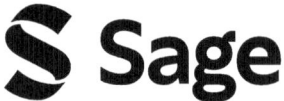

1 Oliver's Yard
55 City Road
London EC1Y 1SP

2455 Teller Road
Thousand Oaks
California 91320

Unit No 323-333, Third Floor, F-Block
International Trade Tower
Nehru Place, New Delhi – 110 019

8 Marina View Suite 43-053
Asia Square Tower 1
Singapore 018960

Editor: Janka Romero
Assistant editor: Hanine Kadi
Production editor: Martin Fox
Copyeditor: Sarah Bury
Proofreader: Thea Watson
Marketing manager: Lucia Sweet
Cover design: Bhairvi Vyas
Typeset by: C&M Digitals (P) Ltd, Chennai, India
Printed in the UK

Library of Congress Control Number: 2024941570

British Library Cataloguing in Publication data

A catalogue record for this book is available from the British Library

ISBN 978-1-5296-8508-4
ISBN 978-1-5296-8509-1 (pbk)

Richard de Visser: For Thom, Felix, and Iris

Susan Ayers: For my grandchildren

LIST OF FIGURES AND TABLES

Figures

Tables

LIST OF LEARNING FEATURES

Highlight Boxes

Research Boxes

Case Studies

Clinical Notes

Activities

GUIDED TOUR

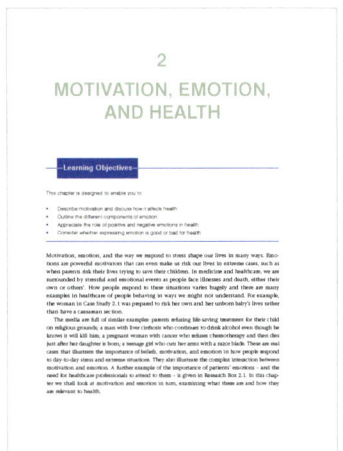

Learning Objectives are given at the beginning of each chapter. These state the most important things we hope you will learn from each chapter.

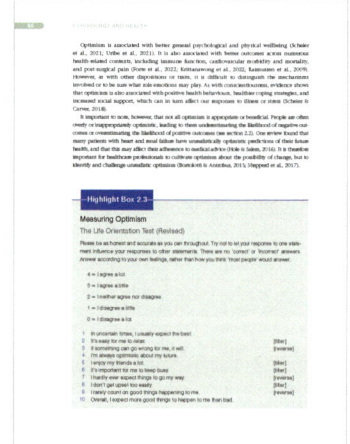

Highlight Boxes are used to illustrate the key concepts described in the text. Some of these are lists of key points, some are descriptions of important issues, and others are diagrams or tables of information.

Figures A variety of figures is used to help you understand the material described in the text. These include photographs, diagrams, flowcharts, and theoretical models.

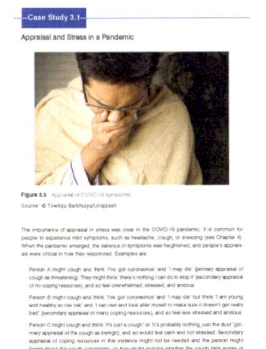
Case Studies are used to illustrate peoples' experiences of the issues described in the text. They also show how psychological theories and techniques can be used in clinical practice to help patients.

Clinical Notes give key recommendations and tips for healthcare practice based on the psychological principles and techniques described in the text.

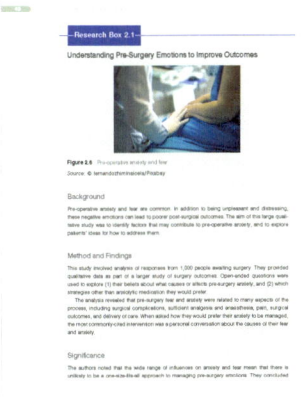
Research Boxes describe a research study that illustrates the psychological concepts or findings described in the text, and gives examples of how different research methods are applied in clinical contexts.

Activities are designed to help you stop and think about the information contained in the text and how it might apply to the real world or to your own life.

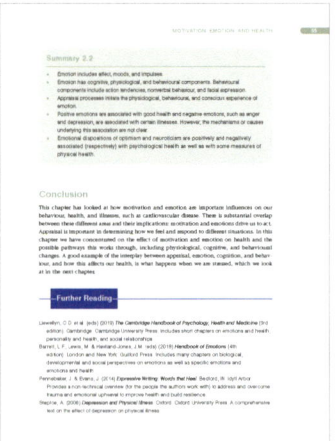

Further Reading At the end of each chapter there are suggestions for further reading, along with brief comments about each resource to help you choose which ones to read.

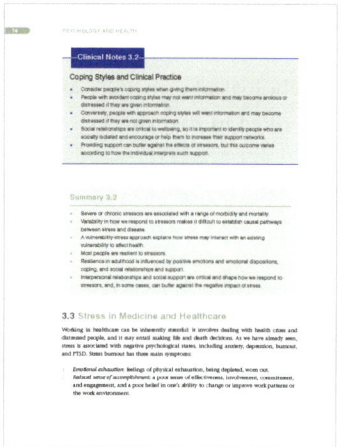

Summaries Each section concludes with a bullet-point summary of the most important psychological theories and applications covered in that section. These summaries relate to the learning objectives and revision questions, so will help you learn and revise.

Revision Questions are included at the end of every chapter to help you learn and revise for exams.

ONLINE RESOURCES

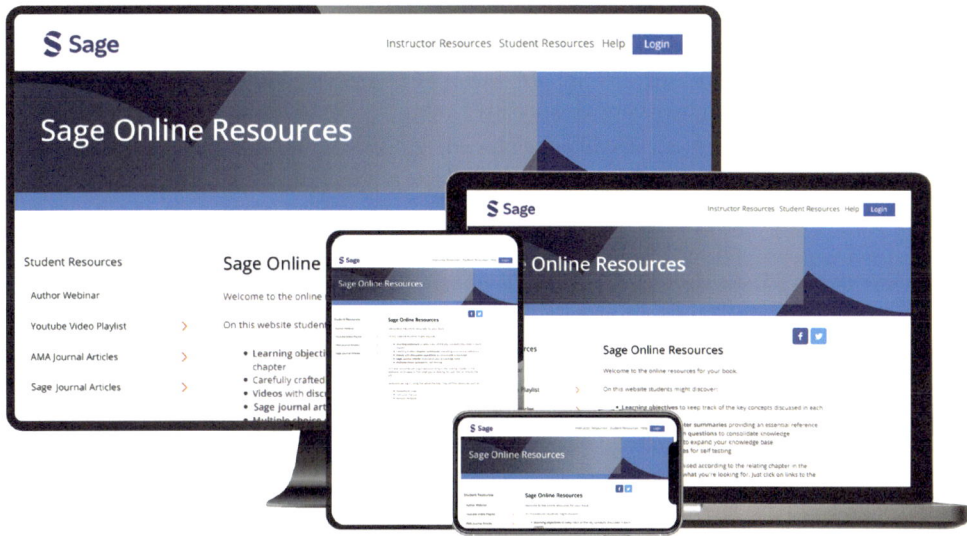

The fourth edition of *Psychology for Medicine and Healthcare* is supported by a range of additional resources for instructors to support teaching, which are available at: **https://study.sagepub.com/devisser-ayers4e**

For Instructors

- A **Teaching Guide** providing you with author-selected journal articles and case studies to use in class or for assignments.
- A **Test Bank** containing multiple-choice questions related to the key concepts in each chapter can be downloaded and used in class, as homework, or in exams.
- A **Resource Pack**, which allows you to upload the Test Bank directly to your university's virtual learning management system.

ABOUT THE AUTHORS

Richard de Visser is Professor of Health Psychology at Brighton & Sussex Medical School. His research interests span a broad range of topics in health psychology, including sexuality and relationships, gender and health, alcohol use, use of health services, and cross-cultural analyses. He has expertise in qualitative and quantitative methods, intervention studies, and mixed-method designs, and he has received awards for his individual and group teaching. Richard is co-editor of *The Palgrave Handbook of Psychological Perspectives on Alcohol Consumption* (2021) and co-author of *Psychology for Medicine and Healthcare* (2011, 2017, 2021).

Susan Ayers is a psychologist specialising in wellbeing and mental health during pregnancy and after birth. She is a professor at City St George's, University of London in the School of Health and Psychological Sciences, a chartered health psychologist, and a cognitive behaviour therapist. Since obtaining her PhD from the University of London, Susan worked at St George's Medical School (London) and Brighton & Sussex Medical School (Sussex) before moving to City (now City St George's), University of London. Susan is co-author of *Psychology for Medicine and Healthcare* (2011, 2017, 2021) and editor of *The Cambridge Handbook of Psychology, Health and Medicine* (2007, 2019). She has given numerous invited lectures and has received awards from the British Medical Association Foundation (2023), the Miriam de Senarclens Foundation (2022), and the Society of Reproductive and Infant Psychology (2012).

ACKNOWLEDGEMENTS

There is more to a book than its contents, and the story behind this one would make a good read in itself. The journey started because we were frustrated by the lack of a comprehensive textbook on psychology for medical students. We happened to mention this in passing to the people at SAGE who harnessed all their enthusiasm and considerable expertise into getting the first edition of this book published in 2011. SAGE started the ball rolling with the first edition and their enthusiasm and subsequent success of the book took us into a second, third, and now fourth edition, so we are grateful for their impetus and help.

This fourth edition gave us the opportunity to make some important changes. The book is used in many countries by people studying medicine and other health professions. The language and examples throughout the book therefore reflect the global community and diversity of healthcare students and professionals using this book. A key addition in this edition is a chapter on diversity, inclusivity, and equality in medicine and healthcare. Some areas of research and understanding have developed rapidly since the first edition, so we've been able to include and update information on issues such as epigenetics, health technology, and psychological intervention. We've expanded important topics that we were only able to cover briefly in previous editions and consolidated some areas so that they are more relevant for students on undergraduate programmes. This fourth edition is accompanied by a range of online resources for instructors, including a test bank of multiple-choice questions, a teaching guide with chapter learning objectives, suggested questions and prompts for the case studies featured in the book, and expanded suggestions for further reading. You can find these at https://study.sagepub.com/devisser-ayers4e.

The real story of this book, however, has always been in the students and health professionals who were so important in making it happen. It was only really when students got involved that the book took on a life of its own. Our students told us what works and what needs to change, what online materials help (or don't). We are truly indebted to the many amazing people who have been an integral part of every edition. Students have given up their summer vacation to help with researching literature, sourcing permissions, developing online resources, and arranging illustrations with the requisite amount of enthusiasm and unbelievable organisational skills to make sure this book was completed. Students also read, re-read, and commented on every chapter through various drafts. They gave us their honest opinions and helped make this book what it is. When we asked for volunteers, we never dreamt so many people would get involved. They told us what they liked and did not like, where we had the tone wrong, what features were missing. We were lucky to have excellent health professional consultants advise us on chapters throughout the book – and with plenty of good humour. We laughed a lot along the way!

We have been humbled by people's enthusiasm, the amount of time they put in, and the expertise they brought to this book. We have been inspired by many of these people and are very grateful for their input. Even now, when celebrating a fourth edition, it feels like a collective journey, which has been a great experience and a testament to the combined efforts of many people who gave their considerable time and energy to get it there. This must clearly include our respective families, who put up with us being total book-bores and still supported us at every step.

1

PSYCHOLOGY AND MEDICINE

┌─ Learning Objectives ─

This chapter is designed to enable you to:

- Understand different definitions of health and discuss their implications for treatment.
- Describe the biomedical and biopsychosocial approaches to healthcare.
- Appreciate the role of psychological and social factors in health and healthcare.

1.1 Psychology, Health, and Medicine

The importance of psychology for health and medicine is increasingly recognised: psychological topics are now part of most training programmes in medicine and other health professions. This development rests on extensive evidence that psychological factors are important in many aspects of physical and mental health – as you will see throughout the course of this textbook.

Yet it has been our experience that there are numerous barriers to students of medicine and other health professions learning about psychological topics. First, psychology is often seen as a 'soft' science. We will come back to this later in the chapter, but we hope that this book encourages the sceptics among you to explore psychology more and to see how relevant it is to your clinical practice. Second, psychology is a wide-ranging discipline that includes many specialisms. As a result, few students or health professionals have the time to become familiar with the extensive evidence base and psychological theories that are available. Table 1.1 shows the different psychological specialisms along with examples of how these are relevant to medicine. Psychology's breadth of scope can make it hard for health professionals to work out which parts are most relevant to clinical practice. Third, being bombarded with psychobabble in the press makes it even more difficult to screen out evidence-based information from popular 'facts'. A further challenge is that psychological and social services are often separate from physiologically-orientated services, such as acute medical wards. This may create a false separation between medical care and psychological or social care. Throughout this textbook we present substantial evidence that healthcare is most effective when this separation is removed through the application of a biopsychosocial approach.

Table 1.1 Specialisms in psychology

Specialism	Focus	Relevance to medicine
Health	Psychological factors and health	Effective health promotion and intervention. Psychosocial influences on health, including resilience
Clinical	Psychological resilience and disorders	Emotions, emotional disorders (psychopathology), and developing effective interventions
Developmental	Change over the lifespan	Typical and atypical aspects of development across the lifespan
Forensic	Criminal and judicial behaviour and systems	Criminal behaviour. Medico-legal investigations and testimony
Social	Social and group processes	How social and group processes influence our own and other people's behaviour in healthcare settings
Biological and neuropsychological	Links between physiological and mental processes	The interaction between physiological processes and psychological experiences, and behaviour
Cognitive	Internal mental processes, e.g. attention, perception, memory	Risk perception and decision making. How memory processes and biases affect treatment and adherence to medication
Occupational	Work, the workplace, and organisations	Work performance and training requirements. How healthcare organisations function
Educational	Learning and education	Improving education and training for health professionals. Health education

This book provides a single, integrated overview of the psychology that is relevant to medicine and healthcare, and considers how this can be applied in practice. This is done in four sections. In this introductory chapter we examine fundamental conceptual issues of what we mean by health and illness, why psychological and social factors are important, and different approaches to medicine and healthcare.

The rest of the book is divided into four sections. Section I focuses on the psychology of health and covers theories and research relevant to most areas of healthcare practice, such as emotions, stress, symptoms, and chronic illness. Section II discusses knowledge from other areas of psychology that is relevant, such as the brain and behaviour, development from infancy to old age, and the effects of social factors on people's behaviour. Section III begins with an overview and the importance of acknowledging and responding to diversity, inclusivity, and equality in medicine and healthcare. It then outlines psychology that is relevant to clinical practice, such as evidence-based practice, communication skills, clinical interviewing, and psychological interventions. Finally, Section IV focuses on psychology that is relevant to different body systems: the immune system, cardiovascular, respiratory, and gastrointestinal health, reproduction and endocrinology, and genitourinary medicine.

Throughout the book you will find clinically-relevant information and tips in the clinical notes boxes. Activity boxes encourage you to apply what you are learning to your own experiences. Case studies also help you to apply what you are learning to clinical scenarios, and help you to understand the impact of illness on individuals. Learning objectives and summary boxes provide easy guides to the main learning points that may prove useful for exams. Revision questions are given at the end of every chapter to help you revise and test yourself. Online supporting resources are available for students and teachers at https://study.sagepub.com/devisser-ayers4e.

1.2 What is Health?

As health professionals, you are embarking on careers that involve helping people to get better. But 'better', like 'health', is not the same for everyone. So how can we decide who to treat and who not to treat? Take a look at the examples in Case Study 1.1 and the definitions of health in Table 1.2.

Health operates on many levels: the physical, subjective, behavioural, functional, and social. One large landmark study found that people think of health in six different ways (Blaxter, 1990):

1 Not having symptoms of illness.
2 Having physical or social reserves.
3 Having healthy lifestyles.
4 Being physically fit or vital.
5 Experiencing psychological wellbeing.
6 Being able to function.

These definitions are not mutually exclusive: they overlap and intersect. Research Box 1.1 provides an illustration of how definitions of health are also shaped by broader social factors.

─Research Box 1.1─

Lay Definitions of Health

Background

The concept of 'successful ageing' is a fundamental concept in gerontology which challenges the misconception that growing older is inevitably linked to physical, cognitive, and social decline and dependence on others. Previous studies had found that the meaning of successful ageing can vary between cultures, so this study aimed to explore the topic among older African American men.

Method and Findings

In-depth individual interviews were conducted with 22 men aged 55–76. They were asked about their definitions of health, whether they consider themselves to be healthy, and what they do to protect their health.

(Continued)

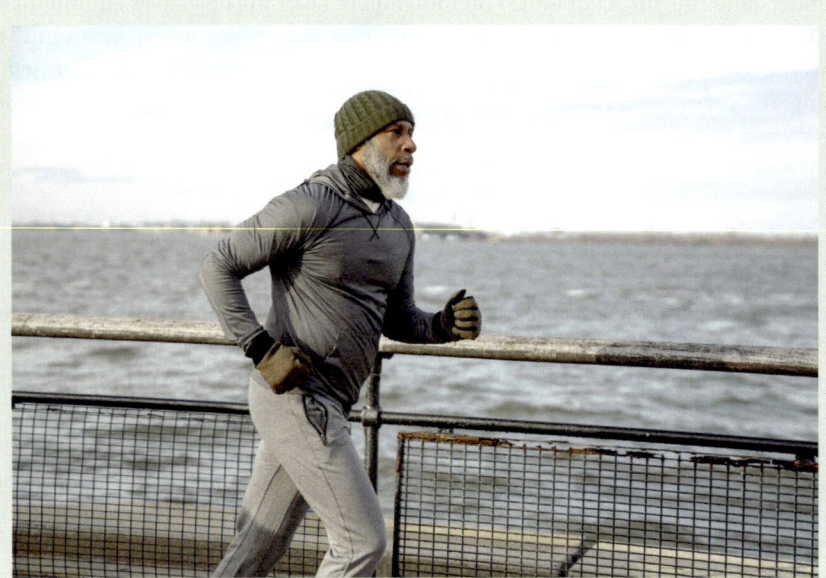

Figure 1.1 Successful ageing

Source: Barbara Olsen/Pexels

Consistent with other similar studies, health is considered to be multifaceted: the absence of disease and disability; the ability to function physically, cognitively, and socially; and living a healthy lifestyle. Assessments of health were made with reference to other African American men, and reflected cultural views of masculinity as potent and productive.

Significance

Like other studies, this study illustrated how lay definitions of health are multifaceted, and reflect a biopsychosocial conceptualisation of health and wellbeing. Whereas the definitions of health and successful ageing were similar in many ways to those expressed in other segments of the population, there were some unique elements that reflected specific cultural influences.

Griffith, D.M., Cornish, E.K., Bergner, E.M., Bruce, M.A. & Beech, B.M. (2018) 'Health is the ability to manage yourself without help': How older African American men define health and successful aging. *The Journals of Gerontology: Series B, 73*(2): 240–247. doi:10.1093/geronb/gbx075.

Which of the various definitions we prioritise will have implications for who receives treatment. Table 1.2 applies these to the cases of a fit young woman with a high risk of breast cancer (Jeeval), a terminally ill man who is living life to the full (David), and a suicidal woman (Karen). It shows, for each one, who would be considered healthy and who would be considered ill using these different definitions. Common sense would suggest that the terminally ill man, David, and the suicidal woman, Karen, are ill and need treatment. Yet David would be classified as ill by physical definitions of health but not by behavioural, functional, or psychosocial definitions. In contrast, Karen would be classified as ill by behavioural, functional, and psychosocial definitions but not by physical ones. In fact, the only definition of health that would classify both of them as ill is the cultural norm for health – in other words, they are both outside the norm within our society for what is regarded as healthy.

Table 1.2 Definitions of health

Definition	Features of definition	Are they healthy or ill?		
		Jeeval	David	Karen
Physical	Absence of disease	Healthy	Ill	Healthy
	Not vulnerable to disease	Ill	Ill	Healthy
	Strong physical reserves	Healthy	Ill	Healthy
	Physically fit, has vitality	Healthy	Healthy	Ill
Subjective	No symptoms of physical illness	Healthy	Ill	Healthy
Behavioural	Living a healthy lifestyle	Healthy	Healthy	Ill
Functional	Able to function in day-to-day life	Healthy	Healthy	Ill
Psychosocial	Psychosocial wellbeing	Healthy	Healthy	Ill
Social	Able to contribute to society	Healthy	Healthy	Ill
Cultural	Matches cultural norm for health	Healthy	Ill	Ill

These cases illustrate that 'health' is not easy to define and is very individual. This may be especially so for people with a comorbidity (i.e. the presence of another illness in addition to a major 'index' chronic condition) or multimorbidity (i.e. the presence of multiple chronic illnesses where there is no major 'index' condition) (Suls et al., 2019). Multimorbidities are becoming more prevalent due to our ageing populations and the increasing prominence of chronic conditions (Mohamud, 2023). They place increased demand on health services (Kabir et al., 2024). Multinational analyses indicate that multimorbidities are more prevalent among people who are less well-off (Ni, 2023) – an issue that is addressed in more detail in Chapter 11. Studies across different countries and age groups indicate that multimorbidities are associated with lower self-rated health, quality of life, and psychological wellbeing (Felez-Nobrega & Kyanagi, 2023; Kader et al., 2024; Thomsen et al., 2023). There is also evidence of the role of depression as a causal factor in the development of multimorbidities, and possible reciprocal relationships between depression and multimorbidity (Birk et al., 2019; Triolo et al., 2020). This highlights the need to screen for and treat depression in those who are at risk of developing multimorbidities. It is notable that physical activity can reduce the impact of multimorbidities on wellbeing (Marques et al., 2018).

Furthermore, research shows that people with a terminal illness generally have a reduced quality of life. Yet quality of life is not a single entity, and although people with terminal illnesses tend to report worse physical symptoms, greater pain and disability, many also report an increased appreciation of life and family, and other positive benefits – as illustrated by David in Case Study 1.1.

In Case Study 1.1, Karen may be particularly at risk, as research shows that young, divorced, or widowed women are most likely to attempt suicide, although men are more likely to succeed at completing suicide. Being depressed is a critical risk factor. In Europe, 28% of people with clinical depression will attempt suicide at some point during their lives (Bernal et al., 2007).

Cases of apparently healthy people being offered interventions for genetic risk of disease are likely to become more common as screening for genetic risk becomes more widespread. Women who have prophylactic mastectomies (like Jeeval in Case Study 1.1) generally report a reduction in cancer-related distress afterwards, although there can be other negative impacts on their lives.

Case Study 1.1

Are These People Healthy or Ill?

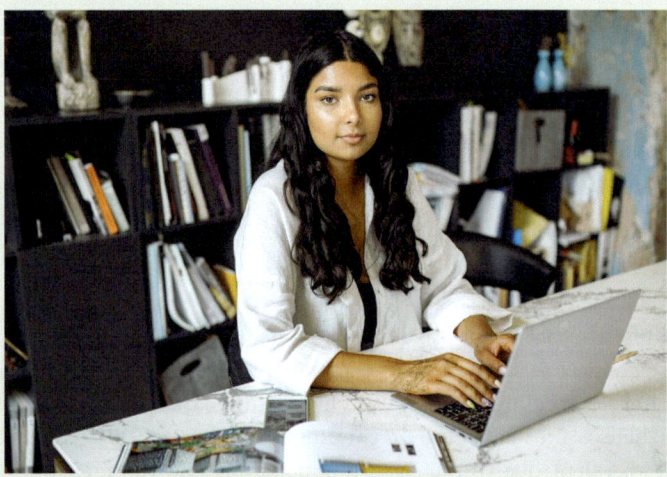

Figure 1.2   Jeeval: Healthy or ill?

Source: © Yan Krukau/Pexels

Jeeval is a university student. She has a healthy diet and is a keen athlete. Her mother died of breast cancer when Jeeval was 13 and Jeeval's older sister has just been diagnosed with breast cancer. Screening shows that Jeeval is carrying a mutation in the BRCA gene, which means she is at higher risk of breast cancer. She has been offered surgery to remove both breasts as a preventative measure.

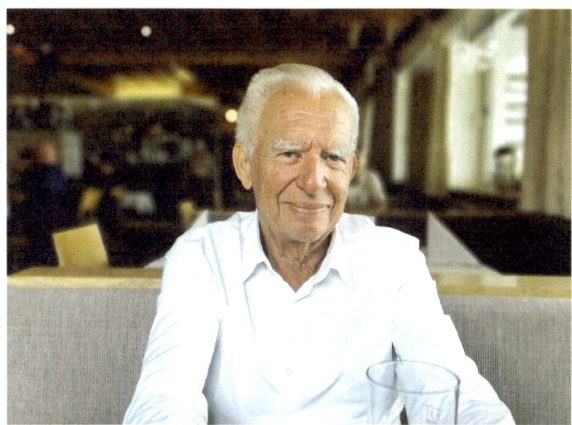

Figure 1.3   David: Healthy or ill?

Source: © Alexandra_Koch/Pixabay

David is a businessman who has taken a sabbatical to ski the 'Swiss Wall', a slope in the Alps which is notoriously difficult. David did it once when he was younger and fitter, but had to stop and inch his way down parts of it. Last week he attempted it and managed to ski all the way down without stopping. He says it was exhilarating. He has terminal liver cancer and approximately six months left to live.

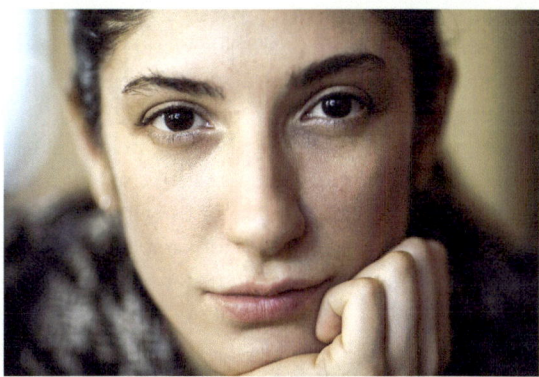

Figure 1.4   Karen: Healthy or ill?

Source: © Engin_Akyurt/Pixabay

Karen is divorced with four children under the age of seven. She works part-time. Her ex-husband has remarried and has a new baby. Karen is upset about her divorce, struggling financially, and finding it hard to maintain another steady relationship. She is depressed and smokes 30 cigarettes a day. Four weeks ago, she took a large number of paracetamol pills with a bottle of wine, but was found by a friend and taken to the emergency department at hospital.

It is clear that health issues are complex and that health and illness are subjective states of well-being. In other words, does the person *feel* or *think* they are healthy or ill? Do they have physical symptoms that *they* believe mean there is a problem with their health? We also need to take account of disease in the form of underlying pathology, although research shows that a physiological basis is not found for many physical symptoms and at least 10% of primary care patients have a history of unexplained symptoms (Haller et al., 2015; Hilderink et al., 2013; Rasmussen, 2020).

Activity 1.1

What is Health?

- How would you rate your own health?

  - Very poor
  - Poor
  - Fair
  - Good
  - Excellent

- What factors were important in helping you decide where to rate your health?

We therefore need to think of health on many levels. The World Health Organization (WHO) defines **health** very broadly as 'a state of complete physical, mental, and social wellbeing and not merely the absence of disease or infirmity' (World Health Organization, 1992). The value of this definition is that it is inclusive, and the emphasis on wellbeing accounts for individual differences in subjective perceptions of health. However, this definition has been criticised for being too broad to be useful and for referring to a utopian 'perfect' state that few of us will reach, even when we feel healthy. Nevertheless, we should not denigrate the aspiration for complete health for all people.

How we define health has wide-ranging implications for the treatments provided by health services. For example, if we aim for health as defined by the WHO, it might put unrealistic pressures on countries to provide social circumstances and medical systems that mean everyone lives in a state of complete wellbeing. Others have pointed out that conceptualising health as complete wellbeing confuses happiness with health (Saracci, 1997). This opens the door to limitless treatments if people view the pursuit of happiness as a legitimate medical goal. The increase in cosmetic surgery and aesthetic procedures to address people's concerns about their appearance is one example of this.

The way we define health has implications for who can be seen as responsible for our health and for which treatments we offer. These implications are more than just medical: they affect society's policies and laws. In the western world, the dominant view is that individuals are responsible for their health by adopting either healthy or unhealthy lifestyles, and much work goes into encouraging people to adhere to guidelines for healthy living. Additional policies to help improve our lifestyles and health include providing fruit for young school children and banning smoking in public places.

A striking example of the effect that our definition of health has on treatment is the increasing numbers of obese children being put into foster care by the authorities in an attempt to combat their obesity. The story of one such girl is given in Case Study 1.2. This course of action rests on a number of debatable assumptions, including the view that: (1) obesity is an illness; (2) obesity is controllable through diet; (3) parental behaviour is the major cause of childhood obesity; and (4) a child's physical health takes priority over the psychological impact of removing that child from their family.

Ultimately, the multidimensional nature of health makes finding an adequate definition difficult. Antonovsky (1987) therefore proposed that we think of **health as a continuum** from optimal wellness to death, as shown in Figure 1.5. Health promotion techniques operate on the wellness side of the continuum to encourage people to choose a lifestyle that optimises their health. Medical treatment focuses on the illness side of the continuum when people show signs or symptoms of illness.

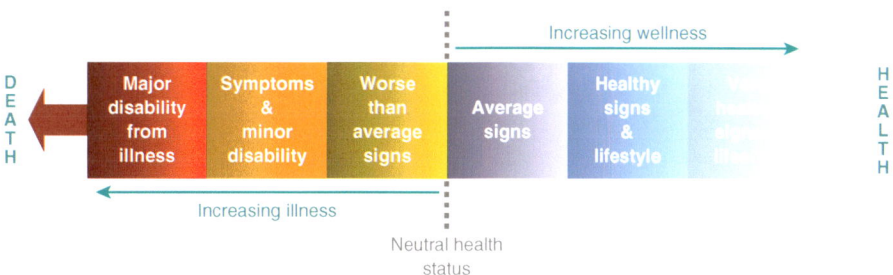

Figure 1.5   Illness–wellness continuum

Source: Antonovsky, 1987 (adapted from Sarafino, 2002)

Case Study 1.2

Obese Child Taken into Care

In August 2000, in a controversial case, the state of New Mexico took legal custody of a three-year-old girl because she was morbidly obese. She was removed from her parents and put in foster care for three months. A gagging order was put on her parents so they could not talk publicly about the case for five months.

She weighed three times more than a normal three-year-old and was 50% taller. She had undergone numerous tests to determine what was causing her increased growth, but doctors could not find a medical cause.

While in foster care, she was put on a strict diet, lost weight, and learned to walk unassisted. It is difficult to gauge the emotional impact of being taken from her parents (e.g. she stopped speaking Spanish, her father's language). After three months of legal and political wrangling, she was returned to her parents, although the state kept legal custody of her for a while, monitoring her progress.

(Continued)

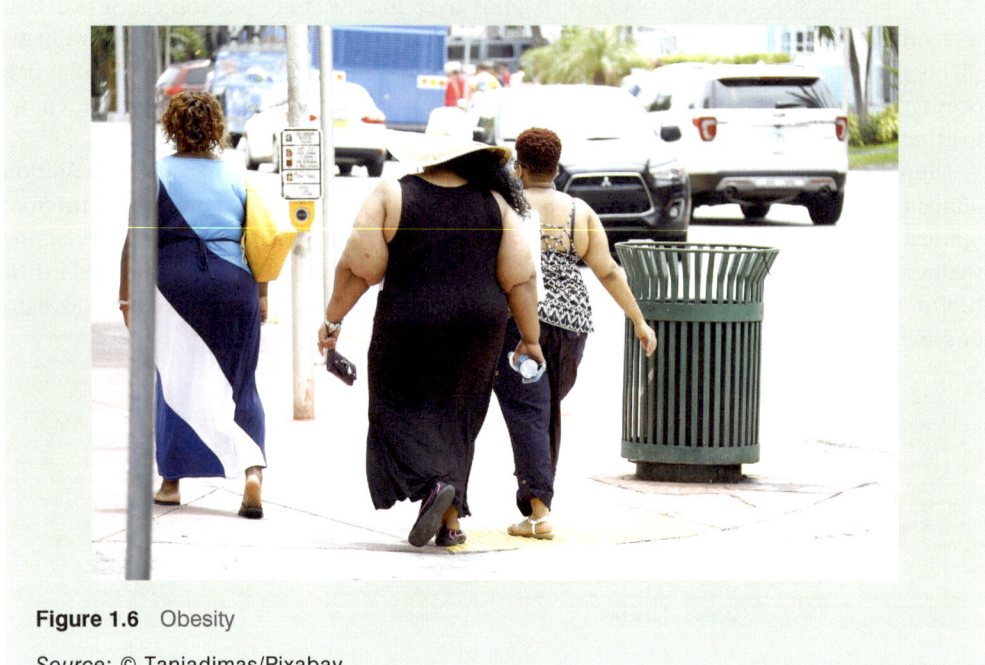

Figure 1.6   Obesity

Source: © Taniadimas/Pixabay

1.3 Why is Psychology Important?

The importance of treating the person and not just the disease is widely recognised. Each person is a unique mix of thoughts, emotions, personality, behaviour patterns, and their own personal history and experiences. Understanding more about people will help us to treat them more effectively. Psychology, however, is a subject that some students think is 'just common sense', 'interesting but I can't see how it's useful', or not 'proper medicine'. Here we will consider each of these objections in turn before looking at the science underpinning the integral nature of body and mind.

1.3.1 'Psychology is Just Common Sense'

Often statements from psychological research coincide with common sense. Examples of these include 'Stress is bad for you', 'A healthy lifestyle is important', and 'People with chronic illness have a worse quality of life'. If this was all we could take from psychology, then most of us would indeed dismiss the subject as mere common sense. The value of psychological research is that:

- It *tests* common-sense views empirically to confirm or disconfirm them.
- It goes *beyond* common sense.
- People don't always act according to common sense.

First, let's look at the empirical testing of common-sense views. Much common sense is in fact contradictory. For example, the proverbs 'Too many cooks spoil the broth' and 'Many hands make light work' contradict each other. In some cases, psychological research has confirmed common-sense views, although in other cases it has rejected them. Examples of common-sense views that have been tested by research are given in Highlight Box 1.1 – take a look at these statements and make up your own mind about whether they are facts or myths.

Highlight Box 1.1

Common Sense: Fact or Myth?

1 Taking vitamin C prevents colds.
2 The majority of domestic violence is committed by men.
3 Being an oldest, middle, or youngest child affects your personality.
4 People with schizophrenia are often violent.
5 Eating fruit and vegetables improves your eye health.
6 Ginger reduces nausea and vomiting in pregnancy.

Sources: 1. Douglas et al. (2007); 2. Breiding et al. (2014); 3. Rohrer et al. (2015); 4. Large et al. (2011); 5. Grover and Samson (2014); 6. Dante et al. (2013).

In fact, statements 1, 3, and 4 in Highlight Box 1.1 have not been supported by research. In contrast, there *is* evidence that antioxidants can reduce the progression and impact of some eye disorders (Evans & Lawrenson, 2017), that ginger can reduce nausea and vomiting in pregnancy (McParlin et al., 2016), and that the majority of domestic violence toward women and men is carried out by men (Breiding et al., 2014). Research therefore not only challenges common sense but also examines the things that go beyond common knowledge, such as why depression puts people at a higher risk of heart disease, whether there are critical periods in development when babies are more sensitive to psychosocial or biological circumstances, and whether therapy for psychological disorders should try to change *what* people think or the *relationship* people have with their thoughts. There are many other examples that you will read about throughout the course of this book.

1.3.2 'Psychology is Interesting but not Useful'

If the goal in medicine and healthcare is to treat people effectively and restore them to health, then what does this involve and how can psychology help? In order to treat people effectively we need to be able to: (1) diagnose the problem accurately; and (2) treat that problem appropriately. Psychology can help in both of these areas. Accurate diagnoses are more likely if we understand how people's experiences shape their perception and reporting of symptoms, and help-seeking behaviours (see Chapter 4). Negotiating an acceptable and effective treatment plan rests on understanding decision-making processes, what makes people more likely to adhere to treatment, and the influence of people's beliefs and emotions (see Chapter 12). In illnesses such as HIV, where there is no complete cure, behaviour change is crucial for limiting the spread of disease (see Chapter 19). Furthermore, research suggests that people would prefer lifestyle modification over medication for conditions such as cardiovascular disease (Jarbøl et al., 2017).

Effective communication skills also help in making an accurate diagnosis and in agreeing appropriate treatment for each individual (see Chapter 13). Thus, understanding psychological and social processes will help us to diagnose and treat people more effectively.

Psychology can also help us to understand psychological *symptoms*, such as anxiety and depression, which can range from mild to severe, as well as *diagnostic disorders*, such as panic disorder, major depressive disorder, or schizophrenia. Psychological symptoms of anxiety and depression account for many consultations in primary care (Slee et al., 2021). However, people with psychological symptoms often present with physical symptoms, leading to under-diagnosis and missed opportunities for treatment (Cepoiu et al., 2008; Jackson et al., 2007; Love & Love, 2019). One study asked primary care physicians in the UK to rate the content of 2,206 consultations and found that, in addition to the 6% of consultations that were booked for entirely psychological concerns, another 30% of consultations were rated as involving some important psychological content (Ashworth et al., 2003).

Evidence shows a strong link between physical health and psychological health: if we concentrate on only one side, we risk missing important information and prescribing ineffective treatments. For example, chronic illness is associated with increased rates of psychological disorders (Lotfaliany et al., 2019; Senra & McPherson, 2021). People with psychological disorders are also at an increased risk of illness. A population-based survey conducted in Australia found that the prevalence of physical illness differed between those who had depression and/or anxiety (Stanton et al., 2019). More specifically, analyses showed that the strongest predictor of chronic illness was having a diagnosis of depression and/or anxiety. As discussed elsewhere in this book, psychological interventions, such as cognitive behavioural therapy (CBT), can be effective in managing or treating illnesses that have physical and psychological components, such as obesity, chronic pain, irritable bowel syndrome, and addiction (see Chapters 15 to 19), as well as psychological disorders, such as bipolar disorder, personality disorder, and schizophrenia (see Chapters 7 and 14).

Although psychological knowledge can help us to be more effective health practitioners, many students are put off psychology because of a sense that it is 'interesting, but there's no right answer'. Psychology can appear abstract or ambiguous, especially in areas where there are many competing theories. The reasons for this are that when studying people, we must deal with numerous outcomes related to behaviour and emotions. Furthermore, these behaviours and emotions are influenced by many different factors. Explanatory theories are therefore tested by using a range of research methods and statistics to try to identify which factors are the most important for specific situations or health issues. This means that psychology will often present students with competing theories and their associated evidence. The ambiguity or uncertainty that this involves may contrast directly with the large amount of physiological and anatomical facts students are required to learn in the first few years of their training.

So psychology requires a different way of thinking, but this method of thinking is a useful skill in itself – and one that is essential in healthcare practice. A lot of healthcare practice is about dealing with uncertainty, often in the face of patients who want certainty. For example, people will rarely present with a clearly defined textbook set of symptoms. In trying to diagnose and treat a person, you will often have to form a hypothesis about what might be wrong, then find a way to test it, and then reformulate your hypothesis if the tests do not confirm it. Understanding the psychosocial context of a person's symptoms and concerns will help you to reach a more probable diagnosis and/or provide reassurance in the face of uncertainty. Furthermore, there are still many medical conditions that do not have suitable tests to confirm them. Examples include chronic fatigue syndrome and irritable bowel syndrome (see Chapter 17). As with psychological learning, these conditions involve a tolerance of ambiguity and an openness to alternative explanations, particularly in the early stages of diagnosis and treatment. Research Box 1.2 provides an example of research that shows the importance of helping students of health professions to learn to anticipate uncertainty and how to manage it.

Research Box 1.2

Learning to Deal with Uncertainty

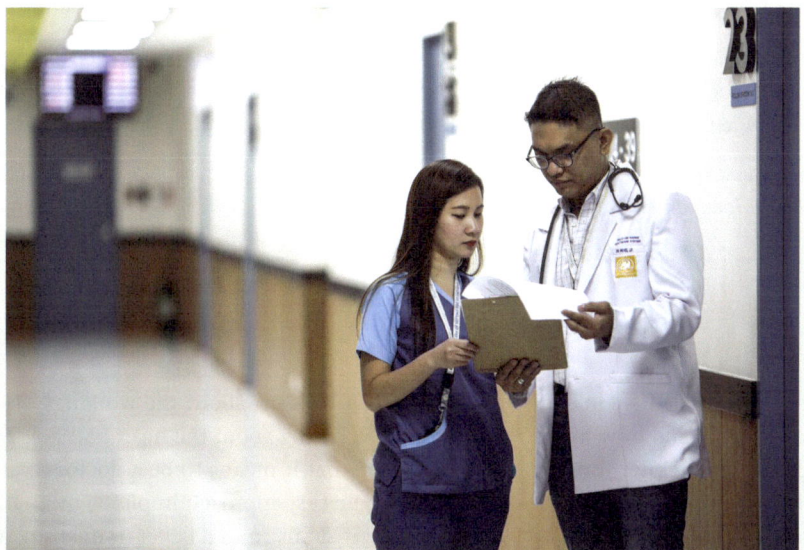

Figure 1.7 Clinical uncertainty

Source: © HalcyonMarine/Pixabay

Background

Simulated consultations are an important part of learning and assessment for students of health professions. However, because they are often simplified to ensure that specific learning outcomes can be assessed, they may not properly prepare professionals for the real-world challenges of complex cases. This is reflected in graduates' reports of feeling underprepared to cope with uncertainty in relation to diagnosis or treatment, particularly in acute settings.

(Continued)

Method and Findings

This study adapted a simulation scenario so that it replicated clinical uncertainty. The simulated patient had a confused history, no clear current diagnosis, ambiguous physiological markers, and no diagnostic investigations were yet available. Forty-five final-year medical students engaged in 'uncertainty' simulations followed by debriefs facilitated by the researchers. Transcripts of the recorded debriefs underwent qualitative analysis.

Students generally considered the 'uncertainty' simulation to be useful, but they found it more challenging than a 'typical' one. Three key themes emerged: (1) students were unfamiliar with uncertainty; (2) students were unsure of how to act in the absence of a diagnosis: some responded with inaction whereas others became fixated on applying potentially incorrect diagnoses; and (3) students were uncertain of what their role was in an uncertain situation but many were also reluctant to seek senior support.

Significance

The researchers suggested that their findings highlight a need for educators to give time, space, and support to allow students to consider appropriate strategies to use to help them better manage uncertainty and complex cases.

Scott, A., Sudlow, M, Shaw, E., & Fisher, J. (2020) Medical education, simulation and uncertainty. *The Clinical Teacher, 17*(5): 497–502. doi:10.1111/tct.13119

1.3.3 'Psychology is not Real Medicine'

Most healthcare students come to their studies keen to learn about the workings of the body, how it goes wrong, and how to fix it. For example, learning about the heart and how to resuscitate people is much closer to the common view of what it means to be a doctor than learning about topics such as health behaviours and stress. The first approach implies a mechanical view of the body and medicine. Such a view is not new: it stems from a belief in dualism, according to which the mind and body are independent. Dualism has its roots in classical philosophy and was reinforced by later thinkers, such as René Descartes (1637). Focusing on the mechanics of the body enabled rapid advances in medicine during the eighteenth and nineteenth centuries. Medical understanding grew exponentially as doctors and researchers focused on increasingly detailed physiological processes and identified the causes of pathology. Treatments also advanced: antibiotics and vaccines were developed and anaesthesia was introduced. The disadvantage of dualism is that it provided the basis for the **biomedical approach** or model, which dominated medicine for centuries. This approach, which is examined later in this chapter, is based on a separation of body and mind that is unhelpful in many ways.

1.4 The Science of Mind and Body

Science has advanced considerably since dualism, and there is now increasing evidence that the mind and body are integrally linked and important in health. Throughout this book there are examples of how our mind influences physiological factors, such as fight-flight stress responses, pain, and physical symptoms. Cognitive science and neuroscience have also challenged dualism by showing that the mind (e.g. thoughts, feelings) is influenced by our body and bodily experiences. Theories of embodied cognition propose that many aspects of cognition are influenced by our bodily state. These cognitive factors include memory making and recall, tasks such as decision making and judgement, as well as higher-level mental constructs such as concepts and language. Bodily factors that influence cognition include the motor system (e.g. movement, posture), perceptual system (e.g. vision, hearing), and physical interactions with others and the environment.

Theories of embodied cognition rest on research from areas like psychology, neuroscience, linguistics, and artificial intelligence. Psychological research has shown that sensorimotor feedback can influence our thoughts and emotions (Niedenthal, 2007). Many of these studies artificially place a person in a particular posture and examine the effect of this posture on thoughts, feelings, and behaviour. For example, research into feedback from facial expressions gets people to activate smile muscles by holding a pencil between their teeth and shows that when people 'smile' they are more likely to rate cartoons as funny, remember positive memories, evaluate stories more positively, and are quicker to perceive things that are congruent with a positive emotional state (Coles et al., 2019). There is also some evidence that facial feedback from smiling may reduce pain and stress responses (M.P. Cross et al., 2023).

The importance of bodily feedback in how we think and feel extends beyond the individual. Social psychologists have illustrated how rapport between people – such as between health professionals and patients – is embodied through mirroring each other's posture and gestures (interpersonal synchrony). A review and meta-analysis of the research on interpersonal synchrony shows that it leads to people having more prosocial attitudes and behaviours, such as perceived affiliation, cooperation, and helping behaviours (Rennung & Göritz, 2016).

Functional brain imaging has identified some of the physiological processes that underlie interpersonal synchrony. There is evidence that animals and humans have mirror neurons which fire both when we carry out a specific act and when we see others performing the same action. So our minds respond to observed movements of others as if we were carrying out the same behaviour. Similarly, recognising someone else's facial expression of an emotion and feeling that emotion ourselves involve overlapping neural circuits in the brain (Bonini et al., 2022).

The science of mind and body has therefore moved beyond simple separation of mind and body to show that they are interdependent and influence each other in numerous ways, as does our environment and the people around us. This science has informed developments in artificial intelligence and robotics. The increasing capacity of, and acceptance of, artificial intelligence has informed the ongoing development and deployment of artificial humans designed to display socio-emotional intelligence, such as virtual characters that facilitate interaction between humans and technology by interpreting and responding to nonverbal cues (Vogeley & Bente, 2010). This is also being used in healthcare interventions, such as using virtual characters to assess and train people with high-functioning autism to recognise nonverbal communication cues (Georgescu et al., 2014). However, it is important to acknowledge the limitations of these systems, and to pay attention to their perceived acceptability and the willingness of both patients and healthcare professionals to use them (Wutz et al., 2023).

1.5 Different Approaches to Medicine and Healthcare

This section outlines and compares two prominent approaches to explaining and treating health and illness, and makes the case for the need to consider not only biological factors and processes, but also psychological and social infleunces.

1.5.1 Biomedical Approach

The biomedical approach to healthcare is based on a dualistic approach to mind and body, so it is not consistent with current science and evidence. The biomedical approach is summarised in Figure 1.8. It assumes that all disease can be explained in terms of physiological processes: therefore, the treatment acts on the disease and not on the person. There is a linear progression of causality from the pathogen to the person and not the other way around. Psychological and social processes are separate and incidental. The person as a whole is therefore not considered by the biomedical approach.

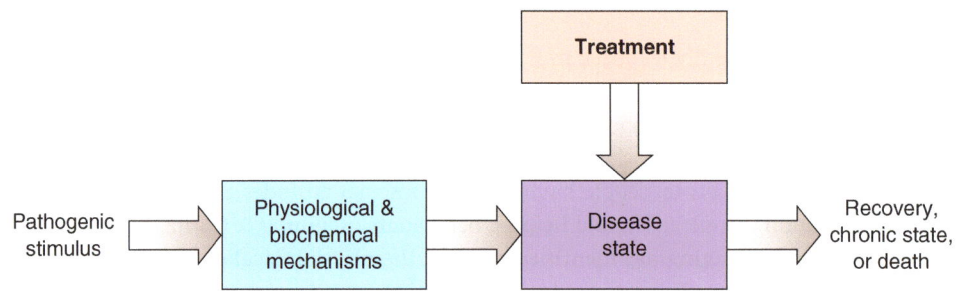

Figure 1.8 Biomedical approach to health (adapted from Lovallo, 2004)

Although the biomedical approach has dominated medicine and led to great advances, it has been criticised for many reasons, in particular that it does not consider the influence of social or psychological factors on health. Historically, the influence of social factors on population health is clear. Let us take the example of infectious diseases. The rapid decline in deaths from infectious diseases in the UK between 1859 and 1978 occurred *before* most vaccines were introduced. Some of this change was the result of more effective treatments, but a lot was due to changes in people's understanding of illness and the effect of lifestyle. For example, in the mid-1800s a physician, John Snow, noticed that patterns of cholera outbreaks clustered around particular water supplies in London. His discovery led to a better understanding of the cause and transmission of cholera as well as social changes, such as an improved water supply and sanitation. More recently, the global COVID-19 pandemic showed how individual and collective actions, such as lockdowns, quarantines, and self-isolation, could reduce or even stop the spread of a virus. The examples of cholera and COVID-19 show how social and cultural change is important and that the reduction of infectious diseases cannot be explained on a purely biomedical basis.

Social factors are just as important today. One of the most consistent findings from public health research is the influence of socioeconomic status (SES) on health. People of lower SES are at more risk of illness (**morbidity**) and death (**mortality**) from a variety of causes (see Chapter 11). This increased risk is partly due to differences in lifestyles. For example, people of lower SES have poorer diets, experience harder working and living conditions, and are more likely to smoke. However, studies indicate that even after these lifestyle factors are taken into account, people of lower SES still remain at an increased risk of poor health.

The role of lifestyle in illness illustrates the importance of psychosocial factors, yet these are not considered by the biomedical model. Understanding and changing health behaviour does more than anything else to reduce morbidity and mortality (see Chapter 5). For example, global data indicate that 22% of all deaths are attributable to poor diets (GBD 2017 Diet Collaborators, 2019). Greater alcohol use is directly related to increased rates of liver disorders and cancers of the GI tract (see Chapter 17). Smoking is directly related to lung cancer and cardiovascular disease – two of the most important causes of mortality in the world.

In addition to lifestyle, individual factors such as personality, health behaviours, and beliefs also have important effects on health. For example, individuals who are higher on the personality trait of conscientiousness are less likely to engage in risky behaviours and more likely to engage in positive health behaviours, so they are therefore also more likely to have better health and to live longer (Milad & Bogg, 2020; Turiano et al., 2015). Stress and depression are strongly implicated in a range of illnesses, including cardiovascular disease: evidence suggests that both of these factors are associated with the onset of heart disease (see Chapter 16).

A good example of the effect of our beliefs on health and illness is the **placebo effect**, whereby people recover because they think they are going to recover, as opposed to recovering because of pharmacological or physical treatment. The placebo effect is typically tested by giving one group of people a fake treatment (placebo group) and comparing their recovery to another group of people given an active treatment (treatment group) or no treatment (control). The placebo effect is the recovery that occurs in the placebo group that is over and above any recovery observed in the control group. The treatment effect is the recovery that occurs in the treatment group that is over and above any placebo effect. For example, a study of surgery for osteoarthritis compared two different types of procedure (arthroscopic debridement or lavage) with placebo surgery where people were anaesthetised and skin incisions made but the arthroscope was not inserted. Those who had placebo surgery showed the same level of improvements up to two years later (Moseley et al., 2002). A review and meta-analysis of this and seven other randomised controlled trials concluded that arthroscopic debridement does not improve pain or functional status more than sham surgery or usual care (Evidence Development and Standards Branch, Health Quality Ontario, 2014). The placebo effect is well established and there is evidence that beliefs are responsible for a large part of it. It is considered in more detail in Chapter 4.

The biomedical approach cannot account for any of these effects of social and psychological factors on health. Even when the biomedical approach dominated healthcare, many health professionals realised that psychological and social factors were still important. However, working within the biomedical framework meant that these factors were not made explicit or used to the advantage of medicine. They therefore remained part of the *art* of medicine rather than the *science* of medicine, although ironically the term 'medicine' comes from the Latin *medici-na (ars)* – the (art of) healing.

—Clinical Notes 1.1—

In Primary Care

- At least 30% of physical symptoms seen in primary care have no identifiable organic cause.
- At least 10% of primary care patients have a history of multiple unexplained physical symptoms.
- Psychological and physical symptoms are highly related. Many people will only mention physical symptoms, so it is important to ask about psychological symptoms as well.
- A large part of 'treatment' effects is due to people believing they will recover rather than the treatment itself.

1.5.2 Biopsychosocial Approach

The **biopsychosocial approach** (Engel, 1977) incorporates biological, psychological, and social factors. This approach was later expanded to include such factors as ethnicity and culture (Suls & Rothman, 2004). A schematic diagram of the biopsychosocial approach is shown in Figure 1.9, which shows the personal and external factors that, according to this approach, affect health.

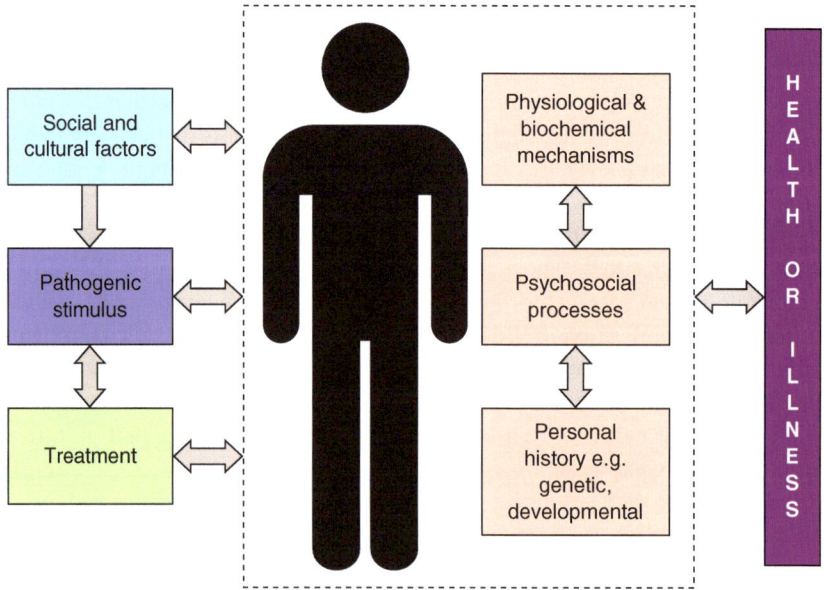

Figure 1.9 Biopsychosocial approach to health

Source: Adapted from Lovallo, W.R. (2004) *Stress & Health: Biological and Psychological Interactions*. Thousand Oaks, CA: Sage

External factors include the sociocultural environment, such as poverty, available support structures, access to healthcare and other facilities, and environmental factors and legislation that affect health. External factors include pathogenic stimuli, which can range from being exposed to a virus, to passive smoking, to living in an area high in radon gas. External factors also include any treatment that the individual receives which can act on the pathogenic stimuli or the person. All of these external factors both influence the person and are influenced by the person.

Internal factors include personal history, psychosocial processes, and physiological and biochemical mechanisms. Personal history involves multiple factors, such as ethnicity, genetic make-up, learned behaviour, developmental processes, and previous illnesses. These factors inevitably influence psychosocial processes such as lifestyle, sociability, personality, mood, perception of symptoms, behaviour, and adherence to treatment. All of these factors influence, and are influenced by, physiological mechanisms.

Consider smoking, for example. Many people report that their first cigarette is fairly unpleasant, so why do people persist in smoking until they are addicted? Most people start smoking in adolescence when it is important for them to gain peer approval and to fit in with group norms. In high-income countries, the prevalence of smoking is often highest in people from deprived backgrounds with a low socioeconomic status (Office for National Statistics, 2022). Thus, a child growing up in a deprived area may be more exposed to others who smoke and more likely to start smoking, which further reinforces the group norm. Without motivation to quit smoking, this child is also unlikely to seek help.

The pathogens in cigarettes mean that, with continued use, smokers are at increased risk of many illnesses, including lung cancer, chronic obstructive pulmonary disease, heart disease, head and neck cancer, impotence, infertility, gum disease, back pain, and Type 2 diabetes (World Health Organization, 2024a). Whether an individual develops any of these illnesses is determined by the other aspects in the biopsychosocial approach, such as their individual vulnerability, physiological processes, other lifestyle behaviours, and exposure to other pathogens. However, to return to our example, not all children in deprived circumstances will smoke. Therefore, the sociocultural environment interacts with the characteristics of each child to determine exposure to the pathogen of cigarettes, the likelihood of seeking treatment, and the risk of disease.

The examples just given show how internal and external factors interact and combine to influence healthy or unhealthy behaviours and outcomes. It is also important to note that some psychosocial phenomena are combinations of internal and external factors. For example, loneliness is an internal experience that arises from a lack of engagement with other people (who would be defined as an external factor). Loneliness is a negative psychological experience that has a significant effect on many health outcomes. For example, a US study that followed over 8,000 people over 10 or more years found that chronic loneliness increased the risk of stroke by over 50% (Soh et al., 2024).

The biopsychosocial approach provides a clear framework that sums up what many health professionals already intuitively know. It is an improvement on the biomedical approach in that it makes the links between psychological and social factors and health explicit. Illness is seen to be caused by many factors at different levels, rather than purely by pathogens, as posited by the biomedical model. Responsibility for health and illness therefore rests on individuals and society rather than on the medical profession alone. Similarly, treatment considers physical, psychological, and social contributing factors as opposed to the physical in isolation. A further comparison of the key features of the biomedical and biopsychosocial approaches is given in Table 1.3.

Table 1.3 Comparison of biomedical and biopsychosocial approaches

	Biomedical	Biopsychosocial
Mind–body relationship	Separate; independent (dualism)	Part of dynamic system; influence each other
Cause of disease	Pathogens	Multiple factors at different levels
Causality	Linear	Circular
Psychosocial factors	Irrelevant	Essential
Approach to illness and treatment	Reductionist	Holistic
Responsibility for health	Medical professionals – e.g. to combat disease	Individuals/society – e.g. healthy lifestyle
Focus of treatment	Eradication or containment of pathology	Physical, psychological, and social factors contributing to illness
Focus of health promotion	Avoidance of pathogens	Reduction of physical, psychological, and social risk factors

The biopsychosocial approach has implications for research, education, and clinical practice. It should lead to more comprehensive research that examines the multiple levels, systems, and factors involved in health. Moreover, in clinical practice, the biopsychosocial approach should result in a more complete understanding of the many factors that can contribute to health or illness. This in turn should lead to a more **holistic approach** – that is, treatment of the whole person. The biopsychosocial approach has already formed the basis for a more person-centred approach to medicine (Borrell-Carrio et al., 2004). It should also lead to better healthcare training, with the inclusion of education about psychological and social factors.

Thus, the biopsychosocial approach is an improvement on the biomedical approach and should result in clear clinical benefits if used. It is therefore puzzling that, more than 40 years after it was proposed, the biopsychosocial approach still is not widely used or practised in medicine or psychology. Although the biopsychosocial approach is taught in most training courses for health professionals, it tends to be taught as a theoretical framework rather than being applied to clinical work.

So we still have a long way to go to properly incorporate the biopsychosocial approach into medicine and healthcare. There are many reasons why this might be. The biomedical approach has been dominant for centuries, and modern medicine and healthcare developed within this framework. Although the biopsychosocial approach may appear simple, in fact the inclusion of all the different elements makes research and medicine more complicated to carry out in practice. In addition, the biopsychosocial approach suggests circular or nonlinear causality. In other words, physical, psychological, and social factors all influence, and are influenced by, each other, and there is rarely a simple and linear cause–effect relationship between one factor and illness. This raises difficulties in clinical practice if we need to choose or prioritise one treatment (see Case Study 1.3). To do this, we have to think in terms of a hierarchy of causes (e.g. one cause is more important than others) and linearity of treatment (e.g. removing this cause will remove illness) (Borrell-Carrio et al., 2004).

Clinical Notes 1.2

In Clinical Practice

- Promoting healthy lifestyles is an important aspect of medicine and has the potential to save thousands of lives.
- People respond differently to illness so it's important not to assume you know how each person feels.
- Tolerance of ambiguity and the ability to test alternative explanations for symptoms are essential clinical skills.
- The holistic approach means we should consider biomedical factors, lifestyle behaviour, psychological factors (e.g. beliefs, emotions, symptoms), and social factors.

Case Study 1.3

Applying a Biopsychosocial Approach

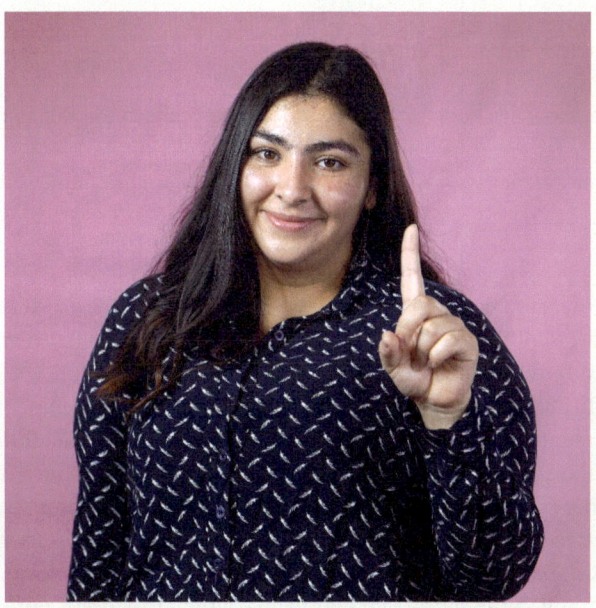

Figure 1.10   Damini's hypertension

Source: © Fernanda/Adobe Stock

(Continued)

Damini has hypertension, which could be due to her high cholesterol, obesity, demanding job, stress of juggling work and home responsibilities, or strong perfectionist tendencies and beliefs about responsibility, which mean she works long hours and is stressed. Which of these explanations we adopt will influence the treatment we offer, but for her it's important that we consider all these factors.

If we take the biological cause (high cholesterol), then we would treat Damini with cholesterol-reducing drugs. If we take the behavioural explanations (obesity), we might offer Damini treatment to lose weight. If we take the psychological explanation (stress and maladaptive beliefs), we might offer Damini stress-management or psychotherapy sessions. Finally, if we adopt the social explanations (work stress and a lack of support), we might refer her to an occupational health worker, counsellor, or a life coach.

In reality, Damini's hypertension will be affected by all these factors, and we need to treat her in the most effective way. To decide this, we would need to consider which treatment will provide the best outcome for Damini at the least cost and time for the health service. What do you think would constitute effective treatment in this case?

Activity 1.2

Different Approaches to Medicine

Reflect on the last time you saw a doctor.

- To what extent was this doctor working with a biomedical framework or a biopsychosocial one?
- How would their treatment have differed if they had altered their framework(s)?

We can see that barriers to applying the biopsychosocial approach include the facts that (1) it is not possible to address all the factors that influence illness, and (2) in order to plan treatment, we need to think in terms of linear causality rather than circular causality. However, this does not mean we should abandon it and return to the biomedical approach, which ignores psychosocial and environmental factors completely. There is, after all, a crucial difference between, on the one hand, recognising all potential determinants and then selectively treating an individual and, on the other hand, focusing only on biomedical factors because that is all we look at. Psychologists also need to be reminded of this. Just as medicine and other health professions err toward biological explanations, psychologists err toward psychological explanations. Very few studies apply a truly biopsychosocial approach – which is perhaps not surprising given the broad range of variables that would need to be measured – and different disciplines use different definitions and measures of the psychological and social variables (Cruwys et al., 2023; Suls & Rothman, 2004).

Therefore, we all need to consciously remind ourselves to explore factors at each level of the biopsychosocial approach when assessing and treating people. This will give us a more complete understanding of the illness, encourage a holistic treatment of the person, include a consideration of potential psychosocial barriers to treatment efficacy, and allow us to change or modify treatments accordingly if our first approach is not as effective as expected.

The tendency to focus on biology or psychology emerges in debates about nature and nurture. Some argue strongly that nature (i.e. genes) is the determinant of behaviour and wellbeing. Others argue just as strongly that nurture (i.e. environment and psychosocial context) is the main determinant. The problem with many **nature–nurture debates** is that health and wellbeing are determined by nature *and* nurture. Furthermore, interactions between nature and nurture are often crucial. As noted in Chapter 7, the likelihood of developing psychological disorders such as schizophrenia may be influenced by a genetic predisposition *and* experiences during pregnancy/birth, early childhood, or later life. Similarly, material presented in Chapter 8 shows how the cognitive potential children inherit in their genes can be optimised or impaired by psychosocial experiences in childhood.

The field of **epigenetics** focuses on how environmental factors – including social contextual factors – regulate the activity and expression of genes (Dieckmann & Czamara, 2024; Xavier et al., 2019). Skin cells, muscle cells, and neurons all contain the same DNA, but they have a different structure and function because their genes are expressed (turned 'on' or 'off') differently. The expression of genes in cells – and the consequences of this – is the key focus of epigenetics. After cells have formed, external factors can influence the expression of their genes. Our physical environments, psychological experiences, and behaviour all influence how our genes are expressed. Various epigenetic processes affect how genes are expressed. One is DNA methylation: the addition of a methyl group to part of the DNA molecule prevents certain genes from being expressed. Another is histone modification: this determines how tightly DNA is wrapped, and influences whether the DNA is accessible to proteins that read genes. Research in humans and non-human animals has provided growing evidence of epigenetic processes across various bodily systems. These include epigenetic modifications to DNA methylation in pancreatic islets, adipose tissue, skeletal muscle, and the liver in Type 2 diabetes (Ling et al., 2022), the effects of stress on DNA expression in immune cells (Glaser et al., 1990; see also Chapters 3 and 15), and the effects of stress and trauma on methylation of serotonin transporter genes (Nikolova & Hariri, 2015; see also the diathesis-stress model of psychiatric disorders in Chapter 7).

There is emerging evidence that environmental influences, such as a lack of nurturing, can lead to physiological changes that can then be passed from parents to children and grandchildren; this is sometimes termed the **intergenerational transmission of vulnerability**. It has led some to suggest that health communication and health education should incorporate epigenetics to explain how parenting practices, lifestyle factors, and social environments affect different people in different ways (Koehly et al., 2021). Better knowledge of epigenetic processes could inform the planning of public health interventions so that they are delivered at key times, when environmental exposures most strongly influence gene expression.

Summary 1.1

- It is difficult to define health. The choice of definition has implications for medical practice and society.
- No single definition of health is adequate and it is perhaps easier to think of health and illness on a continuum from complete wellness to death.
- The separation of psychology and medicine was initially founded on the mind–body divide (dualism).
- Contemporary research challenges dualism by showing that the mind and body are interdependent and influence each other in many ways.
- Medicine was dominated by the biomedical approach for many years, but it assumes a mind–body split so cannot account for contemporary research evidence.
- The more recent biopsychosocial approach has the capacity to unify disciplines in theory and practice, and encourage a holistic approach to medicine.

Conclusion

In this chapter we have looked at how health is difficult to define and how health is subjective in terms of whether people feel or think they are healthy or ill. It is therefore important to consider psychological and social factors for numerous reasons. First, a substantial proportion of people seen by health professionals have no identifiable physical cause for their symptoms. Second, there is substantial evidence for the importance of psychological and social factors in both the onset, spread, and treatment of diseases, such as COVID-19. Third, elements of social diversity and intersectionality are also associated with health and health outcomes.

Historically, the lack of focus on psychosocial factors in healthcare was perpetuated by a widespread belief in mind–body separation (dualism) and the pervasiveness of the biomedical approach. Developments in psychological sciences and neuroscience have shown how the mind and body are integrally linked. Research on embodied cognition and emotion shows how bodily sensations influence our thoughts and feelings, as do the actions of people around us. Epigenetics shows how environmental factors regulate the activity and expression of genes, and there is evidence that psychosocial factors during pregnancy and early childhood influence long-term health and can lead to an intergenerational transmission of vulnerability (see Chapters 8 and 18).

The biopsychosocial approach is consistent with current evidence and shows that we need to consider biological, psychological, social, and macro-cultural factors in health and healthcare. This will lead to a more complete understanding, more accurate and appropriate treatment, and a holistic approach to treating people. The aim of health psychology is to identify and understand the range of biological, psychological, and social factors that influence health and illness, and to use this knowledge to develop effective interventions. In the chapters that follow, attention is given to the four Ps (McKnight et al., 2019): the **predisposing** factors, such as genetics and early life experience that increase susceptibility to illness; the **precipitating** factors, such as unhealthy behaviours that influence whether a predisposition actually leads to illness; the **perpetuating** factors, such as use of healthcare services and adherence to treatment that influence the course of illness or recovery; and the **protective** factors, such as lifestyle and social support that interact with the other three Ps.

Further Reading

Llewellyn, C.D. et al. (eds) (2019) *The Cambridge Handbook of Psychology, Health and Medicine* (3rd edition). Cambridge: Cambridge University Press. Includes short chapters on social, cultural, and ethnic factors and health, health inequalities, socioeconomic status, and medically unexplained symptoms.

Bolton, D. & Gillett, G. (2019) *The Biopsychosocial Model of Health and Disease: New Philosophical and Scientific Developments*. Cham, Switzerland: Palgrave. Available at https://link.springer.com/book/10.1007/978-3-030-11899-0. This open-access eBook addresses the philosophical foundations and clinical utility of the biopsychosocial model in the light of advances that have occurred in the 40 years since the model was first proposed.

White, P. (ed.) (2005) *Biopsychosocial Medicine: An Integrated Approach to Understanding Illness*. Oxford: Oxford University Press. An edited book based on experts discussing the application of the biopsychosocial approach in medicine.

Revision Questions

1 Describe three specialisms in psychology and outline how they are relevant to healthcare.
2 Compare and contrast two definitions of health. What are the implications of each definition for treatment?
3 Compare and contrast the key focal points of physical, subjective, behavioural, functional, and social definitions of health.
4 Why is it important for healthcare professionals to learn to manage uncertainty?
5 What is dualism? How has it influenced medicine?
6 Describe the biomedical approach to medicine and outline the strengths and weaknesses of this approach.
7 Describe the biopsychosocial approach to medicine and outline the strengths and weaknesses of this approach.
8 Compare and contrast the biomedical and biopsychosocial approaches to medicine.
9 How do lay definitions of health align with the biomedical and biopsychosocial approaches to medicine?
10 Outline the concept of epigenetics. Explain its importance for arguments that pit nature against nurture.

SECTION I
PSYCHOLOGY
AND HEALTH

2

MOTIVATION, EMOTION, AND HEALTH

Learning Objectives

This chapter is designed to enable you to:

- Describe motivation and discuss how it affects health.
- Outline the different components of emotion.
- Appreciate the role of positive and negative emotions in health.
- Consider whether expressing emotion is good or bad for health.

Motivation, emotion, and the way we respond to stress shape our lives in many ways. Emotions are powerful motivators that can even make us risk our lives in extreme cases, such as when parents risk their lives trying to save their children. In medicine and healthcare, we are surrounded by stressful and emotional events as people face illnesses and death, either their own or others'. How people respond to these situations varies hugely and there are many examples in healthcare of people behaving in ways we might not understand. For example, the woman in Case Study 2.1 was prepared to risk her own and her unborn baby's lives rather than have a caesarean section.

The media are full of similar examples: parents refusing life-saving treatment for their child on religious grounds; a man with liver cirrhosis who continues to drink alcohol even though he knows it will kill him; a pregnant woman with cancer who refuses chemotherapy and then dies just after her daughter is born; a teenage girl who cuts her arms with a razor blade. These are real cases that illustrate the importance of beliefs, motivation, and emotion in how people respond to day-to-day stress and extreme situations. They also illustrate the complex interaction between motivation and emotion. A further example of the importance of patients' emotions – and the need for healthcare professionals to attend to them – is given in Research Box 2.1. In this chapter we shall look at motivation and emotion in turn, examining what these are and how they are relevant to health.

─Case Study 2.1─

Freebirth or Unassisted Childbirth

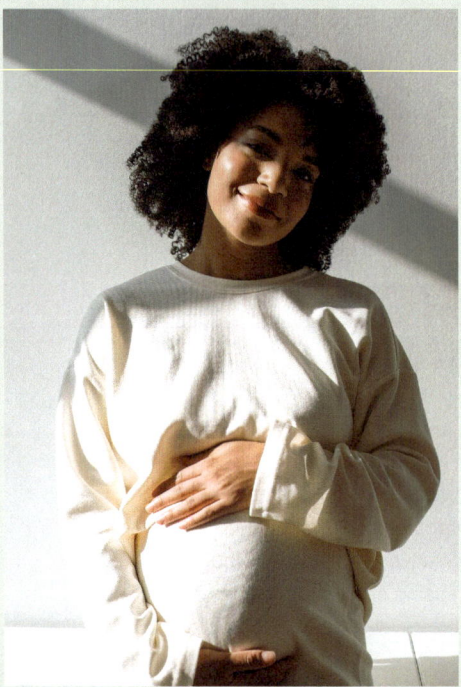

Figure 2.1 Pregnant woman

Source: © Blogcube/Pixabay

Freebirth or unassisted childbirth is where women intentionally give birth without a medical professional being present. This is within women's rights and is legal in most countries. Ms S was a 29-year-old single woman who did not see a doctor for the majority of her pregnancy. When she was 36 weeks pregnant, she registered with a doctor, who found she had severe pre-eclampsia – a life-threatening condition marked by high blood pressure, which can develop very quickly and lead to the death of the mother and baby. Women with this condition are usually admitted to hospital immediately, and the baby is delivered by inducing labour or performing a caesarean section. However, Ms S refused to be admitted to hospital despite two doctors recommending it. She insisted she wanted to give birth without medical assistance and not in hospital. When told that she and the baby might die, Ms S responded, 'so be it'.

The doctors called a social worker, who concluded that Ms S had 'little interest in her own survival and certainly none in the survival of her baby'. The social worker and doctors therefore admitted Ms S to a psychiatric hospital against her will. Although a psychiatrist judged her mentally competent, Ms S was then transferred to a hospital and a court application was made to perform an emergency caesarean section. The court granted the injunction and Ms S was forced to have a caesarean section. Her daughter was born healthy.

Ms S took her case to the High Court. Her admission to hospital and caesarean section were deemed unlawful and she was awarded financial compensation. The judge acknowledged that the social worker and doctors appeared to be well-motivated, but concluded that women have the right to refuse operations, even if they risk their own life or that of their baby. Ms S argued that she did not want a hospital birth because she did not like medical procedures and was prepared to risk both her own and her daughter's lives because she felt so strongly about it.

2.1 Motivation

Motivation is essentially a drive to act. People are motivated to do (or, indeed, not do) things in their life by many different factors. Because of this, theories from various areas of psychology and other disciplines are relevant. These include health behaviour (see Chapter 5) and decision making (see Chapter 12). Some motives are biological – for example, the desire to eat, drink, or reproduce. Others are more psychological and social – for example, the drive for achievement and status. Highlight Box 2.1 gives some examples of biological and social motives, although it is worth noting that the distinction between biological and social motives is not clear-cut. For example, sexual motives can be both biological (the drive to reproduce) and social (e.g. the need for affiliation and nurturance).

Highlight Box 2.1

Examples of Motives

Biological Motives

Hunger

Thirst

Sex

Temperature: need for appropriate body temperature

Excretion: need to eliminate bodily wastes

(Continued)

Sleep and rest

Activity: need for optimal stimulation/arousal

Aggression

Social Motives

Achievement: need to excel

Affiliation: need for social bonds

Autonomy: need for independence

Nurturance: need to nourish and protect others

Recognition: need to be acknowledged positively by others

Dominance: need to influence or control others

Exhibition: need to make an impression on others

Order: need for orderliness, tidiness, organisation

Play: need for fun, relaxation, amusement

(Adapted from Weiten, 2004)

Theories of motivation can be separated into three broad categories, namely drive theories, evolutionary theories, and incentive theories. **Drive theories** use the concept of homeostasis to explain motivation. Homeostasis is a state of physiological equilibrium or stability that organisms strive to maintain. An organism's behavioural and physiological systems operate together to ensure the stability in bodily functions that is necessary to survive. A lack of equilibrium between our current state and our needs creates an internal tension which we are motivated to reduce.

Drive theory is most easily applied to biological drives, such as hunger. When we are hungry, we are motivated to find food and eat. Therefore, we are also more likely to think about food, and to notice food-related stimuli such as advertisements for food (Jonker et al., 2020). Drive theory would predict that once we have eaten, we are no longer motivated to continue eating. However, there are many examples of people continuing to eat when they are no longer hungry or refusing to eat when they are hungry. Dieting provides a good example of where a drive to eat is not acted on (see Chapter 17). In societies where food is abundant, our intake of food is actually dependent on internal cues, such as hunger and satiety, and external cues, such as availability, packaging, and portion sizes, which determine what and how much we eat (Bilman et al., 2017). Thus, drive theory can account for some biological drives and motivation, but is limited in its application to a lot of human behaviour.

Evolutionary theories of motivation argue that social characteristics are shaped by processes of natural selection in the same way as physical characteristics: desirable social characteristics maximise the chances of reproductive success. Thus, social motives, such as the need for affiliation or dominance, are thought to occur because they increase our chances of survival and reproduction. There is some evidence to support this. For example, pair bonding and parental care occur in many species and facilitate reproduction and the survival of offspring. Research suggests that the hormone oxytocin is important in reproductive and social behaviours like bonding, attachment, and love. Oxytocin is released during sexual activity, giving birth, and breastfeeding. It is also released in response to pleasant touch, such as a hug or massage, and can reduce stress (Moberg et al., 2020). Oxytocin is therefore sometimes referred to in the media as the 'love' or 'cuddle' hormone. There is plenty of research demonstrating this effect. For example, parents who have higher levels of oxytocin after birth have better physical and visual contact with their children, are more attuned to the infant's emotions, have a better parent–infant bond, and show more positive caregiving (Shorey et al., 2023).

Incentive theories emphasise the role of external factors that trigger and regulate motivation. For example, a man may not be motivated to seek a relationship until he meets a woman whom he finds particularly desirable. More elaborate incentive theories take into account **expectations** and **values**, which are common in models of health behaviour (see Chapter 5). Expectancies and values allow for the influence of whether people (1) expect to attain their goal, and (2) how important or valuable that goal is to them. Therefore, when a woman meets a person whom she finds very desirable, she will not act on her desire if she thinks (1) that there is no chance that the other person is interested in her, or (2) that she does not really value having a relationship at that stage in her life.

These different theories of motivation are not incompatible. Drive theories emphasise internal states as motivating us, whereas incentive theories emphasise external stimuli and rewards. The two can be thought of as push and pull theories of motivation: internal states push us to act, and external stimuli pull us. However, all these theories are reductionist in one form or another because they concentrate solely on internal, external, or genetic causes. More comprehensive theories have therefore been proposed that incorporate biological, behavioural, cognitive, and social elements of motivation (e.g. Bernard et al., 2005; Pincus, 2024; Toates, 2009).

—Activity 2.1—

Motivation

- How would different theories explain the motives of Ms S in Case Study 2.1? She refused a caesarean even though it put both her own and her baby's lives at risk.

2.2 Motivation and Health

Clearly, motivation is relevant to health and health professionals. Understanding biological motivations can help us to treat abnormal extremes of biological drives, such as obesity, eating disorders, smoking, addiction, risky sexual behaviour, and insomnia. Understanding social motivations can help us to comprehend our own behaviour and what motivates us to work as health professionals. It can also help us to empathise and deal better with other people's behaviour that we might not understand. Knowing more about another person's motives means we can address situations more constructively. Interventions such as motivational interviewing have been developed to treat disorders with a strong motivational component, such as addiction. Motivational interviewing is defined as 'a collaborative conversation style for strengthening a person's own motivation and commitment to change' (Miller & Rollnick, 2013). There is some evidence that it can be effective in encouraging and promoting behaviour change in various domains, including drug and alcohol use, and is an effective adjunct to standard treatment (Bischof et al., 2021; Schwenker et al., 2023).

Motivation is relevant to many health topics. These include smoking, which is discussed in Chapter 5, and obesity, which we look at in Chapter 17. Here we focus on alcohol use because it is a good example of complex motives preventing people from changing their drinking behaviour. Alcohol consumption and alcohol-related problems are high in developed countries. Rates of consumption per capita are shown in Figure 2.2. Alcohol use is causally linked to over 200 disease and injury conditions, and it is the seventh leading risk factor for burden of disease worldwide (World Health Organization, 2018). Alcohol-related diseases account for almost 5% of deaths worldwide, and 5% of the global disease burden (World Health Organization, 2018). Alcohol consumption increases as societies become richer, with the highest consumption of alcohol per capita in Europe, where alcohol-related diseases account for 10% of all deaths. However, the disease burden due to alcohol-related diseases is greater in low- and low-middle income countries (World Health Organization, 2018). Increased alcohol consumption inevitably affects morbidity and mortality. There is more information on alcohol use in Chapter 17.

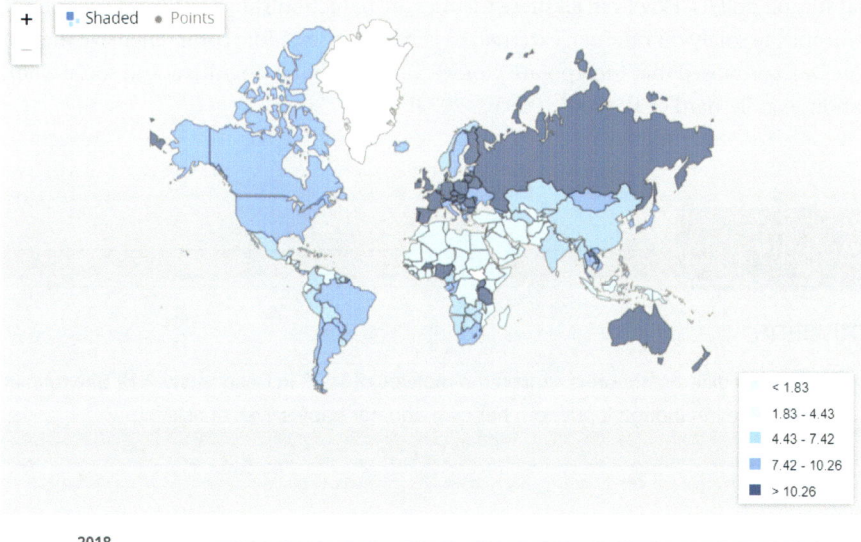

Figure 2.2 Alcohol consumption worldwide

Source: Image courtesy of World Health Organization, Global Health Observatory Data Repository. Shared under the CC BY-4.0 license

The motivation to drink alcohol involves both biological and social factors. As with many activities that become habitual, drinking alcohol is usually pleasurable. For many people, the immediate feeling or reward they get from drinking alcohol outweighs the long-term risks, especially when those risks seem removed or unlikely. The common bias of **health optimism** means that most people will consistently underestimate their own risk of disease compared to others:

this has been observed among people with higher levels of alcohol use (J. Morris et al., 2024). Therefore, the long-term negative consequences are minimised and outweighed by short-term pleasure or gain. Drinking alcohol is also a part of many social rituals and norms. It is also a marker of adulthood in many cultures, and what people drink, where they drink, and how they drink may be important elements of displays of personal image and social status. Changing a habitual behaviour such as alcohol consumption is difficult, particularly when it is longstanding and associated with social events and affiliations. Case Study 2.2 provides an example of using motivational interviewing with a woman who has an alcohol problem.

Healthcare professionals must acknowledge that although we may be motivated by reducing harms to health, the people we work with may have different motives for changing or not changing their behaviour. In the context of alcohol use, avoiding the long-term risks of liver damage and cancer may be key motives for health professionals, but drinkers may be more strongly motivated by other (short-term) concerns. For example, studies of the alcohol abstinence challenge 'Dry January' indicate that many people are motivated to change by short-term outcomes such as better sleep, better concentration, clearer skin, and saving money (de Visser & Piper, 2020). Social motives unrelated to health are also important: fear of missing out on fun social occasions may be a disincentive to drinking less or not drinking. Successful behaviour change campaigns should recognise the diversity of motives for change (and non-change) and tailor support and feedback so that it provides appropriate motivation for each individual (de Visser & Nicholls, 2020). For example, the 'Dry January' campaign allows people trying to drink less to choose motivational messages that focus on how much less alcohol they have consumed, how many calories they have avoided, or how much money they have saved (www.dryjanuary. co.uk). The need to focus on what motivates patients is also addressed in Clinical Note 2.1.

Case Study 2.2

Treating Alcohol Misuse with Motivational Interviewing

Kate is a 37-year-old senior executive in the music industry. She works 12-hour days and finds it hard to unwind. In the evening, she drinks to relax. She often has to entertain clients at lunch and will also drink alcohol on these occasions. Her total alcohol consumption is more than three times the recommended maximum. Kate does not think she has an alcohol problem. Many of her friends and colleagues also drink every day.

Kate has been trying to get pregnant for 10 months without success, and wants fertility treatment. However, heavy alcohol use is associated with decreased fertility, less effective fertility treatment, and greater risk of miscarriage and stillbirth (Van Heertum & Rossi, 2017). Kate needs to reduce her alcohol intake substantially for it to be within safe levels.

Motivational Interviewing

Motivational interviewing rests on the principle of not judging or imposing our own views on Kate but instead trying to understand her situation and helping her to harness her own motivation to change.

(Continued)

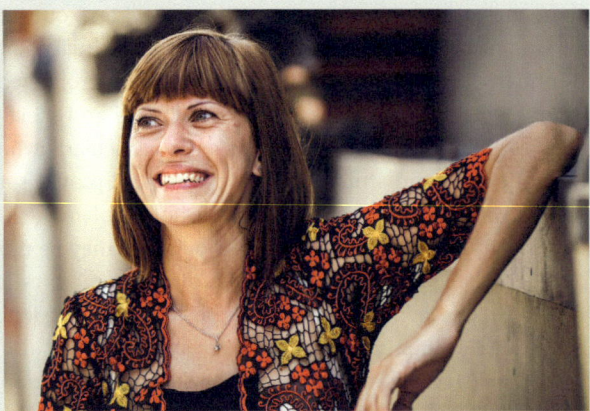

Figure 2.3   Kate: Motivational interviewing for alcohol use

Source: © Artem Beliaikin/Unsplash

1   Exploring Kate's reasons for drinking and whether she has any ambivalence brings up the following:

Motives for drinking	**Motives against**
It helps me relax	I want to get pregnant
I like it – it is my treat	I like it at the time but not afterwards
It switches my brain off	It is not good for me
Entertaining is part of my job	I don't want people to see me as a 'drinker'

2   Making these ambivalent motives explicit leads Kate to re-evaluate her drinking. It also highlights the fact that falling pregnant is the most important motive for her at the moment.

3   Kate sets a goal to stop drinking. Strategies to help her to achieve this are explored. For the first week she decides to replace wine with a non-alcoholic alternative and to join a yoga class to help her relax. An appointment is made for one week later to review her progress and support her.

Clinical Notes 2.1

Using Motivation to Encourage Behaviour Change

- Understanding motivation can help us to treat health problems that involve motivational elements, such as obesity, eating disorders, smoking, addiction, risky sexual behaviour, and insomnia.
- If you ask people about perceived negative behaviours, such as smoking or alcohol intake, they will often under-report their behaviour.

- Educating people about the negative effects of these behaviours can trigger them to try to change.
- However, imposing our views and making people feel judged will not help them to change as much as assisting them to harness their own motivation.
- Try to understand why they behave in this way and empathise with their situation. Focus on what would motivate them to change (or not want to change). Then support them to change their behaviour.
- Help them to believe that they *can* change.

Summary 2.1

- Motivation is a drive to act for a range of reasons, including internal and external factors.
- Theories of motivation include drive theories, evolutionary theories, and incentive theories. More recent theories integrate biological, behavioural, cognitive, and social elements of motivation.
- Understanding motivational processes can help to guide intervention for changing health-related behaviours, such as alcohol misuse.
- Theories of motivation have clinical applications.

2.3 Emotion

Human life involves a wide range of emotions. Indeed, the English language has over 550 words referring to emotion, and the importance of emotions is evident in the widespread use of emojis in electronic communications. Facial expressions are critical in revealing our emotions, as illustrated in Figure 2.4, and the use of emojis shows how indication of emotions through facial expressions has transferred into our non-face-to-face communication.

Our emotions have a huge impact on the quality of our life. For example, severe depression can motivate people to end their life. In healthcare settings where people face stress and personal difficulties, emotion has a huge impact on people's attitude, recovery, and quality of life. For example, one person with terminal cancer may cope with humour and a renewed zest for life, whereas another person with curable cancer may feel devastated, depressed, and convinced they will die.

Emotional disorders such as depression are one of the leading contributors to the burden of disease in the world, and their contribution to the overall global burden of disease appears to be increasing (GBD 2019 Mental Disorders Collaborators, 2022; World Health Organization, 2024b). Emotional disorders also incur huge economic costs due to loss of work, low productivity, incapacity benefits, and absenteeism. Furthermore, mental illness is also frequently implicated in physical and mental disability (Layard, 2006). Much research and theory has therefore concentrated on negative emotions, such as anxiety and depression. The development of **positive psychology** over the last 30 years has encouraged the study of positive emotions, such as happiness, and the effect these can have on our wellbeing. There has also been research

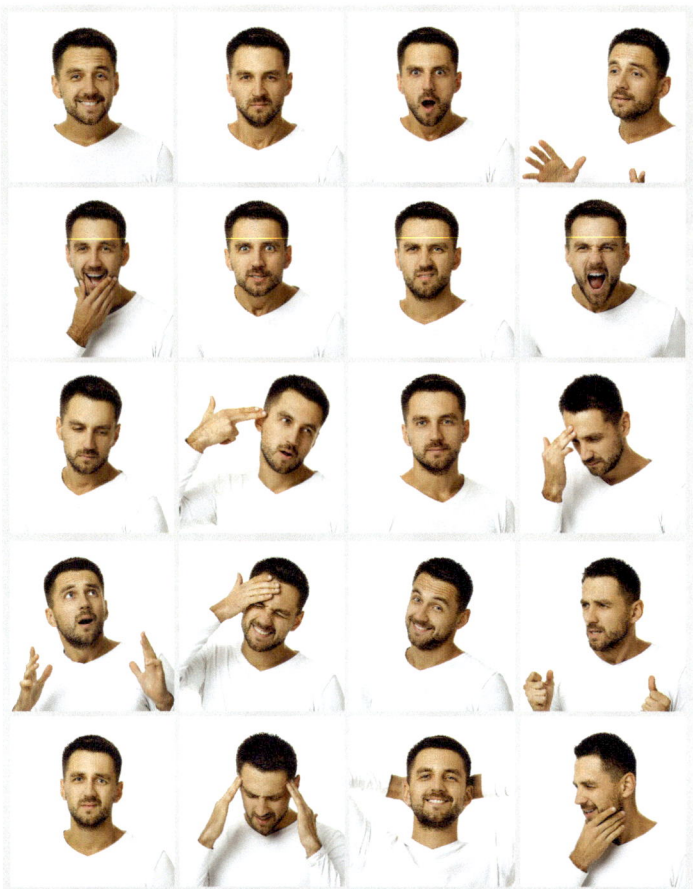

Figure 2.4 Facial expressions and emotions

Source: © producer/Adobe Stock

into normal emotions and their associated physiology as it is thought that they may provide a link between psychosocial factors – such as stress and social relationships – and health. Theories of emotion have therefore emerged from the study of both normal and abnormal emotional processes.

In psychology, the term **affect** is used generally to include **emotions**, **moods**, and **impulses**. The range and complexity of emotional experiences make it difficult to define. It has been debated whether we have basic emotions that are experienced similarly by all humans. Ekman (1999) proposed that there are six basic emotions: happiness, sadness, surprise, anger, fear, and disgust. Research supports this by finding that these emotions have distinct neurobiological underpinnings and are associated with different patterns of brain activity, for example, fear involving activation of the amygdala, and anger involving the orbitofrontal cortex (Celeghin et al., 2017). Others have argued that emotions are constructed from multiple individual and social factors (Barrett, 2017). In addition, some have argued to expand the focus to include interpersonal emotions such as love and jealousy (Sabini & Silver, 2005). However, in the context of health promotion and healthcare, individual-level emotions may be most relevant: Research Box 2.1 highlights the importance of addressing patients' fear, given that surgery-related emotions influence treatment outcomes (Pinto et al., 2013; Riecke et al., 2023).

Most theories of emotion start with the premise that emotion has three core components: cognitive (thoughts), physiological, and behavioural. The **cognitive component** is the conscious experience of emotion, including the meaning we attach to it and the influence of previous experience and knowledge on how we respond. The **physiological component** of emotions is complex and involves the central nervous system, autonomic nervous system, and endocrine system, as well as exteroceptive sensations through sight, smell, touch, etc. The **behavioural component** can be further separated into the nonverbal expression of emotions (facial expression, body posture, etc.) and behavioural responses (e.g. recoiling from something disgusting). The interplay between these three core components is reflected in common phrases such as 'being frozen with fear' or 'blood boiling with anger'. Figure 2.5 shows how these different elements might interact to result in emotional experience.

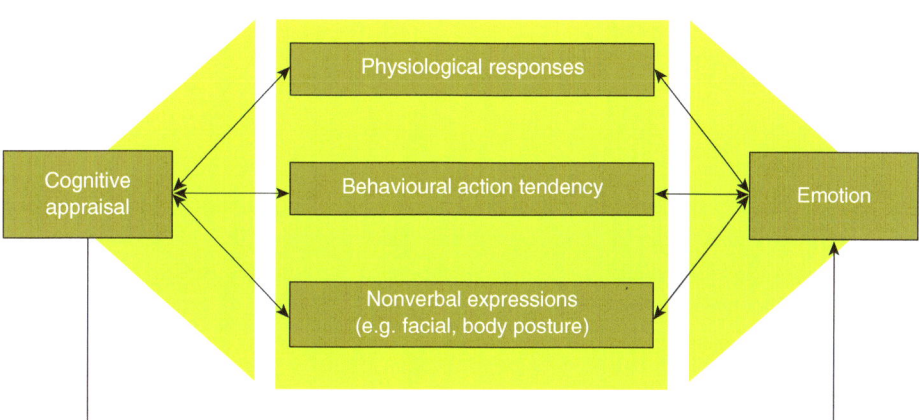

Figure 2.5 Components of emotions

▮Activity 2.2▮

Regulating Your Emotions

Think of the last time you were really upset or angry about something.

*   What things did you do to calm yourself down?
*   Did this involve cognitive factors, taking action, changing behaviour, or social factors?

─Research Box 2.1─

Understanding Pre-Surgery Emotions to Improve Outcomes

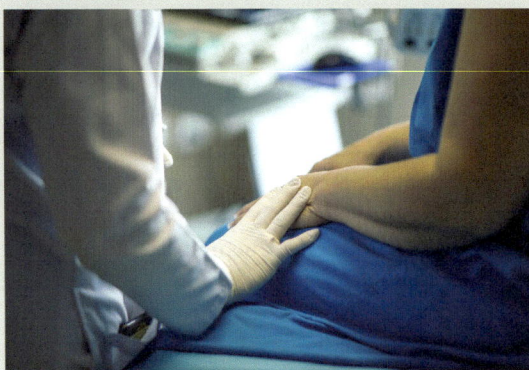

Figure 2.6 Pre-operative anxiety and fear

Source: © fernandozhiminaicela/Pixabay

Background

Pre-operative anxiety and fear are common. In addition to being unpleasant and distressing, these negative emotions can lead to poorer post-surgical outcomes. The aim of this large quali-tative study was to identify factors that may contribute to pre-operative anxiety, and to explore patients' ideas for how to address them.

Method and Findings

This study involved analysis of responses from 1,000 people awaiting surgery. They provided qualitative data as part of a larger study of surgery outcomes. Open-ended questions were used to explore (1) their beliefs about what causes or affects pre-surgery anxiety, and (2) which strategies other than anxiolytic medication they would prefer.

The analysis revealed that pre-surgery fear and anxiety were related to many aspects of the process, including surgical complications, sufficient analgesia and anaesthesia, pain, surgical outcomes, and delivery of care. When asked how they would prefer their anxiety to be managed, the most commonly-cited intervention was a personal conversation about the causes of their fear and anxiety.

Significance

The authors noted that the wide range of influences on anxiety and fear mean that there is unlikely to be a one-size-fits-all approach to managing pre-surgery emotions. They concluded that giving patients the opportunity to discuss their anxiety and fear may improve provider–patient communication and help to reduce anxiety, and they suggested that it should be a standard component of preparation for surgery.

Salzmann, S., Euteneuer, F., Kampmann, S., Rienmüller, S. & Rüsch, D. (2023) Preoperative anxiety and need for support: A qualitative analysis in 1,000 patients. *Patient Education and Counseling, 115*: 107864. doi:10.1016/j.pec.2023.107864

2.3.1 Cognitive Components of Emotion

The *meaning* of a situation is critical to how we respond to it emotionally. For example, if a woman finds a lump in her breast and interprets it as a harmless cyst, she will not be hugely alarmed, whereas if she interprets the lump as cancer, she will be frightened and anxious. Strong negative emotions like this usually motivate people to take action. Reviews of studies of why women delay getting help for breast cancer highlight that how women interpret their symptoms is one of the most important influences on seeking help (Grimley et al., 2020; Khakbazan et al., 2014). Table 2.1 illustrates women's emotional responses to discovering a breast lump and how quickly they went to see their doctor.

Table 2.1   Responses to discovering a breast lump (adapted from Petrie & Pennebaker, 2004)

Visited doctor < 4 days after discovering lump	Visited doctor 7–90 days after discovering lump
'I felt sheer panic, I freaked out' (1 day)	'I felt fine' (7 days)
'I was worried – my hands were shaking' (1 day)	'I'm not a worrier – sometimes I'm too relaxed' (90 days)
'Scared stiff' (3 days)	'Just a little bit worried' (14 days)
'Scared – I even cried' (1 day)	'Just "oh, a lump". I was fairly blasé' (7 days)
'I felt bad – panic and worry' (2 days)	'I didn't think anything of it really' (7 days)
'I was scared, nervous and sweaty' (3 days)	'I wasn't really bothered' (21 days)

The first cognitive element of emotion is how people **appraise** a situation when it occurs, or what immediate meaning they make of it (e.g. whether it is dangerous, challenging, or harmless). A second element is how people **label** their emotional state when it occurs. The physiological arousal experienced with many emotions is similar. For example, sympathetic nervous system arousal occurs when we are anxious and excited, so how we label our emotional state will influence our emotional experience. On a roller-coaster, some people will label the experience exciting or thrilling, but others (including the authors) will label it terrifying and aversive. This leads us to a third important cognitive element, which is whether we **evaluate** our response as positive or negative. Those people who evaluate their experience on the roller-coaster as positive will enjoy it and want to do it again. Helping people to reappraise or re-label their experiences can therefore change the way they feel about it. This is particularly relevant to medicine, which often involves invasive and uncomfortable procedures.

This process of appraisal, labelling, and evaluation shapes our future emotional responses as well. Panic disorder is a good example of this. Around 5% of people experience panic at some point in their lives (Grant et al., 2006). Panic is associated with extreme physiological arousal, which is part of the 'fight-flight' response (see Chapter 3). Although panic is very unpleasant, it is not life-threatening or uncommon. Thus, long-term panic disorder is most likely to develop in people who interpret their initial experiences of panic in a catastrophic way, such as 'I'm going mad' or 'I'm going to die', and who label and evaluate the panic attack as extremely negative (Robinaugh et al., 2019). Under these circumstances, people will worry about having another panic attack. This increases their anxiety levels and physiological arousal, thereby also increasing the likelihood they will experience panic again. In addition, if a person interprets the panic attack as being linked to a particular situation, they will be highly anxious when put in that situation again and may become phobic. For example, if a person has a panic attack in an MRI scanner, they are likely to become more anxious when having another MRI, which in turn increases the likelihood they will experience another panic attack.

The meaning that people attach to their experience of panic can therefore result in them becoming anxious about being anxious, which becomes a self-fulfilling cycle. However, although the cognitive component is *necessary* for emotion, it is not *sufficient* on its own. Emotions are rarely consciously initiated – we cannot force ourselves to feel panic, disgust, or anger. As we have seen in Chapter 1, emotions are also embodied and the physical response that accompanies emotion (as well as motorsensory input from movement, posture, and gestures) is an important part of how we feel.

2.3.2 Physiological Components of Emotion

The physiological components of emotion are initiated in the brain from several structures that form the **limbic system** (see Chapter 7). Elements of the limbic system control the autonomic nervous system and endocrine responses (see Chapter 3), and are involved in learning and modulating emotion. For example, the amygdala is particularly important in fear. If the amygdala is damaged, animals are unable to learn fear when exposed to a threatening object. In people, imaging studies show the amygdala is activated during fear (Celeghin et al., 2017).

─Highlight Box 2.2─

The Case of Phineas Gage

Phineas Gage was working on the railroads in 1848 when a gunpowder explosion drove a large metal rod straight through his head. The rod entered below his left cheek bone and passed through the frontal cortex before exiting and landing many metres behind him. A model of the injury he sustained is shown here. Remarkably, he survived his injury and was conscious moments later.

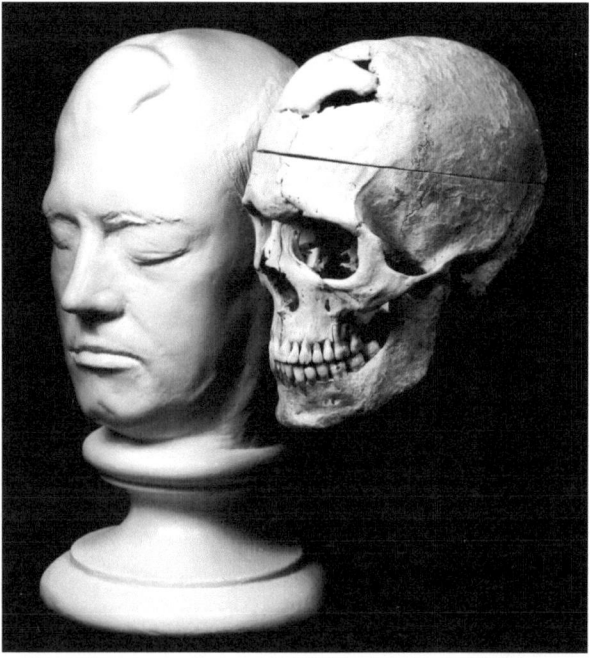

Figure 2.7   Skull of Phineas Gage

Image credit: Warren Anatomical Museum, Centre for the History of Medicine in the Francis A. Countway Library of Medicine

After his injury, Gage is reported to have changed from a hard-working, kind, and likeable man to an impulsive, inconsiderate person who used vulgar language. Up to this point, the frontal lobes were not considered to affect personality or social interaction. Gage became the first medically reported case to indicate the frontal lobes were important. Although there is some debate over whether the damage was exclusively to the left frontal lobe or involved both lobes, it was clear from his case that the frontal lobe was important in the inhibition of inappropriate emotional responses.

Emotion also involves areas of the **frontal cortex**. It is thought that the limbic system provides a fast, emotional response and the cortex then provides a slower, secondary response that elaborates and regulates the more basic emotional processes of the initial response (Dixon et al., 2017). This two-part process explains why we often react or 'feel' before we think. The role of the cortex in inhibiting emotional and behavioural responses was first suspected in the case of Phineas Gage (see Highlight Box 2.2). Research has since indicated that the prefrontal cortex, and orbitofrontal cortex in particular, plays an important role in inhibiting emotional and behavioural responses. For example, damage to the orbitofrontal cortex is associated with increased anger, anxiety, pride, depression, inappropriate crying or laughing, and the impaired filtering of emotional information (Jonker et al., 2015).

2.3.3 Behavioural Components of Emotion

The behavioural components of emotion can be divided into:

- Action tendencies, i.e. the potential or drive to act.
- Nonverbal responses, e.g. posture, gestures.
- Facial expressions.

It is thought that the behavioural components of emotion are part of its purpose. In other words, emotion makes us want to act. This can be clearly seen on the faces of people observing the attack on the World Trade Center on September 11, 2001 (9/11) in Figure 2.8. Thus, emotions are early warning signals that there is something we need to attend to. Research shows that when people experience negative emotions, it narrows their focus of attention onto whatever prompted the negative emotion. Conversely, positive emotions lead to a broadening of attention, promoting broader processing of information and events (Fredrickson, 2004).

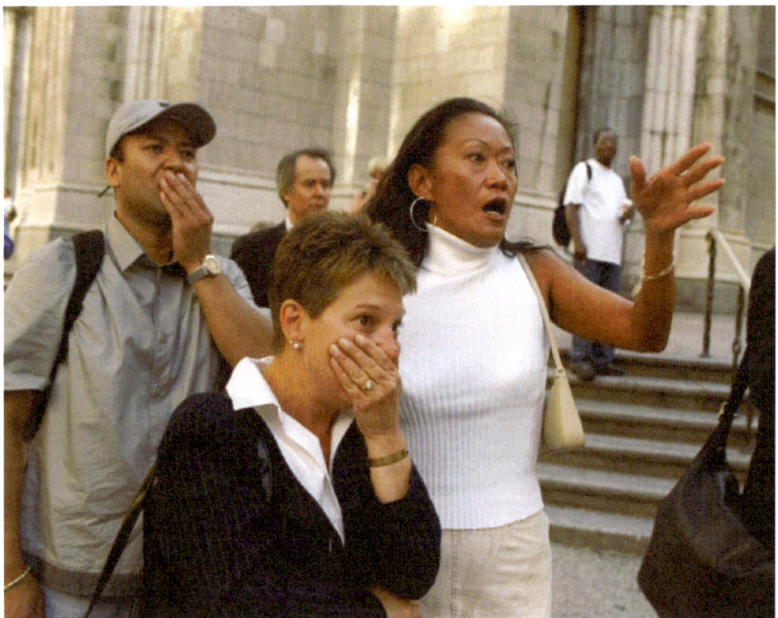

Figure 2.8   Observers of 9/11 attacks

Source: Photograph reproduced courtesy of Associated Press

Emotions therefore direct our attention. The physiological response equips our body for action, and action tendencies provide us with ways to cope with the situation, such as fight or flight if we are under threat. The fight-flight response is certainly observable in extreme situations, but people do not always respond in this way. For example, following the 9/11 attacks, there were reports of people walking in a calm and orderly fashion to get out of the World Trade Center twin towers. Thus, people's responses to threat are more complicated and influenced by social circumstances and norms. Consequently, there has been a substantial amount of research that has examined how people regulate their emotions, and the coping strategies they use to deal with challenging circumstances (Ochsner & Gross, 2005; Yih et al., 2019). We shall return to this in section 2.4 on Emotion and Health.

The behavioural component of emotion also includes the nonverbal expression of emotion in our posture, movements (e.g. clenched fists), and facial expression. Studies of embodied cognition and emotion show that sensorimotor feedback on our bodily state also affects the way we label our emotions. Research where people have been asked to tense certain facial muscles in ways that resemble a 'smile' has shown that people will report more positive emotion in response to stimuli, such as a film clip or photographs, although the effects are not always strong, and they vary from person to person (Coles et al., 2019). According to the **embodied cognition hypothesis**, sensorimotor signals are used by the brain to interpret which emotion is being felt (Niedenthal, 2007).

Activity 2.3

Embodied Emotion and Facial Feedback

Raise your eyebrows and try to be angry.

- What happens?
- Why do you think this is?

2.3.4 Theories of Emotion

Early theories of emotion concentrated on the relationship between different components of emotion. In a 'chicken and egg' type of debate, theorists argued about whether physical responses preceded cognitive appraisal or vice versa. The current consensus is that appraisal processes initiate our physiological, behavioural, and conscious experience of emotion. These appraisal processes can be preconscious or conscious, which fits with the view that the limbic system is a fast-processing system (preconscious appraisal) that is then moderated by the frontal cortex (conscious appraisal).

Substantial evidence confirms that preconscious processing occurs and influences our mood and behaviour. For example, Chartrand, Van Baaren, and Bargh (2006) flashed positive words (e.g. friends, music), negative words (e.g. war, cancer), and neutral words (e.g. plant, building) very quickly on a screen so people could not consciously 'see' them. They found that even though people could not 'see' the words, they reported a more negative mood after being shown negative words. Other experiments have shown that if we 'see' something preconsciously, we are more likely to prefer it or feel good if it is shown to us so we can consciously see it (Monahan et al., 2000), and that we are more likely to trust people we interact with after preconsciously seeing the word 'trust' rather than 'suspicion' (J. Cai et al., 2020).

More recent theories, such as Conceptual Act theory (Barrett, 2017), look at how our emotional experience is constructed from the interaction between various physiological changes and exteroceptive sensations, such as fight-flight, sensory perception of what we see and hear, and cognitive factors such as appraisal, attention, memory, and knowledge.

Another theory divides emotion into positive and negative affect (Watson & Tellegen, 1985). Thus, all emotions can be plotted according to whether they are positive (e.g. pleasurable) or negative (e.g. distressing), and on a second dimension according to intensity (high versus low), as shown in Figure 2.9. This has the advantage of simplifying emotions so that it is easier to look at relationships between emotions, health, and illness. It also accounts for the *intensity* of emotion, which may be important in the effect emotion can have on health. It is quite reasonable to assume that emotion at a low level of intensity (e.g. irritation) will have a different physiological effect and influence on health than a high-intensity emotion (e.g. extreme anger).

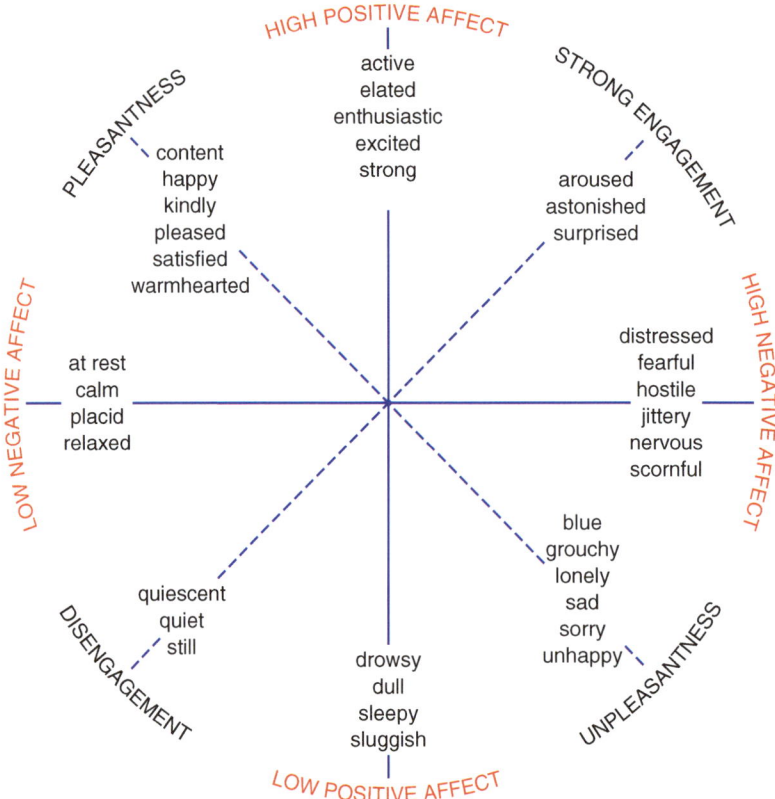

Figure 2.9   Model of positive and negative affect

2.4 Emotion and Health

A good example of the link between emotions and health is the association of psychological disorders such as depression with an increased risk of morbidity and mortality. For example, there is such robust evidence that depression is a risk factor for all-cause mortality and cardiac mortality in people with coronary heart disease that the American Heart Association has identified depression as a specific risk factor for mortality (Lichtman et al., 2014; Shiga, 2023).

In this section, the nature of the relationship between emotions and health is considered in three main ways:

- The association between typical emotions and health.
- The influence of emotional dispositions on health.
- The effect of how people regulate and express their emotions on health.

2.4.1 Emotional States and Health

Laboratory studies show that any acute, strong, or extreme emotion is associated with increased physiological arousal regardless of whether that emotion is positive or negative. This arousal has potentially negative effects on health through influencing systems such as the cardiovascular and immune system. However, studies of people's moods in day-to-day settings suggest that positive emotion in natural settings produces less negative physiological responses than negative emotion (Pressman & Cohen, 2005).

Large-scale epidemiological and survey studies of mood and health generally find that positive mood is associated with better health. People with high positive affect report fewer symptoms or pain and have fewer illnesses, such as strokes, colds, and accidents. In people aged 55 and over, positive affect is associated with longer life (Pressman & Cohen, 2005). Reviews of research evidence have shown that positive affect (e.g. emotional wellbeing, positive mood, joy, happiness, vigour, energy) and positive dispositions (e.g. life satisfaction, hopefulness, optimism, sense of humour) are associated with reduced mortality in healthy people, even after taking into account medical, psychological, and social factors (Chida & Steptoe, 2009; Zhang & Han, 2016). As noted in Section IV of this textbook, positive wellbeing is also associated with reduced mortality in people with various medical conditions.

However, the association between happiness and health does not mean that one causes the other. Better health may mean people are more likely to be happy: happier people may be more likely to *say* they are healthier, have a stronger support network, be more likely to carry out good health practices, etc. Theories of positive affect and health outline several pathways through which positive affect may lead to better health. These include the Broaden and Build model (Fredrickson, 2004), which proposes that positive affect results in: (1) healthier thought processes by broadening attention which promotes more global information processing, connections across concepts, and more forward thinking; and (2) more resilience by enhancing resources, such as coping and social relationships. Cameron, Bertenshaw, and Sheeran (2015) built on this model and other evidence to propose additional pathways, such as increased motivation, more responsiveness to health-related goals, better mood maintenance or repair, physiological arousal, and increased self-control and resilience. They conducted a meta-analysis of 39 experimental studies where positive affect was induced in a laboratory through tasks such as watching positive videos to examine the influence on different aspects of cognition and behaviour. However, the study found no reliable effect of positive mood on health cognitions (e.g. intention to drive safely, intention to refrain from alcohol, risk perceptions, perceived control over health behaviours) or behaviour (e.g. food and alcohol consumption, exercise, smoking). The only reliable effect of positive mood was on choosing healthier food (although not reducing food consumption). It therefore appears that at least part of the effect of positive emotions is direct, rather than an indirect effect explained by different patterns of behaviour.

The role of negative emotions in health has been more extensively researched, with mixed results depending on which outcomes are examined. There is now substantial evidence that some types of negative emotion are associated with specific illnesses. The main examples of this are associations between anger, hostility, and cardiovascular disease (Chida & Steptoe, 2009), and depression and cardiovascular disease (Fiedorowicz, 2014; Prigge et al., 2022; Smaardijk et al., 2020), which are covered in more detail in Chapter 16.

In summary, there is evidence that positive emotions are associated with good health and that specific negative emotions are associated with certain illnesses, but there are many ways in which one may influence the other. This is often the case with links between psychosocial and biological phenomena and explains why we use terms such as **association** or **relationship**, rather than **cause** or **predict**. For example, the association between emotion and health can in part be explained by biased attention, meaning people focus more on their symptoms or, alternatively, mood influencing the way people interpret these symptoms. Possible pathways between emotion and health are summarised in Figure 2.10. The important point to note is that emotion can influence our health through biological, behavioural, and/ or social mechanisms.

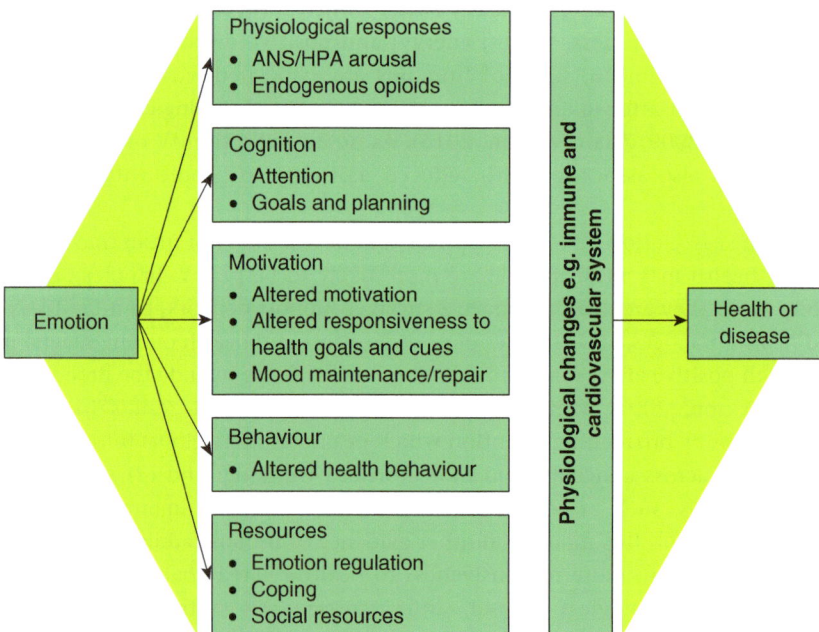

Figure 2.10 Pathways between emotion and health (adapted from Cameron et al., 2015; Pressman & Cohen, 2005)

2.4.2 Emotional Dispositions and Health

Emotional dispositions are personality-like tendencies toward experiencing certain emotions. There are five main personality traits: openness to new experience, conscientiousness, extroversion, agreeableness, and neuroticism (as shown in Table 2.2). Of these, we look at conscientiousness and neuroticism more fully here because they are most consistently linked with health (Heilmayr & Friedman, 2020; Kang et al., 2023; Wettstein et al., 2020). **Conscientious** people are defined as having self-discipline and being efficient, organised, reliable, and responsible. Evidence suggests conscientious people live longer, although this is probably due to the fact that conscientious people are more likely to practise positive health behaviours, such as exercising and attending for health screening, and are less likely to practise negative health behaviours, such as smoking (Hajek et al., 2020). Although conscientiousness is not associated with particular emotions (Heilmayr & Friedman, 2019), it appears to be related to different emotion-regulation strategies, such as problem solving and reappraisal, and less avoidance (Hughes et al., 2020).

Table 2.2 Five main personality traits (OCEAN)

Openness to new experiences	Intellect and interest in culture. Includes characteristics such as being artistic, curious, imaginative, insightful, having wide interests, and being unconventional
Conscientiousness	Dependable with the will to achieve. Includes characteristics such as being self-disciplined, efficient, organised, reliable, responsible, dutiful, and thorough
Extroversion	Outgoing. Includes characteristics such as being talkative, gregarious, enthusiastic, seeking excitement, assertive, and active
Agreeableness	Loving, friendly, and compliant. Includes characteristics such as being sympathetic, appreciative, trusting, kind, forgiving, generous, and altruistic
Neuroticism	Tendency to experience negative emotions. Includes characteristics such as being anxious, tense, self-pitying, worrying, self-conscious, hostile, and vulnerable

Neuroticism is the personality trait with the most obvious emotional component. People who are high in neuroticism experience a wide range of negative emotions, such as low mood, anxiety, guilt, hostility, and fear. People high in neuroticism are at greater risk of mental disorders and some physical illnesses, and they use psychological and physical health services more (Hajek et al., 2021; Lahey, 2009; Willroth et al., 2023). However, it is difficult to know whether this increased risk is due to the personality trait of neuroticism itself, or to components of neuroticism, such as negative affect, depression, anxiety, and hostility. There is also no consistent link between neuroticism and measures of chronic morbidity, such as heart disease, cancer, or mortality (Heilmayr & Friedman, 2019).

Emotional dispositions associated with psychological health are **optimism** and **pessimism**. Optimism is a general disposition toward expecting good things to happen in the future and pessimism is expecting bad things. These are not mutually exclusive, and it is possible to be generally optimistic about most things but pessimistic about others. A commonly used measure of optimism and pessimism is shown in Highlight Box 2.3.

Optimism is associated with better general psychological and physical wellbeing (Scheier et al., 2021; Uribe et al., 2021). It is also associated with better outcomes across numerous health-related contexts, including immune function, cardiovascular morbidity and mortality, and post-surgical pain (Forte et al., 2022; Krittanawong et al., 2022; Rasmussen et al., 2009). However, as with other dispositions or traits, it is difficult to distinguish the mechanisms involved or to be sure what role emotions may play. As with conscientiousness, evidence shows that optimism is also associated with positive health behaviours, healthier coping strategies, and increased social support, which can in turn affect our responses to illness or stress (Scheier & Carver, 2018).

It important to note, however, that not all optimism is appropriate or beneficial. People are often overly or inappropriately optimistic, leading to them underestimating the likelihood of negative outcomes or overestimating the likelihood of positive outcomes (see section 2.2). One review found that many patients with heart and renal failure have unrealistically optimistic predictions of their future health, and that this may affect their adherence to medical advice (Hole & Salem, 2016). It is therefore important for healthcare professionals to cultivate optimism about the possibility of change, but to identify and challenge unrealistic optimism (Bortolotti & Antrobus, 2015; Shepperd et al., 2017).

─Highlight Box 2.3─

Measuring Optimism

The Life Orientation Test (Revised)

Please be as honest and accurate as you can throughout. Try not to let your response to one statement influence your responses to other statements. There are no 'correct' or 'incorrect' answers. Answer according to your own feelings, rather than how you think 'most people' would answer.

4 = I agree a lot

3 = I agree a little

2 = I neither agree nor disagree

1 = I disagree a little

0 = I disagree a lot

1	In uncertain times, I usually expect the best.	
2	It's easy for me to relax.	[filler]
3	If something can go wrong for me, it will.	[reverse]
4	I'm always optimistic about my future.	
5	I enjoy my friends a lot.	[filler]
6	It's important for me to keep busy.	[filler]
7	I hardly ever expect things to go my way.	[reverse]
8	I don't get upset too easily.	[filler]
9	I rarely count on good things happening to me.	[reverse]
10	Overall, I expect more good things to happen to me than bad.	

Scoring

To calculate your score, ignore the fillers (items 2, 5, 6, 8). Reverse your score on negatively worded statements (items 3, 7, and 9). Then total your score. Scores range from 0 to 24: high scores indicate optimism; low scores indicate pessimism.

Source: Scheier, M.F., Carver, C.S. & Bridges, M.W. (1994) Distinguishing optimism from neuroticism (and trait anxiety, self-mastery, and self-esteem): A re-evaluation of the Life Orientation Test. *Journal of Personality and Social Psychology, 67*: 1063–1078. Copyright ©1994 by the American Psychological Association. Reproduced with permission

2.4.3 Emotional Expression, Emotional Regulation, and Health

Research into emotional expression raises a few puzzles. On the one hand, there is a view that not expressing strong emotions is bad for you. Research has found that the suppression of emotion is associated with poorer health, but the evidence is inconsistent (Garssen, 2004). In contrast, we have already seen that anger and hostility, which both involve some expression of these emotions, increase the likelihood of heart disease.

A particularly interesting area of research has looked at the effect of writing about negative or traumatic events on health. This research suggests that writing about negative events can have positive effects on health in some groups of people (Frattaroli, 2006; Mogk et al., 2006; Travagin et al., 2015). It is not clear why emotional expression in this way might lead to better health. Various explanations have been put forward, including that people find more meaning in the experience, that it helps to regulate and decrease negative emotions attached to the event, that people are more likely to talk about it with others, and/or that other people are more supportive when they are told about the event (Doucet et al., 2018).

Emotion regulation is critical in how we respond to stress and control our emotions. Regulation may take two forms. The first is intrinsic regulation, which entails attempting to regulate our own emotions through strategies such as cognitive reappraisal, talking to others, and seeking help from others. The importance of individual differences in emotion regulation is highlighted by findings that difficulties with emotion regulation are more common among people experiencing psychological distress, and people with substance use disorders (Kraiss et al., 2020; Stellern et al., 2023).

The second form of regulation is extrinsic regulation, which is where we attempt to regulate someone else's emotion through strategies such as providing empathy, comfort, or support (Zaki & Williams, 2013). There is now compelling evidence that other people regulate our emotions. For example, the mere presence of another person can reduce negative responses to stress, particularly if that person is a friend or family member (Farley & Kim-Spoon, 2014; Lindsey, 2020). Interpersonal factors are therefore a powerful influence in people's experiences of illness and treatment, when we frequently have to help individuals face challenging circumstances. This may help to explain the clear benefits for mothers and babies that result from continuous social support during labour (see also Chapter 18) (Bohren et al., 2017). Interventions have therefore been developed to help improve emotional regulation in young people and people with difficult emotions, such as those in emotional crisis or experiencing mental illness. This has been done through family therapy, individual or group therapy, and school-based programmes. A review of the evidence concluded that emotion regulation interventions can improve physical and psychological wellbeing in people with existing illness, and that school-based programmes result in improved emotional regulation and emotional competence (Smyth & Arigo 2009; Waxmonsky et al., 2021). An example of how emotion regulation techniques can be used to help people in healthcare is given in Case Study 2.3, which looks at how to help children manage needle procedures more easily (see also Research Box 15.2).

Clinical Notes 2.2

Emotions and Healthcare

- Emotional disorders incur large financial costs, and mental illness is responsible for 40% of disability.
- How people respond to illness is initially determined by how they appraise it.
- Helping people to appraise things more positively can reduce negative emotions and help people to cope.
- Positive emotions have the potential to have a positive influence on health.
- Negative emotions, such as anxiety, anger, and depression, are associated with chronic illnesses such as heart disease. Treating people for problematic emotions can therefore prevent later illness.
- Encouraging optimism can help people if they are facing an essentially controllable or modifiable illness.
- Getting people to write about stressful or traumatic events has the potential to improve health in some people.

Case Study 2.3

Regulating Emotional Responses to Stress in Healthcare

Immunisation is important to protect children and adolescents from serious diseases but it can be painful and distressing. Charlotte is three years old and needs to have a routine vaccination but has reacted badly in the past to injections. She doesn't like coming to the clinic and when she sees the nurse she gets very worked up and distressed.

How can we help Charlotte to regulate her emotional reaction to needles? The following suggestions are based on some of the principles underlying emotion regulation interventions.

1   Select situations that make things less negative

People and places can become associated with negative events. If Charlotte associates the nurse or clinic with pain, she will become distressed even before she enters the clinic. It might help for Charlotte to have her injection in a different place, especially if it is one where

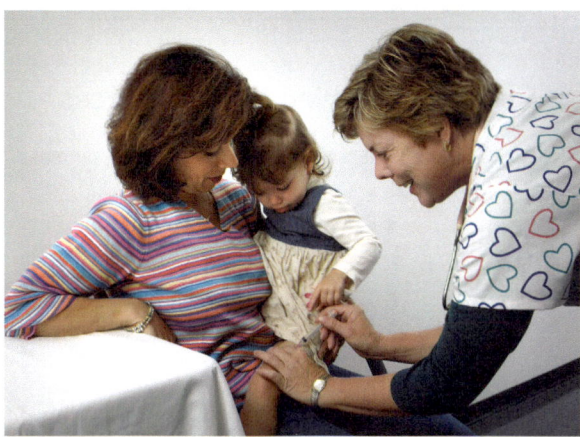

Figure 2.11   Stressful situations in healthcare

Source: © CDC/Unsplash

she feels relaxed and there are things she enjoys, such as music, toys, or something else she finds interesting.

2   **Focus attention away from the situation or emotion**

Encourage Charlotte to concentrate on something else while the injection is being done by distracting her, asking her to focus on another object, or talking about a happy event. Being calm and helping her to cope is much more effective than getting stressed and upset yourself, which often increases distress in others.

3   **Change the way a situation or emotion is appraised**

Charlotte's appraisals need to be changed from negative (e.g. the injection will hurt, it's bad, she doesn't understand why the nurse is hurting her) to positive (e.g. the injection will be over very quickly, the injection will keep her safe for many years, the nurse is there to look after her, after the injection she will feel better).

4   **Regulate physical, behavioural, and emotional responses**

There are many things Charlotte and her parents or carers can do beforehand to help regulate her response to injections. For example, they can explain to her why it's important and good to have the injection. Charlotte and her carers can role-play injecting a teddy and the teddy feeling better afterwards and being protected against diseases. Physical activity before the injection will help Charlotte to be more relaxed. During the injection distraction techniques, such as focusing on teddy or something else in the room, will help. Breathing techniques can also help relaxation. One strategy is to ask Charlotte to take a deep breath, hold it, and let it out when you count to three (and give the injection on three). The injection is timed according to Charlotte's slow breathing on her outbreath, and when she is focusing on her breathing she is less likely to experience a stress response. Using topical anaesthetic cream before the injection may help Charlotte not associate injections with pain and distress.

─Research Box 2.2─

A Music-Based Emotion Regulation App for Distress

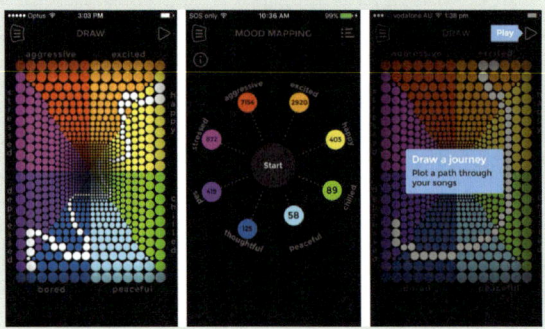

Figure 2.12   The mobile app *Music eScape*

Background

Emotion dysregulation increases the risk of depression, anxiety, and substance use disorders. Music can help to regulate emotions, so these researchers developed a *Music eScape* mobile app to help young people identify and manage negative emotions using music. The app analyses the songs in the user's music library for valence (pleasant to unpleasant) and arousal (very low to very high). These are then plotted onto a circle of eight emotions. Before creating a playlist, users are asked to reflect on their current mood and their desired mood and plot the journey their playlist will support them to achieve.

Method and Findings

This randomised controlled trial (RCT) involved 169 people aged 16–25 years who were experiencing distress. Participants were randomly allocated to access *Music eScape* immediately or wait one month before accessing *Music eScape*. There were no differences in emotional regulation between the groups at one month. However, both groups reported significantly improved emotion regulation skills and wellbeing at two, three and six months, as well as reduced distress.

Significance

Music and apps are accessible ways to help young people to regulate their emotions. This study found no differences in the short term between those using the app and those waiting to use it, but did find improvements in everyone using the app over the longer term. This suggests that people may need time to learn how best to use the app. Another RCT is therefore needed that explores the impact of app use over the longer term.

Hides, L., Dingle, G., Quinn, C., Stoyanov, S.R., Zelenko, O., Tjondronegoro, D., Johnson, D., Cockshaw, W. & Kavanagh, D.J. (2019) Efficacy and outcomes of a music-based emotion regulation mobile app in distressed young people: Randomized controlled trial. *JMIR mHealth and uHealth, 7*(1): e11482.

Summary 2.2

- Emotion includes affect, moods, and impulses.
- Emotion has cognitive, physiological, and behavioural components. Behavioural components include action tendencies, nonverbal behaviour, and facial expression.
- Appraisal processes initiate the physiological, behavioural, and conscious experience of emotion.
- Positive emotions are associated with good health and negative emotions, such as anger and depression, are associated with certain illnesses. However, the mechanisms or causes underlying this association are not clear.
- Emotional dispositions of optimism and neuroticism are positively and negatively associated (respectively) with psychological health as well as with some measures of physical health.

Conclusion

This chapter has looked at how motivation and emotion are important influences on our behaviour, health, and illnesses, such as cardiovascular disease. There is substantial overlap between these different areas and their implications: motivation and emotions drive us to act. Appraisal is important in determining how we feel and respond to different situations. In this chapter we have concentrated on the effect of motivation and emotion on health and the possible pathways this works through, including physiological, cognitive, and behavioural changes. A good example of the interplay between appraisal, emotion, cognition, and behaviour, and how this affects our health, is what happens when we are stressed, which we look at in the next chapter.

──Further Reading──

Llewellyn, C.D. et al. (eds) (2019) *The Cambridge Handbook of Psychology, Health and Medicine* (3rd edition). Cambridge: Cambridge University Press. Includes short chapters on emotions and health, personality and health, and social relationships.

Barrett, L.F., Lewis, M. & Haviland-Jones, J.M. (eds) (2018) *Handbook of Emotions* (4th edition). London and New York: Guilford Press. Includes many chapters on biological, developmental and social perspectives on emotions as well as specific emotions and emotions and health.

Pennebaker, J. & Evans, J. (2014) *Expressive Writing: Words that Heal*. Bedford, IN: Idyll Arbor. Provides a non-technical overview (for the people the authors work with) to address and overcome trauma and emotional upheaval to improve health and build resilience.

Steptoe, A. (2006) *Depression and Physical Illness*. Oxford: Oxford University Press. A comprehensive text on the effect of depression on physical illness.

Revision Questions

1 Describe motivation and give examples of different types of motives.
2 Outline and evaluate three different theories of motivation.
3 Describe the core components of emotion.
4 What are the six basic emotions that are expressed similarly across different cultures?
5 Discuss how the different components of emotion might interact to determine our emotional experience.
6 Outline the effect of positive and negative emotions on health.
7 How might the expression of emotion affect health?
8 Outline the two-factor model of positive and negative affect.
9 Distinguish the various pathways through which emotion may influence health.
10 What personality traits have been associated with health?

3

STRESS AND HEALTH

─Learning Objectives─

This chapter is designed to enable you to:

- Define stress and outline aspects of stress, including (1) appraisal and (2) stress responses.
- Describe physical responses to stress and discuss variations between (1) individuals and (2) situations, in how we respond physically to stress.
- Discuss the relationship between stress and physical health, and outline the factors that protect us or make us more vulnerable to illness following stress.
- Understand some of the psychological consequences of stress, including burnout.

People typically think that stress is bad for us. However, stress is *not* always bad for us – a small amount of stress is necessary for us to confront challenges such as competitions or exams. However, long-term stress does have negative effects, and there is a lot of evidence linking stress to adverse outcomes such as depression, cardiovascular disease, infections, slower recovery, and a worsening of symptoms in many illnesses. In this chapter we explore what stress is, our physical responses to it, how it can affect our physical and mental health, and how we can reduce its harmful effects.

3.1 What is Stress?

The concept of stress originated in physics and mechanical engineering to describe the internal forces in a system caused by external pressures, such as the pressure of water or wind on a bridge. The word **stress** is now widely used to mean many things, including a negative situation, or a feeling of pressure, tension, or negative emotion. According to the psychological definition, stress occurs when perceived demands on us are appraised as exceeding our perceived resources to cope.

Like emotion, stress has many components, so it is necessary to distinguish between stressors and stress responses. **Stressors** are external or internal events that may trigger stress responses. If, for example, you feel stressed because you are sitting an exam, we may say that the exam is an external stressor. If, on the other hand, you feel stressed because you are torn between helping a friend who needs you and revising for that exam, the stress is caused by an internal stressor (your conflicting desires). Stressors can be further divided according to their type or duration, such as acute or short-term stressors (e.g. the death of a relative), chronic or prolonged stressors (e.g. caring for a sick relative), daily hassles (e.g. problems getting to work), traumatic stressors (e.g. an assault), and role strain (e.g. balancing home and work roles). Not everyone responds to the same stressors in the same way.

Stress responses are the various ways we respond to a stressor. They can be divided into cognitive, affective, behavioural, and physiological responses. Interestingly, there is not always a strong association between these different responses. In other words, it is possible for a person to have a strong physiological response to a stressor but report not feeling emotionally stressed. A commonly used questionnaire measure of stress is given in Highlight Box 3.1 so you can consider how stressed you are.

—Highlight Box 3.1—

How Stressed Are You?

Complete the questionnaire in Table 3.1 for an indication of your current levels of stress.

Table 3.1 'How stressed are you?' questionnaire

During the last month how often have you...	Never	Almost never	Sometimes	Fairly often	Very often
Been upset because of something that happened unexpectedly?	0	1	2	3	4
Felt that you were unable to control the important things in your life	0	1	2	3	4
Felt nervous and 'stressed'?	0	1	2	3	4
Felt confident about your ability to handle your personal problems?	4	3	2	1	0
Felt that things were going your way?	4	3	2	1	0
Found that you could not cope with all the things that you had to do?	0	1	2	3	4
Been able to control irritations in your life?	4	3	2	1	0
Felt that you were on top of things?	4	3	2	1	0
Felt angered because of things that were outside of your control?	0	1	2	3	4
Felt difficulties were piling up so high that you could not overcome them?	0	1	2	3	4

Scoring

Add your scores together. Scores range from 0–40. The average score for people aged 18–29 is around 14; aged 30–44 is 13; >45 years is approximately 12.

Source: Cohen, S., Kamarack, T. & Mermelstein, R. (1983) A global measure of perceived stress. *Journal of Health and Social Behaviour, 24*: 385–396. Copyright © 1983 American Sociological Association. Reproduced with permission.

3.1.1 Physical Responses to Stressors

Understanding physical responses to stressors is critical to explaining the link between stress and disease. Our understanding of physical responses to stressors initially comes from research in the 1950s detailing the physiological fight-flight response. The **fight-flight response** involves the sympathetic branch of the **autonomic nervous system** as a fast, first-wave response, and the endocrine pathways of the **hypothalamic-pituitary-adrenal** (**HPA**) axis as a slower, second-wave response. The sympathetic nervous system (SNS) and HPA responses are illustrated in Figure 3.1. The SNS directly activates body systems to prepare the body for immediate action. The adrenal medulla is stimulated to produce stress hormones such as **adrenaline** (epinephrine) and **noradrenaline** (norepinephrine). This causes stimulation of the heart and lungs and the diversion of energy away from unnecessary functions, such as saliva production, digestion, and reproduction.

At the same time, the HPA axis is activated so the hypothalamus releases corticotrophin releasing factor. This sets off a cascade of endocrine events culminating in the release of cortisol and other hormones from the adrenal cortex. **Cortisol** is a steroid and is a critical stress hormone. It results in an increase in blood sugar levels and metabolic rate, hence further supporting the body in the need for fight or flight. It also influences the regulation of blood pressure, the immune system, and the inflammatory response. Normally, the HPA axis works as a negative feedback loop so the presence of cortisol in the bloodstream triggers the hypothalamus to stop producing corticotrophin releasing factor. Thus, cortisol will usually return to normal levels within an hour of the end of the stressor event. However, under prolonged periods of stress, the HPA axis can become dysregulated and result in chronically elevated levels of cortisol. In the long term this has negative effects, such as the accumulation of abdominal fat and the wasting of bone and muscle tissue. The effects of excess cortisol are illustrated by Cushing's syndrome, where there is overproduction of cortisol (hypercortisolism). People with Cushing's syndrome have large amounts of fat on their abdomen and face, perspiration, thinning of the skin, stretch marks, and facial hair. In some cases, it also leads to sleep problems, reduced sexual function, reduced fertility, increased depression, and anxiety; but the syndrome is not *caused* by stress.

Our understanding of physical responses to stressors has developed substantially since the fight-flight responses were first identified. It is now clear that physiological responses to stressors vary according to the characteristics of a situation. Research with animals shows that stronger physiological stress responses occur in situations that are novel, unpredictable, or uncontrollable. Research examining this in humans is broadly consistent with the findings from animal research. It has been acknowledged for some time that unpredictability is related to more stress and higher cortisol levels (Evans et al., 2002), and that a lack of control is associated with greater stress and a more negative impact on health (Walker, 2001). A study of over 5,000 retired adults in the USA found that the effect of chronic stress on physical frailty was fully mediated by perceived control (Mooney et al., 2016). In other words, a high sense of control cancelled out the expected effect of chronic stress on frailty.

This has led to the view that it is important to empower people and encourage them to have as much perceived control as possible. Although this is usually true, there is not a simple blanket effect of perceived control on health, and the effect of perceived control can be moderated by a number of factors. For example, another study of over 6,000 adults in the USA found that stronger beliefs of control over one's life were associated with less risk of dying prematurely for people with low levels of education, but not for those with high levels of education (Turiano et al., 2014). It is also important to note that if a situation is essentially uncontrollable, encouraging someone to

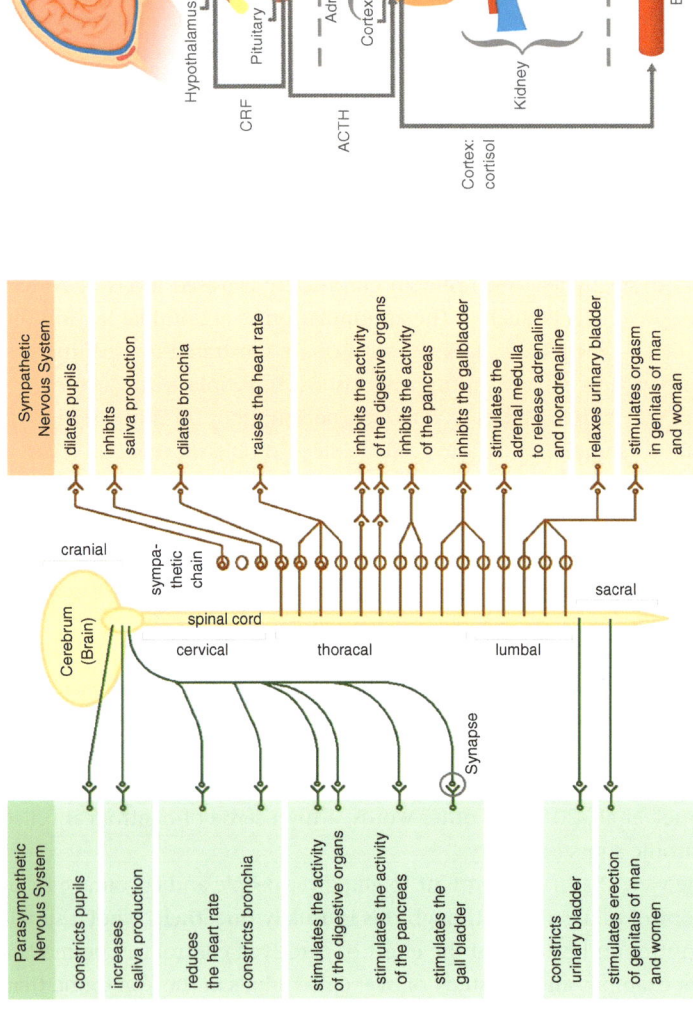

Figure 3.1 Fight-flight responses to stressors

Source: The Autonomic Nervous System courtesy of Geo-Science-International/Wikicommons, shared under the Public Domain. Response to Stress courtesy of Campos-Rodriguez, R. et al./Wikicommons, shared under the CC BY 3.0 license

strive for control might result in more stress. This has important implications for uncontrollable situations in healthcare, such as births that involve obstetric complications that women cannot predict or control. In these circumstances, it may be unhelpful to encourage women to strive for control, and perhaps more emphasis should be placed on supporting them through such events and focusing on those aspects of the experience that they can control.

People also vary in *how* they respond physiologically to stress. Some individuals are more responsive than others. This is called **stress responsivity** or **reactivity**. Studies of twins, epigenetic studies, and animal studies indicate that stress responsivity is partly genetically determined, but that the early environment is critical in altering and shaping our physical and behavioural responses to stressors. Babies of mothers who had high levels of stress and anxiety during pregnancy are more responsive to stressors, show more anxiety and fearfulness, and are more likely to have cognitive and attentional problems (Juruena et al., 2020; Lautarescu et al., 2020). This is referred to as foetal programming, and it makes sense from an evolutionary perspective, because offspring born into a stressful or dangerous environment may need exaggerated stress responses to survive (see also Chapter 18).

The environment is important in shaping infants' stress responses. Animal studies show that offspring of more nurturing mothers have reduced HPA axis responses to stress through less corticotrophin releasing factor (see Figure 3.1) and enhanced negative feedback (Champagne & Meaney, 2001). In addition, the mere presence of the mother alters and reduces their offspring's physiological responses to stressors (Debiec & Sullivan, 2017).

It is apparent that individuals vary in their levels of stress responsivity and that this is determined by **nature and nurture**. Classic studies conducted in the 1990s showed that young children differ in their levels of cardiovascular and immune responsivity to stressors, but showed how their responses to stress are also affected by the context in which they grow up (Boyce et al., 1995). These findings have since been replicated in many studies: children who are more responsive to their environment have the best outcomes if they are raised in a positive environment, and worse outcomes if they are raised in a negative environment. This is found for both physical and psychological health outcomes (Del Giudice et al., 2011; Ellis & Del Giudice, 2019) (see also Chapter 8).

The fight-flight response provided the initial basis of our understanding of physical responses to stressors. However, the matter is more complex than this. In particular, there is more variation between individuals than the above explanations imply. There is also evidence that fight-flight is only one way of responding to stressors and that an alternative response is a **tend and befriend** response, where animals and humans take care of their offspring (tend) and seek out others for safety and comfort (befriend) (Taylor, 2012). In non-human animal studies, tend and befriend responses are more commonly displayed by females, so it has been argued that fight-flight responses may be more relevant to males. However, humans' behavioural responses to stress (such as whether we run away or stay with the group) are influenced by many factors, including social and cultural norms, so there is not a consistent gender difference in whether men and women show fight-flight or tend-befriend responses (Bedrov & Gable, 2023).

The biological basis of the tend-befriend (or affiliative) response to stressors is thought to be the hormone oxytocin in conjunction with endogenous opioids. There is substantial evidence from animal studies for the importance of oxytocin and opioids in affiliative behaviours. For example, administering oxytocin and/or opioids leads to an increase in maternal and other prosocial behaviours (Lim & Young, 2006). If male animals are injected with oxytocin and then subjected to stressors, they are more likely to nurture any young animals present and to show tending behaviours (Taylor, 2012).

There is also accumulating evidence from research with humans that oxytocin and opioids are involved in affiliative behaviours and attachment to others (Carter, 2021; Tolomeo et al., 2020). This may include attachment behaviours (see section 8.1.1) (Plasencia et al., 2019). For example, rises in oxytocin and endogenous opioids occur in women during labour, breastfeeding, and in both men and women during sexual activity, which are presumably to increase affiliation and bonding. Increased oxytocin is also observed in people who are socially isolated or those with poor quality relationships – presumably because they need to seek social affiliation (Taylor et al., 2009). The opioid system is involved in reducing physical pain but also in reducing separation distress. Researchers have therefore argued that coping with social pain (as in loss and separation) might be based on similar physiological mechanisms to physical pain, but there is debate about the strength of the associations (Persson et al., 2019; Sturgeon & Zautra, 2016).

The tend-befriend response also reduces the negative effects of stressors. Oxytocin is associated with reduced physiological stress responses and psychological distress. Studies administering oxytocin to animals show that it reduces fearful behaviour and increases exploration. In humans, oxytocin is associated with decreased SNS and HPA activity (Taylor, 2012). It is therefore thought that, although fight-flight responses are good for acute resolution of threatening events, tend-befriend responses and social affiliation can buffer against the long-term negative impact of stressors on health. This is consistent with the extensive literature showing the importance of social support in health (see section 3.2.2). Figure 3.2 summarises how affiliative responses might decrease stress responses.

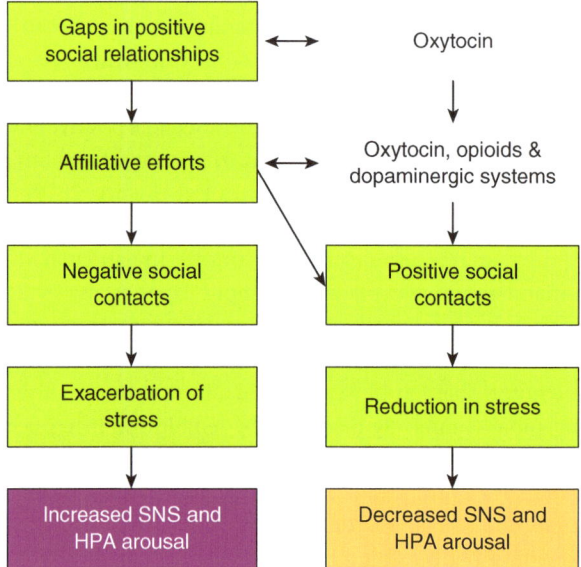

Figure 3.2 Affiliative responses to stressors (adapted from Taylor, 2006)

It can be seen that the fight-flight response to stressors is well established, but is not the only biobehavioural response to stressors. Tend-befriend responses and the importance of affiliation and social relationships illustrate the notion that physical responses to stressors will differ according to circumstances, the individual, and the social context.

Clinical Notes 3.1

Stress and Health

- People vary in how responsive they are to stress, and stress is subjective.
- Severe or chronic stressors are associated with poor health, so helping people to manage and reduce their stress has the potential to reduce illness in the long term.
- The physical symptoms of stress will vary between individuals – some may experience cardiovascular symptoms, such as palpitations, whereas others may experience gastrointestinal symptoms.
- In uncontrollable circumstances, such as an emergency, it may be more helpful to support people through it and to focus on the things they can control rather than encourage them to strive for control over every aspect.

3.1.2 Stress and the Immune System

Stress has various effects on the immune system, depending on the demands of the situation. Both the SNS and the HPA axis affect the immune system. The SNS increases immune system activity, particularly large granular lymphocyte activity, such as natural killer cells. However, the HPA axis suppresses some immune activity through the production of cortisol, which has an anti-inflammatory effect and reduces both the number of white blood cells and the release of cytokines (see Chapter 15).

Different types of stressors make different demands on the body, and the immune response to stress has developed to reflect this. A review and meta-analysis of over 300 studies of stress and immunity showed that immune responses vary according to whether the stressor is acute (lasting a few minutes), a brief naturalistic stressor, a sequence of stressors, or a chronic long-term stressor (Segerstrom & Miller, 2004). Short stressors, such as giving a presentation, lead to an acute increased immune response and redistribution of cells to provide an immediate defence against injuries and the broad risk of infection. This response is rapid, and the immune system quickly returns to baseline levels. Brief stressors that continue for several days, such as studying for exams, have a different effect on the immune system and influence the function of the immune system with a switch away from cellular immunity, which protects against injury or damage, to humoral immunity, which protects against infection. This means that the body will be more able to coordinate responses against infections, and might explain why students often get sick after exams – during the stressful revision period they have increased immunity against infections which disappears when the exams are over. Chronic stressors, such as unemployment or caring for a relative with dementia, have a negative impact on almost all aspects of immune functioning, with poorer immune function overall. This makes a person more likely to get ill, particularly if they are already vulnerable (e.g. elderly people) or have a pre-existing disease (Segerstrom & Miller, 2004).

Activity 3.1

Memory for Stressful Events

- Can you remember how many stressful events you have been through in the last year?
- Can you remember how intense the stress was, or how long it lasted?
- How accurate do you think you can be? Are there things you might have forgotten?
- What do you think affects whether you remember stressful events or not?

3.1.3 Stress as a Person–Environment Interaction

It is now widely accepted that how we respond to stressors depends on the interaction between a person and their environment. Interactional or transactional explanations of stress provide a more complete account of the different processes involved in stress. This approach argues that stress occurs when a person appraises the demands of a situation as being greater than their perceived ability to cope with these demands (Lazarus & Folkman, 1984). Appraisal processes are central and explain why there is so much variation in how different people respond to stressors.

The interactional approach outlines three processes of appraisal:

1. *Primary appraisal*: the demands of a situation are evaluated as benign or stressful (i.e. challenging, threatening, or potentially involving harm or loss).
2. *Secondary appraisal*: a person evaluates their resources and capacity to cope.
3. *Reappraisal*: after applying a coping strategy (or strategies) a person reconsiders the situation. This may lead to reappraisal of a stressor as less or more stressful than originally thought, depending on the effect of their coping responses.

There is a wealth of evidence for the importance of appraisal in how we respond to stressors. A meta-analysis of 81 studies of people with chronic pain or who had pain induced in laboratory experiments showed that in both these situations appraisals of pain as threatening were associated with greater pain, reduced tolerance of pain, and more passive coping. In people with chronic pain, appraisal of the pain as threatening was also associated with more impairment and psychological distress. In contrast, appraisals of pain as challenging were associated with more pain tolerance and active coping (Jackson et al., 2014). The importance of primary appraisal is illustrated throughout this book (see, for example, the discussion in Chapter 2 of responses to discovering a breast lump). Case study 3.1 gives examples of primary and secondary appraisal. A strength of the interactional approach is the recognition of the appraisal–coping–reappraisal cycle. The constant interplay between appraisal, coping, and reappraisal means that stress is conceptualised as a dynamic process. It is also important to note that this dynamic process is a biopsychosocial phenomenon: differences in appraisal and coping between countries and cultures indicate that our appraisal and coping response are learnt, and therefore possible to change (Sharma et al., 2020).

Case Study 3.1

Appraisal and Stress in a Pandemic

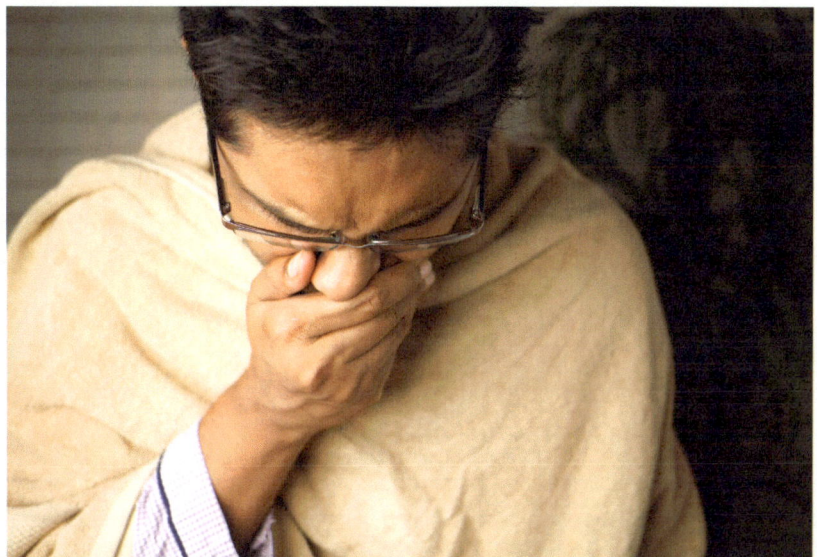

Figure 3.3 Appraisal of COVID-19 symptoms

Source: © Towfiqu Barbhuiya/Unsplash

The importance of appraisal in stress was clear in the COVID-19 pandemic. It is common for people to experience mild symptoms, such as headache, cough, or sneezing (see Chapter 4). When the pandemic emerged, the salience of symptoms was heightened, and people's appraisals were critical in how they responded. Examples are:

Person A might cough and think 'I've got coronavirus' and 'I may die' (primary appraisal of cough as threatening). They might think 'there's nothing I can do to stop it' (secondary appraisal of no coping resources), and so feel overwhelmed, stressed, and anxious.

Person B might cough and think 'I've got coronavirus' and 'I may die' but think 'I am young and healthy so low risk' and 'I can rest and look after myself to make sure it doesn't get really bad' (secondary appraisal of many coping resources), and so feel less stressed and anxious.

Person C might cough and think 'it's just a cough' or 'it's probably nothing, just the dust' (primary appraisal of the cough as benign), and so would feel calm and not stressed. Secondary appraisal of coping resources in this instance might not be needed and the person might forget about the cough completely; or they might monitor whether the cough gets worse or goes away over time.

The interactional model as originally proposed is not without problems, but elements of it are now widely accepted, such as the importance of the interaction between the person and environment, the central role of appraisal, and that coping and other psychosocial factors moderate how we respond to stressors. A biopsychosocial approach to stress incorporates all these elements and is illustrated in Figure 3.4.

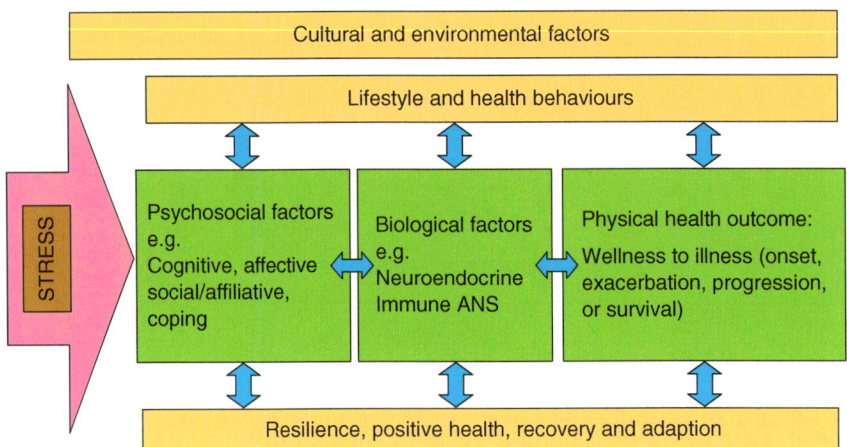

Figure 3.4   Biopsychosocial approach to stress (adapted from Turner-Cobb & Katsampouris, 2019)

Summary 3.1

- The stress process involves (1) stressors and (2) stress responses.
- Stress responses include physiological, behavioural, emotional, and cognitive changes.
- Stress occurs when the perceived demands of a situation are appraised as exceeding a person's perceived resources and ability to cope.
- Appraisal is therefore central to whether a person feels stressed or not.
- Physical stress responses involve the sympathetic nervous system, HPA axis, and immunological changes.
- The fight-flight response is not the only biobehavioural response to stressors. The tend-befriend response is an affiliative response to stressors which is more common in female animals and underpinned by oxytocin and endogenous opioids.
- Physical stress responses vary according to the characteristics of the stressor, with novel, unpredictable, and uncontrollable stressors associated with greater stress responses.
- Individuals vary in the strength and nature of their physical responses to stressors (stress responsivity).

3.2 Stress and Health

The sections above have addressed some conceptual issues related to stress, and explored some of the effects of stress in some bodily systems. This section gives greater attention to how stress affects health, and the various factors that can reduce stress or the effects of stress.

3.2.1 Links between Stress and Health

There is plenty of evidence that stress is associated with morbidity and mortality. For example, studies of bereavement show that older people are more likely to die in the year after their spouse dies than other people of the same age and health (Subramanian et al., 2008). The impact of stress on physical health varies for different illnesses. There is good evidence that prolonged stress (whether measured in terms of stressors or the subjective experience of stress) results in increased episodes of infectious illnesses like colds, a greater risk of cardiovascular disease, slower wound healing, and worsening of auto-immune conditions such as asthma, rheumatoid arthritis, inflammatory bowel disease, and HIV/AIDS (Alexander & Turnbaugh, 2020; Bierstetel et al., 2021; Haykin & Rolls, 2021). Examples of research in these areas can be found throughout Section IV of this book. Similarly, the association between stress and poor mental health is well recognised. Chronic or severe stress can lead to a number of mental health problems, including anxiety, depression, burnout, and post-traumatic stress disorder (PTSD).

However, as with our emotions, it is difficult to establish the definitive pathways between stress and health. There are three main issues. The first is the huge variation in how people respond to stressors. Why is it that if we put two people in the same circumstances, one person becomes stressed and the other does not? Or that one person develops heart disease and another remains healthy? Some of these differences can be accounted for by differences in appraisal and stressor characteristics, as we have already seen, but the effect of stress is also influenced by many other factors, such as an individual's resilience, coping responses, and social support.

The concept of allostasis and **allostatic load** is one way to explain how stress might lead to disease (McEwen, 1998). Allostasis refers to the process of regulating our physiological state to achieve stability, or homeostasis. This is done through physiological systems, such as the autonomic nervous system, HPA axis, neuroendocrine and immune systems, or through changing behaviour. In the short term, these changes are adaptive because they maintain physiological stability while adapting to changing external circumstances. However, frequent or chronic activation of these systems results in a high allostatic load (or strain) on the body. This cumulative allostatic load can lead to an imbalance in allostatic systems and disease. Different types of allostatic load have been proposed. A prolonged response is where physiological systems remain in a continually high state, which results in long-term strain on the body. An inadequate response is where one allostatic system does not respond adequately so other systems have to overcompensate. Alternatively, if people are exposed to repeated acute stressors, there can be a lack of adaption, with repeatedly high physiological stress responses (Guidi et al., 2021; McEwen, 1998). Allostatic load is usually measured by a combination of biomarkers from the cardiovascular, metabolic, immune, and neuroendocrine systems.

A review of the evidence for allostatic load shows that it is associated with a range of social and environmental factors associated with health, and with health disparities between certain groups. Factors associated with allostatic load include ethnicity, socioeconomic status, social relationships, gender, lifestyle factors, exposure to stressors, and genetic factors. Higher allostatic load is also associated with worse health outcomes, and higher all-cause mortality (Beckie, 2012; Guidi et al., 2021; Parker et al., 2022). The concept of allostatic load is therefore useful in that it provides a framework through which the interaction between the environment and individuals' biobehavioural responses can lead to poor health outcomes. The use of combined measures from multiple physiological systems has also broadened the focus onto systemic responses to stressors and the impact this has.

However, a second issue is that it is usually not possible to say whether an illness is due (1) entirely to stress or (2) entirely to other factors (i.e. not at all to stress). Illnesses often have multiple causes, ranging from the genetic and biological to the environmental. The role of stress will also vary widely in different illnesses. A traumatic stressor may cause PTSD but only exacerbate the symptoms of asthma. The contribution of stress to illness will therefore vary widely between individuals, circumstances, and illnesses.

A third issue is that the effect of stress on health can be due to behavioural, emotional, or physical responses to stressors. For example, people who are stressed are also more likely to smoke, drink alcohol, or have a poor diet (Deasy et al., 2015; Hill et al., 2022; Sahani et al., 2022). The physical response to stressors is therefore not the only pathway between stress and disease.

3.2.2 Vulnerability and Resilience

We have already seen how some people are more vulnerable to poor health. Examples include the health disparities observed between different groups, such as people from disadvantaged socioeconomic groups or other minoritised groups (see Chapter 11). The vulnerability-stress model (sometimes called the diathesis-stress model), shown in Figure 3.5, summarises how vulnerability factors interact with stressors to influence whether someone develops disease. This model is also often used to describe the development of psychological distress and psychiatric conditions (see Chapter 7).

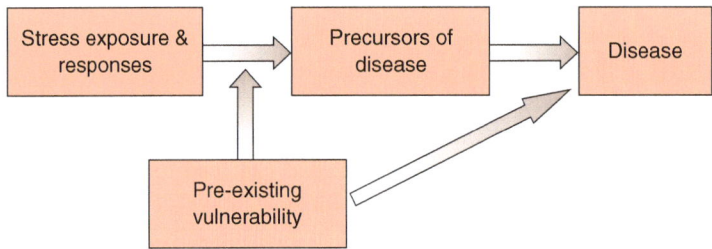

Figure 3.5   Pathways between stress and disease (vulnerability-stress model)

It is also clear that some people are very resilient in the face of stressors and remain in good health despite adverse circumstances. This is illustrated by the research described earlier (section 3.1.1) in which the more resilient children had similar health outcomes regardless of whether they were raised in positive or adverse environments (Boyce et al., 1995). Even in the face of significant adversity, such as chronic or terminal illness, many people can adapt and find happiness and personal growth (see Chapter 6 and section 15.4.2). This kind of resilience has been classified as people showing swift recovery from stressful events, having sustainability of purpose in the face of adversity, and growth or new learning from adversity (Mesman et al., 2021; Zautra & Reich, 2010).

Research suggests that the majority of people are resilient. For example, trauma and adversity are common and at least 50% of people will experience trauma or adversity in their lifetime. However, the prevalence of PTSD in the general population is approximately 10%, suggesting that most people who experience a traumatic event recover (Horn et al., 2016). A review of factors associated with resilience identified those in Highlight Box 3.2 as being important in developing resilience during childhood and remaining resilient in adulthood (Horn et al., 2016; Mesman et al., 2021). However, it is important to note that whereas resilience is commonly thought of as a characteristic of individuals, it is important to think of how contextual and environmental factors interact with individual characteristics (Ungar & Theron, 2020).

─Highlight Box 3.2─

Psychosocial Factors Associated with Resilience

Table 3.2 Factors associated with resilience in children and adulthood (adapted from Horn et al., 2016)

Childhood	Adulthood
Positive bonds with caregivers	Positive emotions, optimism
Consistent parenting	Active coping
Self-regulation of emotions	Cognitive reappraisal
Intelligence and problem solving	Altruism
Mastery	Mastery
Positive friendships	Social support
Motivation for achievement	Facing fears
Meaning	Meaning, sense of purpose

Here we focus on a few of the factors associated with resilience, namely (1) emotion and emotional disposition, (2) ways of coping, and (3) social relationships and social support.

Emotion and Emotional Disposition

As we saw in Chapter 2, positive emotions and positive emotional dispositions have a powerful influence on health, and thus are important in resilience. A range of positive emotional states (e.g. emotional wellbeing, positive mood, joy, happiness, vigour, energy) and positive dispositions (e.g. life satisfaction, hopefulness, optimism, sense of humour) are associated with reduced mortality in healthy people and in people with chronic illness (Chida & Steptoe, 2009). Having an optimistic disposition is associated with reduced mortality, increased survival, fewer physical symptoms, lower risk of cardiovascular disease, and improved physiological functioning (including immune function) (Amonoo et al., 2021; Rasmussen et al., 2009). This may be due to direct effects of positive moods and/or indirect effects, whereby more optimistic people are more likely to begin or continue healthy behaviours and cease or reduce unhealthy behaviours. Optimism and hope can also reduce the risk of developing post-traumatic stress disorder (PTSD) following traumatic events (Gallagher et al., 2020).

The role of negative emotions and emotional dispositions as a vulnerability factor is not as straightforward. There is now substantial evidence that some types of negative emotion are associated with specific illnesses. The main examples are associations between stress, anger, hostility, depression, and cardiovascular disease (see section 16.1.1) (Osborne et al., 2020; Prigge et al., 2022; Smaardijk et al., 2020). Depression is a clear vulnerability factor and is associated with a wide range of morbidity and mortality. For example, depressed people are between 50% and 100% more likely to develop cardiovascular disease than healthy people (Lett et al., 2004; Trajkova et al., 2019).

Neuroticism has been identified as a vulnerability factor for poor health. Neuroticism entails a wide range of negative emotions, including anxiety, worrying, low mood, and negative emotions such as guilt, hostility, and fear. People higher in neuroticism generally report more pain and somatic symptoms and are at greater risk of psychological disorders (Contrada & Goyal, 2005). For example, a large prospective study of over 20,000 adult twins in the USA, who were followed up over 25 years, found that, after controlling for genetic vulnerability in twins, those who were high in neuroticism were significantly more likely to report musculoskeletal pain, headaches, migraine, chronic fatigue, colitis, irritable bowel syndrome, gastroesophageal reflux disease, and cardiovascular disease (Turk Charles et al., 2008). However, there is also no consistent link between neuroticism and measures of chronic morbidity, and when combined with conscientiousness, neuroticism may result in healthy worrying (Friedman, 2019). As in other contexts, focusing on single personality traits may obscure the diversity of various intersecting variables.

Activity 3.2

Being More or Less Responsive to Stress

- Do you know anyone who gets stressed very easily?
- Which kind of factors do you think influence why they are so responsive to stress?
- How much of it is due to stressors, social circumstances, the person's resources, vulnerability or resilience, their appraisals, or the coping strategies they use?

Coping

As we saw earlier when looking at the interactional model of stress, coping is a vital part of how we respond to stressors. How we cope with stressors partly determines our physical and emotional responses. People who appraise an event as challenging have smaller cortisol responses than people who appraise it as threatening. Research on coping defines it as *any* attempt to cope with a stressor, irrespective of whether it is successful. This covers a huge range of coping actions and there has been an extensive debate over how to best conceptualise different coping strategies. Categories that are widely used distinguish between emotion-focused and problem-focused coping, or between approach and avoidant coping. **Emotion-focused strategies** are those that concentrate on reducing distress (e.g. not thinking about it, seeking emotional support) whereas **problem-focused strategies** concentrate on dealing with the problem (e.g. information seeking, problem solving).

In the context of healthcare, the distinction between approach coping and avoidant coping may be more useful. **Approach coping** strategies are efforts to deal with the situation proactively: they are predominantly active strategies, so they share some overlap with problem-focused strategies. **Avoidant coping** strategies do not address the problem directly (e.g. denial, not wanting to talk about it), so they are predominantly emotion-focused. The important point for health professionals is that a person who predominantly uses avoidant coping may find it very difficult to discuss their illness, the side effects of treatment, or any potential complications. Conversely, someone who uses approach coping will want to know about their illness, and be involved in finding solutions: they may come to consultations armed with extensive information gathered online!

In general, coping strategies that enable a person to feel more in control (mastery) increase positive emotions and decrease negative emotions, and are associated with resilience and better health. For example, finding meaning or benefit in adverse events is associated with resilience. A review of the literature on people with cancer showed that those who found some benefit in having cancer had better immune function (Pascoe & Edvardsson, 2013).

However, it is not possible to say that one coping style is always better than another. Under certain circumstances, avoidant or passive coping strategies may be good for reducing anxiety and distress in the short term. This can be helpful before an operation because it keeps anxiety levels down and once the operation is over the stressor is over. However, for someone with a chronic illness, avoidance can lead to a lack of adherence to treatment regimens and compound illness problems.

Research Box 3.1

Physical Activity May Alleviate the Impact of Racial Discrimination on Allostatic Load

Background

Racial discrimination is a stressor that has been linked to biological dysfunction as reflected in allostatic load. There is evidence that physical activity can reduce the harmful effects of stress, but there was a lack of evidence as to whether regular physical activity may buffer the impact of racial discrimination on allostatic load.

Method and Findings

This study explored the associations between physical activity, racial discrimination, and allostatic load among 150 Indigenous adults in Canda. The index of allostatic load was a combination of measures of blood pressure and body mass index, and analysis of neuroendocrine and immune function based on saliva samples. Participants self-reported their experiences of racial discrimination and physical activity.

For the whole sample, those who reported more racial discrimination also had higher allostatic loads. However, this association was only significant among people who were insufficiently active. Among people who were sufficiently active, allostatic load was not significantly related to experiences of discrimination.

(Continued)

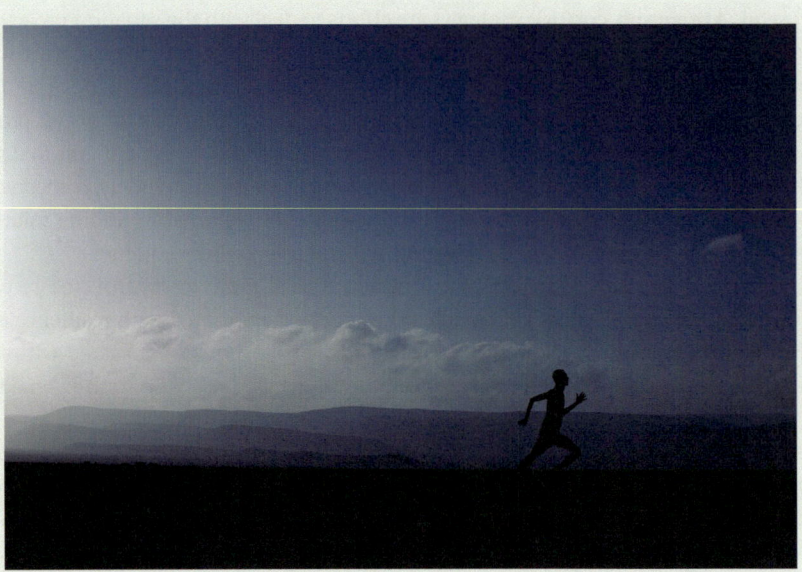

Figure 3.6   Running to alleviate stress

Source: © Pixabay

Significance

This study indicates that physical activity can reduce the harmful physiological effects of racial discrimination. The authors note that whereas physical activity can help to buffer the effects of racism on the health of minority populations, there is also a need to address the overarching problem of racism.

Copeland, J.L., Currie, C.L. & Moon-Riley, K.C. et al. (2021) Physical activity buffers the adverse impacts of racial discrimination on allostatic load among Indigenous adults. *Annals of Behavioral Medicine, 55*: 520–529. doi:10.1093/abm/kaaa068

Activity 3.3

Coping Strategies

- Which kind of coping strategies do you tend to use?
- Can you think of anyone who is clearly an avoidant-coper or an approach-coper?
- How well does this coping approach work for them in different situations?

Social Relationships and Social Support

Interpersonal relationships are vital to our quality of life and health. Negative relationships involving abuse or conflict are some of the most potent stressors. Traumatic events that involve intentional harm from another person, such as rape, assault, or torture, are much more likely to cause PTSD than traumatic events such as natural disasters (Charuvastra & Cloitre, 2008). However, better social support and social relationships can reduce the risk of PTSD, and strong support in one domain (e.g. from friends) may counter unsupportive relationships in other domains (e.g. family) (Hansford & Jobson, 2022).

Social relationships also shape the way we respond to stressors. As noted above, early mothering influences the way young animals respond physiologically and behaviourally to stressors. In humans, social bonds are very influential in shaping a child's stress responses. Attachment theory (see Chapter 8) proposes that babies are born with an instinct to seek their parents or significant others when they experience stressors or are in danger. In extreme situations, such as children being abandoned or abused, children are more likely to develop insecure and chaotic responses to stressors. Parents also shape their children's responses to stressors. Studies of parents and children exposed to the same stressor show that their responses are very similar. There is evidence of links between parental anxiety and the likelihood of their children displaying anxiety (Subar & Rozenman, 2021; van der Bruggen et al., 2008). It has also been shown that interventions designed to promote positive parenting improve resilience in children and young people (Wolchik et al., 2009).

It is well established that social relationships are associated with better health outcomes in both healthy people and those with chronic diseases. A review and meta-analysis of over 300,000 people showed that having stronger social relationships is associated with a 50% increase in survival rates regardless of age, sex, initial health status, or the cause of death (Holt-Lunstad et al., 2010). Conversely, loneliness, social isolation, and living alone are associated with a 26–32% increased risk of premature mortality (Holt-Lunstad et al., 2015). The negative health effects of social isolation and loneliness are comparable to, or greater than, other well-known risk factors, such as smoking, exercise, and hypertension (Uchino et al., 2019).

However, although there is extensive evidence of the importance of social networks and relationships in health, the impact of an act of support on perceived stress is more complex. Laboratory experiments that induce stress by asking people to undertake social speaking or difficult arithmetic tasks show that having someone present can reduce SNS and HPA axis responses, although this finding is not consistent and varies according to factors such as culture, gender, and the nature of the relationship (Hennessy et al., 2009). Similar beneficial effects (but also with variation) have been observed when pets are present (Schreiner, 2016).

Thus, social relationships are critical to health. Having a strong support network and positive relationships has a positive impact on health, and being socially isolated has a negative impact on health. Receiving support during a stressful event can buffer against the effects of stress, but this outcome varies according to a number of factors, such as individual and cultural differences in how support is interpreted. Some have therefore argued that the effect of support on health may be more the result of feeling that other people are close and available to support us if we need it, rather than the actual support received during stressful events (Taylor, 2020).

─Clinical Notes 3.2─

Coping Styles and Clinical Practice

- Consider people's coping styles when giving them information.
- People with avoidant coping styles may not want information and may become anxious or distressed if they are given information.
- Conversely, people with approach coping styles will want information and may become distressed if they are not given information.
- Social relationships are critical to wellbeing, so it is important to identify people who are socially isolated and encourage or help them to increase their support networks.
- Providing support can buffer against the effects of stressors, but this outcome varies according to how the individual interprets such support.

Summary 3.2

- Severe or chronic stressors are associated with a range of morbidity and mortality.
- Variability in how we respond to stressors makes it difficult to establish causal pathways between stress and disease.
- A vulnerability-stress approach explains how stress may interact with an existing vulnerability to affect health.
- Most people are resilient to stressors.
- Resilience in adulthood is influenced by positive emotions and emotional dispositions, coping, and social relationships and support.
- Interpersonal relationships and social support are critical and shape how we respond to stressors, and, in some cases, can buffer against the negative impact of stress.

3.3 Stress in Medicine and Healthcare

Working in healthcare can be inherently stressful: it involves dealing with health crises and distressed people, and it may entail making life and death decisions. As we have already seen, stress is associated with negative psychological states, including anxiety, depression, burnout, and PTSD. Stress burnout has three main symptoms:

1   *Emotional exhaustion*: feelings of physical exhaustion, being depleted, worn out.
2   *Reduced sense of accomplishment*: a poor sense of effectiveness, involvement, commitment, and engagement, and a poor belief in one's ability to change or improve work patterns or the work environment.

    Depersonalisation: having an unfeeling, impersonal approach to co-workers or patients, cynicism, and a lack of engagement with the job or people.

Burnout can be conceptualised as one end of a continuum. At the opposite end, engagement is characterised by high levels of vigour, dedication, and absorption, and is associated with good performance (Montgomery & Maslach, 2019). In contrast, burnout is associated with high job dissatisfaction, poor performance, absenteeism, and staff turnover. In addition, symptoms of exhaustion are associated with many other physical symptoms, such as headaches, gastrointestinal disorders, hypertension, colds or flu, and sleep disturbances (Leiter & Maslach, 2000).

    Burnout is a particular problem for doctors, nurses, and student health professionals. Reviews across these various populations indicate that more than one-quarter report burnout (Balendran et al., 2021; Li et al., 2018; Naji et al., 2021; Pradas-Hernández et al., 2018). A European survey of family doctors in 12 countries found that high levels of burnout were associated with poor job satisfaction, stronger intentions to change job, more sick leave, being younger, being male, and using alcohol, tobacco, and psychotropic medication (Soler et al., 2008). Burnout also varies according to country and region. In one meta-analysis, burnout in doctors in the USA was associated with work–life conflict and poor coping strategies, whereas in Europe, burnout was associated with negative attitudes to work (R.T. Lee et al., 2013). In another meta-analysis, burnout among Asian nurses was most strongly influenced by person-related factors such as personality and empathy, whereas burnout among European nurses was influenced more by work-related factors (Ma et al., 2023). Lifestyle and health behaviours are also affected: a study of burnout in seven European countries found that burnout led to more fast-food consumption, less exercise, and greater use of alcohol and painkillers. These associations remained even after controlling for individual differences and country of residence (Alexandrova-Karamanova et al., 2016).

    Although there is some evidence that interventions to prevent and reduce burnout among undergraduate and graduate medical education trainees can be effective, there is a need for well-designed studies that are conducted with a specific focus on prevention (Anger et al., 2024; Walsh et al., 2019). Research Box 3.2 gives an example of a study that used a team-based programme designed to promote physical activity as a way of improving quality of life and reducing burnout among physician trainees.

    Risk of burnout operates at three levels: individual (healthy lifestyle/behaviours, adequate coping), the individual and the environment (social support structures, relationships, improving person–organisation fit), and at the organisational level (adequate working conditions, organisation of work, work design). Interventions to prevent burnout should therefore be aimed at all three levels. However, although there is evidence for individual risk factors for burnout, there is more substantial evidence for the importance of organisational risk factors (Montgomery & Maslach, 2019). The six main organisational factors associated with burnout are shown in Highlight Box 3.3. Ways to change these to engender a positive organisational culture and staff engagement have also been proposed. There is some evidence that interventions such as Civility, Respect and Engagement in the Workplace (CREW) promote change and a work culture that is more empowering for staff (see Research Box 3.2).

—Highlight Box 3.3—

Workplace and Burnout

Evidence suggests that burnout is more likely in jobs that involve:

- High workload
- Lack of control
- Insufficient rewards
- Absence of fairness
- Value conflicts
- Poor sense of community

(Leiter & Maslach, 2004)

—Research Box 3.2—

Impact of a Team-Based Exercise Programme on Quality of Life and Burnout among Physician Trainees

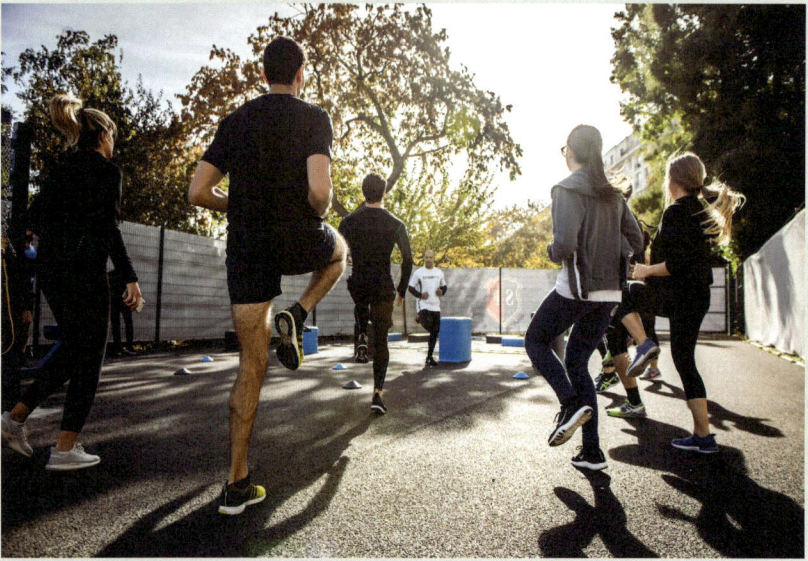

Figure 3.7   Exercise to reduce burnout

Source: © Gabin Vallet/Unsplash

Background

Burnout is common in healthcare professions, and is a particular problem among trainees due to long work hours, clinical responsibilities, academic demands, and sleep deprivation. Regular physical activity is known to provide benefits for physical and psychological wellbeing, and this study was designed to explore whether it could reduce the risk of burnout.

Method and Findings

This study evaluated the impact of an incentivised physical activity programme run over 12 weeks. Incentives were awarded for self-reported exercise and gym attendance, completion of surveys and physical assessments, and improvements in objective markers of fitness. Participants were also encouraged to form teams to provide mutual motivation and support. The participants were 532 residents and fellows at a single site: 174 took part in the challenge, and 358 did not. Although 1,060 people were invited, only 230 enrolled in the programme.

Among participants, there was high satisfaction with the exercise programme. At the 12-week follow-up, participants reported greater engagement in fitness and strength training and better quality of life, and there was a significant association between greater physical activity and better quality of life. Scores on three markers of burnout were lower among participants than non-participants, but these were not statistically significant differences.

Significance

This study indicated that residents and fellows could be incentivised to engage in physical activity, and that this could lead to improvements in their quality of life. The use of incentives and teams appears to have facilitated continuation with the programme among those who enrolled, but there is a need to find ways to encourage more people to engage with the programme.

Weight, C.J., Sellon, J.L., Lessard-Anderson, C.R., Shanafelt, T.D., Olsen, K.D. & Laskowski, E.R. (2013) Physical activity, quality of life, and burnout among physician trainees: The effect of a team-based, incentivized exercise program. *Mayo Clinic Proceedings, 88*(12): 1435–1442. doi:10.1016/j.mayocp.2013.09.010

Students training in medicine and other health professions also face many stressors. These include keeping up with coursework and exams, dealing with death, suffering, and difficult ethical issues, performing intimate examinations of others, and demanding work hours. Longitudinal studies that have followed medical students over time have identified some characteristics that are associated with stress and burnout later in life. One UK study followed medical students over a 12-year period, and found that those who were disorganised, had poor time management skills, felt overwhelmed, and were unsure of the demands of different tasks were more likely to report stress and burnout in the years following graduation (McManus et al., 2004). Another study with a shorter study period found that burnout during the one-year follow-up was associated with poor support, employment during studies, depression, poor quality of life, more stress and fatigue, and experiencing the learning environment less positively (Dyrbye et al., 2010). A more recent study with three rounds of data collection found that students who were more resilient at enrolment were less likely to experience burnout during the two-year study period (Q. Wang et al., 2022). Learning positive ways to manage stress is therefore extremely important for health professionals. These include using appropriate support and learning positive stress management techniques. The remainder of this chapter focuses on how to manage stress, and Case Study 3.2 below shows how the interactional model of stress can be used to help a student cope with exam stress.

3.4 Managing Stress

Understanding the processes of stress provides a basis for helping people to manage stress more effectively. Most stress management interventions aim to reduce arousal and build coping skills so that the person is able to manage stress better. There are many different approaches to stress management, which can broadly be divided into two main categories: (1) those that focus on physical and mental relaxation, such as relaxation exercises, meditation, mindfulness, and yoga; and (2) those that focus on cognition and behaviour, such as psychoeducation, cognitive restructuring, assertiveness training, and stress inoculation. More information about relaxation, mindfulness, and cognitive behavioural therapy (CBT) is given in Chapter 14. Interventions such as stress inoculation are based on exposing people to potential stressors and training them in skills (e.g. skills drills) so they become 'inoculated' against these stressors and are able to work effectively under potentially stressful conditions. For example, paramedic training will often include rehearsals or 'mock ups' of major road traffic accidents, so that when paramedics are in a real accident situation they are equipped with the right knowledge and actions to deal with it effectively.

Building resilience is frequently suggested as a preventative strategy against burnout among doctors and health professionals. This is a broad approach that can draw on many of the techniques described in Case Study 3.2 to help an individual to cope better with stress and to recover more quickly. Research referred to in section 3.3 showed that resilient students are less likely to experience burnout, but also found that one consequence of burnout is lowered resilience (Q. Wang et al., 2022). It is therefore important to prevent a downward spiral of eroding resilience, and to support the development and maintenance of resilience in all students. The dynamic and evolving nature of resilience was observed in a qualitative study of physicians in Canada (Jensen et al., 2008). In that study, the four main aspects of resilience in physicians were:

1   Attitudes and perspectives, which included valuing the physician role, maintaining interest, developing self-awareness, and accepting personal limitations
2   Balance and prioritisation, which included setting limits, taking effective approaches to continuing professional development, and honouring the self
3   Practice management style, which included sound business management, having good staff, and using effective practice arrangements
4   Supportive relations, which included positive personal relationships, effective professional relationships, and good communication.

Cognitive-behavioural stress management programmes focus on appraisals and coping responses to help people to manage stressors and perceived stress better. These can be useful to assist people who are coping with illness. Stress management techniques have therefore been widely implemented and evaluated for people with cardiovascular disease, cancer, and chronic headaches – but with mixed results. The evidence suggests that stress management has positive effects on psychological outcomes, such as reducing depression, increasing self-esteem, and improving quality of life, and cortisol levels, but psychological and educational interventions have less obvious positive impact on morbidity or mortality (Anderson & Taylor, 2014; Antoni et al., 2023; Horn, Stangl et al., 2023; Rogerson et al., 2024).

One particular type of stress management programme, called critical incident debriefing, has proved controversial. Debriefing was initially developed to help people to deal with very stressful or traumatic events and prevent the development of PTSD. Debriefing programmes vary but they usually involve one session within four weeks of the event, during which a person is encouraged to talk about their thoughts and feelings during the event and their symptoms since the event. The therapist will then educate the person about responses to traumatic events in an attempt to normalise these experiences. Reviews have found a lack of clear evidence that early interventions of debriefing reduce the symptoms of PTSD or depression, and have highlighted a need for better quality research (Roberts et al., 2019).

Case Study 3.2

Managing Stress in Medicine and Healthcare

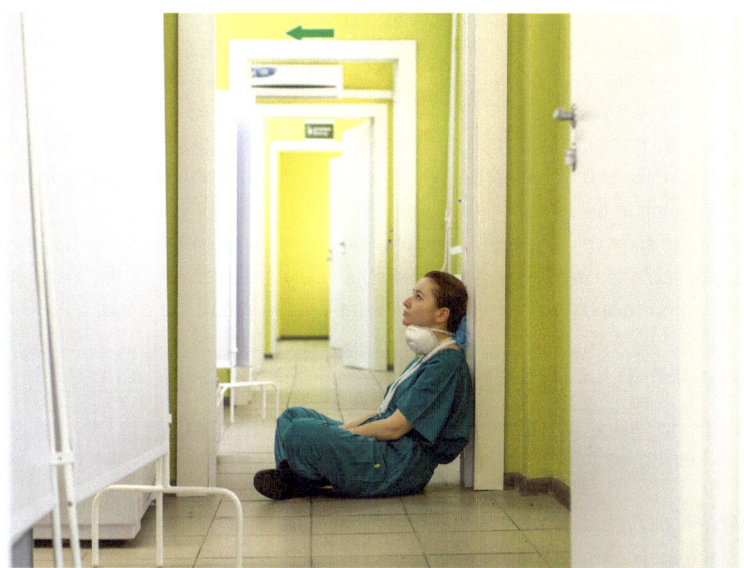

Figure 3.8 Stress in medical students

Source: © Vladimir Fedotov

Isha is a medical student approaching the end of her first year. Before medical school Isha was a straight-A student. Since she has been at medical school her results have varied. She has passed everything but has lost confidence. Isha finds the constant assessments at medical

(Continued)

school really hard. She feels tired, tense, and is finding it difficult to concentrate on her studies. She is beginning to doubt whether medicine is the right career for her.

Stress management involves education about stress and coping, exploring each person's unique way of dealing with stressors, and facilitating more adaptive coping. When based on the interactional model, stress management looks at demands, appraisal, coping resources, and strategies to manage stress. Here, the interactional model of stress management is applied to Isha's situation.

Demands

The demands of medical school on Isha can be explored in order to make them explicit. For example:

- *What are the triggers to this situation?* For example, assessments.
- *What demands does it place on Isha?* The exams make Isha feel not good enough, and she has lost confidence.
- *How real are these demands?* Are they based on fact or Isha's fears?

Appraisal

This stage looks at Isha's appraisals and how the demands of medical school affect her feelings and ability to cope. For example:

- *When she is feeling unable to cope, what thoughts are going through her head?* This question would emphasise the role of appraisal in how Isha feels. Her appraisals include: 'I am going to fail', 'I'm not good enough'.
- *How can she think differently to help her to feel and cope better?* This question highlights appraisals and coping strategies that might be more adaptive: 'Exams are hard but it's not only me who finds exams hard', 'If I fail, it's not the end of the world'.

Resources to Cope

This stage involves exploring with Isha which resources she can use to help her to cope better. It includes helping her to draw on existing coping strategies and to learn new ones. For example:

- *What support is available?* Support includes other students, teachers, friends, family, and health professionals. *How can she use this support now?*
- *How has she coped with difficult situations in the past?* This question would raise Isha's awareness of which coping strategies are available to her.
- *What worked and what didn't work?* This question would help Isha to realise which coping strategies are adaptive or maladaptive in different situations.
- *How can she use these strategies to cope now?* This could help Isha to realise that she has the resources to cope and that these resources should reduce her feelings of helplessness and encourage her to use strategies that will help her to feel better.
- *What new coping strategies might help her now?* This question would encourage Isha to learn and use new ways of coping.

Managing Stress

Drawing on the previous stages, some practical steps and strategies are explored to help Isha to manage now and in the future. To some extent, managing stress is very individual. For example, Isha may realise that talking to other students really helps because it normalises a certain amount of anxiety and worry. Or she may realise that in a previous stressful situation she was able to think about it differently and 'talk' herself out of her fears.

Interventions to prevent work stressors and perceived stress in health professionals have mixed results. Some interventions have good results in particular settings. For example, an intensive training programme for oncology nurses to help improve attitudes, communication skills, and reduce perceived stress led to nurses having better communication skills with patients, reporting less stress, and patients being more satisfied with their care (Delvaux et al., 2004). Reviews of mindfulness interventions to help nurses cope with stressors and perceived stress found that they lead to improved wellbeing, reduced anxiety and depression, and improved performance at work (Guillaumie et al., 2016; Karo et al., 2024). Mindfulness-based interventions have also been found to decrease stress, anxiety, and depression in health profession students, and to improve their mood, self-efficacy, and empathy (McConville et al., 2017). A Cochrane review concluded that individual-level stress interventions can lead to enduring reductions in stress among healthcare workers (Tamminga et al., 2023).

—Clinical Notes 3.3—

Looking After Yourself

- Studying and working in healthcare can be stressful. It is therefore really important that you are aware of your own stress levels and take steps to look after yourself.
- Recognise the signs and symptoms of stress in yourself and take steps to manage your stress.
- Avoid trying to 'go it alone'. Use the formal and informal support resources that are available to you, such as student counsellors (at university) and colleagues (in practice). There are also organisations that provide support where health professionals can talk through stressful or difficult issues and their wellbeing, for example Doctors' Support Network, Balint groups.
- If you have symptoms of burnout or other psychological problems, seek help as soon as possible, before the problem becomes chronic or severe.
- Skills in organisation, time management, and finding positive ways of dealing with stressors are worth developing early in your career.

Summary 3.3

- Severe or chronic stress is associated with psychological problems such as anxiety, depression, burnout, and PTSD.
- Burnout occurs when people feel exhausted, depersonalised, and have a poor sense of personal accomplishment.
- Health professionals are at increased risk of burnout and stress-related psychological problems, particularly in demanding specialties such as intensive and palliative care.
- Understanding stress processes is important for the development of interventions that help people to manage stressors more effectively.
- Stress management interventions are generally associated with increased psychological wellbeing, but evidence of their effect on physical health outcomes is mixed.

Conclusion

It is clear that we need to take a more sophisticated approach than thinking there is a simple dose–response relationship between stress and illness. As we saw in Chapter 2 on emotion, some negative emotions, such as depression and anger, are associated with illnesses such as heart disease. However, as this chapter on stress has shown, we need to account for individual differences in many factors, including pre-existing vulnerability and resilience, exposure, health behaviour, and social and environmental factors, in determining whether a person under stress will become ill and the type of illness they may suffer.

In the previous chapter and this one we have concentrated on the effects of motivation, emotion, and stress on health. In trying to explain the mechanisms underlying the associations between emotion, stress, and health, we have primarily concentrated on physical and behavioural pathways. However, emotion and stress will also influence symptom perception, help-seeking, and illness behaviour. In the next chapter we examine the role of symptom perception and illness beliefs in more detail.

Further Reading

Llewellyn, C.D. et al. (eds) (2019) *The Cambridge Handbook of Psychology, Health and Medicine* (3rd edition). Cambridge: Cambridge University Press. Includes short chapters on stress, coping, personality, emotions, physical activity, social factors, social relationships, psychoneuroimmunology, and burnout in health professionals.

Cooper, C.L. & Campbell Quick, J. (2017) *The Handbook of Stress and Health*. Malden, MA: Wiley Blackwell. A comprehensive book covering all aspects of stress and health.

Hill-Rice, V. (2012) *Handbook of Stress, Coping, and Health*. London: Sage. A comprehensive book that covers various models of stress, coping, and health, with a particular focus on their relevance to nursing and related fields of healthcare.

Medical School Council and General Medical Council (2022) *Achieving Good Medical Practice: Guidance for Medical Students*. Manchester: General Medical Council. Includes a section on why it is important for medical students to look after their psychological wellbeing and provides advice on how to address concerns.

Revision Questions

1 How is stress defined in psychology?
2 Outline the different elements of the interactional model of stress.
3 Describe the physiological responses to stress.
4 What factors explain differences in how people respond physiologically to stress?
5 Outline the vulnerability-stress model of how stress influences health.
6 Discuss some of the factors that can moderate the effect of stress on health.
7 Define 'coping' and describe two different ways in which coping strategies have been classified.
8 Outline the evidence that social support affects health.
9 What is stress burnout and how does it affect health professionals?
10 Describe two types of stress management intervention and briefly discuss the evidence that they are effective.

4

SYMPTOMS, PAIN, AND ILLNESS

┌─Learning Objectives─

This chapter is designed to enable you to:

- Discuss the role of psychological factors in physical symptoms.
- Describe the multidimensional nature of pain and the role of psychological factors in the perception of pain.
- Outline placebo and nocebo effects and how they affect illness and recovery.
- Describe the different representations of illness and explain how these affect the psychological and physical outcomes of illness.
- Understand how these principles can be used in clinical interventions to improve health.

Understanding symptoms is fundamental to providing good healthcare. Symptoms are a sign that something may be wrong. They motivate people to seek help from healthcare services, they help doctors and other health professionals to diagnose the problem, and they give an indication of whether a treatment is working and people are getting better. All of this would be fairly straightforward if there were a simple relationship between having symptoms and having a disease, or the severity of symptoms and disease. However, the relationship between symptoms and disease is not always simple or straightforward.

First, symptoms are remarkably common. Surveys of the general population indicate that around 90% of people report at least one physical or psychological symptom, and that most of these people report multiple symptoms (Petrie et al., 2014; Sætre et al., 2024; Wilson et al., 2023). The most commonly-reported symptoms include back pain, fatigue, headache, runny or stuffy nose, abdominal bloating or pain, and joint pain. However, it is important to note that most people with symptoms do not consult doctors, and instead ignore the symptoms, treat themselves, or rely on a natural recovery. The observation that only one-third of people see their doctor for symptoms that they experience means that relevant diagnosis may be delayed, and that the symptoms presented to health professionals are only the 'tip of the iceberg' of a larger symptom burden (Sætre et al., 2024).

Thus, symptoms are often also ambiguous: they are strongly influenced by psychological factors, such as the degree of attention we pay to symptoms, how they are interpreted, and beliefs about illness and healthcare. The previous chapters have described how the perception of symptoms is influenced by emotion and stress, and how motivation determines whether people will act on them and in what way. In this chapter, we examine more specifically how people perceive symptoms and illness, including pain, which is a primary symptom of many disorders. Placebo and nocebo effects demonstrate the importance of beliefs in the perception of symptoms and illness. These show that in some cases people recover because they believe they will recover, or feel ill because they believe they will get ill.

Symptoms are not only a sign of the *onset* of illness but also indicate the *progression* of illness. Chronic illnesses, such as rheumatoid arthritis or multiple sclerosis, involve remitting or slowly worsening symptoms and disability. Perhaps unsurprisingly, appraisals and beliefs about symptoms play an important role in how people adjust to chronic illness and predict further symptoms, distress, and disability. For example, a person who believes that their illness is uncontrollable, incurable, and disrupts every area of their life will be highly distressed and focused on their symptoms, worrying about whether the disease is getting worse. In contrast, a person who believes their illness is controllable and requires adjustment but does not disrupt every area of their life will be less distressed and less focused on their symptoms. As we have seen in previous chapters, distress such as anxiety or depression is in turn associated with poorer health and slower recovery. Thus, negative beliefs, distress, and negative interpretation of symptoms can become a vicious downward spiral, which is often seen in people with chronic pain. This chapter therefore examines the perception of symptoms, pain, placebo and nocebo effects, and how beliefs about symptoms and illness influence the experience and progression of chronic pain.

4.1 Symptom Perception

Symptoms are defined as subjective physical or mental experiences, appraised and defined by the person as reflecting an altered physical or health state (Riegel et al., 2019). Therefore, as with emotion and stress, appraisal and interpretation are central. For example, a racing heartbeat just before giving a presentation could be interpreted as nerves (unusual, transient, not harmful) or a possible heart problem (unusual, potentially chronic, harmful). Symptoms of a myocardial infarction (MI) may differ for women and men, and are also experienced and interpreted differently by women and men (Blakeman & Prasun, 2022; van Oosterhout et al., 2020). This affects how women respond to these symptoms, which may cost them their life if medical treatment is delayed. Evidence shows that women suffering a heart attack can take up to twice as long to get to hospital as men. The main reasons that women delay getting treatment include experiencing different symptoms from those typically associated with a heart attack, not perceiving symptoms as severe, having other illnesses, incorrectly attributing or labelling symptoms as due to something else, and women believing that they are less likely than men to have a heart attack (Lefler & Bondy, 2004; van Oosterhout et al., 2020).

How people appraise and interpret symptoms is therefore critical. Unfortunately, people are generally not very good at interpreting their physical state accurately. This has important implications for treatment. For example, people with asthma are expected to monitor their symptoms and use inhaler medication when they need it. However, most people with asthma are unable to detect changes in their lung function reliably (Janssens et al., 2009; Still & Dolen, 2016). Similarly, the majority of people with diabetes are not able to accurately estimate their blood glucose (Frankum &

Ogden, 2005). There are some exceptions to this general pattern. Some people are more accurate at detecting symptoms than others, and most people can accurately perceive extreme symptoms or physical changes that need immediate action, such as a bad injury or strong pain.

4.1.1 Psychological Factors and Symptoms

Psychological factors can affect the perception and interpretation of symptoms in a number of ways, including (1) the role of *attention* in whether people notice their symptoms, (2) the effect of the *environment* on symptom perception and interpretation, (3) *individual differences in the interpretation* of symptoms, and (4) the *influence of emotions* on symptom perception and interpretation.

Attention and the Environment

The degree of attention we pay to our internal physical state has a strong influence on the perception of symptoms. Most theories of attention assume we have a limited capacity to pay attention to different stimuli at the same time. Therefore, changes in our internal states have to compete with what is going on around us for attention. There are many examples of injured people doing remarkable things, such as soldiers fighting on or athletes continuing to compete. Similarly, some enduringly painful activities are enjoyed by many people, such as long-distance running and cycling races (see Case Study 4.1). This can be explained on different levels. Physiologically, the release of endogenous opioids such as endorphins reduces the level of pain we feel. Psychologically and socially, the demands and rewards of a situation mean that people are less likely to attend to their physical symptoms, or that the painful symptoms are overridden by the situational demands and goals.

Research confirms the importance of attention in the perception of symptoms. People are more likely to report symptoms if they are in boring environments. More symptoms are reported by people who are unemployed, living alone, or who are put in boring situations in laboratory research (Broadbent & Petrie, 2019). People also report more symptoms if they are instructed to attend to their internal physical stimuli rather than to external stimuli. For example, in one study, listening to music while walking on a treadmill resulted in women paying less attention to the exercise and bodily cues, and rating the exercise as less demanding (Silva et al., 2016). However, this effect is not simply the result of listening to any music. In a subsequent study, performance in strength tests was greatest and perceived exertion was least when people listened to their preferred music than when they listened to no music or music that they did not prefer (Silva et al., 2021). The implications for healthcare are that taking a person's attention away from internal stimuli by using strategies such as distraction toward preferred sensory stimuli can lower the perception of symptoms. Attention is covered in more detail in Chapter 10.

Case Study 4.1

Tour De France Winner On the Incredible Pain of Racing

Geraint Thomas was the surprise winner of the Tour de France in 2018. In an interview, he talked about the pain of cycling races. He described the pain of cycling being different from high impact sports like boxing, and how cycling involves pain over long periods on a daily basis.

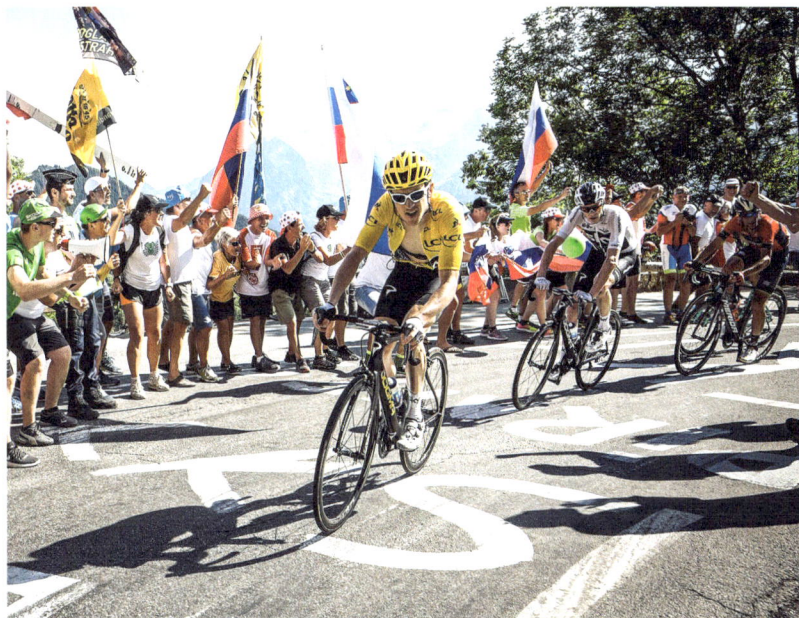

Figure 4.1   Geraint Thomas winning the 2018 Tour de France

Source: © Konstantin Kleine/Wikimedia Commons

Interestingly, he referred to the mental suffering or pain being as bad as the physical pain. He said how gruelling it is to be cycling for hours, day after day, and that 'You always have that devil on your shoulder saying "why don't you just take that shortcut home?"'.

Ultimately, however, he reported enjoying the suffering, and even described it as being addictive. When he doesn't ride his bike, he misses his muscles aching and the intense tiredness after hours of cycling. He said that after 'six or seven hours on the bike you feel wasted, but it's a nice feeling too. In a sadistic sort of way'. This suggests that, for him, knowing that the pain is for a purpose makes it worthwhile.

Individual Differences in the Interpretation of Symptoms

People differ in the amount of attention they pay to internal states, and also to which types of symptoms they are more likely to attend. Most people have sets of beliefs, or **schemas**, about their vulnerability to certain illnesses, which symptoms indicate potential illnesses, and which illnesses comprise a threat to their overall health. Schemas are mostly developed during childhood and are not always rational. Events in adulthood may lead to schemas changing or being modified. Schemas we have about our health and illness will therefore be influenced by our past experience of illness and others' attitudes to illness – particularly those of our parents.

Schemas usually operate unconsciously to influence what symptoms people attend to and how they interpret them. For example, in one study, healthy volunteers were shown either a neutral TV programme or a programme on the negative effects on health of being exposed to

Wi-Fi. Afterwards, volunteers were exposed to sham Wi-Fi and asked to rate various physical sensations. Volunteers who had watched the programme on the negative effects of Wi-Fi on health rated their physical sensations as more intense and were more anxious about being exposed to Wi-Fi (Bräscher et al., 2017). A similar phenomenon is apparent in the finding that up to one-third of medical students worry that they have an illness they have just studied. This is probably because they scan their symptoms for any that fit with the illness they are learning about (Broadbent & Petrie, 2019).

Thus, the perceived cause of symptoms is important. The process of interpreting the cause of something is called **attribution**. At a very basic level, people can attribute the cause of their symptoms to somatic causes, psychological causes, or environmental causes. If a middle-aged woman feels hot and faint, she could attribute these symptoms to menopause (somatic), being upset or embarrassed (psychological), or the room being too hot (environment). Within each category there are potentially many explanations. The attribution that a person makes affects the action they then take. For example, an aching muscle could be attributed to exercise (somatic but benign) or to the start of flu (somatic and threatening), and this will influence whether someone seeks help for a symptom.

Research into attribution indicates that people have different **attributional styles**. Individuals may be more or less likely to attribute events internally (to themselves) or externally (to the environment or others). In relation to symptoms, it is possible that some individuals who have an internal/somatic attribution style may also have increased healthcare use in response to symptoms.

The Influence of Emotion

Emotion, which was covered in Chapter 2, is strongly associated with the perception and reporting of symptoms. Strong emotion is accompanied by physiological changes that can be misinterpreted as symptoms. There is a large amount of evidence that negative emotions or emotional dispositions are related to increased reports of symptoms, pain, disability, and psychological distress. In part, this is due to negative emotions making people more likely to notice symptoms and interpret them as threatening. Research into anxiety shows that it leads to a narrowing of attentional focus and a bias towards the perception of threat. Anxiety therefore makes people hypervigilant, so they will scan themselves and the environment for any potential threat, including threats to health (Shi et al., 2022). In addition, some people are very sensitive to the physiological symptoms of anxiety and do not tolerate them well. High anxiety sensitivity is associated with more fearful appraisal of pain, reduced tolerance of pain, and more pain-related disability (Ocañez et al., 2010).

Research has also shown that inducing negative moods in people leads to similar effects. In such studies, negative moods are usually induced by showing people upsetting videos or asking them to recall difficult episodes from their past. Such research finds that people report more symptoms and think they are more vulnerable to illness when they are in a negative mood. People are also more likely to attribute the cause of symptoms to illness. For example, one study surveyed people a week after a vaccination and found that those with high negative affect reported more symptoms from the vaccination than people who were low in negative affect (Petrie et al., 2004). Our emotional state and dispositions therefore influence our attention to symptoms, appraisal, and interpretation of symptoms.

—Clinical Notes 4.1—

Symptoms

- There is no straightforward relationship between the number and severity of reported symptoms and disease.
- Most people are inaccurate at estimating their physical state, so do not rely on self-reported measures of physical processes such as lung function, blood glucose, or blood pressure.
- Getting people to focus on external stimuli (e.g. distraction) is a useful technique for reducing symptoms such as pain. It is particularly useful for brief painful procedures, such as injections or venepuncture.

4.1.2 Effects of Symptom Perception on Health

The misperception of symptoms potentially compromises the effectiveness of healthcare services through:

- Delay in seeking help if symptoms are interpreted as non-threatening.
- Overuse or underuse of healthcare services if symptoms are interpreted wrongly.
- Compromised treatment if people self-treat or do not adhere to a treatment because they misattribute the cause of symptoms.

For example, someone may stop taking medication, such as antibiotics, because they feel a bit better but are not 'cured'. This is an obvious waste of resources and undermines effective treatment. Adherence is discussed further in Chapter 12.

Understanding the processes that affect symptom perception can therefore help us to design more effective interventions, particularly for chronic illnesses where people have to adhere to intensive treatment regimes. For example, interventions have been developed to increase awareness of blood glucose in people with diabetes. These interventions include education about symptom recognition, biases, and management, and lead to better metabolic control of diabetes than standard educational interventions (Kim & Lee, 2016; Tan et al., 2015).

4.1.3 Medically Unexplained Symptoms

Many people have persistent symptoms that do not have an identifiable physical cause. Medically unexplained symptoms (MUS) are defined as persistent bodily symptoms with functional disability but no known explanatory structural or other pathology (Chalder & Willis, 2019). Diagnostically, MUS have been classified as **somatoform disorders** or somatic symptom disorders (American Psychiatric Association, 1994, 2013). These disorders include conditions where the cause is poorly understood, such as irritable bowel syndrome, fibromyalgia, chronic fatigue syndrome, non-cardiac chest pain, and chronic pain, as well as those with a clear psychological component, such as hypochondriasis. For some of these conditions, the terms

functional disorder or functional somatoform disorder may be used to reflect the lack of obvious structural differences or disease (Burton et al., 2020). The use of these various terms is perhaps a reflection of how MUS challenge the assumption of the biomedical approach that there must always be identifiable physical causes of ill-health.

MUS are common, but their precise prevalence is difficult to determine due to differences in diagnostic criteria, or a lack of clear diagnostic criteria. However, one review suggested that it is likely that more than one-quarter of patients in primary care have at least one MUS (Haller et al., 2015). MUS can be distressing for patients, and they are associated with a greater use of healthcare services (Jadhakhan et al., 2022). The absence of effective treatment in many cases results in repeated attendance, which can be frustrating for patients, and incurs costs for healthcare services.

MUS are strongly associated with psychological disorders such as anxiety or depression, illustrating the close relationship between negative emotions and physical symptoms discussed in the previous section. Indeed, some have even suggested that severe MUS should be interpreted as indicators or symptoms of depression and anxiety (Smith, 2020). The close association between psychological symptoms and MUS highlights the limitations of taking a purely biomedical approach to these conditions, but it is also important not to consider MUS as simply the result of individual psychological processes: from a biopsychosocial perspective, it is also important to consider social contextual factors.

The importance of factors other than individual physiology or psychology is indicated by the observation that MUS are more common in women, in lower socioeconomic groups, and among people with a history of adversity or trauma. Symptoms may also run in families – there is some evidence that the children of parents with MUS are more likely to report symptoms themselves (Shraim et al., 2013). Research Box 4.1 illustrates the wide variations in how patients understand and experience MUS.

Research Box 4.1

Patients' Experiences of Medically Unexplained Symptoms

Background

To provide appropriate care and treatment for medically unexplained symptoms (MUS), healthcare professionals need to understand patients' experiences. The aim of this study was to synthesise the findings of qualitative studies of living with MUS to identify common issues to address in interactions with patients.

Method and Findings

The authors conducted a qualitative meta-summary of interview-based studies of adolescents' and adults' experiences of living with, and seeking treatment for, MUS. The 23 studies included articles that presented the experiences of 445 people with MUS.

Eight themes were found. The three most common themes were: (1) the need to feel understood, (2) the search for explanations, and (3) disappointment in healthcare. People with MUS noted that even if diagnosis and treatment are not available, it is important that they are listened to and that their experiences and concerns are taken seriously.

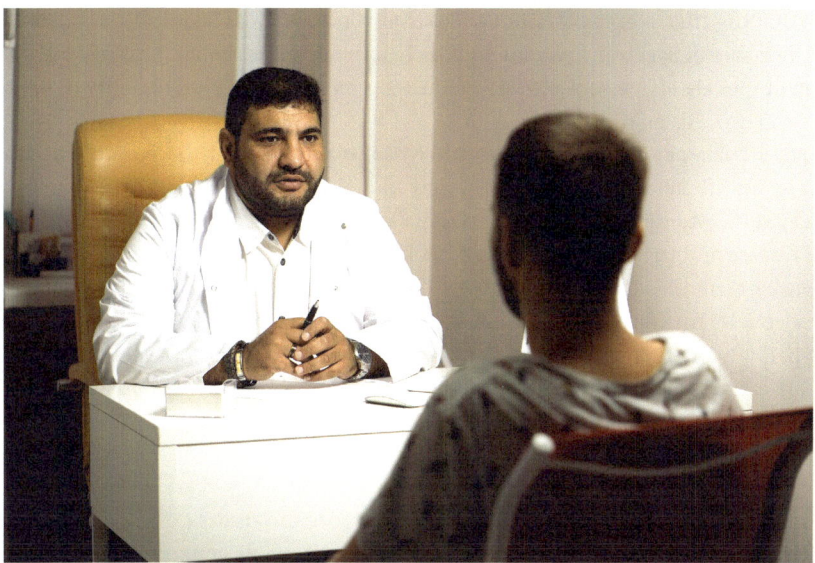

Figure 4.2 Listening to a patient with medically unexplained symptoms

Source: © Maximilianovich/Pixabay

Significance

Although many themes were common across studies and across interviewees, the analysis also revealed considerable variability in attitudes towards formal diagnoses, expectations of healthcare professionals, and capacity to cope with illness. It is important for healthcare professionals to understand this diversity and to respond to the concerns and needs of each patient.

Polakovská, L. & Řiháček, T. (2022) What is it like to live with medically unexplained physical symptoms? A qualitative meta-summary. *Psychology and Health, 37*(2): 580–596. doi:10.1080/08870446.2021.1901900.

Research indicates that symptoms and disability are perpetuated by both cognitive and behavioural factors, such as increased attention to symptoms, fear and avoidant coping, and attribution of symptoms to physical causes (Chalder & Willis, 2019). There is also considerable overlap of symptoms between different conditions, such as chronic fatigue and irritable bowel syndrome, despite different aetiological pathways. Chalder and Willis (2019) outlined a model of MUS that shows how predisposing vulnerability (e.g. childhood abuse, neuroticism), precipitating factors (e.g. life events, stress, viral infections), and perpetuating factors (e.g. a focus on symptoms, attribution, catastrophic misappraisal, rumination) may interact to perpetuate the disorder. They used this model to propose an individualised treatment based on cognitive behavioural therapy (CBT). Given the close association between medically unexplained symptoms and psychological factors, it is perhaps unsurprising that psychotherapy is associated with a reduction in symptoms and disability (Kaur et al., 2022; van Dessel et al., 2014). One review indicated that the effectiveness of behavioural interventions for MUS is influenced by the quality of the relationship between the patient and the healthcare professional (Leaviss et al., 2020). Self-help programmes are also associated with reduced symptoms and better quality of life compared to usual care (van Gils et al., 2016).

MUS are a challenge for doctors and other health professionals because of the uncertainty about cause, and therefore treatment. A review of 13 studies of doctors' experiences with MUS found a key difficulty for doctors was the lack of congruence between the dominant biomedical model of disease and the reality of trying to help people suffering from chronic symptoms with no known biomedical pathology or cause (Johansen & Risor, 2017). Doctors reported feeling stuck, inadequate, frustrated, and powerless to help, which could lead to a difficult relationship with the patient. Doctors had to work flexibly and use a more psychosocial approach through establishing a good relationship, alliance, and partnership with the patient. This led to positive experiences of mutual trust and validation. Part of this process was doctors learning to balance the 'ideal versus real', where the ideal is biomedicine as a learnt discipline in which all symptoms can be attributed to known causes, and the real is experience-based knowledge.

MUS highlight the limitations of a biomedical approach to disease. The classification systems used in healthcare services are diagnostic, and they require some certainty about physical cause. This has led to proposals for new classification systems that, instead of focusing on physical disease, focus on a range of prognostic factors, such as symptom characteristics (e.g. number, multi-system, frequency, severity), concurrent psychological disorders, and sociodemographic characteristics (e.g. female, low socioeconomic status) (Rosendal et al., 2017). These characteristics can be used to group symptoms according to whether they are likely to be self-limiting, recurrent, persistent symptoms, or symptom disorders (Rosendal et al., 2017). In the next section we look at the symptoms of pain and how psychological knowledge and research can help to provide effective treatments for chronic pain, which in many cases is a type of medically unexplained symptom.

Summary 4.1

- Understanding symptoms is fundamental to good healthcare.
- Symptoms are subjective physical or mental experiences, appraised and defined by the person as reflecting an altered physical or health state.
- Symptoms can be a sign of the onset and progression of a disease. However, there is not a straightforward relationship between symptoms and disease.
- How people appraise and interpret their symptoms affects whether they take appropriate action and receive appropriate treatment.
- Psychological factors affect the perception and interpretation of symptoms through variables such as attention, beliefs, or schemas about illnesses and individual vulnerability.
- Negative mood is associated with heightened symptom perception.
- Medically unexplained symptoms are common. They illustrate the importance of psychosocial factors in the onset, perpetuation, and treatment of such symptoms.

4.2 Pain

Pain is a common symptom and often an important signal that the body has been damaged or that something is wrong. In rare cases of congenital insensitivity to pain, children have a reduced ability to feel pain and are unable to recognise physical damage or danger. These children are at risk of a range of problems, including biting off parts of their tongue, being prone to eye infections following damage by foreign objects, and suffering bone fractures or burns.

Pain has been defined as a distressing experience that is associated with actual or potential tissue damage and which has sensory, emotional, cognitive, and social elements (Williams & Craig, 2016). A number of distinctions are important in understanding pain. First, it is important to distinguish between nociception, sensation, and suffering. **Nociception** is the stimulation of peripheral pain receptors, which send pain messages to the central nervous system. The **sensation** of pain is how this is interpreted and it is influenced by many factors, including attention, schemas, and emotion. **Suffering** refers to the perceived pain, distress, and disability that can arise from pain and other related factors.

Second, it is important to distinguish between pain threshold and pain tolerance. The **pain threshold** is the point at which a stimulus becomes painful and is similar for most people, regardless of their gender, ethnicity, or culture. **Pain tolerance** is the degree to which a painful stimulus can be tolerated, and it varies widely between individuals, cultures, and contexts. For example, music and humour can increase people's tolerance of pain. Research shows that simply listening to music or watching a funny film increases pain tolerance (Lee, 2016; Pérez-Aranda et al., 2019). Indeed, music is increasingly used to help people undergoing difficult procedures or with severe illnesses. For example, a Cochrane review of music therapy for people with cancer found that it reduces pain and anxiety, increases mood and quality of life, and has positive effects on heart rate, respiratory rate, and blood pressure (Bradt et al., 2016).

Acute pain is necessary to protect us from damage or infection: when we experience acute pain, we usually do something about it. These actions can include ceasing the activity that results in pain, resting, and seeking treatment.

Chronic pain is somewhat different: it is pain that persists for a prolonged period. In addition to being an unpleasant experience in itself, it can also detrimentally affect people's engagement in various activities. Chronic pain can incur huge treatment costs and have broader indirect costs related to lost work productivity. Reviews of studies of the general population in various countries indicate that chronic pain is common: approximately 25% of adults report chronic pain, many of whom report that it is moderately or severely disabling (Ekholm et al., 2022; Mills et al., 2019; Santiago et al., 2023).

Prolonged aches or pains are usually a signal that a part of our body is damaged or healing. However, if pain continues for three months or longer, it is possible that the original physical damage has healed but that pain pathways have become over-sensitised or dysregulated so that pain is still felt in the absence of physical injury. Research has shown that after three months of stimulation to a pain pathway, molecular changes occur in the ribonucleic acid (RNA) in the neurons of the spinal cord. Thus, pain neurons adapt and change in the face of constant stimulation. Similarly, imaging research has shown extensive cortical reorganisation in response to chronic pain and that some maladaptive coping strategies, such as thinking the worst (catastrophising), can affect this (Gracely et al., 2004; Henn et al., 2023). This has implications for the treatment of chronic pain. Rather than taking a 'wait and see' approach, early intervention is important to prevent changes to the neural pathways.

How we view pain has implications for our understanding and treatment of it. Biological explanations of pain assume that pain results from physical damage. Treatment will therefore comprise analgesia to numb the pain and, if possible, surgery to repair the damage. However, as we have seen above, there can be many instances where pain occurs in the absence of physical injury. Pain is increased by negative emotion, cognitive processes, and behaviour, such as inactivity.

Overall, it is clear that pain is highly subjective and influenced by many factors, including biological, psychological, and social factors. The range of factors that can affect pain perception is illustrated in Figure 4.3. The point at which a person complains of pain will vary according to the immediate context, their background and characteristics, and what they have learned from others about pain expression. The implication for healthcare is that each person's pain should be treated *as needed*, without referring to stereotypes about how much pain they 'should' be in.

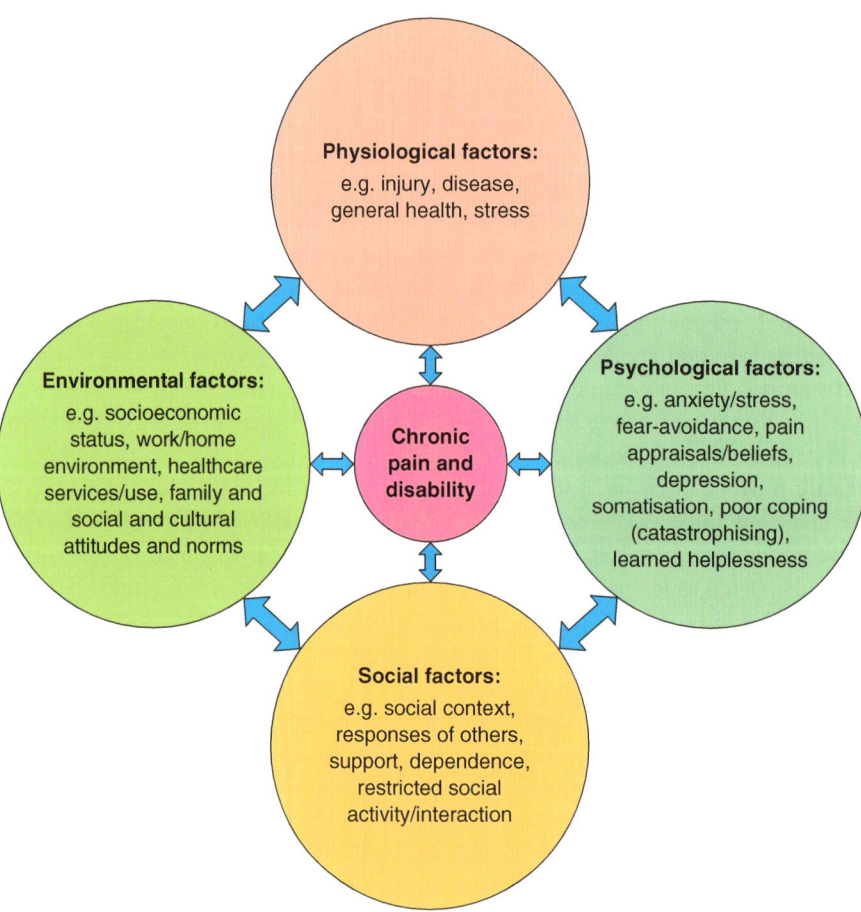

Figure 4.3 Biopsychosocial model of pain (adapted from Stinson et al., 2016). Copyright Elsevier (2016).

4.2.1 Theories of Pain

Historically, pain was viewed from a biomedical perspective: pain was considered to be a direct result of injury, and the severity of the pain would be proportionate to the severity of the injury. A wealth of evidence has since emphasised the importance of a biopsychosocial understanding of pain, such as that shown in Figure 4.3. A biopsychosocial approach acknowledges that pain occurs within a social context and that there are different aspects to it: biological factors, such as injury, genetics, immune and central nervous system responses; psychological factors, such as emotional, cognitive, and behavioural responses; and social factors, such as support from others, reactions of others, and cultural norms for expressing pain. In many ways, this is similar to the models of emotion in Chapter 2, which also highlight the interdependence between physical sensations, thoughts, and emotion.

Theory has made a significant contribution to our understanding of how psychological and physical factors interact in the perception of pain. Historically, the **Gate Theory of pain** (Melzack & Wall, 1965) was seminal in our understanding and is based on the notion of a synaptic gate between peripheral nerves and neurons in the spinal cord, as illustrated in Figure 4.4. Pain signals from peripheral nerves compete with other neural signals to get through the gate. The gate can be open or closed by physical factors (e.g. counter-stimulation of other peripheral nerves, endogenous opioids) or by psychological factors (e.g. attention, downward stimulation from the brain, moods). This theory therefore provides a basis on which to understand the interplay between physical and psychological factors in pain. It also accounts for the phenomenon of pain being reduced through touch, such as when a child is hurt and someone 'rubs it better'. This theory was later expanded into the *neuromatrix* model, where pain is considered to be due to interacting neural networks with somatosensory, limbic, and cognitive components (Melzack, 1999).

The advantage of the Gate Theory is that it provides a physiological explanation for how psychological factors affect pain perception. It also makes it clear that pain is not simply physical or psychological, but a combination of both. However, evidence for this theory is mixed. There is a large amount of supporting evidence showing that psychological factors influence pain but the physiological evidence for Gate Theory is less consistent (Mendell, 2014). It has also been noted that theory may over-simplify the process and the detail of the neural architecture. However, as a conceptual model, Gate Theory is an important and useful part of pain management programmes because it helps people with chronic pain to understand how their mental attitude and behaviour can influence their pain. This can help them to feel less helpless and more in control. It provides them with knowledge about the things they can do that can open or close the gate, such as those shown in Highlight Box 4.1, so they can actively work to reduce their pain by increasing those things in their life that will close the gate.

Since Gate Theory was proposed, more has become known about psychological processes and pain. Theories that address the psychological component of a biopsychosocial approach include the role of conditioning, cognitive-behavioural models, and functional-contextual approaches in chronic pain. **Conditioning** approaches to chronic pain focus on the role of operant conditioning in experiences of pain and behavioural responses to pain (Adamczyk et al., 2019). Although the initial behavioural response may be triggered by injury, this approach focuses on how long-term pain behaviours are shaped by how others respond to these behaviours. If behaviours are reinforced, then they are more likely to continue, whereas behaviours that are not reinforced or are punished are likely to stop. Thus, long-term behavioural responses to pain are contingent on reinforcement

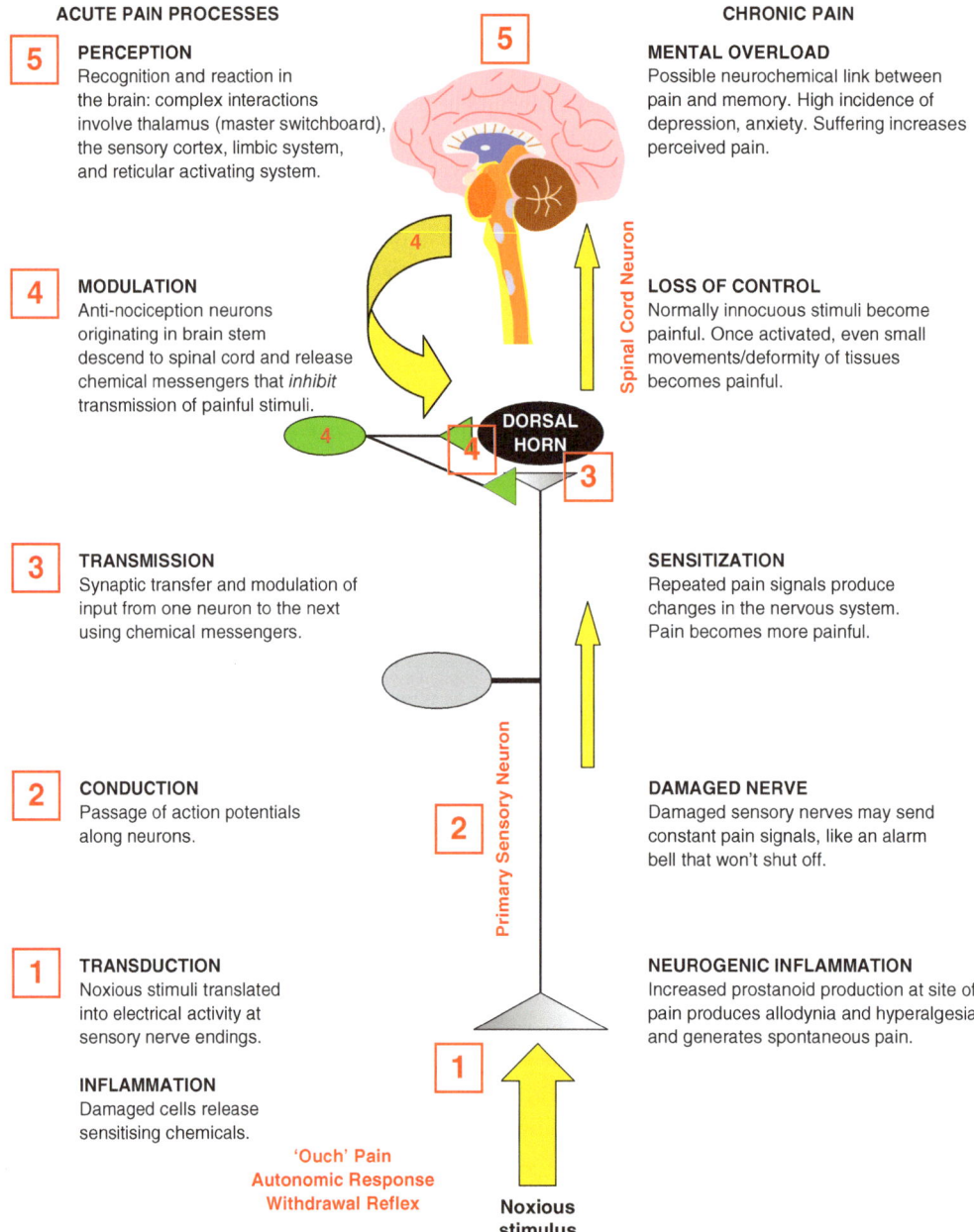

ACUTE PAIN PROCESSES

5 **PERCEPTION**
Recognition and reaction in the brain: complex interactions involve thalamus (master switchboard), the sensory cortex, limbic system, and reticular activating system.

4 **MODULATION**
Anti-nociception neurons originating in brain stem descend to spinal cord and release chemical messengers that *inhibit* transmission of painful stimuli.

3 **TRANSMISSION**
Synaptic transfer and modulation of input from one neuron to the next using chemical messengers.

2 **CONDUCTION**
Passage of action potentials along neurons.

1 **TRANSDUCTION**
Noxious stimuli translated into electrical activity at sensory nerve endings.

INFLAMMATION
Damaged cells release sensitising chemicals.

'Ouch' Pain
Autonomic Response
Withdrawal Reflex

5

DORSAL HORN

Spinal Cord Neuron

Primary Sensory Neuron

Noxious stimulus

CHRONIC PAIN

MENTAL OVERLOAD
Possible neurochemical link between pain and memory. High incidence of depression, anxiety. Suffering increases perceived pain.

LOSS OF CONTROL
Normally innocuous stimuli become painful. Once activated, even small movements/deformity of tissues becomes painful.

SENSITIZATION
Repeated pain signals produce changes in the nervous system. Pain becomes more painful.

DAMAGED NERVE
Damaged sensory nerves may send constant pain signals, like an alarm bell that won't shut off.

NEUROGENIC INFLAMMATION
Increased prostanoid production at site of pain produces allodynia and hyperalgesia and generates spontaneous pain.

Figure 4.4 The psychophysiology of pain (Whitten et al., 2005)

Reproduced courtesy of Christine Whitten MD

from others (see Chapter 10 for more information on conditioning). There is evidence to support this. For example, one study of children with chronic pain showed that when parents responded maladaptively to the child's pain, their children reported increased symptoms and disability (Claar et al., 2008). This occurred regardless of whether parents' responses were positively reinforcing (e.g. paying more attention to the pain, granting special privileges) or negatively reinforcing (e.g. criticism, discounting the pain). Behavioural interventions for chronic pain therefore aim to reduce symptoms and disability through training health professionals and family members to reinforce 'well' behaviours, such as increased functioning, and to ignore pain behaviours, such as verbal or nonverbal expressions of pain or disability (Scott & McCracken, 2018). Reviews of published research do not provide convincing evidence for the effectiveness of behavioural therapies, but this is in some part due to the need for better quality research in this domain (Williams et al., 2020). Behavioural interventions alone may not be effective treatments for chronic pain.

─Highlight Box 4.1─

Factors That Open or Close the Pain 'Gate'

Table 4.1   Opening or closing the pain 'gate'

	Factors that tend to open the gate	Factors that tend to close the gate
Physical	Further injury	Appropriate use of medication
	Inactivity/poor physical fitness	Heat/cold
	Long-term drug and alcohol use	Massage
Behavioural	Poor or too little pacing of activity, i.e. doing too much	Exercise
		Relaxation training
	Poor sleep	Meditation
Emotional	Anxiety, depression	Laughter/humour
	Stress, distress	Love
	Hopelessness/helplessness	Pleasure/happiness
Cognitive	Focusing on the pain	Focusing on other things, e.g. hobbies
	Worrying about the pain	Distraction
	Catastrophising (thinking the worst)	Positive coping strategies
	Focusing on the negative consequences of pain	
	Wishing it would go away	

Cognitive-behavioural approaches to chronic pain incorporate behavioural factors, such as operant conditioning, as well as individual factors, such as perceived pain, pain-related beliefs, cognitions, and emotions. There are many approaches within this category, one of which is the **fear-avoidance model**. The fear-avoidance model suggests that if people catastrophise about their pain (e.g. focus on how awful it is, feel helpless and out of control), it leads to greater fear of pain, greater focus on pain, and restricted functioning, such that people actively avoid any activity that may increase their pain. This avoidance leads to disuse, disability, and depression, as shown in Figure 4.5 (Crombez et al., 2012).

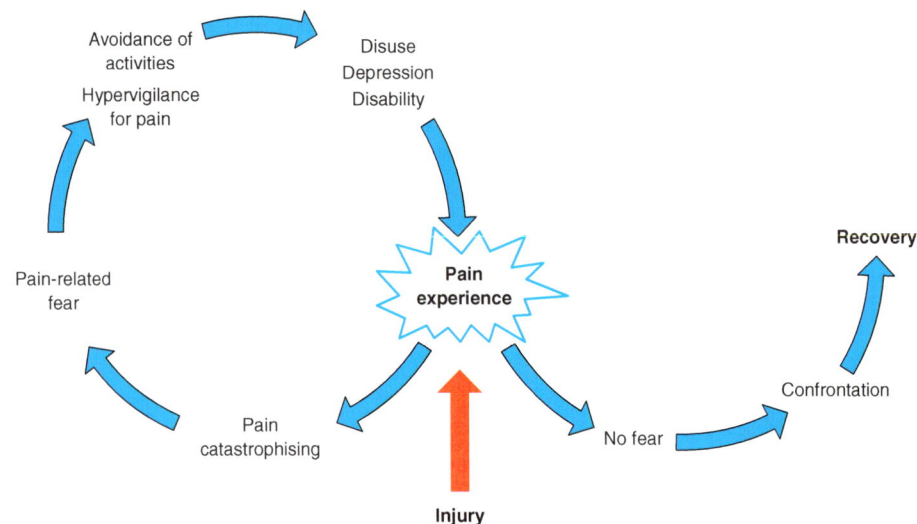

Figure 4.5 Fear-avoidance model of pain (Crombez et al., 2012)

Cognitive behavioural therapy (CBT) for chronic pain draws on these and other approaches to identify and change maladaptive thinking, emotional and behavioural responses, and coping styles. CBT for pain management might involve education about the role of psychological factors in pain, examination of current appraisals, beliefs, and responses to pain, and exploration of more adaptive ways of thinking and coping. People are taught coping strategies such as relaxation, distraction, or stress management. Functioning is increased through setting goals and gradually increasing activity. CBT is an effective treatment for chronic pain. A review of 75 randomised controlled trials with over 9,000 participants showed that CBT led to small but significant improvements in pain, disability, and distress (Williams et al., 2020).

The **functional-contextual approach** to chronic pain (McCracken & Morley, 2014) was developed in line with third wave CBT, particularly **acceptance and commitment therapy (ACT)**. The functional-contextual approach focuses on the *processes* and *function* of thoughts and behaviours, rather than the *content* of thoughts (e.g. pain-beliefs), which is the focus of standard CBT. The contextual aspect of this model is a focus on psychological flexibility, which is the function and workability of responses to pain and whether people's responses to pain are consistent with their values and goals in life. The focus of treatment is therefore to improve functioning and quality of life, rather than specifically targeting pain. This is done through a range of techniques, such as accepting chronic pain, identifying life values, and using mindfulness and cognitive defusion to help people manage their pain and live according to their values and goals. More information on ACT, mindfulness, and other techniques is given in Chapter 14. Meta-analyses suggest that ACT may be an effective way to alleviate pain and disability, and to enhance emotional functioning. It appears to be superior to mindfulness-based interventions (Veehof et al., 2016). However, a more recent review noted that to be more certain of the efficacy of ACT, there is a need for more evidence from high-quality studies (Williams et al., 2020).

The **communal coping model (CCM)** is also a social-contextual approach (Thorn et al., 2003). The CCM looks at the relationship between pain and catastrophising thoughts and behaviour. It suggests that some people may be predisposed to dealing with distress by catastrophising in order to communicate their distress and attempt to increase social proximity and support from others. In this way, it is similar to operant conditioning approaches, because the behaviour of others is important. However, like the functional-contextual approach, it looks at the social function of catastrophising behaviour to the person in chronic pain. The CCM distinguishes between pain severity, the emotional components of pain, catastrophising thoughts, catastrophising behaviour, and reinforcing or solicitous behaviours of others (Thorn et al., 2003). For example, a study of 105 married couples found that the spouses of people experiencing chronic pain changed their behaviour during and after elevated pain catastrophising episodes (Burns et al., 2015). This finding confirmed the hypothesis that pain catastrophising is a coping response that elicits assistance or empathic responses from others.

4.2.2 Biopsychosocial Approach to Pain Management

The section on theories of pain showed how different theories have led to the development of various treatments for chronic pain. Because pain is multidimensional, interventions need to tackle the physiological, psychological, and social factors involved in chronic pain. Interventions and management programmes should therefore involve physicians, physiotherapists, psychologists, and specialist nurses working together to use pharmacological, behavioural, and psychological techniques. The aim of these programmes is to assist people in effectively *managing* their pain so that they can lead a functional and positive life. These programmes are usually effective, particularly if they involve a psychological component such as CBT or ACT. Psychological components include educating people about the different dimensions of pain and how vicious cycles can arise, such as the fear-avoidance cycle shown in Figure 4.5. People are encouraged to take control of their life and through a process of empowerment to become more active. This can then lead to a positive cycle of less fear, less focus on the pain, and therefore less pain.

Pain management programmes are usually effective and reduce pain, depression, or other negative emotion and abnormal pain behaviours. They can also lead to more successful coping, increased activity, and improved social functioning (Morley, 2007). Programmes vary widely in their specific approaches and in how the members of interdisciplinary teams work together (Connell et al., 2022). Case Study 4.2 illustrates a broad approach.

─Case Study 4.2─

Treating Chronic Back Pain

Robert works as a laboratory technician and has chronic lower back pain following a work-related accident three years ago. In the last six months the pain has become constant and gets much worse when Robert is driving or sitting. Robert's back occasionally 'goes into spasm'. When this happens, he feels semi-paralysed and has to lie down on the floor until the attack passes. This has only happened twice but Robert is very worried and frightened of the possibility of another attack.

(Continued)

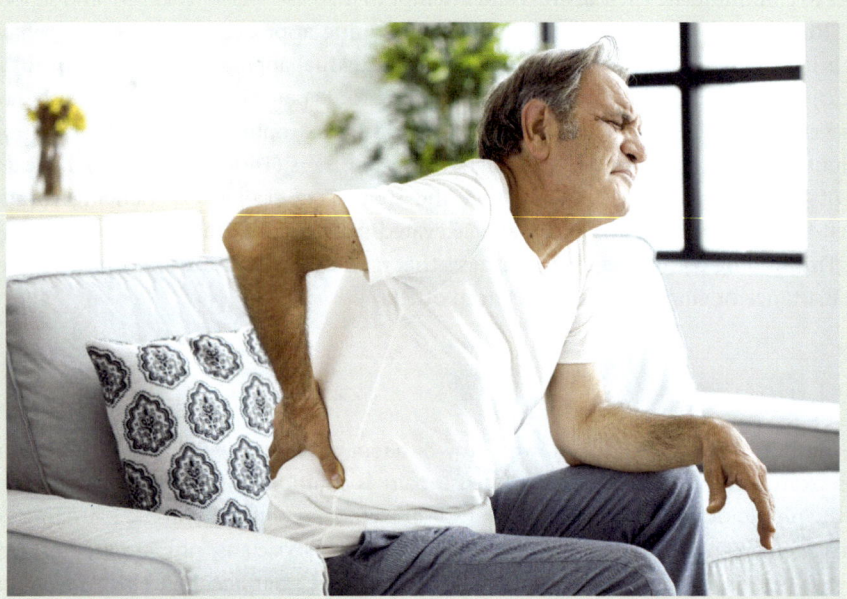

Figure 4.6 Robert's lower back pain

Source: © sebra/Adobe Stock

Robert is on long-term sick leave. He does not go out much because he is worried that he will have another attack and collapse. Robert is depressed and says the pain has taken over his life. He uses a number of pain relief medications every day, but says it doesn't help. He is physically inactive.

Treatment

In a typical pain management programme, Robert would be seen by a physician to rule out any physical cause for his pain and agree an effective approach to analgesia. A physiotherapist would work with Robert to do exercises that strengthen his back. The physiotherapist might also help Robert to gradually increase his activity levels each week.

Psychological treatment might involve education about the psychological aspects of pain to help Robert to understand how his actions and thoughts affect his pain. He would be encouraged to manage his pain, rather than allowing it to control him. A traditional CBT approach might involve deconstructing the pain by monitoring pain-related thoughts and behaviour, and increasing Robert's awareness of pain processes. Robert might complete a pain diary to identify any pattern to his symptoms, the effect it is having on his life, and how his pain is linked to triggers such as stress, thoughts, emotions, and general activity levels. Maladaptive thought processes or behaviours would be identified, and Robert would be encouraged to change them. Robert would be taught coping strategies, such as relaxation techniques, mindfulness, positive self-talk, and setting and achieving personal goals.

This approach should help Robert to exercise and go out more often, which in turn should reduce his fear and avoidance of activity, and help him to feel more in control of his pain. Providing Robert with positive coping strategies may consolidate his feelings of control and empowerment, and help him to have a better quality of life.

Summary 4.2

- Pain is a common symptom: approximately 25% of the adult population is estimated to suffer from chronic pain.
- Pain is multidimensional: it involves nociception, pain sensations, thoughts, emotions, pain behaviours, and suffering.
- Attention, anxiety, and distress are associated with increased pain.
- The Gate Theory of pain provided a physiological explanation for the influence of psychological factors on pain.
- Pain management programmes help people to cope better with chronic pain. They are often effective at reducing pain, depression, negative emotion, negative coping, and maladaptive pain behaviour, and increasing activity, positive coping, and social functioning.

4.3 Placebo and Nocebo Effects

Placebo and nocebo effects provide clear examples of the effect of beliefs on symptoms. The term 'placebo' is Latin for *I shall please*. A **placebo effect** occurs when people are given a fake treatment that has no active ingredient but they report an improvement in health. Placebo effects are not limited to fake drugs but can also occur in response to fake surgery. For example, a review comparing arthroscopic procedures (debridement or lavage) for osteoarthritis of the knee with sham surgery (where incisions were made but no debridement or lavage was done) revealed that people who have sham surgery have comparable pain and functioning after the surgery than those who had real surgery (Evidence Development and Standards Branch, Health Quality Ontario, 2014). Similarly, a placebo effect can occur with an active drug, where part of the drug effect is due to the active ingredients and part due to a placebo effect. For example, studies have been conducted where people consent to having medication administered intravenously without their knowledge so they do not know when, or if, they are being given medication. Comparing their responses to people who know when they receive medication shows that a substantial proportion of the effects of morphine on pain, beta-blockers on heart rate, and diazepam on anxiety are due to the placebo effect (Benedetti et al., 2003; Colloca et al., 2004). Furthermore, reviews of studies of the effect of antidepressant medication on depression suggest that they may not be any more effective than placebos (Mallery et al., 2019). For example, one study of the general population found that a placebo could duplicate 80% of the effect of antidepressants. In people with extremely severe depression, antidepressants had a small effect on recovery, but this seemed to be mainly due to these people being less responsive to placebos rather than being more responsive to antidepressants (Kirsch et al., 2008).

Some people respond to placebos more strongly than others, and some illnesses are more amenable to placebos. Evidence suggests that placebo effects are most powerful for conditions with psychological components, such as pain, depression, asthma, and insomnia. Placebos are not effective for disorders with a clear simple biological basis, such as anaemia and infections (Wampold et al., 2005). The characteristics of placebos affect how well they work. For example, injections have a larger effect than pills, fake morphine has a larger effect than fake aspirin, and placebo effects are larger if the doctor or health professional expresses a belief that it will work (Kirsch, 2019).

The **nocebo effect** is a counterpoint to the placebo effect. The term 'nocebo' is Latin for *I shall harm*. The nocebo effect occurs when people develop symptoms that fit their beliefs even when they have not been exposed to a pathogen. For example, Lorber, Mazzoni, and Kirsch (2007) asked students to inhale an inert substance, which they said was a toxin that could result in particular symptoms. In addition, half the students watched another person, who was secretly a research confederate, inhale the substance first and show these symptoms. All students who inhaled the placebo reported the symptoms they were told they might have, and women were particularly influenced if they saw the confederate display symptoms. Nocebo effects with demonstrable physical changes have also been observed. For example, giving people with asthma a sham inhaler, which they are told contains an allergen, leads to bronchoconstriction, even when they are given harmless nebulised saline (Colloca & Miller, 2011). In another study, people who read a medication information sheet that listed various side effects were significantly more likely to report those side effects than people who did not read about them (Mondaini et al., 2007).

There is substantial evidence for placebo and nocebo effects (Kirsch, 2019). The prevalence and strength of placebo effects is the reason why placebo-controlled trials are needed when testing new treatments, whether they are drugs, physical interventions, or psychological therapies. For a treatment to be considered effective, it must have an effect that is clearly better than a placebo effect.

Although the importance of placebo and nocebo effects is evident, what is less clear is the mechanisms through which these effects are produced. Explanations include conditioning (including modelling) and the effect of expectations. **Classical conditioning** occurs when a stimulus (in this case an active drug or treatment) is paired with a response (an improvement in health) and over time becomes associated with a neutral stimulus that also occurs in this context (pills, injections, the actions of health professionals). The neutral stimulus then becomes a conditioned stimulus, which results in some of the changes observed to the initial active stimulus. **Modelling** occurs when one observes the effect in someone else and learns it. These types of learning are covered in more detail in Chapter 10.

Another key explanation is that placebos work through a person's **expectations** – they expect to get better or worse, so they do. There is evidence that both classical conditioning and expectations can contribute to the placebo effect, and that these are not incompatible (Kirsch, 2019). Because there may be more than one process or mechanism underlying placebo effects, an integrated framework has been proposed where the placebo response is thought to be a learned response, where a variety of cues trigger expectations that generate placebo or nocebo effects via the central nervous system. These can be verbal, conditioned, or social cues, such as being influenced by what health professionals say about the placebo, as well as by observation of others' responses. Evidence from neurological studies supports the role of the central nervous system in the placebo effect. A review of functional magnetic resonance imaging (fMRI) studies of responses to placebo analgesia found reduced activity in the brain regions that are associated with pain perception (Atlas & Wager, 2014; Skyt et al., 2020). Genetic research into possible determinants of why people are more or less responsive to placebos suggests genetic variation in various neurotransmitter systems may be involved (Colagiuri et al., 2015).

4.3.1 Using the Placebo Effect in Clinical Practice

The placebo effect has many clinical implications. The first is that the effect of many active drugs can be increased by the way they are presented – both in form (e.g. pill or injection) and in manner (e.g. with belief and conviction). A health professional who encourages people to believe treatments will work can harness the placebo effect in addition to the drug. The second implication is that placebos can result in a positive change without any negative side effects, so are useful treatments for those conditions that are amenable to placebos, such as depression. In fact, surveys of health professionals in different countries show that up to 80% of doctors and even more nurses have used placebos, such as saline injections (Fässler et al., 2010). However, if we use these strategies, we must be mindful of the ethical and legal issues. People should be encouraged to have positive expectations, but within realistic limits. The dilemma when using placebos is how to do so without using deception, although research suggests that placebos can be effective even when people know they are placebos (Carvalho et al., 2016; Carvalho et al., 2021). Kirsch (2019) recommends using treatments that do not have active components only where there is some evidence that they may be effective, such as some complementary therapies or physical exercise.

─Clinical Notes 4.2─

Pain and Placebo

- Pain is subjective so each person's pain should be treated *as needed*, without reference to stereotypes about how much pain they 'should' have.
- Chronic pain results in extensive neural changes that may be difficult to reverse, so we should intervene as early as possible to avoid these.
- A substantial proportion of the effects of medication on some illnesses is due to placebo effects.
- To use the placebo effect to increase the effect of treatments, express confidence that treatments will work to increase people's positive expectations.
- Conversely, if you tell people to expect negative side effects or symptoms, they will be more likely to experience them (the nocebo effect).

Summary 4.3

- A placebo effect occurs when someone's health improves in the absence of any active substance or treatment.
- A nocebo effect occurs when someone reports symptoms in the absence of any active pathogen.
- These effects can account for a substantial proportion of recovery, particularly in illnesses with strong psychological components, such as asthma and depression.
- The extent of the placebo effect varies between individuals.
- Placebos are thought to work through a combination of expectations, classical conditioning, and modelling.
- The placebo effect can be used in clinical practice to aid recovery, but consideration should be given to ethical issues.

4.4 Illness Beliefs and Representations

Earlier in this chapter we looked at the effect of unconscious schemas on the perception of symptoms. In addition to this, people hold conscious beliefs about illness which will shape their behaviour in response to symptoms. Beliefs about illness will determine the action a person chooses to take, which information they give to a health professional, the kind of treatment they want, whether they adhere to that treatment, and their emotional, behavioural, and cognitive responses to the illness. Illness beliefs are not necessarily accurate or coherent. **Illness representations** are people's organised sets of beliefs about the experience, impact, effect, and outcome of an illness. They are unique to each individual and are shaped by many factors, including their personal history, experience of different illnesses, and social and cultural learning.

Five main dimensions of illness representations have been identified: identity, timeline, cause, control, and consequences (Leventhal et al., 1984; Leventhal et al., 2016). Here we will outline each of these in more detail. The concept of **illness identity** refers to the way a person labels the illness and symptoms, such as what they believe multiple sclerosis is and what it involves. People will have mental models of which symptoms go with different illnesses. If more of their various symptoms match a person's model of a particular illness, then they are more likely to diagnose themselves as having that illness. For example, a headache could be due to many things, such as a hangover, tension, migraine, brain tumour, or meningitis. A self-diagnosis of meningitis is more likely if a person experiences a headache, stiff neck, and a rash. Making a self-diagnosis is important in seeking help. Research shows that people are more likely to attend a doctor if they have self-diagnosed a specific illness (Asghari et al., 2022; Simons et al., 2015).

The **timeline** is the length of time that a person believes the illness will last and the pattern it will take, for example chronic, acute, remitting, or cyclical. This affects their adjustment to the illness and adherence to treatment. For example, people who believe their illness is chronic report more disability and distress compared to other people with the same illness who believe it is acute or cyclical (Millar et al., 2005).

The **cause** is what a person thinks caused their symptoms or illness. It overlaps with the attributions and interpretation of symptoms discussed earlier. However, it may not be medically accurate. For example, stress is commonly believed to cause a range of illnesses, including cancer, diabetes, multiple sclerosis, and arthritis (Cameron & Moss-Morris, 2004).

Beliefs about **control** concern whether the person believes their illness can be prevented, controlled, or cured. People who think their illness is controllable are more likely to take an active part in their treatment and rehabilitation. Conversely, thinking an illness is uncontrollable is associated with using passive coping strategies (e.g. avoidance) and poorer mental health outcomes (Dempster et al., 2015; Hudson et al., 2014; Richardson et al., 2017). In a chronic or terminal illness, we should therefore encourage people to focus on those aspects of their illness they can control, such as their symptoms, disability, and the timeline.

Beliefs about **consequences** are concerned with the effect of the illness, for example physical, psychological, social, and economic effects. Perceived consequences are usually closely linked to the severity of someone's symptoms, so asymptomatic illnesses, such as hypertension, are often viewed as having no consequences (Rivera et al., 2020).

Figure 4.7 shows how illness representations can affect the way a person copes with their symptoms, illness, and treatment (Leventhal et al., 1984). This is known as the **self-regulation model of illness behaviour** because it accounts for how people self-manage their illness based on their personal beliefs. The strengths of this model are that it recognises the importance of appraisal, emotion, and coping in managing illness. Case Study 4.2 illustrates how illness beliefs can affect perceptions of chest pain. A difficulty with the illness representations model is that severe illnesses like cancer are more likely to result in negative illness representations, for example being chronic, uncontrollable, and having severe consequences. A key question is therefore whether illness representations can affect a person's adjustment over and above the severity of the illness itself. Many studies have shown that this is the case. Beliefs about the consequences of chronic diseases such as rheumatoid arthritis and multiple sclerosis are associated with poorer psychological outcomes, reports of more symptoms, and an increased use of health services (Rivera et al., 2020).

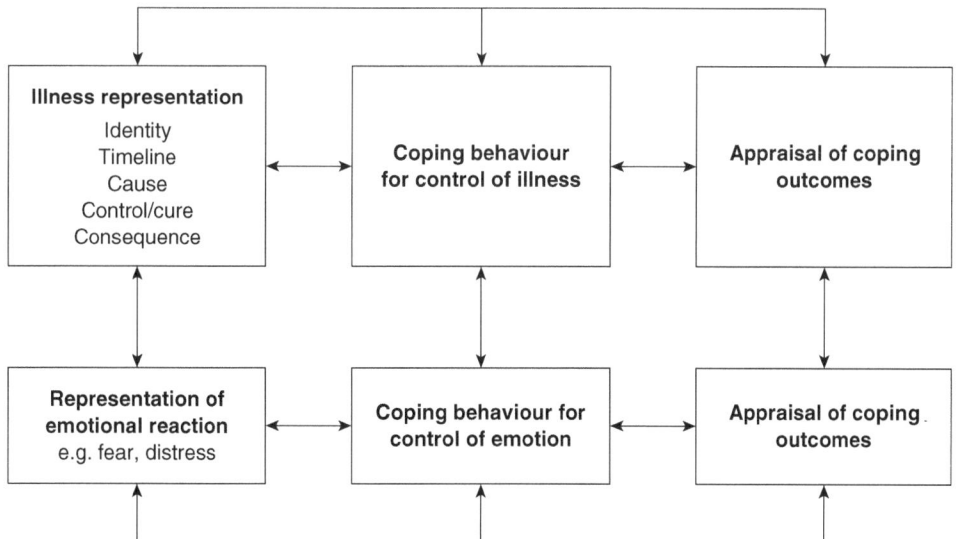

Figure 4.7   Self-regulation model of illness cognition and behaviour

Source: Used with permission of Taylor & Francis Informa, from Leventhal et. al, 1984

Case Study 4.3

The Self-Regulation Model and Chest Pain

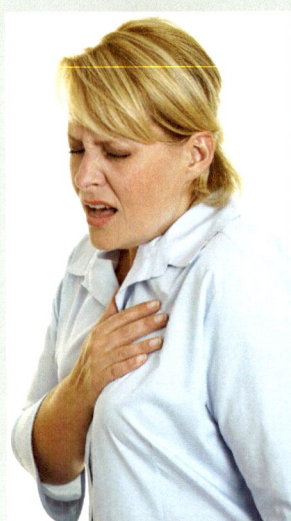

Figure 4.8   Tanya's chest pain

Source: © Robert Kneschke/ Adobe Stock

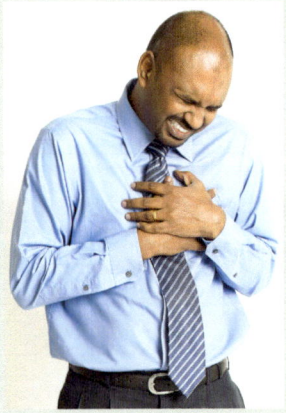

Figure 4.9   Vinay's chest pain

Source: © WONGSZE FEI/ Adobe Stock

The self-regulation model illustrates how symptoms, such as chest pain, will be perceived and interpreted by a person on the basis of their illness representations, which in turn will influence their coping behaviour. The symptom will also evoke an emotional reaction that will lead to coping strategies to control that emotion. Both the emotional and cognitive strands will influence each other. Coping and reappraisal can then lead to an adjustment of beliefs, emotions, and coping responses and so on, as illustrated below.

Tanya is 46 years old and has a pain in her chest one evening after she has eaten a large dinner and had an argument with her husband. Tanya's uncle died of a heart attack a few years ago, aged 65. Tanya thinks that men are particularly vulnerable to heart attacks but women are not (identity). Tanya knows that indigestion or heartburn can also cause pain in the chest (cause). She also knows that arguments and stress can lead to an upset stomach (cause). She therefore interprets this pain as indigestion, which will pass if she relaxes (consequences). She makes herself a calming cup of tea and goes to lie down (coping response).

Vinay is 48 years old and has a pain in his chest one evening after he has eaten a large dinner and had an argument with his wife. Vinay's uncle died of a heart attack a few years ago, aged 65. Vinay knows that men in their 40s are particularly vulnerable to heart attacks (identity) and that they can be caused by stress (cause). He therefore immediately interprets this pain as a possible heart attack with potentially fatal (consequences). He becomes very anxious and upset and feels his heart pounding. He calls an ambulance to take him to hospital immediately (coping response).

—Activity 4.1—

Illness Representations

Think of a person you have seen who was particularly upset by their illness.

- What sort of beliefs did they have about their illness identity, timeline, cause, control, and consequences?

4.4.1 Applications to Clinical Practice

Illness representations have many implications for clinical practice. Managing an illness which seems abstract is harder than managing an illness when a person has concrete experience of it. In other words, people are less likely to adhere to treatment for an illness when there are no concrete symptoms. This can be the case in asymptomatic illnesses such as hypertension, or illnesses that do not have regular symptoms, such as diabetes or HIV. This links to the issue of motivation: if people do not have symptoms, they may be more likely to favour an immediate reward (such as sugary food for people with diabetes) over the long-term consequences.

People can also have beliefs and representations about treatment procedures that will affect how likely they are to adhere to particular treatments. For example, the use of corticosteroids will not be effective if a person associates it with the steroids used by body builders and is put off by this association. Some people may also worry about the addictive properties of certain drugs and will therefore not take them. For example, a survey in Germany found that 80% of people believed antidepressants were addictive (Althaus et al., 2002). For this and other reasons, around half of people prescribed antidepressants for Major Depressive Disorder do not take them as prescribed, and many discontinue using them within months of starting them (Dell'Osso et al., 2020).

The self-regulation model of illness beliefs can therefore be useful when treating people. By exploring and changing a person's illness beliefs, we can maximise the chances of them managing their illness appropriately, both through changing their lifestyle and adhering to treatment. These types of intervention are broadly referred to as **self-management interventions** because they target people's beliefs and coping strategies in order to help them manage their illness and treatment effectively. Research has shown that self-management interventions are usually effective at promoting the positive self-management of diabetes, asthma, HIV, and cancer (Barakou et al., 2023; Gonzalez et al., 2016). Research Box 4.2 gives one example of a study that found that interventions based on self-regulation principles can be an effective way to increase physical activity among previously insufficiently active people with cancer.

─Research Box 4.2─

Self-Regulation-Based Intervention to Increase Physical Activity in People with Cancer

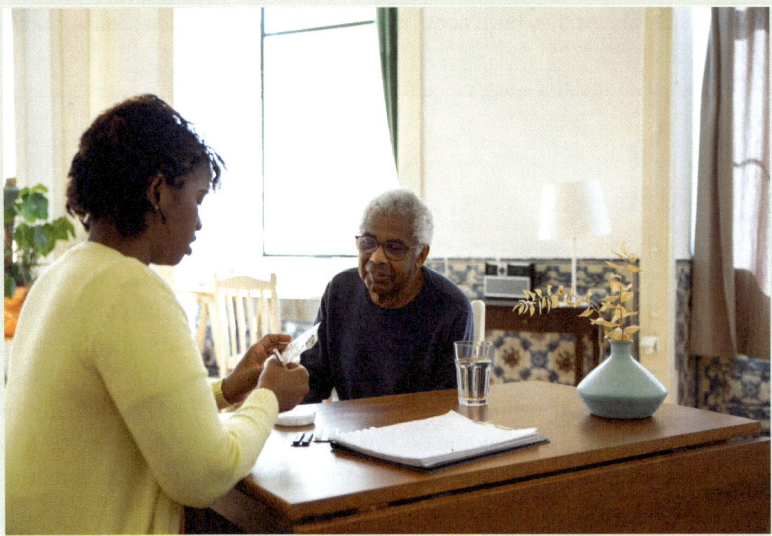

Figure 4.10   Intervention to increase physical activity

Source: © Kampus Production/Pexels

Background

Physical activity (PA) can provide various benefits for people with cancer: improved quality of life, better physical functioning, and fewer treatment side effects. Because few people with cancer adhere to PA guidelines, it is important to develop and test interventions to increase PA. This study examined whether a behaviour-change intervention focusing on self-regulatory strategies could increases PA levels.

Method and Findings

Seventy-two ambulatory cancer patients were randomly allocated to a four-week intervention group or an active control group. The active control group completed stress management training. The intervention group received a one-hour counselling session designed to focus on applying the self-regulation principles of goal-setting, action planning, coping planning, and self-monitoring. Both groups had weekly telephone follow-ups. Participants gave self-reports of PA and also wore accelerometers to measure PA.

People in the PA self-regulation group had bigger increases in PA immediately after the intervention and at ten-week follow-up. All patients reported reductions in perceived stress.

Significance

This study shows how a PA intervention based on self-regulation principles can increase levels of PA in insufficiently active people with cancer. The results also suggested that the intervention was most successful when participants used peer support. This highlights the importance of the social context in individual treatment and rehabilitation.

Ungar, N., Sieverding, M., Weidner, G., Ulrich, C.M. & Wiskemann, J. (2016) A self-regulation-based intervention to increase physical activity in cancer patients. *Psychology, Health & Medicine, 21*(2): 163–175. doi:10.1080/13548506.2015.1081255.

—Clinical Notes 4.3—

Illness Representations

- How a person thinks about their illness will affect their distress, symptom perception, and disability.
- Self-management interventions can educate people and help them to think about their illness in more adaptive ways.
- To help people manage their illness better we need to help them:

  - Correct any misperceptions about the cause of their illness (and therefore future risk).
  - Focus on an aspect of their illness that they can control, such as treatment adherence or symptom management.
  - Reduce their perceptions of severe consequences through education and joint treatment plans. In cases of terminal illness, this may involve tackling worries about pain relief and dying.

Summary 4.4

- Beliefs about illnesses affect how people appraise symptoms, interpret symptoms, whether they seek help, and their adherence to treatment.
- Illness representations include illness identity, timeline, cause, control, and consequences.
- Illness representations are associated with both the psychological and physical outcomes of illness.
- The self-regulation model explains how illness representations can interact with coping to determine health outcomes.
- Illness representations can be used to develop effective self-management interventions for chronic illnesses that will help people to cope with and manage their illness and treatment more effectively.

Conclusion

In this chapter we have seen how the perception of symptoms is strongly influenced by psychological factors, including attention, emotions, beliefs, and environmental factors. The importance of psychological factors in the outcome of illnesses has been illustrated by placebo and nocebo effects, which can be substantial. Research and theory in this area are therefore highly relevant to clinical practice and have been used to develop effective treatments, such as pain management programmes and self-management programmes, in order to help people to manage their symptoms and illnesses more effectively.

Further Reading

Llewellyn, C.D. et al. (eds) (2019) *The Cambridge Handbook of Psychology, Health and Medicine* (3rd edition). Cambridge: Cambridge University Press. Includes short chapters on pain, pain management, placebo and nocebos, and illness representations.

Cameron, L.D. & Leventhal, H. (2003) *The Self-Regulation of Health and Illness Behaviour*. London: Routledge. Includes more in-depth information on illness beliefs and self-regulation, with chapters on the theory of self-regulation, illness representations, social and cultural influences, and interventions.

Creed, F., Henningsen, P. & Fink, P. (eds) (2011) *Medically Unexplained Symptoms, Somatisation and Bodily Distress: Developing Better Clinical Services*. Cambridge: Cambridge University Press. An edited collection that provides an overview of the conceptualisation of medically unexplained symptoms (MUS) and their epidemiology, but usefully gives most attention to treatment in different groups and in different contexts.

Revision Questions

1   What is a symptom? How accurate are people at detecting changes in physiological states (e.g. blood pressure)?
2   Discuss the role of two psychological factors in the perception of physical symptoms.
3   Outline how medically unexplained symptoms (MUS) affect people and their interactions with healthcare professionals.
4   What is the difference between a person's pain threshold and pain tolerance? Briefly outline the role of psychological factors in both.
5   What is the Gate Theory of pain? How has it helped our understanding of the interplay between psychological and physical factors?
6   What is the communal coping model of pain? What implications does it have for treatment?
7   What is a placebo effect? What factors affect how strong it is?
8   What is a nocebo effect? What is the evidence that it affects symptom perception?
9   Describe the five main dimensions of illness representations.
10 Describe a self-management intervention based on the self-regulation model.

5

HEALTH AND BEHAVIOUR

━━━| **Learning Objectives** |━━━━━━━━━━━━━━━━━━━━━━━━━━

This chapter is designed to enable you to:

- Discuss the importance of health behaviour and of health behaviour change.
- Outline different models of health behaviour.
- Understand how to apply these models in clinical practice to help people to change.

Understanding and changing health behaviour effectively would do more than anything else to reduce morbidity and mortality in our society. The leading global risks for mortality in high-, middle-, and low-income countries are high blood pressure, tobacco use, high blood glucose, physical inactivity, and being overweight (World Health Organization, 2020a). These raise the risk of chronic diseases such as heart disease, diabetes, and cancers. Globally, the vast majority of premature deaths are caused by non-communicable diseases, including cardiovascular disease, cancer, diabetes, and chronic respiratory diseases (World Health Organization, 2020a), which in turn are predominantly caused by lifestyle and health-related behaviour. These non-communicable diseases have become a major focus of concern and action for the World Health Organization, other international organisations, and national governments (Sustainable Development Solutions Network, 2012; World Health Organization, 2023a).

5.1 Predicting and Changing Health Behaviour

If we want to change behaviours that affect health, then we first need to clarify what we mean by 'health behaviours'.

5.1.1 What Are Health Behaviours?

Numerous lifestyle factors affect morbidity and mortality. At the global level, the World Health Organization has noted that noncommunicable diseases (NCDs) are responsible for

74% of all deaths worldwide. Key NCDs include cardiovascular disease (including heart disease and stroke), cancer, diabetes, and chronic lung disease. These NCDs share five major risk factors: tobacco use, physical inactivity, alcohol use, unhealthy diets, and air pollution. These risk factors cause metabolic and physiological changes such as high blood pressure, being overweight/obesity, high blood glucose levels, and high blood fat levels (hyperlipidaemia). Other influences on morbidity and mortality, which are linked to sanitation and safety, may be beyond the direct control of individuals but they highlight that psychosocial factors are important, and that a purely biomedical approach to health (section 1.5.1) is unwarranted.

Our health is affected by a range of behaviours, which can be categorised as health protective behaviours and health risk behaviours. **Health protective behaviours** consist of things like exercise, a good diet, and adequate sleep. These behaviours are linked to a lower risk of a wide range of illnesses. Health protective behaviours also include **screening behaviours**, such as attending regular screening checks for hypertension and dental checks, and self-monitoring behaviours, such as checking testicles or breast tissue for abnormal growths. **Health risk behaviours** include things such as smoking, use of alcohol or other drugs, unsafe sex, and risky driving. These behaviours are known to increase the risk of specific negative health outcomes.

We need to understand why people choose to behave in ways that harm their health if we are to help them to change. This is not simple: behaviour is determined by many factors, including individual differences, social surroundings and influences, and cultural factors. To have effective health promotion programmes we need to know the main determinants of specific behaviours in different groups of people. For example, young people may be more motivated to eat a low-fat diet and regularly brush their teeth to improve their appearance rather than to improve their health, so only emphasising the health benefits of these behaviours may not result in significant change in this group. The range of factors that influence health behaviour is shown in Table 5.1. Research and theories of health behaviour try to identify the most important causes of behaviour so that interventions can target those factors which are most likely to result in change.

Table 5.1   Factors that influence health behaviour

Biological factors	Sex
	Age
Psychological factors	Cognitive factors: attitudes and beliefs
	Motives
	Conditioning
	Modelling of behaviour
	Emotional state
	Self-esteem
Social factors	Demographic characteristics
	Financial/employment status
	Legislation
	Economics
	Healthcare provision

5.1.2 Theories of Health Behaviour

Many theories of health behaviour have been proposed. Social cognitive models focus on the interplay between social and cognitive factors, such as individual beliefs and attitudes, and social pressures and norms. These models are based on the *expectancy-value* principle, which assumes that a behaviour is most likely to be maintained or changed if (1) a person expects it to result in certain outcomes and (2) the person values these outcomes as important or positive. These models account for a large amount of the variance in people's behaviour. Many theories integrate additional factors, such as an individual's readiness or motivation to change.

This chapter discusses four models of health behaviour: two social cognitive models and two integrative process models. We examine the evidence for these models and explore how we can use them in clinical practice to help people to change their behaviour. We use a case study to illustrate how each model can be adopted to help someone to stop smoking.

Predicting and Changing Health Behaviour

The social cognitive models that have been most widely used in the study of health behaviour are the Health Belief Model and the Theory of Planned Behaviour. Examples of integrative process models are the Transtheoretical Model and dual process models. These models are not necessarily in competition. Although one model may be more successful at predicting a particular type of behaviour, aspects of all of these models can be used in clinical practice.

Summary 5.1

- Lifestyles and health behaviours are key risk factors for the major causes of disease and death globally.
- 'Health behaviours' is a term used to describe protective behaviours, risk behaviours, and use of health services.

5.2 Social Cognitive Models of Health Behaviour

Various social cognitive models have been proposed as alternatives to the biomedical model. In this section, we describe and apply two of the most prominent social cognitive models.

5.2.1 The Health Belief Model

The Health Belief Model (HBM: Rosenstock, 1974) is shown in Figure 5.1. It suggests that the likelihood of someone changing their behaviour is primarily determined by the perceived threat of their current situation, coupled with an evaluation of the outcome if they change. Perceived threat is a combination of perceived susceptibility to negative consequences and the perceived severity of these consequences for the person. For example, if a person thinks they are not susceptible to coronavirus, then obviously coronavirus will not be a threat to them, so they are unlikely to take preventative action. Another person may think they are susceptible to coronavirus but that coronavirus is not severe enough for them to do anything about it. Perceived susceptibility and severity combine to produce a level of perceived threat that motivates people to take action or change their behaviour. However, it is clear from the HBM – and other evidence (Ruiter et al., 2014) – that fear and threat are not sufficient to change behaviour.

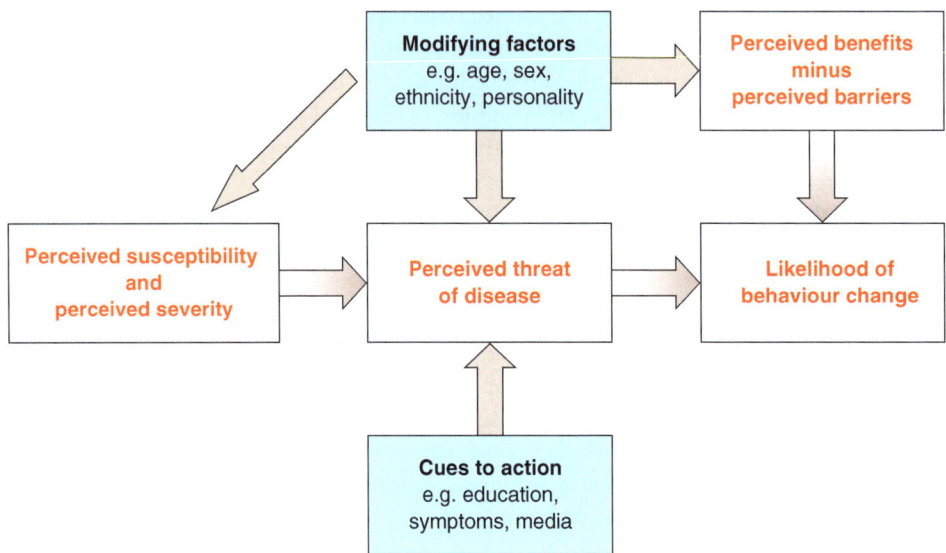

Figure 5.1   The Health Belief Model

Even when the perceived threat is high, people may not change their behaviour. An additional factor that influences behaviour is how a person evaluates the outcome. This evaluation is affected by perceived benefits and perceived barriers. Perceived benefits are what a person thinks they will gain from the behaviour or behaviour change. These can be positive gains or the removal of negative factors. For example, getting tested for coronavirus can mean that the illness is treated in its early stages, or that the threat of the illness is removed. Perceived barriers are things that make it difficult for a person to carry out the behaviour. For coronavirus screening, this might include not being able to afford to take time off work to self-isolate if the test comes back positive, testing facilities being a long distance away, or a lack of transport.

The HBM explicitly recognises the importance of cues to action that prompt people to change. These can be internal cues such as perceived symptoms. They can also be external cues such as health promotion, the advice of a health professional, or warning labels of products. For example, the illness or death of a public figure can provide strong cues to act that may be wide-reaching through extensive media coverage. Celebrity disclosures of medical conditions are often followed by increases in people seeking information or help for those conditions (Kamiński & Hrycaj, 2024). Smoking research has indicated that an effective trigger in persuading someone to quit smoking is for a health professional to tell a person that they should give up. Even brief, simple advice from a physician can make it more likely that a smoker will quit and remain a non-smoker 12 months later (Stead et al., 2013). Furthermore, providing behavioural support or additional counselling can boost the impact of advice from physicians.

However, cues to action are not always necessary for change. If an individual has a sufficient perceived threat and positive evaluation of the outcome of the change, then they will often change without needing a cue. In other cases, cues can be the final trigger that will tip the balance between a perceived threat and barriers, and will prompt someone to act (Holliday et al., 2021; Lindson et al., 2021).

Revisions of the HBM have included health motivation as a factor. This relates to how much a person is concerned about their health and prepared to consider behaviour change. Research has given less attention to health motivation and cues to action than other model components, but it may have important effects on behaviour (Conner, 2019). Chapter 2 (section 2.2) focuses on the influence of motivation, and Chapter 14 (section 14.3.1) outlines the behaviour change process of motivational interviewing.

The HBM has been researched in relation to many health behaviours (see Figure 5.2), including breast self-examination, flu vaccinations, diabetes management, medication for hypertension, and cancer screening. Reviews of the evidence for the HBM have been generally positive and find that perceived barriers, benefits and cues to action are often the most important factors in determining change (Jones et al., 2014; Ritchie et al., 2021; Sanaei Nasab et al., 2019). It should be noted that different components of the HBM may be more important for different behaviours. When changing risky behaviours, the perceived benefits of behaviour change may be most important, whereas adherence to treatment may be more strongly affected by perceived barriers, such as cost and side effects. Furthermore, different HBM components may be more important at different stages of behaviour change processes, with information provision being more influential early on, and cues to action being more important for maintaining behaviour change (see also section 5.3).

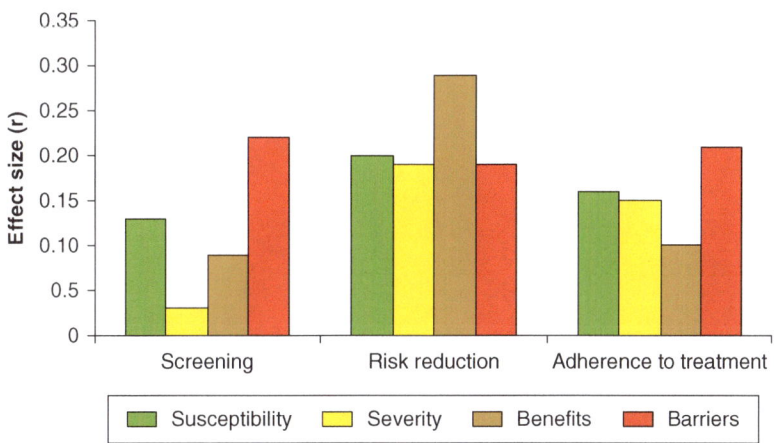

Figure 5.2 The Health Belief Model and different types of behaviour (adapted from Harrison et al., 1992)

Interventions Using the Health Belief Model

To use the HBM in clinical practice, health professionals explore people's perceived susceptibility, severity, benefits, and barriers, and also provide cues to action. People's perceptions of threat and benefits can be improved through education. Problem solving and action plans can be used to reduce perceived barriers. Using the HBM to design interventions has proved very effective (Conn et al., 2016; Khalil et al., 2024; Zhang & Zhao, 2021).

Case Study 5.1 shows how we might use the HBM to help someone to give up smoking. It illustrates how the model may be implemented as a guide if we wish to help people to change a risky health behaviour.

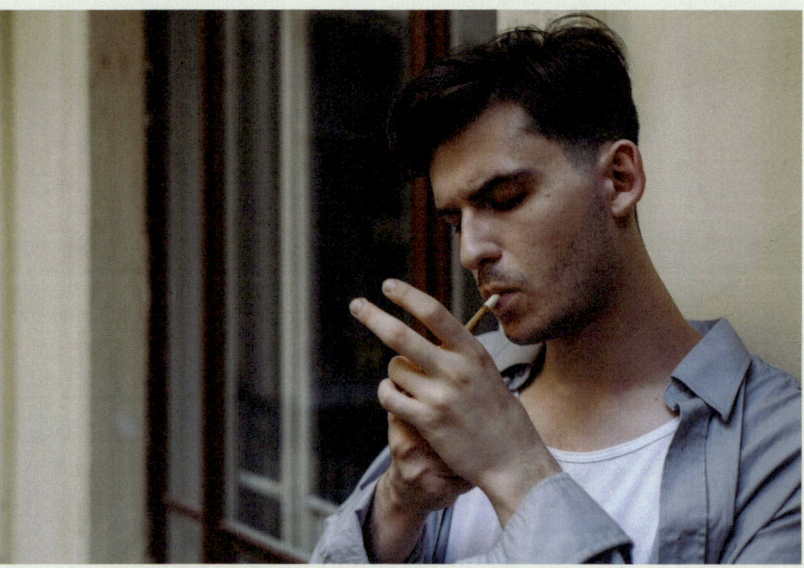

Figure 5.3   The Health Belief Model for Daniel's smoking

Source: © Ron Lach/Pexels

Daniel has smoked 20 cigarettes a day since he was 15 years old. He coughs every morning and gets breathless easily. Although he has a family history of asthma, he has never been checked for asthma.

Cues to Action

Explore whether anything has triggered him to consider giving up smoking:

- Has anything made you think about giving up smoking?

If so, capitalise on this by reinforcing it. Give him positive feedback if he has thought about giving up smoking.

Health Motivation

Explore how motivated or concerned he is about his health:

- How concerned are you about your health? (abstract health concern)
- How important is it to you to stay healthy/not to get ill? (concrete health concern)

Susceptibility and Severity

Explore the perceived susceptibility and severity:

- How do you think smoking is affecting your health? (current susceptibility)
- How might it affect your health in ten years' time? (future susceptibility)
- What would it be like if that happened to you? (severity)

Educate about the negative effects of smoking to increase the perceived susceptibility and severity:

- Smokers are more likely to have heart disease, a stroke, circulation problems, lung cancer, and many other cancers.
- The toxins in cigarettes put huge strain on your body.
- Other effects of smoking are gum disease, a poor sense of smell, reduced fertility, skin ageing and tooth discolouration.

Perceived Benefits and Barriers

Explore the perceived benefits and barriers:

- What are the pros and cons of smoking for you? (current benefits and costs)
- Is there anything stopping you from giving up smoking? (current barriers)

(Continued)

Problem solving to reduce barriers:

- How can you/we change this? What steps can you/we take to help you to give up? (reducing current barriers and focusing on taking action)

Educate about the positive benefits if Daniel gives up smoking now, to increase the perceived benefits:

- If you give up smoking you will improve your health and live longer.
- Your risk of heart disease drops dramatically in the first year after quitting.
- You will feel healthier, and because smoking damages the skin, you might look better too.
- You will save a huge amount of money!

5.2.2 The Theory of Planned Behaviour

The Theory of Planned Behaviour (TPB: Ajzen, 1988) was first proposed to explain all kinds of social behaviour, not just health behaviour. As shown in Figure 5.4, the theory is based on the assumption that a person's **intention** will be the strongest determinant of how they will actually behave.

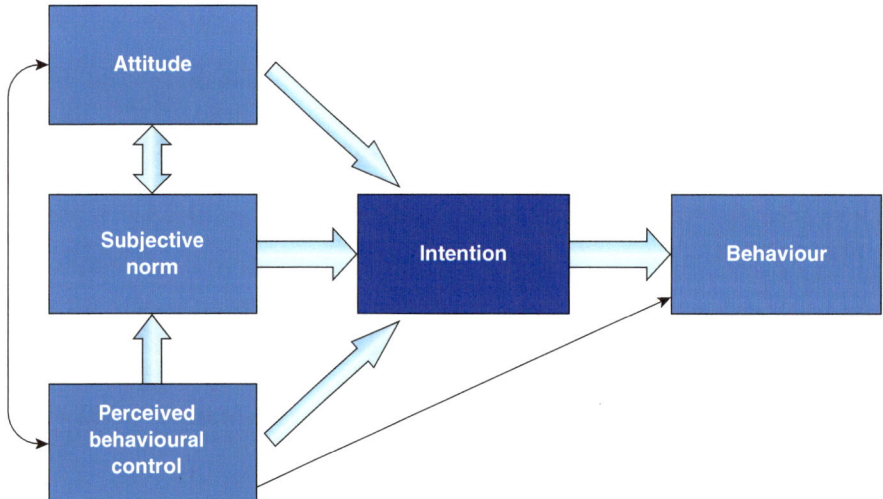

Figure 5.4   The Theory of Planned Behaviour

Intentions are thought to be determined by other social cognitive factors. One is a person's attitudes toward the behaviour (see Chapter 9). This is influenced by their *beliefs about the outcomes of the behaviour* (e.g. the pros and cons) and their *evaluation of these outcomes* (e.g. whether these are positive or negative). Consider our case study. If a person believes that smoking will keep them thin and reduce stress (pros), and that these outcomes are the most important to them (evaluation of outcome), then they will not be motivated to quit.

A second factor that determines intentions is the subjective norm, which is the perceived social norm about the behaviour in a person's environment. This is influenced by the *perceived beliefs of others* about the behaviour and the person's *motivation to comply* with these beliefs. It is important to acknowledge that a person may respond differently from the norms of different groups. For example, young people are often strongly motivated to comply with the norms of their friends. Family-based interventions for young people are therefore less likely to be successful than interventions targeted at peer groups.

Activity 5.2

Social Norms Versus Attitudes

- Has there ever been a time when you have been persuaded to do something against your better judgement because everyone else was doing it? For example:

  ○ Drinking and driving.
  ○ Drinking too much.
  ○ Smoking or other drug use.

- What do you think is more powerful: your own attitudes or social pressure/group norms? Why is this?

A strength of the TPB is that it takes account of the importance of social influences as well as how much control a person believes they have over their behaviour. Research has shown that control beliefs are indeed important in behaviour change (Hagger et al., 2022). The TPB accounts for control quite broadly in the form of **perceived behavioural control**. The link between perceived behavioural control and intentions is via the amount of overall control people believe they have over their behaviour and changing this behaviour. If a person believes they do not have any control over their smoking, then they will not intend to quit. The direct link between control and behaviour is thought to be due to an *actual* lack of control over the factors needed to support or change a behaviour, rather than a *perceived* lack of control. An actual lack of control might involve not having suitable transport to attend a smoking cessation clinic, not being able to afford nicotine replacement therapy, or living in an environment where many other people also smoke.

There are numerous ways in which we can look at control. For example, we can distinguish between an internal **locus of control**, where people believe they can control their behaviour or the outcome of events, or an external locus of control, where people believe that other people or fate are controlling the outcome of events (see Chapter 9). This is very relevant to health promotion and healthcare. For example, a person with an external locus of control is more likely to expect health professionals to sort out their illness. A person with an internal locus of control will be more proactive and likely to make lifestyle changes or adhere to treatment because they believe they have control over the outcome of their illness. This is a useful characteristic to look out for in clinical work because it can help to develop a more effective treatment plan for each individual. For example, a person with diabetes who has an external locus of control might be more effectively treated with regular outpatient appointments to monitor their progress and adjust their medication, whereas someone with a more internal locus of control may feel better able to self-manage their treatment. Using different terminology, but a similar conceptualisation of control, research has also found that strong intentions to engage in heathy lifestyle behaviours are more likely to be found among people who believe that their health is malleable than people who believe that they cannot affect their health (Bunda & Busseri, 2019). The TPB therefore proposes that attitudes, subjective norms, and perceived behavioural control are the major determinants of intentions. The relative importance of these three factors will vary according to different behaviours and individuals. There is evidence to support the value of the TPB across a range of health behaviours, including health risk behaviours, uptake of screening and treatment, and adherence to treatment (C. Adams et al., 2022; Hagger et al., 2022; Ritchie et al., 2021). Although TPB components predict around half of the variance in intentions for a wide range of health behaviours, the TPB is slightly less successful at predicting actual behaviour. However, this may not be a surprise to anyone who has failed to keep a New Year's resolution: although many of us intend to live healthier lifestyles, this does not always mean we will do so!

Researchers have endeavoured to improve the TPB by adding such factors as **habit**, or recent past behaviour, **anticipated regret** about changing a behaviour, and **moral norms** as predictors of intentions. To explain why intentions do not always predict behaviour, some researchers have expanded the model by adding **implementation intentions**, which are specific plans for carrying out the relevant behaviour, for example, 'I will take a healthy lunch to work rather than relying on unhealthy snack foods' (Cooke et al., 2023; Gollwitzer & Sheeran, 2006). These additions appear to be useful, particularly the implementation intentions. However, they have not added greatly to the predictive power of the model.

Clinical Notes 5.1

Changing a Health Behaviour

- Information (education) from a health professional is a strong trigger for a behaviour change.
- Models of health behaviours are useful guides for clinical practice when helping someone to change their behaviour (see case studies).
- It is important to identify barriers to change: even when people are motivated to change, perceived and actual barriers can prevent it from happening.
- Explore how a person's social environment and norms may facilitate or prevent a behaviour change.
- If a person thinks they have no control over a behaviour, they will not attempt to change. Re-education and support can help to increase a person's perceived control.
- Helping someone to develop a plan for how they will change their behaviour makes it more likely that they will succeed.

Interventions Using the Theory of Planned Behaviour

Reviews of the evidence indicate that interventions based on the TPB can lead to significant behaviour change (Lareyre et al., 2021). Research Box 5.1 presents one well-designed study that used the TPB to develop a structured intervention: different sessions emphasised different elements of the TPB, and participants were helped to apply techniques for setting goals and making plans to reach them. Case Study 5.2 illustrates how the TPB might be used as a guide for intervention in clinical practice. Next, we look at a completely different type of model, which focuses on the *processes* of change rather than on the factors that determine behaviour.

Research Box 5.1

Reducing Waterpipe Smoking Using the Theory of Planned Behaviour

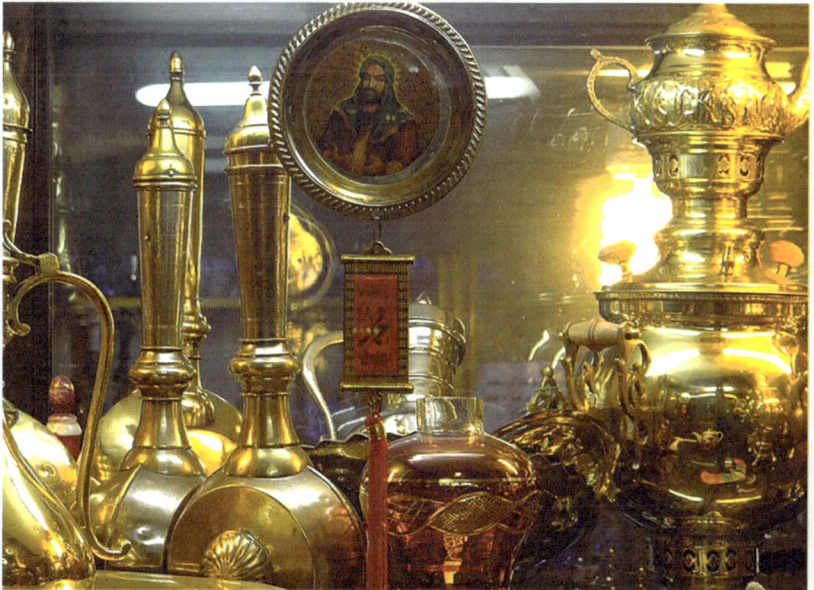

Figure 5.5 Waterpipes in Iran

Source: © Adam Jones/Wikimedia Commons

Background

The Theory of Planned Behaviour (TPB) suggests that healthy behaviour can be promoted by changing attitudes, normative beliefs, and feelings of control. This study looked at whether an

(Continued)

intervention based on an extended version of the TPB. Which included a measure of habit, could encourage women to stop smoking a waterpipe (also known as a hookah or shisha).

Method and Findings

The study recruited 448 women aged 15+ years who were regular waterpipe smokers living in Bandar Abbas city in Iran. Half were allocated to the control group, and half received the extended TPB intervention. The 14-session intervention ran over three months and focused on waterpipe smoking cessation. It included lectures, collaborative discussions, question-and-answer sessions, brainstorming activities, role-play, and peer education. After assessment at baseline, follow-up measures were taken at three months (i.e., post-intervention), and then after six months, and 12 months.

Women in the intervention group recorded significant improvements in attitudes, norms, perceived behavioural control, and intentions for cessation of waterpipe use. Furthermore, they reported significant reductions in waterpipe smoking: one year after enrolling in the study, 44% of women in the intervention group had ceased waterpipe use compared to 7% in the control group.

Significance

This study shows that interventions based on the TPB can change the key components of the model, and that such changes are followed by sustained changes toward healthier behaviour.

Shahabi, N., Shahbazi, S., Kakhaki, H.E.S. & Mohseni, S. (2024) The effectiveness of a theory-based health education program on waterpipe smoking cessation in Iran: One year follow-up of a quasi-experimental research. *BMC Public Health, 24*(1): 664. doi:10.1186/s12889-024-18169-7.

Case Study 5.2

Using the Theory of Planned Behaviour to Stop Smoking

Alex has smoked 20 cigarettes a day since she was 15 years old.

Attitudes

Explore her attitudes toward smoking:

- What do you think about smoking? (general attitude)
- Is smoking a good or bad thing for you? In what way? (evaluation of attitude/behaviour)

Educate about the negative effects of smoking to try to change her attitude from positive to negative.

Social Norms

Explore the norms of important people around her:

- What do your friends/family/partner think about smoking? (general norm)
- What do your friends/family/partner think about *you* smoking? (specific norm)
- Whose opinion is most important to you? (with whom is she motivated to comply?)
- Would you like to give up smoking for [person]? (motivation to comply with norms)

Discuss the pros and cons for her if she were to comply with different norms.

Intentions

Explore whether she intends to quit smoking:

- Have you ever thought about giving up smoking? (previous intention)
- Do you intend to give up smoking in the next few months? (current intention)

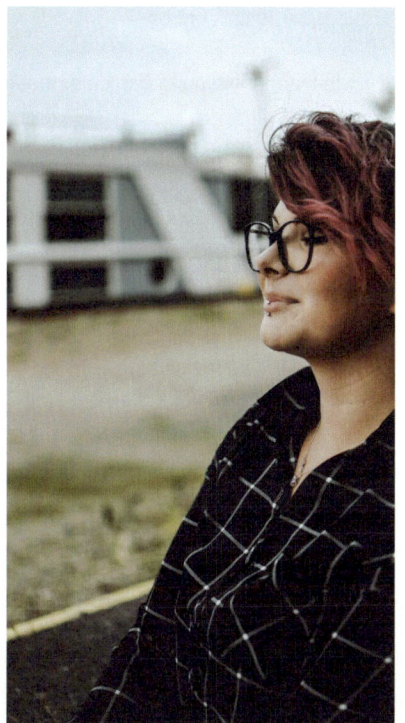

Figure 5.6 The Theory of Planned Behaviour for Alex's smoking

Source: lilartsy/Unsplash

Perceived Behavioural Control

Explore how much control she thinks she has over quitting smoking.

- Do you think you can give up smoking? (perceived control over quitting)

If she indicates low control, explore the reasons for this, for example:

- What makes you think you can't give up?

Normalise the difficulty in quitting:

- Many people find it hard to give up.

Increase the perceived control:

- Most people are successful if they keep trying.

(Continued)

Explore the actual control:

- Is there anything in particular that stops you from trying to quit?

Implementation Intentions

If she is ready to try quitting, discuss the steps she can take to give up smoking:

- What steps are you going to take to give up smoking? (concrete plans)

Discuss how these steps can be modified in order to increase the chances of success, for example:

- Nicotine replacement and smoking cessation groups.
- Setting personal goals about quitting and setting rewards for not smoking.

Summary 5.2

- Social cognition models of health behaviour take an expectancy-value approach and include the Health Belief Model and the Theory of Planned Behaviour.
- The Health Belief Model states that health behaviour change is determined by the threat of illness (perceived susceptibility and severity) balanced by the perceived benefits and barriers to change. Triggers or cues to action can also be important in some cases.
- According to the Theory of Planned Behaviour, health behaviour is determined by intentions, which in turn are determined by attitudes towards the behaviour, social norms, and perceived behavioural control.
- Social cognition models help to explain many health behaviours, and interventions based on these models are effective for changing behaviour.

5.3 Process Models of Conscious Behaviour Change

Social cognitive models are good for explaining what may influence behaviour or the initiation of behaviour change, but they do not provide clear accounts of processes of change or maintenance of change. You may know from your own experience that intending to change your behaviour does not guarantee lasting behaviour change. Furthermore, many smokers try to quit smoking after a heart attack but relapse over time. Process models attempt to explain what is required for people to initiate and maintain behaviour change, and to manage relapses.

5.3.1 The Transtheoretical Model

The Transtheoretical Model (TTM: Prochaska & DiClemente, 1983) was an early attempt to integrate models of health behaviour and psychotherapy to produce an effective model for behaviour change. The model is often referred to as the 'Stages of Change' model. The stages that characterise this model are illustrated in Figure 5.7. It includes four components: (1) the stages of change, (2) decisional balance, (3) confidence and temptation, and (4) processes of change.

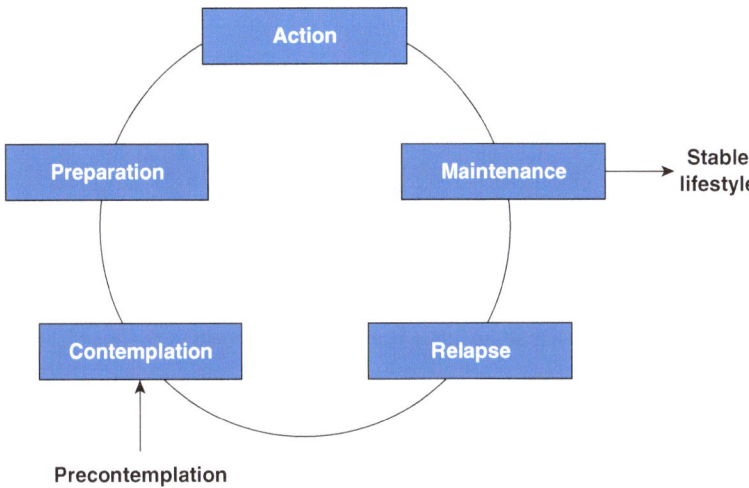

Figure 5.7 The Transtheoretical or 'Stages of Change' Model

The TTM posits that people go through **stages of change** in their behaviour. In *precontemplation*, a person is not even considering changing their behaviour. In *contemplation*, they begin to consider changing. If they want to change, then this leads into *preparation*, where the individual plans how to change. The final two stages are *action*, where the person makes the initial change in behaviour, and *maintenance*, when the behaviour change is consolidated and maintained in the long term. An important aspect of the TTM is the inclusion of relapse, based on the understanding that people often relapse back to previous behaviour and may have to go through the cycle a few times before the new behaviour becomes permanent. The advantage of the model is that it normalises relapse and encourages people not to see relapse as a failure but to keep trying to change their behaviour. In clinical practice, health professionals can emphasise the normality of relapse and explore what a person has learned from the relapse, and how it can be used to increase their chances of success next time around.

Decisional balance involves exploring the relative pros and cons of behaviour change. People are asked to write down the pros and cons of changing their behaviour in a decisional balance task – which has parallels to identifying the barriers and benefits in the HBM. This task can help people to clarify whether there are more pros than cons (or vice versa) and might prompt them to consider changing their behaviour (i.e. to move from precontemplation into contemplation).

Confidence refers to a person's belief in their ability to change. It overlaps with perceived behavioural control from previous models. **Temptation** relates to factors that may tempt a person to continue with an unhealthy behaviour in particular circumstances. It can be seen to relate to the concept of 'cues to action' in the HBM and 'implementation intentions' in extensions of the TPB. For example, in our case studies, people may want to give up smoking but find it difficult to resist smoking when they are out socially with friends who are smoking.

The fourth aspect of the model is that it specifies the **processes of change** that can be used to help people to change their behaviour. These include consciousness raising, replacing smoking with other behavioural responses (counter-conditioning), helping a person to plan rewards (reinforcement), and using social support (helping relationships).

Activity 5.3

Changing Your Own Behaviour

- Do you have a bad habit or behaviour you would like to change?
- If so, what stage do you think you are at?
- How could you use the Transtheoretical Model to help yourself to change that behaviour?

A key strength of the TTM is that it recognises that people may be at different stages of readiness for change, and that interventions should be tailored to their particular stage. For example, if in our case study a person had never thought of giving up smoking (precontemplation), there would be little point in trying to develop an action plan with them. It might make more sense to educate them about the dangers of smoking and encourage them to think about quitting (contemplation). Another strength of the TTM is the inclusion of relapse. This is particularly important in addictive behaviours, where relapse is common.

Clinical Notes 5.2

Working with Resistance and Relapse

- Whether a person is ready to change will affect the type of approach you should take.
- If a person has not considered changing, educate them about the negative impact of their current behaviour and encourage a change.
- Looking at the pros and cons of the current behaviour can also get people thinking about changing.
- Help people to plan how they are going to change and build in rewards to reinforce the new behaviour.
- Relapse is a common part of behaviour change and not a failure. Explore why relapse happened and work out how to avoid it happening again the next time.

Interventions Using the Transtheoretical Model

There is some evidence that behaviour change interventions based on the TTM may be effective, but there is a need for well-designed intervention studies to provide a stronger evidence base (Imeri et al., 2022; Rodrigues et al., 2023; Siewchaisakul et al., 2020). There is, however, less clear evidence that interventions targeting people in particular stages are more effective than interventions that do not target such stages. However, this is not to say that interventions based on the model – or stages of the model – have been completely unsuccessful (Siewchaisakul et al., 2020). Furthermore, the TTM does provide a way to think about how the other models of behaviour – and the component of these models – may operate at different stages, and many studies have combined the TTM with other models (Rodrigues et al., 2023). In other words, the TTM is not an alternative to other models, but it may provide a framework in which to place their components. Case Study 5.3 illustrates how we might use the TTM in clinical practice (see also Case Study 2.2 and Chapter 14 (section 14.3.1) on motivational interviewing).

─Case Study 5.3─

Using the Transtheoretical Model to Stop Smoking

Huang has smoked 20 cigarettes a day since he was 15 years old.

Stage of Change

Identify which stage he may be at:

- Have you ever thought about giving up? (contemplation)
- Have you ever planned to give up, or tried to give up? (preparation and action)

Decisional Balance

Explore his perceived pros and cons of smoking. This is best done by writing them down and then looking at the list together:

- What are the positive things for you about smoking? (pros)
- What are the negative things for you about smoking? (cons)
- Looking at this list, what does it make you think about your smoking?

Confidence

Explore how confident he is that he can control his smoking:

- How much do you think your smoking is under your control?
- How confident are you that you can reduce or quit smoking?

(Continued)

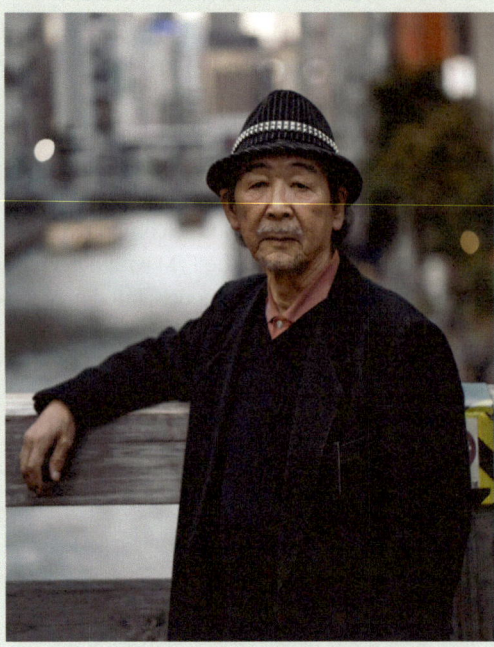

Figure 5.8 The Transtheoretical Model for Huang's smoking

Source: Ash Edmonds/Unsplash

Temptation

Explore which situations are particularly tempting for him to smoke and how this might affect a relapse:

- Are there certain times or situations when you find it difficult not to smoke?
- How can you prevent this from happening if you give up smoking?

Processes of Change

Use any of the processes to plan with him how he can quit smoking. For example:

- Is there someone who can help you quit, or give up with you? (helping relationships)
- Can you do something instead of smoking that distracts you and makes you feel better, for example, exercise? (counter-conditioning)
- It is important to reward yourself to continue not smoking – especially in the beginning. What would be a good reward for you? (reinforcement)

5.3.2 Other Process Models

The TTM proposes specific pathways of behaviour change and provides a framework in which the components of social cognitive models like the HBM and TPB may be placed. Other models expand on social cognitive models by focusing on what people need and what they need to do in order to initiate and maintain behaviour change. For example, the Information-Motivation-Behavioural Skills (IMB) model proposes that people will change their behaviour if they possess information about their unhealthy behaviour and healthier options, if this information motivates them to want to change their behaviour, and if they develop the skills required to carry out the new behaviour. The IMB model was originally designed to explain safer sexual behaviour (Fisher & Fisher, 1992), but has been shown to be useful across health behaviours, such as interventions designed to reduce alcohol intake (de Visser, 2015), and to prevent diabetes during pregnancy (Motahari-Tabari et al., 2023).

The Capability-Opportunity-Motivation model (COM-B) was proposed as the core part of a 'behaviour change wheel' (Michie et al., 2011). Like some social cognitive models and the IMB, the COM-B emphasises the importance of motivation to change. Similar to the IMB, it also highlights the need for people to have the capability to change (i.e. the requisite behavioural skills). A key addition of the COM-B is that people must create, or be provided with, opportunities to try out and establish their new behaviour. Examples of such opportunities include campaigns such as Dry January (de Visser & Piper, 2020) and Stoptober (J. Brown et al., 2014). The COM-B is nested within a broader Theoretical Domains Framework (TDF), which acknowledges that social contextual factors can have a strong influence on whether individuals who wish to make healthy lifestyle choices are able to carry out their intentions (Cane et al., 2012). Evidence is accumulating to confirm the value of using the TDF and COM-B when designing health behaviour interventions (C.E.B. Brown et al., 2024; Buchanan et al., 2021).

Summary 5.3

- The Transtheoretical (or Stages of Change) Model of behaviour change is an integrative theory that focuses on the stages and processes of change, rather than the determinants of health behaviour.
- Models such as the IMB and COM-B highlight the need to develop skills and maintain motivation at different stages of the behaviour change process.

5.4 Non-Conscious Influences on Health Behaviour

Models such as the HBM, TPB, and TTM identify targets for interventions focused on individuals' knowledge, beliefs, or skills. However, in many instances, the behaviour and health of individuals is strongly influenced by the beliefs, attitudes, motivations, and intentions of other people. For example:

- A person's ability to carry out their intention to use a condom may come to nothing if their partner refuses to use one.
- A child's intention to have an active lifestyle may be thwarted by their parents' willingness or capacity to provide the necessary opportunities.

- An adult who needs to change their diet after myocardial infarction may find this difficult in a family that shares meals and prefers less healthy food.

Some work has focused on dyads or larger groups (Balantekin, 2019; Carr et al., 2019; Ukai et al., 2022), but there is a need for further exploration of how the behaviour of individuals is influenced by things other than conscious decision making. Many of our health-related behaviours are habitual – or at least not the result of conscious deliberation every time we do them. For example, it is unlikely that whether you brushed your teeth this morning was the result of you working through the HBM: evaluating your susceptibility to tooth decay and gum disease; considering the severity of these outcomes; weighing up the benefits of brushing your teeth against the costs. It may have been more strongly influenced by whether brushing your teeth is part of your morning routine. Many behaviours are strongly determined by what we have done in the past, especially if they have formed into habits (Hagger et al., 2018; Hamilton et al., 2020; Orbell & Phillips, 2019). Similarly, at least some of the behaviour of health professionals has been shown to be habitual rather than reasoned (Potthoff et al., 2019). These observations highlight the importance of trying to establish healthy habits, so that they become the default pattern, and incorporating habits into models of behaviour (Potthoff et al., 2022).

Activity 5.4

Decisions and Habits

Think about the most recent time you brushed your teeth.

- To what extent was this the result of deliberate decision making?
- To what extent was this a habitual behaviour?

5.4.1 Dual Process Models

Although the HBM, TPB, and TTM have a very strong influence on health behaviour research and intervention development, there is growing awareness of how they are limited by only including conscious processes of rational decision making. Evidence shows that, at best, only around half of the variability in health-related behaviour is explained by the constructs defined in social cognition models (McDermott et al., 2015; Ritchie et al., 2021; Starfelt Sutton & White, 2016). This suggests an equally important role of other influences on behaviour. Dual process theories argue that health behaviours result from two different processes: (1) reflective, conscious, controlled processes, and (2) impulsive, unconscious, automatic processes (Hofmann et al., 2008; Kahneman, 2003; Strack & Deutsch, 2004).

Figure 5.9 provides an illustration of a dual process model. Whether we eat a delicious dessert will be influenced by the balance of automatic unconscious processes, such as salivation (which may be innate reflexes or conditioned responses; see Chapter 10, section 10.3), and conscious deliberation. The model proposes that we are more likely to be influenced by impulsive processes if eating dessert after a meal is habitual, if we associate eating dessert with improving our mood, or if we are preoccupied with other thoughts or demands. Another important boundary condition is intoxication from alcohol or other drugs, which may help to explain why an intention to stay sober formed at the start of a night out gets worn down by each drink we have. These boundary conditions can be considered to interact and overlap with temptation and confidence (see TTM) and cues to healthy and unhealthy action (see HBM).

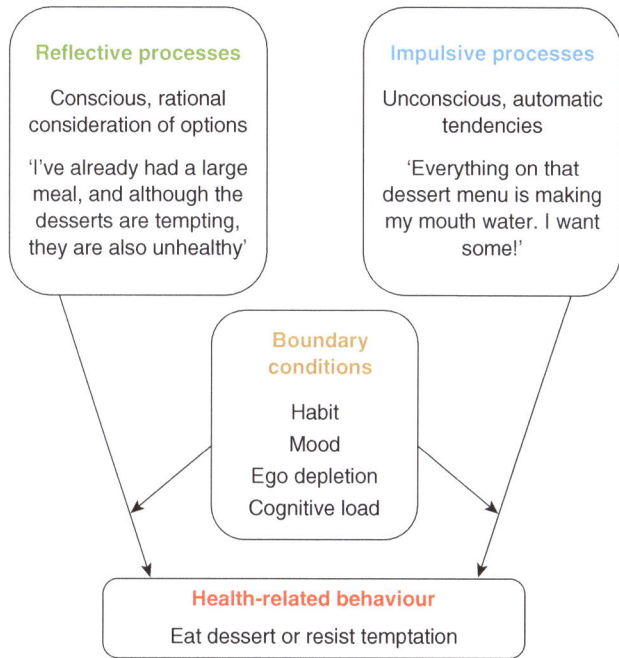

Figure 5.9 A dual process model of health-related behaviours

There is a large body of work highlighting the importance of impulsivity in health-related behaviour, although much of it was conducted without reference to dual process models (Carr et al., 2021; Sliedrecht et al., 2021). We now have evidence of the value of dual process models across various health-related behaviours. Notably, evidence from systematic reviews suggests that interventions focused on food-related impulsivity may be an important part of effective interventions to treat binge eating (İnce et al., 2021). Furthermore, there is evidence that professional practice in healthcare is affected by both reflective and impulsive influences and processes (Presseau et al., 2014). In line with these models, research evidence suggests that over-burdened health professionals may be less likely to engage in thorough rational consideration of treatment options.

Case Study 5.4 outlines some of the approaches that may be used to change behaviour according to dual process model principles. The procedures used to identify and change reflective precursors are similar to those for other models. There is also a need to identify boundary conditions and triggers for unhealthy behaviour. When it comes to addressing impulsive processes, various approaches may be used that involve counter-conditioning to learn new responses (Hofmann et al., 2010), approach/avoidance training to learn how to overcome automatic tendencies (Loijen et al., 2020), attentional bias modification to refocus attention away from triggers of the undesired behaviour (Todd et al., 2023), and mindfulness-based therapy to better understand emotional states and how to respond to them in healthy ways (Howarth et al., 2019).

Activity 5.5

Helping Others to Change

- If you wanted to help a friend to become more physically active, how would you use these models?
- What four things do you think would be most appropriate and useful for this person?
- How would you incorporate them into a behaviour change programme?

Case Study 5.4

Using a Dual Process Model to Stop Smoking

Poppy has smoked 20 cigarettes a day since she was 15 years old.

Reflective processes explore what she thinks, believes, and feels about smoking, and how she plans to change her behaviours:

- Drawing on the HBM (Case Study 5.1), explore Poppy's motivations for smoking or quitting, her perceptions of smoking-related disease susceptibility and severity, and the perceived benefits and barriers to smoking or quitting. Also explore her cues to action (i.e. her triggers for smoking or not smoking).
- Drawing on the TPB (Case Study 5.2), explore Poppy's attitudes toward smoking and not smoking, her subjective norms for smoking and not smoking, and her perceived behavioural control over smoking. Also explore her intentions and how she plans to implement them.

Impulsive processes explore the extent to which smoking is affected by automatic and habitual processes:

- How habitual is Poppy's smoking? In which situations does smoking always seem to happen automatically (e.g. with coffee, after a meal)?
- How automatic is her smoking? How often does she find herself with a lit cigarette without consciously being aware of lighting it?

Boundary conditions identify situations and moods that trigger smoking or the urge to smoke:

- Do particular moods, emotions, or people trigger Poppy's smoking (e.g. feeling stressed? Feeling unhappy? Being with friends who smoke?)

When situational cues and boundary conditions have been identified, different approaches can be used to help Poppy to become more aware of her behaviour, and to substitute alternative responses:

- Some techniques involve substituting the automatic behaviour of smoking with alternative automatic responses.
- Alternatively, some techniques involve mindfully drawing conscious attention to unconscious processes, and making the decision to smoke (or not) a thought-through process.

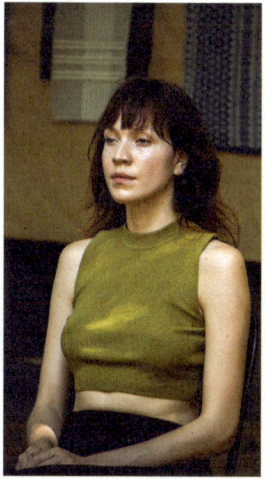

Figure 5.10 The dual process model for Poppy's smoking

Source: © Adarsh N/Pexels

Summary 5.4

- Dual process models emphasise that, although conscious decision making is important, it is not the only influence on health-related behaviours. Habits, emotions, and unconscious processes are also important.
- Each model of behaviour – and each type of model – results in slightly different approaches to intervention, but aspects of all these models can be combined in clinical practice to encourage behaviour change.

Conclusion

There is good evidence that the HBM and TPB can explain some of the factors that determine health behaviour, and that interventions based on these models are effective at changing behaviour. There is less evidence to support the effectiveness of interventions based on the TTM or dual process models.

Each of these models has its own strengths and limitations. It should also be apparent that, although the models possess different concepts and underpinnings, many of the questions in the different case studies are similar and overlap. Thus, in clinical practice, aspects of all these models can be mixed and used effectively to encourage people to change unhealthy behaviours. To aid choices of strategies, a taxonomy of behaviour change strategies has been developed

(Abraham & Michie, 2008). It can be used to synthesise evidence, implement effective interventions, and test theory (Michie et al., 2015).

It is probable that different aspects of the models described above and different behaviour change strategies will work better for different health professionals and different people, and may be more effective for some conditions or situations than others. Despite differences between models, a common implication is that we need to explore each person's beliefs and reasons for behaving in the way they do in order to be most effective in supporting them to change and develop an appropriate plan of change.

Further Reading

Llewellyn, C.D. et al. (eds) (2019) *Cambridge Handbook of Psychology, Health and Medicine* (3rd edition). Cambridge: Cambridge University Press. Includes short chapters on models of health behaviour, health behaviour change interventions, health promotion, motivational interviewing (often used to change addictive behaviours), physical activity interventions, and implementing changes in practice.

Anisman, H. (2016) *Health Psychology*. London: Sage. A textbook designed to introduce undergraduate students to the broad field of health psychology, it includes chapters on lifestyle factors and behaviour change.

Ogden, J. (2019) *Health Psychology* (6th edition). New York: McGraw-Hill. Now in its sixth edition, this book provides a wide-ranging introduction to health psychology. It covers factors that influence susceptibility to disease and illness as well as the psychological experience of being unwell.

Revision Questions

1   What are health behaviours? How can they be categorised?
2   What biological, psychological, social, and societal factors influence health behaviours?
3   What is the expectancy-value principle? How is it relevant to health behaviour change?
4   Outline the Health Belief Model. How effective is it for behaviour change?
5   Outline the Theory of Planned Behaviour. How effective is it for behaviour change?
6   What is locus of control? How is it relevant to clinical practice?
7   Outline the Transtheoretical Model. How effective is it for behaviour change?
8   Outline the key principles of dual process models. How can they be used to promote health behaviour change?
9   Compare and contrast two models of health behaviour change.
10 Choose one model of health behaviour change and explain how you would use it to help someone to stop unhealthy snacking.

6

CHRONIC ILLNESS, DEATH, AND DYING

Learning Objectives

This chapter is designed to enable you to:

- Understand the experience of chronic or terminal illnesses.
- Outline some of the psychosocial interventions to help people to adjust and cope with chronic illness.
- Understand the difficulties of palliative care, in particular the tension between helping a person have a good death and euthanasia.
- Describe the processes of normal bereavement and pathological grief.

As societies become more successful at treating disease and delaying death, the proportion of people living with long-term illnesses increases. Chronic illnesses or long-term conditions are illnesses that cannot be cured so need to be managed with drugs and other treatments. In developed countries, approximately one in three people have a chronic illness at any given time. Although chronic illnesses are more common among older people than younger people, many young people report health conditions lasting for at least one year. For example, UK data indicate that the proportion of people living with a chronic condition is 24% among people in their early 20s, 29% among people in their early 40s, and 52% among people in their early 60s (Office for National Statistics, 2020). Many of us will have a chronic illness at some point in our lives.

Treatment of chronic illness presents health professionals with a particular challenge: it requires a change from focusing on a cure to focusing on helping people to manage their symptoms. The implications of this are examined later when considering quality of life for people with chronic and terminal illnesses. Chronic illnesses raise some of the most difficult ethical issues in medicine. For example, how do we decide who gets a transplant and who does not, when should we stop resuscitation or turn off a life-support machine, and what is the doctor's role in cases of assisted suicide?

Chronic diseases vary hugely. They include disorders such as epilepsy, arthritis, cancer, diabetes, chronic fatigue syndrome, asthma, hypertension, liver disease, and dementia. Seven of the top ten causes of death worldwide are non-communicable diseases that are typically chronic in nature (World Health Organization, 2020a). In high-income countries, there is an even lower proportion of deaths attributable to communicable diseases and more are lifestyle-related diseases: chronic diseases account for over three-quarters of deaths. Interestingly, deaths that receive a lot of media attention, such as those from homicide, are much less likely. For example, homicide accounts for the deaths of 12 people in every one million in the UK (UN Office on Drugs and Crime, 2023).

Given the wide range of chronic illnesses, it is difficult to generalise about the role of psychosocial factors. In previous chapters (Chapters 2, 3, and 5) we have seen how psychosocial factors such as social support, lifestyle, stress, and negative emotion can affect the onset and prognosis of illness. We have also seen the importance of beliefs, attention, and behaviour in how we interpret symptoms and what we do about them (Chapters 2 and 4). The role of psychosocial factors in specific illnesses is covered in the chapters on different body systems in Section IV. In this chapter we will focus on the experience of chronic illness: the impact of chronic illness, how people adapt and cope, and whether psychosocial interventions can help. In the second half of the chapter, we will look at the impact of terminal illness, coping with dying, the effect of death on others, bereavement, and dealing with death in medical practice.

6.1 Chronic Illness

The onset and diagnosis of a chronic illness brings with it profound changes in a person's life that can lead to reduced quality of life and wellbeing. The onset and diagnosis of chronic illness raise significant challenges, including:

- Adjusting to symptoms and disability.
- Maintaining a reasonable emotional balance.
- Preserving a satisfactory self-image and sense of competence.
- Learning about symptoms, treatment procedures, and self-management.
- Sustaining relationships with family and friends.
- Forming and maintaining relationships with healthcare providers.
- Preparing for an uncertain future.

The enormity of these tasks, coupled with the emotional distress brought on by chronic illness, means that people are at high risk of depression. For example, studies of people with multiple sclerosis show that 27% are severely depressed and 35% have severe anxiety (Peres et al., 2022). Furthermore, psychological distress appears to be more common among those living with MS for longer periods of time.

The crisis theory of chronic illness is a seminal theory which proposed that we need a social and psychological equilibrium in our lives, similar to physiological homeostasis (Moos & Schaefer, 1984). This is similar to the concept of **allostatic load** in stress and how we respond to stress (see Chapter 3). The diagnosis of an illness can put someone in an extreme state of disequilibrium, which is accompanied by negative emotions such as fear, anxiety, and depression. Because people cannot remain in a state of disequilibrium, some resolution must be found. People in disequilibrium are more susceptible to outside influence, such as the actions of health professionals. In chronic illness, people's equilibrium may be very fragile and can be destroyed at any moment by even small setbacks or other stressful events. This explains why people may overreact to seemingly minor setbacks or difficulties.

Crisis theory is a useful analogy for the challenges of chronic illness. Theories of stress and coping (Chapter 3) are also useful in understanding people's responses. For example, the demands of illness are more likely to overwhelm a person if they have existing psychological problems, make negative or catastrophic appraisals, and have poor coping skills and resources. Case studies illustrating how our understanding of stress can be used to help people cope with difficult events are given in Chapters 3 and 14. More recent theories of chronic illness have focused on self-care and management of the illness. The middle-range theory of self-care outlines how important self-care is to maintaining health in both health and illness. Self-care includes self-care *maintenance*, such as regular exercise, self-care *monitoring*, such as routine testing, and self-care *management*, such as use of medication. People's detection, interpretation, and response to symptoms informs these processes of self-care at different stages, as shown in Figure 6.1 (Riegel et al., 2019).

6.1.1 Impact of Chronic Illness

Common emotional responses to illness are denial, anxiety, and depression. **Denial** is a psychological defence that helps people to avoid thinking about the illness and its consequences. People may refuse to accept that they have an illness, play down the severity of it, or insist that they will recover, and that the illness will be cured. Denial is not helpful in the long term because it interferes with adherence to treatment and self-management. However, denial can be helpful in the short term, particularly if people are physically weak and not able to cope with the full psychological consequences of the illness. In these circumstances, denial can help to keep fear and anxiety lowered until the person feels more able to cope with the emotional consequences of the illness. For example, one review of the use of denial by people with cancer found that denial gradually reduced over the course of the illness, and that the effect of denial on psychological factors could be positive or negative depending on the types of strategies used (Vos & de Haes, 2007). More specifically, using passive escape strategies to avoid the issues is associated with poorer outcomes than using more active distraction strategies to create a positive outlook.

Anxiety and depression are common in people with chronic illness. The substantial overlap between chronic illness and mental health is illustrated in Figure 6.2, which shows that many of the people with chronic illnesses also have a mental health problem. Similarly, if looked at the other way, many of the people with a mental health problem have another chronic illness (Naylor et al., 2012). The issue of comorbidities is also addressed in Chapter 1.

Reviews of research indicate that depression and anxiety are more common across a range of chronic conditions than among the general population (Aw et al., 2023; Lord et al., 2023; Senra & McPherson, 2021; Zamani & Alizadeh-Tabari, 2023). Depression and anxiety may be present before illness, or can be a response to illness, or both. As explained in Chapter 2, there is strong evidence that positive and negative emotions are associated with health. Both anxiety and depression are associated with physiological states that might affect the course of chronic illness. Anxiety is associated with the sympathetic nervous system and HPA axis arousal, and depression is associated with neuroendocrine changes that can affect inflammatory and immune pathways (see Chapters 3 and 15). For example, depression is associated with an increased risk of cardiovascular disease and mortality from a wide range of other illnesses (see Chapters 15–18). Anxiety is associated with more frequent or severe symptoms in disorders such as asthma or irritable bowel syndrome (see Chapters 16 and 17).

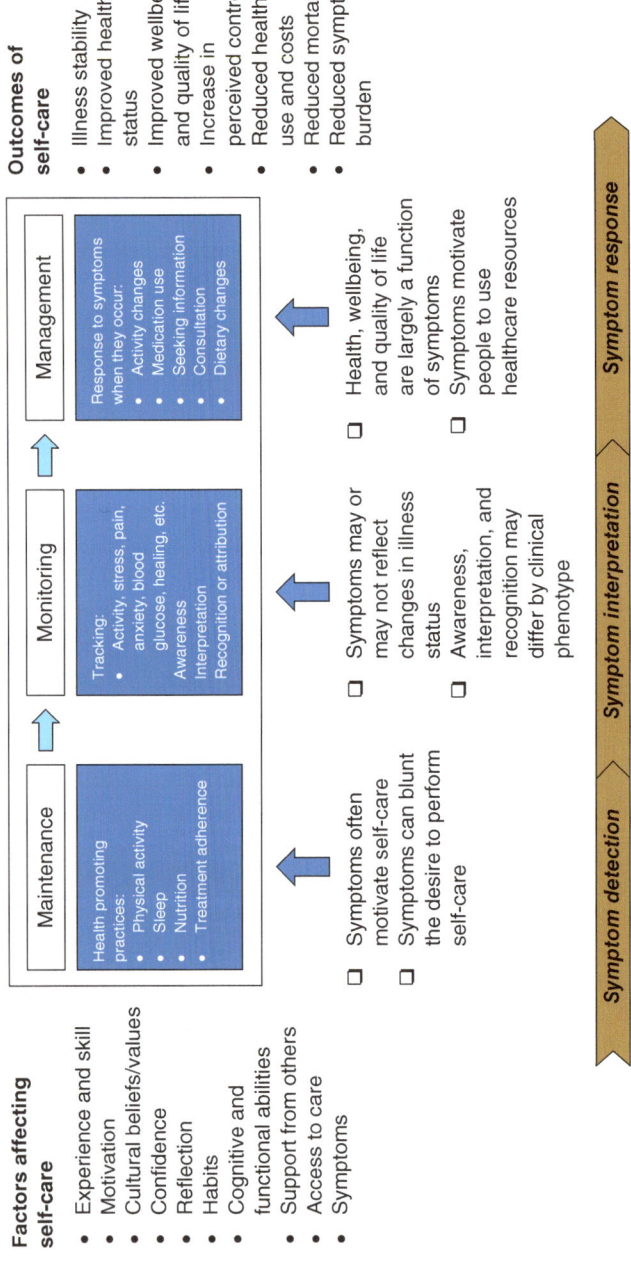

Figure 6.1 Middle-range theory of self-care of chronic illness (Riegel et al., 2019)

Source: Riegel, B., Jaarsma, T., Lee, C.S. & Strömberg, A. (2019) Integrating symptoms into the middle-range theory of self-care of chronic illness. *ANS: Advances in Nursing Science*, 42(3): 206–215. doi: 10.1097/ANS.0000000000000237

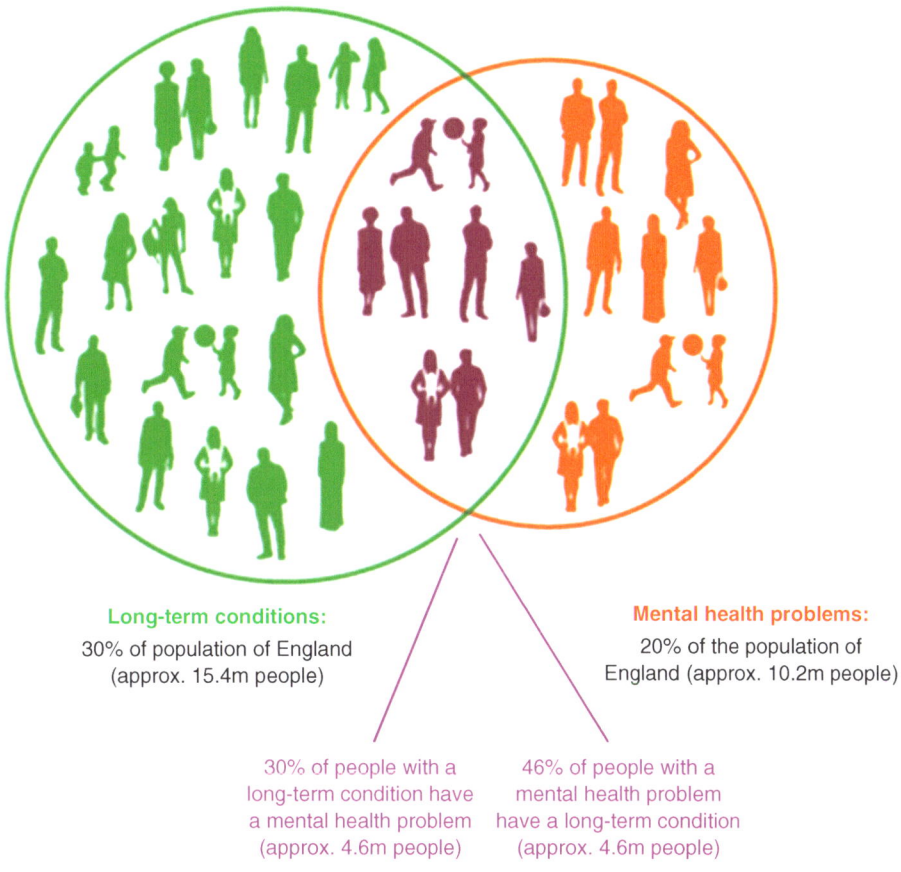

Long-term conditions:
30% of population of England
(approx. 15.4m people)

Mental health problems:
20% of the population of
England (approx. 10.2m people)

30% of people with a
long-term condition have
a mental health problem
(approx. 4.6m people)

46% of people with a
mental health problem
have a long-term condition
(approx. 4.6m people)

Figure 6.2 The overlap between long-term conditions and mental health problems (Khan, 2015)

Although anxiety and depression are often comorbid (occurring together), they stem from different types of appraisals. Anxiety is a response to threat. In chronic illness it is likely to be a threat to a person's wellbeing, work, self-image, etc. Anxiety can increase in medical settings because of potentially threatening events, such as getting test results, having painful procedures, dependence on health professionals, and uncertainty about the course of the illness. For example, a review of anxiety related to dental procedures found that it was associated with the severity of the procedure and expectations and experience of pain, among other things (Astramskaitė et al., 2016). Similar issues are addressed in Chapter 2 and Research Box 2.1. Depression, on the other hand, is usually a response to loss, failure, or helplessness. In chronic illness this will include a loss of health or physical capacity, a loss of social status, a failure to meet healthy standards, and helplessness in the face of illness (Adejumo et al., 2024; Yayan & Rasche, 2023).

Learned helplessness is a seminal theory of depression that proposes that when people believe they have no control over events they can become hopeless, helpless, and subsequently depressed (Seligman, 1975). It is particularly relevant to chronic illness. If people believe they have no control over their illness or outcome, it can lead to detachment, withdrawal, and depression (see illness representations in Chapter 4). Self-management programmes and cognitive behavioural therapy (CBT) can help to deal with negative emotions and expereinces by encouraging people to identify and challenge maladaptive beliefs, educating them about the importance of psychosocial factors, and empowering them to manage their illness.

In chronic illnesses, the emphasis of treatment is on improving **quality of life** rather than curing the illness. However, there are tensions between improving quality of life on the one hand, and the side effects of medical treatments that can decrease quality of life on the other. There is also the controversial issue of the point at which gains in quality of life are worth expensive treatments, such as those for advanced cancer. Finding treatments that maximise physical wellbeing and quality of life can therefore be difficult.

The measurement of quality of life in chronic illnesses is therefore critical to inform healthcare guidelines. However, it is also fraught with problems. Self-report measures typically ask people about pain, disability, restricted functioning or roles, mental health, energy, and overall ratings of health. Unsurprisingly, research using these measures has found that people with chronic illnesses report a poorer quality of life, and that quality of life is affected by deterioration in, or exacerbation of, the chronic physical condition (Hurst et al., 2020; Khan et al., 2024). Measures of quality of life are often not specific to the illness being studied and do not consider changes in people's goals and priorities during illness. For example, standardised measures of pain may be interpreted differently by people with chronic illness. Similarly, some domains of life may be more or less important to someone with a chronic illness.

Specialised measures of quality of life in chronic illness have therefore been developed (Palamenghi et al., 2020). Some of these are patient-generated indexes, where people list five domains of life that are important to them and then rate how much each domain has been affected by their illness (Tang et al., 2014). Research using these measures shows that people generate a wide range of domains, including some not encompassed in traditional quality of life measures. Such domains include memory, writing, and sexual function. Domains may also change over time as people adjust to continuing disease and incapacity. This type of measure is moderately related to global measures of quality of life, life satisfaction, and mental health, but only weakly associated with health and functional status (Wettergren et al., 2009). General quality of life is usually strongly predicted by psychological functioning (Gil-González et al., 2020; Gurková et al., 2023). Research Box 6.1 focuses on how people from less well-off backgrounds face additional burdens from chronic illness that can further impair their quality of life.

⌐Research Box 6.1⌐

Low Socioeconomic Status Adds to the Burden of Chronic Illness

Background

It is known that people of lower socioeconomic status (SES) have worse chronic disease outcomes than better-off people. However, little is known about how people of low SES experience their chronic illness or how it affects their quality of life. Such knowledge could allow healthcare professionals to better meet patients' needs.

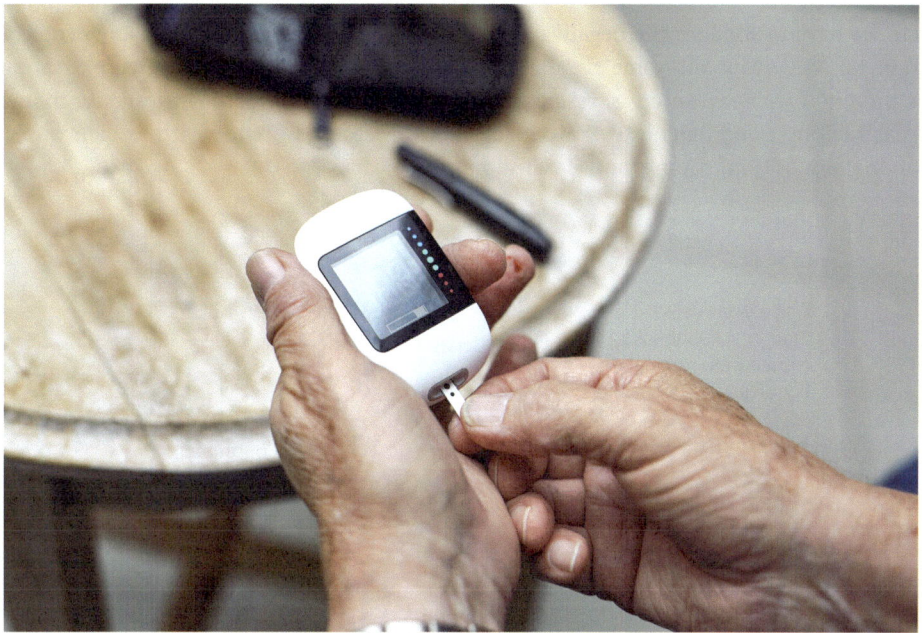

Figure 6.3 Chronic illness
Source: © Sweet Life/Unsplash

Method and Findings

This qualitative study entailed in-depth interviews with 15 Belgian adults aged 38–83 years, who had chronic physical and/or psychological conditions. The analysis identified six major experiences that were organised into a conceptual model of how low SES affects quality of life. Participants experienced chronic illness as an additional burden to existing economic and social disadvantage, and in some cases, it reduced their capacity for paid work. In addition, social exclusion and a lack of resources makes it harder for people to obtain informal support, and reduces their ability to meet the costs of treatment and other care.

Significance

The results of this study highlight that it is important for health professionals to understand that patients' needs go beyond the chronic disease itself. The experience of 'cumulative disadvantage' can impair patients' capacity to engage in activities that maintain or improve their physical health and quality of life.

Van Wilder, L., Pype, P., Mertens, F. & Rammant, E. et al. (2021) Living with a chronic disease: Insights from patients with a low socioeconomic status. *BMC Family Practice, 22*(1): 233. doi:10.1186/s12875-021-01578-7.

6.1.2 Finding Meaning and Benefit

So far, we have focused on the negative aspects of chronic illness. However, many people with chronic illnesses adapt and some even report positive changes to their lives. Figure 6.4 summarises the interplay between crisis, resilience, and growth that can occur in response to a crisis such as the onset and diagnosis of a critical illness. Factors associated with resilience include emotional disposition, coping, and social support (see Chapter 3).

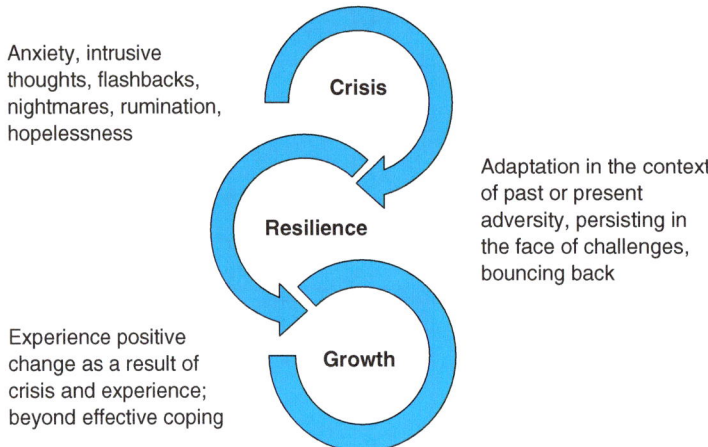

Figure 6.4   Crisis, resilience, and growth

Positive responses to illness are referred to as stress-related growth, post-traumatic growth, or benefit-finding (Tedeshi & Calhoun, 2004). Three areas of positive changes can occur:

1   *Enhanced relationships*: people need support from others, and positive interpersonal experiences may strengthen their appreciation of relationships.
2   *A changed view of themselves*: people may develop a greater sense of personal resilience and strength, an acceptance of their vulnerabilities and limitations, or a heightened awareness of the fragility of life.
3   *Changed life philosophy*: the concern that illness might result in incapacity and a shorter life can lead to changes in priorities and values, a different approach to life, and a greater appreciation of living.

These positive changes can lead to a whole new approach to life. Reviews across various conditions, including living with HIV/AIDS, surviving cancer, or experiencing the COVID-19 pandemic, have shown that many people report post-traumatic growth. Some studies have found that benefit finding or post-traumatic growth is linked to more marked increases in positive aspects of wellbeing than reductions in negative wellbeing (Moore et al., 2023; Pięta and Rzeszutek, 2022; A.W. Wang et al., 2023).

6.1.3 Illness as a Story: Narratives in Medicine

The events of chronic illness and the positive and negative changes that occur become part of people's story, or narrative, about themselves (see Case Study 6.1). Books, internet sites, and blogs provide millions of examples of people writing about their experiences of illness. Stories or narratives have numerous functions (Greenhalgh, 2016). Illness narratives:

- Transform events and construct meaning from the illness.
- Help people to reconstruct their history to incorporate the illness and reconstruct their identity to retain a sense of self-worth in the face of illness.
- Help people to explain and understand their illness.
- Relate the illness to their values and life priorities.
- Make illness a collective experience.

The importance of illness narratives is reflected in **narrative-based medicine** (Zaharias, 2018), in which the emphasis is on listening to people's narratives and using them to improve clinical care. In diagnosis, narratives are useful because they provide an insight into someone's experience of ill-health. However, it has been noted that a focus on the diagnostic usefulness of narratives may prioritise the needs of healthcare professionals rather than patients (Morrison, 2023).

Giving attention to the experiences conveyed in patient narratives can encourage empathy and understanding between doctor and patient. Narratives encourage a holistic approach to treatment. Talking through illness narratives can prove therapeutic or palliative for people. In patient education, narratives are memorable, grounded in experience, and encourage reflection (Barber & Moreno-Leguizamon, 2017). The use of narratives can therefore be helpful both for patients and doctors at many stages of illness (see Chapter 13).

Case Study 6.1

Narratives of Illness

Running for Life

Brooks Williams (Figure 6.5) was diagnosed with cystic fibrosis at 5½ months old. He says:

When I was 21, I had a serious bout of pneumonia: my lung function was down to 40% and I was coughing up lots of blood. After I was released, I was told that due to scarring in my lungs I might never make a full recovery. It made me realise how quickly my health could take an irreparable turn, and this fear is what made me start running seriously. I started running to live and I attribute my improved health to running. My doctor told me not many people with cystic fibrosis try running marathons, so I'm a guinea pig.

(Continued)

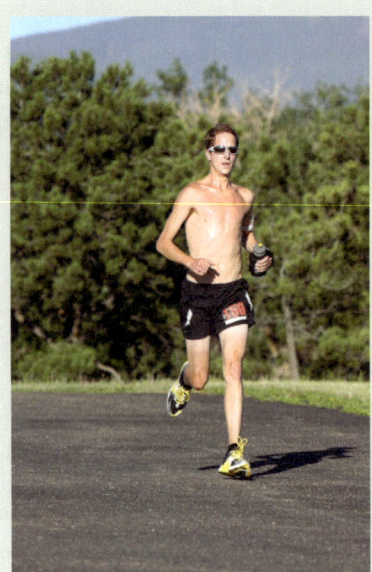

Figure 6.5   Ultramarathoner Brooks Williams

Source: Reproduced with permission of Brooks Williams, www.brookswilliams. blogspot.com; photograph reproduced courtesy of Thomas Dewane

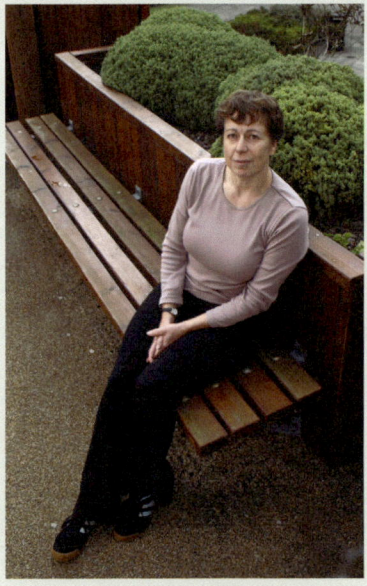

Figure 6.6   After a diagnosis of multiple sclerosis

I have been running for 13 years now and have completed numerous ultramarathons of 50 or 100 miles. My personal best for a 100-mile ultramarathon was in the Rocky Raccoon race in Texas which I completed in 14.9 hours and finished 4th overall. I think only half of finishing is down to your physical conditioning – the rest is down to mental fortitude.

Reactions, Struggles, and Changing Priorities

Ten years ago I was diagnosed with multiple sclerosis – I was going blind and was scared to death. I had young kids and, more than anything, I was scared I would never see them again. All I knew about MS was the worst, so I was convinced I'd become totally handicapped and have a terrible life. However, the treatment worked well, and my sight came back, although I have other side effects to deal with. My hands and feet are numb, and I am allergic to some drugs so can't take them – so it is an ongoing process of trying different drugs and finding out what works.

I try to look on the bright side – I have a great husband, good friends, and God. On good days I can see how wonderful life is. On bad days I try not to take anything for granted and concentrate on what I can do, rather than what I can't. I am excited by the new drugs they are working on and pray for a cure. I take each day at a time and am thankful for what I have. (Anonymous; Figure 6.6)

Acceptance of Death and Strength in Existential Issues

My dad died of cancer when I was young, so I was really scared of cancer. When the doctor told me I had cancer I was shocked and frightened. I was so scared of dying – I had young children so was really worried about what would happen to them. It took a while to get my head around it, but eventually I realised that we all have to die sometime. I can't run away from it – none of us can. I feel connected to all the people who died before me and those who will die after me. I am just a small part of a big circle of life.

I am doing everything I can to get rid of the cancer because I don't want to die, but I am not worried anymore. I enjoy my time with family and friends. I know my children will be okay because other people will be there for them. My experience of cancer has been a revelation, and I have a very different perspective now. I'm not afraid of dying. I think nature has its own way of making it all right because who wants to live in pain? I see that my life has been good – it has been a privilege. (Anonymous; Figure 6.7)

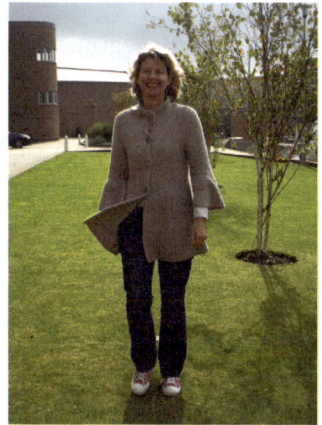

Figure 6.7   After a diagnosis of cancer

—Activity 6.1—

Using Narratives in Medicine

Think about a patient you saw recently. How much do you remember about:

- The clinical details?
- The person and their story?
- How might listening to their narrative have helped you to understand – and remember – what was important to them?

Summary 6.1

- Chronic illnesses affect approximately one in three people in developed countries and account for over three-quarters of deaths.
- The onset and diagnosis of a chronic illness brings with it profound changes in a person's life which can lead to reduced quality of life and wellbeing.
- Common emotional responses are denial, anxiety, and depression. Depression and anxiety may be a response to the illness, present before the illness, or both.
- The relationship between quality of life and physical health is not straightforward, which is partly due to variations between illnesses and how quality of life is measured.
- Many people with chronic illness are resilient and report positive life changes, such as enhanced relationships and a changed view of themselves and their philosophy of life.
- Illness narratives are important in how people make sense of their illness and adjust to them. Narrative-based medicine uses narratives to improve diagnosis, treatment, and education.

6.2 Psychological Intervention

The previous section highlighted the importance of psychological factors in chronic illness. Psychological interventions for chronic illness are usually associated with improvements in psychological wellbeing, quality of life, coping, the self-management of illness, and general functioning (Catanzano et al., 2020; Yan et al., 2020). However, there is little evidence that they affect morbidity or mortality. Information is given elsewhere on specialist interventions (CBT, stress management, and support in Chapter 14; self-management in Chapter 4). The interventions we look at here are relaxation training and expressive writing, which are both easy to learn and use.

Relaxation training can take many forms, including physical relaxation techniques such as progressive muscle relaxation, mental relaxation techniques such as meditation, or a combination of both (see Highlight Box 6.1). Relaxation is useful for coping with pain (Kwekkeboom & Gretarsdottir, 2006), reducing anxiety and depression, and coping with nausea and the side effects from treatment (Tian et al., 2020; Vambheim et al., 2021; van Dixhoorn & White, 2005). However, relaxation training is not effective for all components of all illnesses. For example, relaxation training for people with asthma is associated with improved quality of life but there is little reliable evidence that it improves lung function (Yorke et al., 2015).

The internet can also be a significant resource for people with chronic illness. It provides easy access to information, blogs, and online support, and interventions can be delivered via the internet. Online, electronic, or digital cognitive therapy treatments for anxiety and depression are already widely used, with evidence showing that these interventions are effective (Foroushani et al., 2011; Mamukashvili-Delau et al., 2022; Newby et al., 2016; Pennant et al., 2015). Various online support groups for illnesses are also widely available, and there is emerging evidence of their potential to improve various psychosocial outcomes (Hossain et al., 2021; MacLachlan et al., 2020).

Expressive writing offers a simple intervention for chronic and terminal illness. People are asked to write for 15 minutes every day for three or four days about things they find (or have found) stressful or very upsetting. It is important that people write about their thoughts and feelings and do not just describe factual events. Evidence suggests that this type of intervention can have small but significant effects on psychological wellbeing, physical health, general functioning, and health service use in some groups (Frattaroli, 2006; Meads & Nouwen, 2005; Mogk et al., 2006). There is also evidence that expressive writing can have physical and psychological benefits for the informal carers of people with chronic conditions (Riddle et al., 2016). Writing interventions are easy to use in clinical practice, following the instructions given above and with suitable guidance and encouragement. The importance of guidance and encouragement was highlighted in a review showing that the input of facilitators or guides is a determining factor in whether expressive writing interventions are effective (Nyssen et al., 2016).

—Highlight Box 6.1—

Three-Minute Relaxation Exercise

1   Make sure you are sitting comfortably and are as relaxed as possible.
2   Ask yourself, **what am I experiencing right now?** What body sensations do you have? What thoughts are going through your mind? What sounds can you hear? Just observe all these experiences without trying to change them. (*1 minute*)

3   **Focus on your breathing**. Breathe slowly and deeply: count to 4 as you inhale, then count
     to 4 as you exhale. Focus on the physical sensations of breathing, such as the movement
     of your stomach as your breath goes in and out. Let all thoughts go. (*1 minute*)
4   **Expand your awareness** to the sensations throughout your body. If you have strong
     feelings, it's OK, just allow yourself to feel them. Breathe with the feelings. If you have
     worries, try saying to yourself '*let it go*' when you breathe out. (*1 minute*)

(Adapted from www.cci.health.wa.gov.au)

Clinical Notes 6.1

Treating Chronic Illness

- Be alert to depression or anxiety in people with chronic illness and treat it appropriately.
- When adjusting to illness, people may have a fragile psychological equilibrium and react
  strongly to minor setbacks or difficulties.
- Reactions and adjustment to illness vary hugely, so do not assume you know how a person
  thinks or feels about their illness.
- Helping people to consider positive life changes since an illness can reduce distress.
- Listening to people's narratives helps us to know and treat them better.

Summary 6.2

- Psychological interventions for chronic illnesses include relaxation, stress management,
  self-management, expressive writing, and support interventions.
- Psychological interventions are associated with better psychological wellbeing, quality
  of life, general functioning, self-management of illness, as well as less pain and reduced
  symptoms and healthcare use.
- There is no consistent evidence that psychological interventions for chronic illness
  influence morbidity or mortality, as this is likely to vary across individuals and illnesses.
- The internet and mobile technology have become a significant resource for people with
  chronic illness, providing access to information, blogs, and online support.

6.3 Death and Dying

The way we die has changed substantially over recent generations. At the beginning of the twentieth century most people died at home and their bodies were laid out for friends and family to
see, touch, and mourn. By the 1960s, the majority of deaths in developed countries occurred in

hospitals. For example, in England, 57% of deaths between 2001 and 2010 happened in hospitals, 19% at home, 17% in care homes, and the rest in hospices or elsewhere (Gao et al., 2014). Although it appears that most people would prefer to die at home, the majority will die in an institution (Hoare et al., 2015), with less well-off people more likely to die at home (Davies et al., 2019). Death is therefore much less visible in our society, which means it is perceived as less 'normal' or acceptable.

The fact that most deaths in our society occur in hospitals raises various tensions and ethical issues. Healthcare staff are trained to save life, rather than to support death. Medical technology is rapidly advancing to help people live with severe disease. People have increasing expectations about their ability to survive, which can make it harder to come to terms with dying. As health professionals, it is often difficult to decide the point at which we stop prolonging life and support someone to die. On which criteria should we base these decisions? How much autonomy does the person have in decisions about dying? In this part of the chapter, we look at death and bereavement from the perspective of the individual and family. We then consider death in medical practice, including palliative care, assisted suicide, and decisions to end life.

6.3.1 Dying and the End of Life

For most of us who are healthy, when and how we will die remains unknown. Deaths in modern society can be divided according to three main patterns: a gradual death typified by a slow decline in ability and health; a premature death through accidents or illness; or a catastrophic death through sudden and unexpected events. For most terminal illnesses, people will be aware that they are going to die for some time before their actual death.

Activity 6.2

How Long Will You Live?

- Life expectancy counters or 'death clocks' use a combination of questions about lifestyle to estimate your lifespan. These are just for entertainment as they are estimates based on information about the association between lifestyle factors and mortality. See: www.livingto100.com and www.myabaris.com/tools/life-expectancy-calculator-how-long-will-i-live/

As illustrated in Case Study 6.1, responses to illness are very individual. Table 6.1 summarises some of the main challenges of terminal illness for an individual. It is also common for honest and open communication between terminally ill people, family, friends, and health professionals to break down because of taboos about death, worries that others do not want to talk about it, or finding it difficult to talk about (Dobrina et al., 2016). The combination of the impact of terminal illness and difficulties in communicating can result in reduced or impaired social interaction. Dying has subsequently been referred to as a 'falling from culture' as terminally ill people become increasingly isolated (Seale, 2008).

Table 6.1 Challenges of terminal illness

Illness-related	Self-concept	Social
• Illness symptoms and disability • Continuous treatment and side effects • Possible invasive surgery • Decisions whether to continue treatment • Threat of death	• View of self as patient • View of self as terminally ill • Changes in physical function due to illness or treatment, e.g. tremors, pain • Changes in appearance • Changes in mental function, e.g. cognitive ability	• Depression or anxiety leading to withdrawal • Preparing for loss and withdrawing from others • Mental or physical decline leading to shame, embarrassment, or concern about the impact on others • Worries about being a burden on others • Feeling bitter, angry, or resentful of healthy people

Doctors and other health professionals may also find it difficult to 'diagnose' death and discuss prognosis in terminal illness, and people may have false optimism about their prognosis. This may help them in the short term, but it makes it harder to accept death if it comes quickly. Barriers that make it hard for health professionals to diagnose dying include:

- Hope that the person will get better.
- Lack of a definitive diagnosis.
- Pursuing unrealistic or futile treatments.
- Disagreements about the person's condition.
- Failure to recognise the severity of an illness.
- Lack of knowledge about specific care.
- Poor communication skills.
- Concerns about withholding treatment.
- Fear of foreshortening a person's life.
- Concerns about resuscitation.
- Cultural and spiritual barriers.
- Medico-legal issues.

Facing death and dying among their patients can affect how healthcare professionals and students envisage themselves and their own mortality. This underlines the need for appropriate, responsive, and flexible support systems to ensure that the problems they face can be addressed early. To do so, there must be effective training and structured support mechanisms (Ho et al., 2020).

Activity 6.3

Diagnosing Dying

- What do you think people should be told about their illness?
- Should people always be given a complete and honest prognosis?
- Are there reasons why we should withhold information?

6.3.2 Responses to Terminal Illness

Death is the ultimate existential crisis: we are forced to confront our very existence. Existentialism assumes that most personal crises are prompted by realising our mortality. Therefore, people will tend to question their purpose in life, the meaning of their life, the values they have held, the foundations of their life, their relationships with others, and their religious beliefs. The realisation of mortality may make people feel alone and isolated.

One of the most influential views of dying was put forward by the psychiatrist Kübler-Ross (1969), who proposed that people go through five stages:

1   *Denial*, where the person uses denial to adjust to the fact that they are dying without being emotionally overwhelmed.
2   *Anger*, which stems from a frustration at dying and is often directed at those closest to the person. Questions like 'why me?' are common. Understanding that the person is angry at dying (not at people around them) can help carers to cope with angry outbursts.
3   *Bargaining*, where people try to make a deal with God or medical professionals so that they live, promising good behaviour in return for their life.
4   *Depression*, which occurs when the person realises there is nothing that can be done. This is seen as 'anticipatory grief', where people prepare for, and mourn, their own death.
5   *Acceptance*, where the person accepts their death with calmness and peace.

We now know that people with terminal illness do not go through discreet or consecutive stages of tasks or emotions (Daniel, 2023). People may experience any of these feelings concurrently or move between them. Many people never reach the stage of acceptance, and anxiety and a fear of death are common. Many people fear death, pain and suffering, loneliness, and the unknown. Fear of death is higher in younger people, people with poorer physical or psychological health, and people with lower life satisfaction or less of a sense of purpose in life (Neimeyer et al., 2004; Surall & Steppacher, 2020). Depression is common among people in palliative care, and it is an area where psychological intervention may help: interventions based on cognitive behavioural therapy, mindfulness, and meaning-making have been linked to reductions in depression and anxiety symptoms (von Blanckenburg & Leppin, 2018). Palliative care therefore often includes counselling alongside physical and pharmacological therapies. Research Box 6.2 gives an example of focused narrative therapy with people in palliative care to reduce symptoms of depression.

—Research Box 6.2—

Narrative Intervention for People in Palliative Care

Background

Narrative therapy helps a person to gain understanding and knowledge, and to establish the implications and meaning of their illness and life course, therein reducing distress.

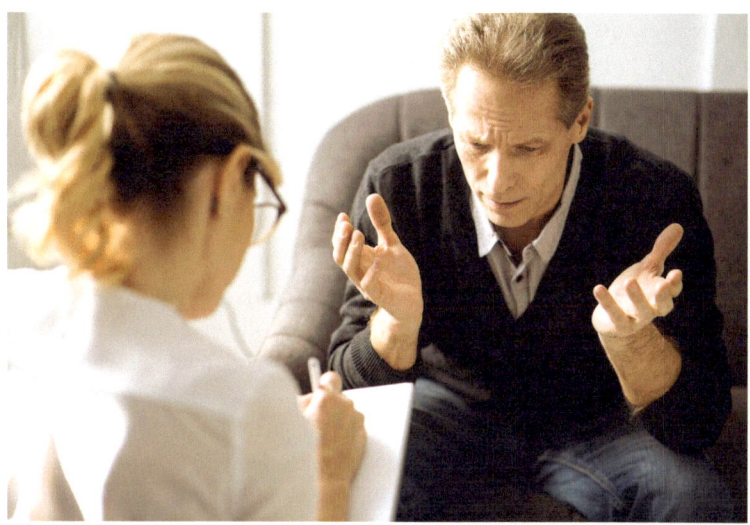

Figure 6.8   Narrative therapy

Source: © Viacheslav Iakobchuk/Adobe Stock

Method and Findings

People receiving palliative care in a hospice who had moderate or severe depression were randomised to focused narrative therapy (n = 33) or usual care (n = 24). All participants had advanced life-limiting cancer. Narrative therapy comprised a single, semi-structured narrative interview of up to one hour where people were encouraged to reflect on their psychological wellbeing, sense of meaning, and coping resources. Depression and physical symptoms were measured before and after treatment. People taking part in narrative therapy had a greater reduction in depression six weeks after treatment than the control group.

Significance

This study suggests that focused narrative therapy can reduce depression in people in palliative care. A large randomised controlled trial with a longer follow-up period is needed to confirm whether this finding is observed in other samples.

Lloyd-Williams, M., Shiels, C., Ellis, J. et al. (2018) Pilot randomised controlled trial of focused narrative intervention for moderate to severe depression in palliative care patients: DISCERN trial. *Palliative Medicine, 32*(1): 206–215.

6.3.3 Bereavement

Dying does not occur in isolation, but affects family, friends, and the community. In this section we will consider the process of bereavement, the impact of bereavement on health, and normal and pathological grief processes.

Process of Bereavement

Bereavement involves loss, grief, and mourning. **Loss** occurs when a person or object we are emotionally attached to becomes permanently unavailable. Loss is an integral part of terminal illness – people lose the ability to function physically, occupationally, and at home. **Grief** is a normal reaction to loss. It involves emotional reactions (e.g. anger, guilt, anxiety, sadness, despair), physical reactions (e.g. changes in appetite, sleep, somatic complaints), and social reactions (e.g. changes in social functioning, inability to work). **Mourning** is the process through which people adapt to loss.

How we grieve and mourn is strongly influenced by cultural customs and rules. What happens after death is prescribed by society. For example, work regulations affect the process and length of mourning. In the UK, health service workers are allowed three days' paid leave following a bereavement. Compare this with specific cultural and religious values, such as Hindu funeral rituals, which can last up to 13 days.

The symptoms that people can experience during bereavement are set out in Table 6.2. Although there are individual differences in how people grieve, 85% of people will usually adjust by the second year of bereavement (Figure 6.9). The duration and severity of a person's grief depends on:

- How attached they were to the deceased person.
- The circumstances of the death and situation of loss.
- How much time they had to work through anticipatory mourning.

Table 6.2   Responses to loss (adapted from Bonanno & Kaltman, 2001; Payne et al., 1999)

Physical	Behavioural	Emotional	Cognitive
Fatigue	Irritability	Depression	Lack of concentration
Sleep pattern changes	Restlessness	Anxiety	Shorter attention span
Aches and pains	Searching	Hypervigilance	Memory loss
Appetite changes	Crying	Anger/hostility	Confusion
Digestive problems	Social withdrawal	Guilt	Preoccupation
Shortness of breath	Inability to fulfil normal roles	Pining/yearning	Helplessness/hopelessness
Palpitations		Emotional loneliness	
Restlessness		Social loneliness	Sense of disrupted future
Increased vulnerability to illness		Feeling detached or distant	Search for meaning
			Disturbances of identity

Bereavement is associated with an increased risk of illness and mortality, particularly in older adults who lose their spouse. This is probably due to a range of factors, such as stress (see Chapter 3), depression (see Chapter 2), and lifestyle (Chapter 5).

What we classify as 'normal' during bereavement will depend on the theoretical view we take. Historical views focused on the *work* of grieving. Traditionally, bereavement was seen as a time

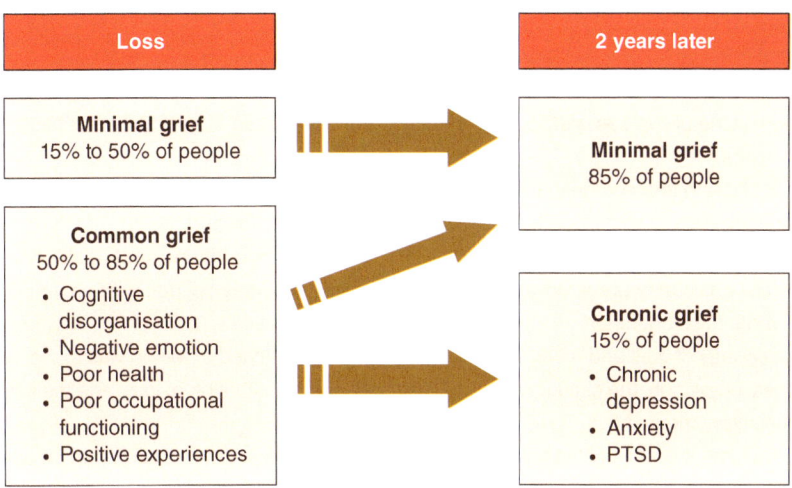

Figure 6.9 Responses to bereavement (adapted from Bonanno & Kaltman, 2001)

during which people would work through unresolved conflict or issues to do with the deceased, accept the reality of their loss, adjust to life without them, and emotionally detach from them to continue living (Worden, 2018). Stage theories emphasise the different stages a person will go through, such as numbness, yearning, despair, and recovery (Buglass, 2010). Stress theories emphasise stress and coping with bereavement as a dynamic process involving changes in orientation toward loss or restoration (Stroebe et al., 2007). When people are orientated toward loss, they will be preoccupied with their loss, think about and yearn for the deceased person, and enact behaviours such as seeking out common places or searching for the deceased loved one. When orientated toward restoration, people will adjust their lifestyle, cope with day-to-day life, build a new identity, distract themselves from painful thoughts, and take over the tasks and roles that the deceased person used to do. It is now accepted that there are multiple dynamic pathways through grief that involve making sense of the bereavement, taking meaning from it, and learning from it (O'Connor & Seeley, 2022). It is also important to acknowledge the possibility of forming continuing bonds whereby, despite the person being dead, the relationship is still meaningful (Hall, 2014).

In pathological or chronic grief, people are severely affected and can develop mental health problems, such as depression or anxiety disorders. Pathological grief affects around 15% of people, and is more likely if the death was sudden or unexpected, if the deceased was a child, and/or there was a high level of dependency in the relationship. Risk is also increased if the bereaved person has a history of psychological problems, poor support, and additional stressors, such as financial difficulties. There is emerging evidence that in-person, online, or app-based interventions can reduce symptoms of grief in bereaved adults, but there is a need for more studies with larger samples (Harrop et al., 2020; Zuelke et al., 2021). Support appears to help bereaved people generally but cannot remove the grief (Stroebe et al., 2007). This suggests that for most people bereavement is a process they must go through and, although support or intervention may be a comfort to them, it will not 'solve' their grief.

Summary 6.3

- Death is the ultimate existential crisis, when people are forced to confront and question their existence.
- Fear of death is common in terminal illness, especially in people who are younger, have worse physical health, low life satisfaction, anxiety, or depression.
- Honest communication between terminally ill people, family, friends, and health professionals may break down, and health professionals may collude with patients to promote false optimism.
- The severity of grief and mourning will depend on how attached a person was to the deceased person, the circumstances of the death and the situation of loss, and the extent of anticipatory mourning.
- Bereavement is associated with an increased risk of illness and mortality, particularly in older adults who lose their spouse.
- 15% of people develop chronic grief. This is more likely if the death was sudden, unexpected, or of a child, if there was high dependency in the relationship, or if the person has a history of psychological problems, poor support, and additional stressors.

6.4 Death and Healthcare Practice

In the 1960s, hospital patients with terminal illnesses were usually not told they were dying but were instead heavily sedated and kept separate from other patients (Glaser & Strauss, 1966). Hospices and palliative care today are founded on the idea that people with terminal illness should have compassionate care that addresses the medical, psychological, social, and spiritual aspects of dying (see Highlight Box 6.2). Palliative care focuses on relieving symptoms such as pain, rather than curing disease. Painful or invasive treatments are usually discontinued, and greater emphasis is placed on the person's psychological wellbeing. The person is given as much control and choice as possible. Honest communication is emphasised, and the family is encouraged to be involved. Palliative care is increasingly provided to people in their own homes by specialist nurses or multidisciplinary teams. Dying at home or in a hospice is associated with better control of pain and symptoms and greater satisfaction on the part of the main carer (e.g. spouse). It has been noted that when healthcare professionals discuss end-of-life concerns proactively, many patients choose more comfort-focused care and receive care that is more aligned with their wishes, values, and goals (Buss et al., 2017). However, evidence for the large and widespread benefits of palliative care is not conclusive: whereas specialised palliative care results in small but significant improvements in overall quality of life, the effects on pain and psychological wellbeing are less clear (Gaertner et al., 2017). It appears that people with cancer and those who receive earlier specialised palliative care may experience greater benefits.

—Highlight Box 6.2—

Aims of Palliative Care

1   To provide relief from pain and other distressing symptoms.
2   To affirm life and regard dying as a normal process.
3   To intend to neither hasten or to postpone death.
4   To integrate psychological and spiritual aspects of patient care.
5   To offer a support system to help patients to live as actively as possible until death.
6   To offer a support system to help the family cope during the person's illness and in their own bereavement.
7   To use a team approach to address the needs of patients and their families, including bereavement counselling if needed.
8   To enhance quality of life and positively influence the course of illness.
9   To be applied early in the course of illness, in conjunction with other therapies that are intended to prolong life, such as chemotherapy or radiation therapy, and to include those investigations that are needed to better understand and manage distressing clinical complications.

(World Health Organization, 2020b)

Working in palliative care puts considerable strain on staff, and burnout rates are high (see Chapter 3). A systematic review found that at least one quarter of oncologists and oncology nurses have symptoms of burnout (HaGani et al., 2022). Burnout appears to be even more common among palliative care specialists (Horn & Johnston, 2020). The inability to cure people and the fact that every patient dies can be unrewarding and frustrating. Health professionals may detach or withdraw from patients to protect themselves emotionally. Others may focus their attention on people who will benefit from medical intervention. The risk of burnout appears to be greater among professionals who are younger, who work in smaller teams, work for longer hours, or who are facing greater administrative or regulatory demands (Horn & Johnston, 2020). The risk of burnout can be reduced if people engage in health-promoting non-work activities such as eating well, being physically active, getting better sleep, avoiding alcohol or other drugs, and engaging in mindfulness practices or similar activities. Organisations may be able to reduce the risk of burnout by ensuring adequate staffing, manageable shift patterns and durations, and reducing administrative burdens.

Palliative care implicitly supports the idea of a 'good death', which is one where the person is psychologically prepared, physically comfortable, and able to die in the best way possible. There has been extensive debate over the notion of a 'good death' and how far we should go to help people achieve this. This is the focus of the next section.

─Clinical Notes 6.2─

Working with Terminally Ill People

- Talk to people about their illness and treatment.
- Involve them in decisions wherever possible.
- Try to address their fears and reduce anxiety.
- Be calm and mindful when with a terminally ill person – even if you don't feel this way.
- Empathise (e.g. 'that sounds …', 'I can imagine …') but do not say you 'know' or 'understand'.
- If they are angry, do not take it personally – it may be anger and frustration at their illness.
- Help them to make the most of the time they have left in the best way for them.
- Help them and their family to work through anticipatory loss and grief.
- Help them to die with dignity. If possible, this should be where and how they wish.

6.4.1 Euthanasia and Assisted Suicide

Euthanasia comes from the Greek words for 'good death'. Voluntary euthanasia is when death is hastened at the dying person's request and with their consent. Involuntary euthanasia is killing a person who has not specifically requested assistance in dying. It occurs in situations such as brain-death or coma, where family and/or doctors withdraw life support. The way in which euthanasia is done can be active or passive. Active euthanasia involves an active acceleration of death through the use of drugs or by other means. Passive euthanasia involves the withdrawal of treatment so that the person dies. It is relatively common in critical care settings as it involves any situation where life support is removed. Passive euthanasia is therefore already practised in countries where active euthanasia is illegal. Assisted suicide is a form of active voluntary euthanasia where someone assists a chronically or terminally ill person to die by suicide in as painless and dignified a way as possible.

Some of the ethical arguments for and against euthanasia are given in Highlight Box 6.3. Euthanasia and assisted suicide are currently illegal in many countries, including most states in the USA, and much of Europe. Other countries have decriminalised euthanasia, for example the Netherlands, Belgium, Switzerland, and Canada. All Islamic doctrines forbid euthanasia, but if the patient has fatal illness and death is imminent, then withholding or withdrawing a futile medical treatment may be considered permissible (Madadin et al., 2020).

Attitudes and laws on euthanasia are increasingly challenged by pressure groups, and people with terminal illness who fight for the right to take their own life. Medical opinion is also slowly changing, with many professional organisations changing their stance from explicitly opposing assisted suicide to being neutral.

─Highlight Box 6.3─

Arguments For and Against Euthanasia

Arguments for euthanasia:

- People should have the right to decide when and how to die.
- It allows people to have a good quality of life when they are alive.
- People will die in less pain and with dignity.
- The alternative is a protracted death with poor quality of life.
- Most people are in favour of euthanasia.
- It happens anyway.
- Passive euthanasia already occurs, so is there any difference between passive and active euthanasia?

Arguments against euthanasia:

- Sanctity of life.
- Intentional killing is not allowed.
- A cure may be found.
- People who chose euthanasia are depressed and/or not given adequate care.
- Good palliative care means euthanasia is unnecessary.
- Legalising killing leads to reduced respect for human life, and this is potentially damaging for society.
- Voluntary euthanasia will lead to the involuntary euthanasia of people who do not want it but cannot express this wish.

(Adapted from *Campaign for Dignity in Dying*: www.dignityindying.org.uk)

─Activity 6.4─

Involuntary Euthanasia

Consider the scenarios below and think about what you would do:

- In intensive care, you have a 78-year-old woman on life support with no hope of recovery. The family are unsure what to do. There is a 21-year-old car accident victim who has just

(Continued)

arrived and needs intensive care, but you have no bed available. He will probably not survive the journey if you send him to the nearest alternative hospital.

- A terminally ill 34-year-old man is in the advanced stages of cancer. He looks uncomfortable and is having trouble breathing. His relatives are very distressed. Should he be given a drug that will settle his breathing but will also mean he dies quicker?

- A 60-year-old woman collapses in the Accident and Emergency department and is being actively resuscitated when the medical team find out she has advanced bowel cancer and has refused chemotherapy. Should they stop resuscitation?

Studies of healthcare professionals' experiences of patient requests for euthanasia or assisted dying have revealed the challenges that often arise. For example, a survey that was sent to all registered physicians in Finland indicated that 16% had received a request for euthanasia or physician-assisted suicide (Piili et al., 2024). Despite the clear interest among patients, euthanasia is illegal in Finland, but assistance in suicide is not mentioned in Finnish law, and the potential consequences for physicians assisting suicide are unknown as the issue has never been tested in a court of law. As a result, many physicians have found themselves in the difficult situation of having to manage such a request themselves by suggesting an alternative to the request, enabling care and support, ignoring the request, giving a reasoned refusal, complying with the request, or considering the request as a possibility. A review of qualitative studies of physicians' responses to legal requests for a hastened death indicated that their individual decisions were influenced by various factors that included relevant policies, the nature of the patient request, their professional identity, their personal values and beliefs, their commitment to patient autonomy, the doctor–patient relationship, and their own emotional and psychological reactions (Patel et al., 2021).

Support from professional bodies could be helpful in these contexts, but such bodies may be reluctant to be seen to endorse illegal activity. A review of 150 medical and surgical professional societies in the USA revealed that less than 10% have position statements on assisted dying and euthanasia (Barsness et al., 2020). Given the apparent increase in public support (Campaign for Dignity in Dying, 2019; Emanuel et al., 2016), many health professionals are active campaigners for legal euthanasia (see Case Study 6.2).

Case Study 6.2

Helping People to Die

Michael Irwin is a former doctor and medical director of the United Nations. He has campaigned to highlight the plight of people who are terminally ill and wish to die by suicide. At present, British people with chronic or terminal illnesses must travel abroad if they wish to die by suicide. British law means that people who assist and accompany people to the clinic can be prosecuted. So far, hundreds of people have travelled to Switzerland for assisted suicide but most

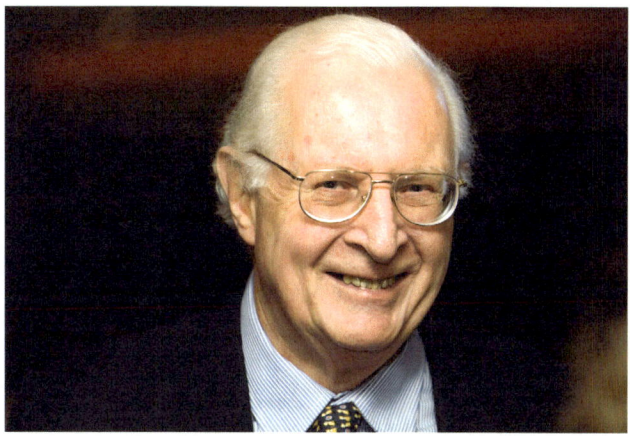

Figure 6.10 Dr Michael Irwin

Source: © Photo courtesy of the National Secular Society/Flickr

friends or relatives who accompany them have not been prosecuted. However, a few people have been investigated or arrested.

One such case is a man who undertook assisted suicide at a Swiss clinic in 2007 with Dr Irwin's help. Dr Irwin helped pay for the trip and was present at the assisted suicide. Dr Irwin and the man's partner were arrested and held on bail for more than five months. Dr Irwin has been completely open about his involvement. He provided police with a diary of his trip that detailed how the suicide was conducted.

Dr Irwin has been investigated before for his involvement in assisted suicide. He spent two years under investigation after accompanying a woman with a severe degenerative disease to Switzerland to die by suicide. However, police did not have enough evidence to press charges. In 2003, he was held on bail for three months because he admitted helping a person with cancer die because the patient was too ill to swallow the pills that Dr Irwin had provided for him.

Dr Irwin has publicly stated that he intends to help other terminally ill people to end their lives.

I've done this before and I would do it again if someone is terminally ill. It's so wrong that people have to travel abroad to die when they could die here at home with dignity. I say to the police 'arrest me'.

In countries where euthanasia is not illegal, most guidelines insist that physicians are involved. For example, the guidelines in the Netherlands state that a doctor must ensure the request for terminating life is made voluntarily by the person. They must also establish that the person's situation means they are in unbearable suffering with no prospect of improvement. The procedure of euthanasia must include the consultation and agreement of two doctors. Euthanasia can only be conducted on request and must be assisted by a doctor, and the death must be reported to the appropriate authorities as euthanasia or physician-assisted suicide.

—Clinical Notes 6.3—

Dealing with Death

- When people are grief-stricken, the priority is to calmly support them (e.g. through touch or gentle words).
- If they are very distressed, a useful technique is to get them to talk about something specific (but relevant). This will focus their mind and should reduce their immediate distress.
- Working with people who are dying is emotionally draining. It is OK to cry and be upset by their circumstances.
- Make sure you look after yourself. Use whatever support is available, whether it is informal (e.g. peers, family) or formal (e.g. colleagues), and maintain activities that nourish you (e.g. exercise, music, being with friends).
- Be self-aware. If you start to feel overwhelmed or burnt out, then get help straight away.

Summary 6.4

- Palliative care is founded on providing terminally ill people with compassionate care that addresses the medical, psychological, social, and spiritual aspects of dying.
- Palliative care implicitly supports the notion of a 'good death', but there is often tension between this and the ethical, moral, or legal opposition to euthanasia.
- Euthanasia can be voluntary (death is hastened at the person's request) and involuntary (enabling or causing death in a person who has not requested it).
- Methods of euthanasia can be active (e.g. accelerated by drugs) or passive (e.g. the withdrawal of life-sustaining treatment).
- Assisted suicide is a form of active voluntary euthanasia which is legal in only a few countries.
- Research suggests that many medical professionals in palliative care are asked by patients to assist death. Staff may therefore face difficult ethical and moral decisions while being professionally unsupported.
- In countries where euthanasia is legal, most guidelines state that physicians must be involved in (1) establishing that assisted suicide is appropriate and (2) assisting death.

Conclusion

This chapter has addressed the challenges of chronic and terminal illness, including the significant impact these illnesses can have on the lives of people and their family. The final section illustrated that these illnesses are a challenge for health professionals, confronting us with difficult ethical and moral decisions as we care for people who are dying. In a medical system founded on saving life, it can be hard to accept that sometimes there is nothing to do except support a person's death. The negative impact of the coronavirus pandemic and deaths among health professionals drew attention to some of the difficulties we face dealing with death and dying, particularly when family members are not able to be with their loved ones (Preti et al., 2020; Stuijfzand et al., 2020). Supporting people to have a 'good death' is needed more than ever under these circumstances. As one doctor observed:

> In my office adjacent to the medical intensive care unit, I have a growing file of letters from relatives of patients we have treated, thanking us for our care. But the majority of these letters are not from families of patients who survived. Rather, most come from people who have lost a loved one, from the bereaved survivors of patients who died in our intensive care unit. Yet they are deeply grateful for what we did. At first, I found these letters ironic and odd. I expected and basked in appreciation for lives saved. But the ones about lives we could not save – those I had trouble understanding. And I feel guilty. I read the letters over and over, wondering what the writers meant to me …
> Saving deaths, I have come to realize, is as important and rewarding as saving lives.
> (Nelson, 1999: 776–777)

Further Reading

Llewellyn, C.D. et al. (eds) (2019) *Cambridge Handbook of Psychology, Health and Medicine* (3rd edition). Cambridge: Cambridge University Press. Includes brief chapters on many topics in this chapter, including chronic illness, health status and quality of life, stress and crisis management, and peer support interventions.

Fallon, M. & Hanks, G. (eds) (2013) *ABC of Palliative Care* (2nd edition). Oxford: Blackwell. An edited collection that covers the medical and psychological aspects of palliative care and includes chapters on managing physical symptoms and pain, communication, interacting with carers, and bereavement.

Sage, N., Sowden, M., Chorlton, E. & Edeleanu, A. (2008) *CBT for Chronic Illness and Palliative Care: A Workbook and Toolkit*. Chichester: John Wiley & Sons. A practical introduction and guide to help health professionals understand CBT methods and how to use them when caring for people with chronic or terminal illness.

Revision Questions

1   Outline the common emotional responses to chronic illness. Discuss how these may affect health.
2   Describe a psychological intervention for people with chronic illness. Discuss the evidence for its effectiveness.
3   What is narrative-based medicine? How can it improve clinical care?
4   What challenges does terminal illness raise for individuals?

5   Why might health professionals find it difficult to 'diagnose' death and discuss this prognosis with people with terminal illness?

6   Outline Kübler-Ross's stages of dying. Discuss how accurate and useful they are in clinical practice.

7   Describe the processes of normative or typical bereavement and how they compare to pathological grief.

8   What are the common symptoms of bereavement?

9   What are the different types of euthanasia? What type of euthanasia is assisted suicide?

10 Outline the main ethical arguments for and against euthanasia.

SECTION II
BASIC FOUNDATIONS OF PSYCHOLOGY

7

THE NERVOUS SYSTEM, NEUROLOGY, AND PSYCHIATRY

──Learning Objectives──

This chapter is designed to enable you to:

- Describe the organisation of the nervous system.
- Outline explanations of the importance of sleep and the implications of poor sleep.
- Appreciate how predisposing, precipitating, and perpetuating factors influence the development of psychiatric disorders.
- Outline the major features, causes of, and treatment options for common psychiatric and neurological disorders.
- Outline the methods used for identifying and treating psychiatric illnesses and neurological disorders.

7.1 Components of the Nervous System

Health professionals need to be able to recognise the physical and psychological aspects of normal and abnormal neurological and psychological functioning. A key part of this is understanding typical or healthy nervous system structure and function.

7.1.1 Organisation of the Nervous System

There are two major divisions of the nervous system: the central nervous system and the peripheral nervous system (see Figure 7.1). The central nervous system (CNS) consists of nerves in the brain, brainstem, and spinal cord. Afferent nerves carry nerve impulses towards the CNS; efferent nerves carry impulses away from the CNS.

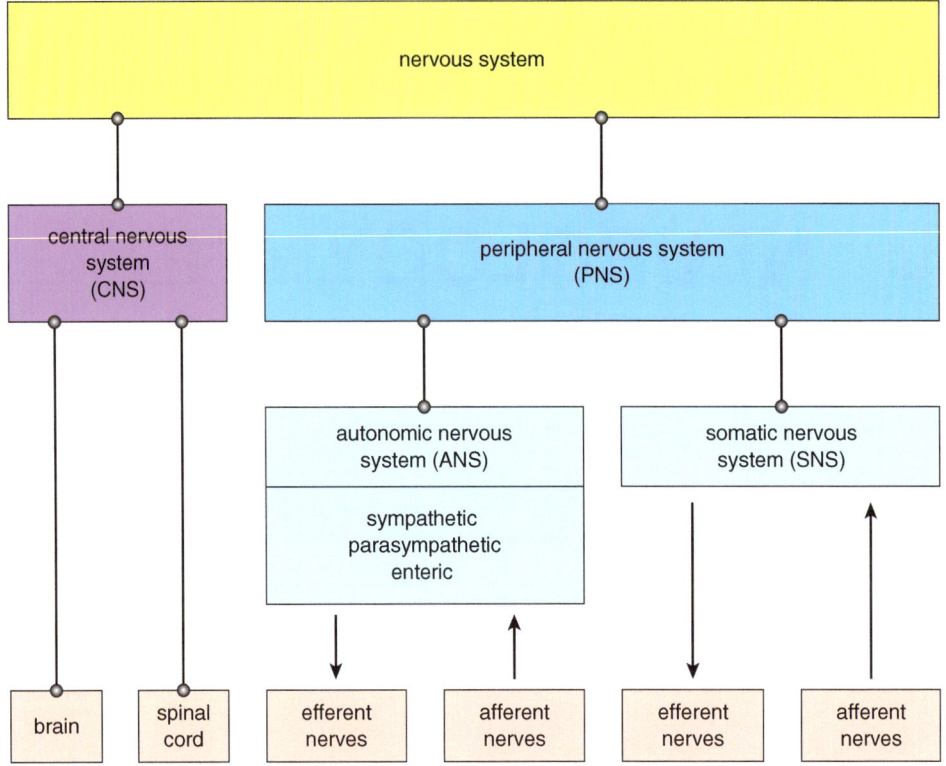

Figure 7.1   Organisation of the nervous system

The peripheral nervous system (PNS) consists of nerves that lie outside the CNS. It has two components: the automatic nervous system and the somatic nervous system. The **autonomic nervous system** (ANS) consists of nerves that regulate processes that are not normally under voluntary control. It comprises *sympathetic* and *parasympathetic nervous systems*. In general, the sympathetic system prepares the body for action – e.g. opening airways, increasing heart rate, and inhibiting digestion. The parasympathetic system tends to work in the opposite way to produce relaxation – e.g. slowing heart rate and promoting digestion. The *enteric nervous system* controls the gastrointestinal system, and is often considered as part of the ANS.

The somatic nervous system (SNS) receives sensory information (what we see, hear, smell, touch, and taste) and relays it to the CNS via afferent nerves. The CNS acts on this sensory information and sends motor signals (e.g. to catch a ball) via efferent nerves to the skeletal muscles.

7.1.2 Neurons and Neurotransmitters

Neurons are the functional units of the nervous system: they process and transmit information. Within neurons, messages are sent as electrical signals called action potentials. Between neurons, they are sent through the release of neurotransmitters into synapses between neurons.

When an action potential reaches the end of a nerve's axon, it triggers the release of neurotransmitters that bind to specialised receptors on the postsynaptic membrane. The response may be the generation of an action potential in a neuron, modification of neurotransmitter release, contraction of a muscle, or release of a hormone. Whereas neurotransmitters within the CNS are involved in direct one-to-one neuron-to-neuron communication, neuromodulators secreted by some neurons diffuse through large areas of the nervous system and affect multiple neurons. Neuromodulators influence the brain's overall levels of activity.

Many neurotransmitters and neuromodulators have been identified. Some are briefly described below and referred to later in the chapter; more detail is available elsewhere (e.g. Carlson & Birkett, 2021).

Acetylcholine influences contraction of voluntary muscles, and is involved in the regulation of attention, memory, and sleep. Acetylcholine-releasing neurons die in people with Alzheimer's disease.

Dopamine is involved in the control of movement. For example, dopamine deficits in Parkinson's disease affect movement, but the dopamine precursor levodopa (L-Dopa) is an effective treatment.

Noradrenaline (norepinephrine) appears to be involved in learning and memory. Noradrenaline deficiencies occur in people with Alzheimer's disease and Parkinson's disease, and are often observed in depression.

Serotonin is implicated in sleep, mood, depression, and anxiety. Drugs that supplement or alter the action of serotonin can relieve the symptoms of depression and anxiety disorders.

Disruptions to neurotransmitter or neuromodulator activity may impair memory and cognition and are implicated in a range of psychiatric disorders.

7.1.3 Brain Regions

The major divisions of the brain are shown in Figure 7.2. The cerebral cortex is the largest part of the human brain and is involved in 'higher' brain functions. It is thought to be responsible for the evolution of intelligence. In each hemisphere, the cerebral cortex is divided into four sections, or 'lobes' that have different functions – the frontal, parietal, occipital, and temporal lobes. The corpus callosum connects the right and left hemispheres.

The **frontal lobes** are involved in reasoning, planning, problem solving, aspects of speech, movement, and emotions. They also play an important part in long-term memory by processing messages from the limbic system (see below). The **parietal lobes** are important for integrating sensory information from various parts of the body and are also important for movement, orientation, recognition, perception of stimuli, and manipulation of objects. The most important functional aspect of the **occipital lobes** is that they contain the primary visual cortex. The **temporal lobes** are the location of the primary auditory cortex and the areas that specialise in language comprehension and speech production. They also contain the hippocampus, which plays a key role in long-term memory.

The **basal ganglia** are involved in motor control, cognition, emotions, and learning. Disorders linked to the basal ganglia include cerebral palsy, Huntington's disease, and Parkinson's disease.

The **limbic system** lies buried within the cerebrum. It is referred to as the 'emotional brain', and is important for the formation of memories.

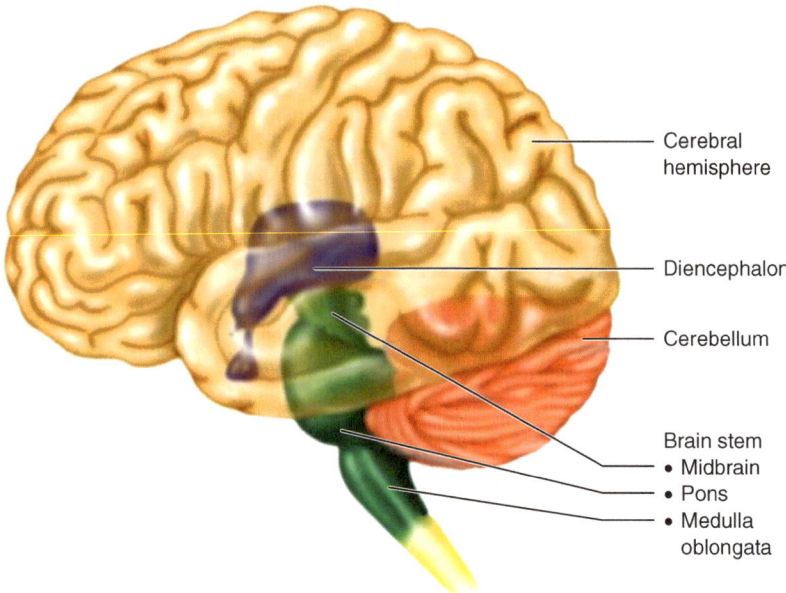

Cerebral hemisphere

Diencephalon

Cerebellum

Brain stem
• Midbrain
• Pons
• Medulla oblongata

Figure 7.2 Anatomy of the brain

Like the cerebrum, the **cerebellum** has a highly folded surface and is divided into two hemispheres. Its functions include the regulation and coordination of movement, posture, and balance.

The term 'brain stem' is often used to refer to the midbrain, pons, and medulla. Collectively, these structures are responsible for basic vital functions, such as breathing, heartbeat, and blood pressure. The **pons** is involved in the regulation of consciousness, sleep, and sensory processing. Some structures within the pons are linked to the cerebellum and therefore influence movement and posture. The **medulla oblongata** is responsible for maintaining vital body functions, such as breathing and heart rate.

Luria's (1973) functional model provides a useful summary: the brainstem regulates the arousal of the brain and muscle tone; the posterior areas of the cortex are involved in processing sensory information; and the frontal lobes and prefrontal lobes are involved in planning, executing, and monitoring behaviour. Disruptions to normal functioning in different brain regions are related to different disorders and diseases.

Summary 7.1

- The frontal lobes are involved in reasoning, problem solving, movement, and emotions.
- The temporal, parietal, and occipital lobes all have specialised capacities for processing and integrating sensory information.
- The brain stem and cerebellum regulate basic functions like breathing, and heart rate. The limbic system is known as the 'emotional brain', and is also important for memory.
- Disruptions to normal functioning in different brain regions are related to different disorders and diseases.

7.2 Movement, Sleep, and Biological Clocks

All muscular activity is influenced by the nervous system. Smooth muscle cells may contract spontaneously, but their rate of contraction is influenced by the ANS. Reflexes in skeletal muscle are coordinated via the spinal cord without control by the brain. Voluntary skeletal muscle activity is controlled by the CNS.

Motor neurons control muscle movement. A single impulse from a motor neuron produces a single twitch in a muscle fibre. A rapid series of action potentials causes a muscle to produce a sustained contraction (rather than twitches). The overall strength of a muscle contraction depends on how many motor units fire and how rapidly they do so.

7.2.1 Voluntary Control of Movement

Voluntary movement is initiated in the primary motor cortex, which is a band of neurons in the frontal lobes organised like a map of the body. However, this 'motor homunculus' is not a scale model of the body. Instead, the size of each region indicates the level of innervation and reflects the degree of control of fine movements: the hands and fingers occupy more space than the rest of the arm.

In addition to these cortical areas, other brain regions are important for controlling motor function. Extensive damage to the cerebellum results in a loss of ability to control movements, and difficulty in maintaining posture. The basal ganglia also modulate movement. Damage to the basal ganglia causes severe motor deficits such as Parkinson's and Huntington's disease (see section 7.4).

─Case Study 7.1─

Parkinson's Disease

Beth is married with four adult children. When she was in her late 30s, she began to experience tremors in her arm. She was diagnosed with Parkinson's disease aged 44 years, and is treated with L-Dopa. Before she takes her medication and sometimes between doses, Beth often feels 'dull' and is often barely able to move and communicate properly.

> You can't think straight … it's a horrible feeling, you feel as if, er, you you're not connecting, you know, that's all I can explain it, your brain isn't telling your body what to do.

Overcoming her reduced capacity to control her movements requires purposeful effort: she talks herself through sequences of actions, such as walking or eating. Whereas she used to enjoy being active and 'never felt tired', Beth now feels fatigued doing things that used to be easy. Parkinson's disease has led to profound changes in how she sees herself and how others see her:

(Continued)

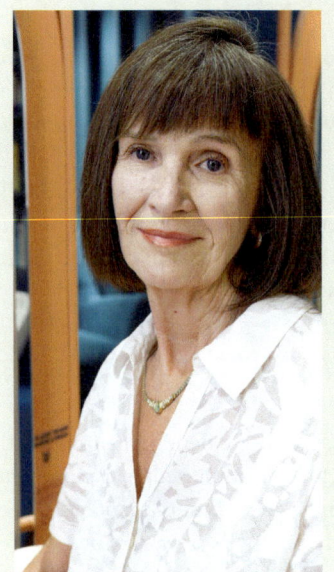

They think that you're senile because you're moving like this and … finding things hard to do like take a top off a bottle.

These changes to daily activities and quality of life are soul-destroying: Beth feels 'young at heart' but appears to others to be an 'old lady' who cannot manage. However, her efforts to avoid negative evaluations from others by concealing her muscle tremors usually only make the situation worse:

I try and stop myself from moving. So I hold my arm, or I put my arms to the back and clasp my fist … but I look worse when I disguise it because I'm doing contortions.

To minimise such experiences, Beth adheres to her medication regimen. It lets her achieve daily activities at the right times, but it also limits her capacity to be spontaneous. She therefore feels empowered, but also disempowered by medication.

(Adapted from Bramley & Eatough, 2005)

Figure 7.3 Beth and Parkinson's disease

Source: © Artem Podrez/ Pexels

7.2.2 Sleep and Biological Clocks

When we are asleep our brains are not simply at rest: important activities are going on, although the levels of activity differ during sleep and wakefulness. Typically, people progress through Stages 1–3 of increasingly deeper sleep before entering Rapid Eye Movement (REM) sleep, which is when dreaming typically occurs. This progression usually takes around 90 minutes. In Stage 3, there are slow, synchronised waves of neural activity. In contrast, REM sleep is characterised by high frequency, desynchronised activity that is more similar to wakefulness. Levels of neural firing, blood flow, and oxygen consumption increase to waking levels, but a marked loss of skeletal muscle tone means that movement is restricted.

Why Do We Dream?

There is no definitive explanation of why we dream, but research shows that the body tries to ensure a certain amount of REM sleep by entering REM sleep more rapidly, and 'catching up' on REM sleep on subsequent nights. This may be because REM sleep appears to be important for consolidating learning and memory (Tsunematsu, 2023).

Why Do We Sleep?

Sleep seems to serve a restorative function. The primary function of slow-wave sleep in Stage 3 appears to be to allow the brain to rest. Short or disrupted sleep is linked to impairments in cognitive performance (Kecklund & Axelsson, 2016; Lowe et al., 2017), mood (Palagini et al., 2019), and immune function (Besedovsky et al., 2019), and a greater risk of disorders of the neurological, cardiovascular, respiratory, gastrointestinal, and endocrine systems (Liew & Aung, 2021).

Research highlights how sleep deprivation and fatigue due to working long shifts significantly impairs healthcare professionals' mood, alertness, and professional practice (Scholliers et al., 2023; see also Research Box 7.1). Such evidence supports calls for legislation to limit health professionals' working hours.

—Research Box 7.1—

Sleep Deprivation and Errors in Healthcare

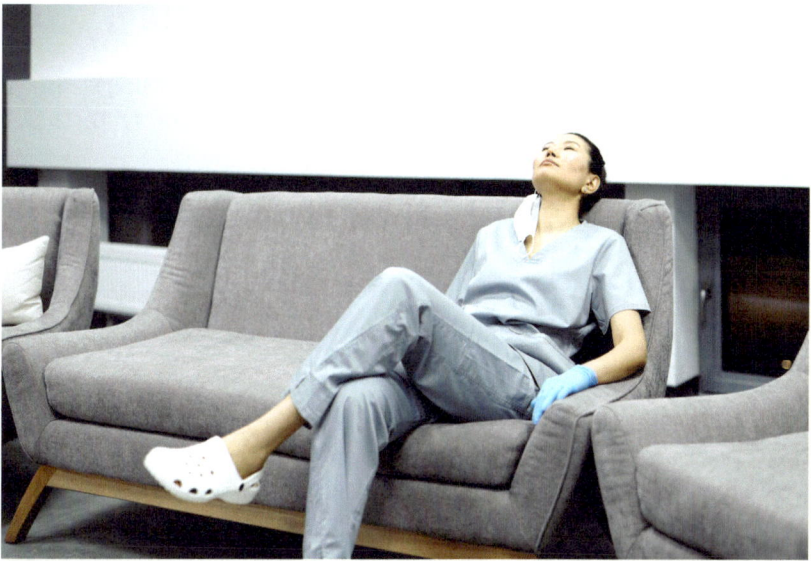

Figure 7.4 Sleep deprivation in nurses

Source: © Cedric Fauntleroy/Pexels

Background

Sleep deprivation can lead to lapses in attention and poorer problem solving, so it is important to understand how sleep deprivation affects patient care errors among health professionals working night shifts. This is important because shift work can affect the timing, duration, and quality of sleep.

(Continued)

Methods and Findings

This study involved 289 experienced nurses employed full-time on night shifts in three hospitals. Any nurses with existing sleep disorders were excluded from the study. Analyses focused on the total number of hours slept in the last 24 hours, and nurses' reports of how many hours they needed to feel rested.

More than half (56%) of the sample reported being sleep-deprived. More patient care errors were made by nurses who had shorter sleep duration or felt sleep-deprived. It is important to note that the analyses took into account years of nursing experience, length of time on night shift, and length of time worked in the unit, so it is likely that errors were actually due to sleep deprivation rather than a lack of experience.

Significance

Improved sleep among night shift nurses may reduce patient care errors. More broadly, there is a need for interventions and shift patterns that increase the quality and quantity of sleep among health professionals working night shifts.

Johnson, A.L., Jung, L., Song, Y., Brown, K.C., Weaver, M.T. & Richards, K.C. (2014) Sleep deprivation and error in nurses who work the night shift. *Journal of Nursing Administration, 44*: 17–22.

—Clinical Notes 7.1—

Sleep Deprivation in Medicine and Healthcare

- For your own sake, and for the safety of your patients, ensure that you get enough sleep.
- Sleep disruption caused by shift work can impair physical and psychological health.
- Be aware of how sleep deprivation impairs learning and memory.
- Be aware of the effects of sleep deprivation on your own performance.
- These issues are important while you are a student, and will remain important throughout your working life.

7.2.3 Why Do We Sleep When We Do?

Sleep has a restorative function, but we do not simply sleep more when we have been more active, or sleep less when we have been inactive (e.g. Atoui et al., 2021; Ryback & Lewis, 1971). Rather than being responsive to activity levels, sleep patterns are determined internally and follow a circadian (literally 'about a day') rhythm. The body also has circadian rhythms for body temperature and hormone secretion. These rhythms are determined by the **suprachiasmatic nucleus** (**SCN**) in the hypothalamus. In the case of sleep, the SCN produces a circadian rhythm via the output of melatonin. Increased melatonin output occurs during darkness and causes drowsiness.

The rhythms provided by the SCN are around 24 hours long. They are kept in this pattern by the daily cycle of daylight and darkness. Jet lag occurs when there is a rapid desynchronisation of the rhythms of the SCN and external patterns of light and darkness. A similar desynchronisation happens among shift workers. Jet lag and shift work are associated with disrupted sleep, fatigue, and impaired cognitive function. Exposure to bright light at key times can make it easier for people to adjust to shift work or to recover from jet lag (Lam & Chung, 2021). Melatonin-analogue drugs can also be used to treat the range of symptoms associated with shift work and jet lag (Arendt, 2018; Carriedo-Diez et al., 2022). A simple explanation is that they move the hands of the circadian clock to better match the new time zone.

Clinical Notes 7.2

Self-Treating Insomnia

- Only go to bed when you are sleepy.
- Set your alarm for a normal waking hour and get up at the same time every day – regardless of how much you have slept.
- Avoid alcohol, caffeine, or nicotine after 6 pm and do not eat a large meal late at night.
- Keep your bedroom for sleeping and sex: do not work in your bedroom.
- If you wake in the middle of the night for more than 20 minutes, get up and do something else. Only go back to bed when you feel sleepy.
- Do not worry about how much sleep you are getting: watching the clock can make it worse.

Summary 7.2

- All muscular activity is influenced by the nervous system.
- Damage to neurons in any of the areas involved in the control of movement can lead to severe motor impairments.
- Sleep is not a period of complete rest for the brain: it consists of several phases, and each is characterised by specific patterns of neural activity.
- The body tries to ensure a certain amount of REM sleep, possibly because dreaming during REM sleep is important for memory consolidation.
- Sleep deprivation affects cognitive function and numerous aspects of physical and psychological wellbeing.
- The timing of sleep is determined by circadian rhythms controlled by the suprachiasmatic nucleus.

7.3 Psychiatric Disorders

Many people attend primary care with complaints that are primarily psychological rather than physical. Furthermore, many physical illnesses have psychological symptoms, and physical symptoms are part of common psychological disorders, such as depression and anxiety (Kitselaar et al., 2023). Disease classification systems such as the *Diagnostic and Statistical Manual of Mental Disorders* (DSM) (American Psychiatric Association, 2022) and the *International Statistical Classification of Diseases and Related Health Problems* (ICD) (World Health Organization, 2024g) define psychiatric disorders as:

- Categorical (one does or does not have the condition).
- Distinct (the condition does not overlap with another condition).
- Independent (having one condition does not affect having another condition).

However, clinical experience and empirical research indicate that these assumptions are not always justified (Krueger & Eaton, 2015). Many psychiatric disorders present with combinations of similar symptoms and comorbidity is also common (Dalgleish et al., 2020). It may therefore be helpful to think of psychiatric disorders as networks of symptoms rather than clear diagnostic entities, and to take a transdiagnostic approach that is focused less on diagnosis and more on the effective treatment of symptoms (Dalgleish et al., 2020; Pearl & Norton, 2017).

┌Activity 7.1┐

What is a Psychiatric Disorder?

Take a few minutes to write your own definition of what a psychiatric disorder (or mental illness) is.

- At what point does abnormal behaviour constitute illness?
- Do psychiatric disorders always have a physiological cause?

7.3.1 Models of Psychiatric Disorders

Different scientific approaches to explaining psychological disorders vary in terms of the importance they assign to biomedical and psychosocial factors.

Biomedical Explanations

According to the biomedical model, psychiatric disorders result from dysfunctions in the biochemistry and physiology of the brain and body, or from damage to the brain. The implication of biomedical models is that if we identify the biological causes of psychiatric disorders, we should be able to develop effective treatments. Although this model is useful for some disorders, it cannot explain all disorders.

Psychological Explanations

Psychological models argue that people's experiences – and responses to them – may cause psychiatric disorders without there being any physiological abnormality. **Psychoanalytic** approaches explain psychiatric disorders as the result of the interplay between conscious and unconscious responses to experiences, rather than abnormalities in brain functioning. Psychoanalytic therapies seek to identify and address these unconscious processes (see Chapter 14). **Learning theory** approaches argue that many psychiatric disorders result from maladaptive learning. Treatment based on this approach is informed by operant and classical conditioning (see Chapter 10) to 'unlearn' maladaptive responses. **Cognitive behavioural** approaches are based on the idea that psychopathology arises when people acquire irrational beliefs or dysfunctional ways of thinking about themselves, their behaviour, or other people's responses to them. Cognitive behavioural therapy (CBT) is aimed at challenging and changing maladaptive patterns of thinking (see Chapter 14).

Psychosocial Models

Psychiatric disorders often involve biomedical, psychological, and social factors. The biopsychosocial model (see Chapter 1) recognises that physiological and psychosocial factors are involved in the onset and progression of psychiatric disorders (Savulescu et al., 2020). It also emphasises the importance of social responses to psychiatric disorders: do we lock 'mad' people in asylums or provide care for 'ill' people in the community?

Rather than assuming that all cases of a particular psychiatric disorder are explained by a single cause, it is important to think of how various factors combine to affect the onset and course of a disorder. These are often referred to as the three Ps: predisposing, precipitating, and perpetuating factors (see Figure 7.5).

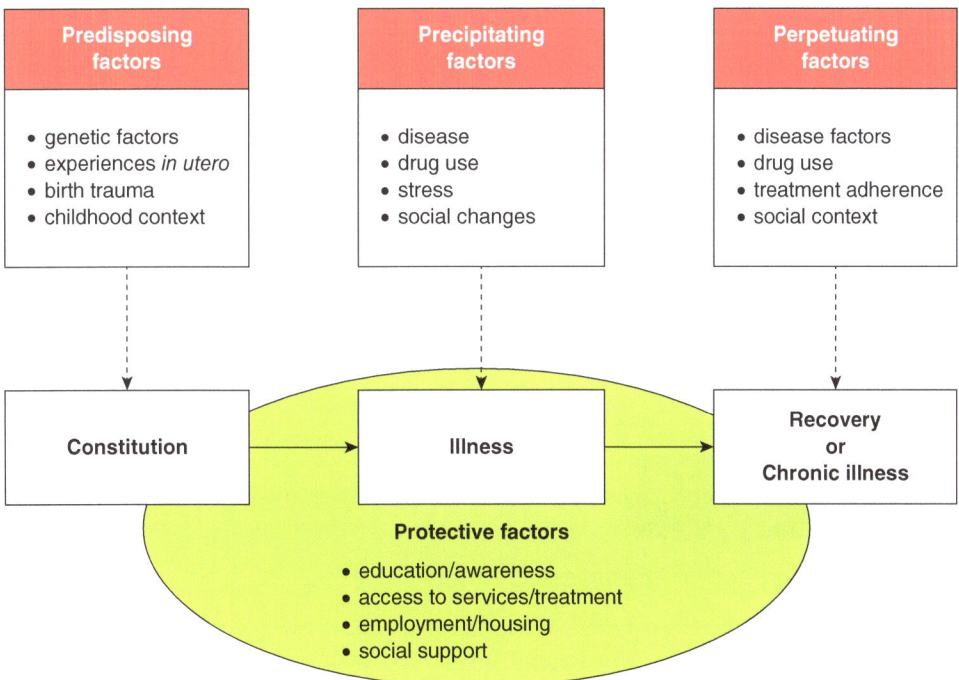

Figure 7.5 Predisposing, precipitating, perpetuating, and protective factors in psychiatric disorders (adapted from McKnight et al., 2019)

Predisposing factors are things that make people more susceptible to mental illness. Genetic factors, experiences *in utero*, a difficult birth, and adverse childhood experiences, such as neglect and abuse, can increase the risk of some mental disorders.

Precipitating factors are events or experiences that influence whether a predisposition to a psychiatric disorder is 'activated'. Not every person with the same predisposing factors will develop a psychiatric disorder – precipitating factors may interact with predisposing factors to bring about psychopathology. Precipitating factors that influence the onset of psychiatric disorders include diseases such as brain tumours and strokes (L. Liu et al., 2023; Ribeiro et al., 2022), use of psychoactive substances, and psychosocial factors such as traumatic events or social isolation (Z. Chen et al., 2023; D'Souza et al., 2022; Tortella-Feliu et al., 2019). The interaction between predisposing factors and precipitating factors is often referred to as a **diathesis-stress model**: diathesis refers to predisposing factors and stress refers to precipitating factors (see Chapter 3).

Perpetuating factors act after the onset of a psychiatric disorder to prolong its duration. Sometimes diseases are self-perpetuating. For example, non-adherence to treatment can prolong illness (McGrady & Pai, 2019) and maladaptive coping behaviours may perpetuate anxiety disorders or depression (Spătaru et al., 2024). Social factors may also prolong illness. For example, a reluctance to give up secondary gains from the sick role (see Chapter 9) may prolong illness.

Consideration should also be given to an important fourth P: **protective factors**, such as education, resilience, and social support, which reduce the likelihood of onset or progression of symptoms (McKnight et al., 2019). One aim of health psychology is to identify and understand the four Ps and to develop effective interventions.

7.3.2 Classifications of Psychiatric Disorders

Definitions of psychiatric disorders change over time to reflect changes in our understanding of different psychiatric disorders and their causes, and changes in social attitudes (see Highlight Box 7.1).

There are two major systems for classifying mental disorders. The American Psychiatric Association's DSM is the standard classification of mental disorders used by clinicians in the USA (DSM-5-TR: American Psychiatric Association, 2022). It is widely used in clinical practice in many other countries, and in academic research. The World Health Organization's ICD classifies all diseases, including psychological illnesses (ICD-11: World Health Organization, 2024g). There is also a simplified version of the ICD for disorders most commonly seen in primary care with materials that help to identify symptoms and develop management plans (ICD-10-PHC: World Health Organization, 1996).

─Highlight Box 7.1─

How Are Psychiatric Disorders Defined?

Definitions of psychiatric disorders are not fixed. This is reflected in the need for regular revisions to diagnostic classification systems such as the ICD and DSM. Definitions of psychiatric disorders often reflect contemporary social issues. For example, until 1973, homosexuality was included as a mental disorder in the American Psychological Association's classification of mental disorders. This was

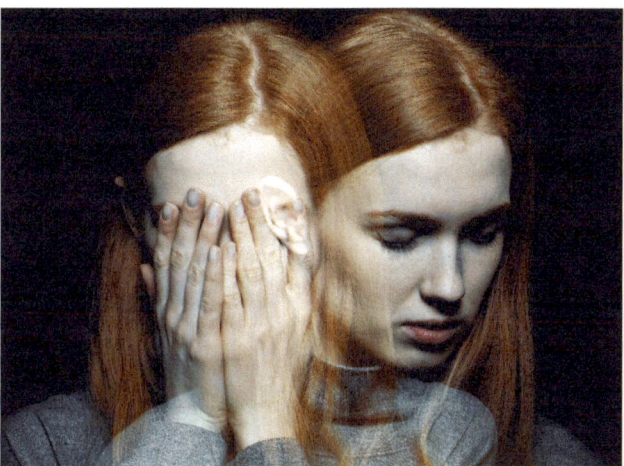

Figure 7.6 Controversies in defining psychiatric disorders

Source: © Photographee.eu/Adobe Stock

controversial because defining homosexuality as a disorder implied that it was something that should be cured, rather than a normal form of sexuality. Debate about pathologising homosexuality continued after 1973 because of the inclusion of a new disorder called 'Sexual Orientation Disturbance'. Part of this debate focused on whether the psychological 'disturbance' observed in some homosexual people was a consequence of their sexuality *per se*, or a reflection of society's discrimination and prejudice towards homosexual and bisexual people.

Here we introduce four common psychiatric conditions that are likely to be seen in primary care because of their prevalence or their chronicity. For each of them, we outline the key features, treatment, and prognosis. They are presented here as distinct disorders because this is how they are officially recognised in the DSM and ICD, in epidemiology, and in insurance coverage for treatment. However, as noted earlier, the assumption that these conditions are categorical, distinct, and independent may not be justified (Dalgleish et al., 2020).

Mood Disorders

We all experience variations in mood, but when such changes in mood are long enough and intense enough to interfere with normal activities and relationships they can be considered as mood disorders. The DSM and ICD distinguish between different manifestations of depression, mania, and combinations of **mania** and **depression**, such as **bipolar disorder** (sometimes referred to as manic depression). Depression not related to, or associated with, other conditions is sometimes called unipolar depression.

The key features of depressive disorders are low mood and a loss of interest in pleasurable activities (anhedonia). Other symptoms are pessimism, lack of energy, poor concentration, low self-esteem, and changes in sleep, appetite, and activity. The key features of mania are elevated mood, hyperactivity, impulsive behaviour, lack of concentration, increased appetite, and increased libido. Bipolar disorder consists of alternating periods of mania and depression. The changes between these states can be relatively rapid (within a few hours) but usually occur over a longer period.

Mood disorders result from an interaction between genetic, physiological, and experiential factors. Reviews indicate evidence of a genetic predisposition to depression and bipolar disorder (Amare et al., 2020). Physiological processes are also important, for example, changes in the levels of neurotransmitters such as dopamine, serotonin, and norepinephrine (Jiang et al., 2022).

Psychological factors are also important. Stressful experiences can affect the development of mood disorders (Chesnut et al., 2021). However, physical activity offers protection against the development of depression (Pearce et al., 2022). There are many theories of the aetiology of depression. Beck's (1967) cognitive theory of depression and Seligman's (1975) theory of learned helplessness highlight the importance of negative thinking in the onset and progression of depression (see Chapter 6). Psychoanalytic explanations of depression view it as a response to a real or symbolic loss of a loved person or object.

Various effective treatments for depression are available. It is recommended that antidepressant drugs are used only for major depression, but not moderate or mild depression (Cipriani et al., 2018). Depression responds well to psychotherapy and interventions that are designed to enhance social support. Psychotherapies do not appear to be as successful in bipolar disorder as they are in unipolar depression.

Case Study 7.2

Depression

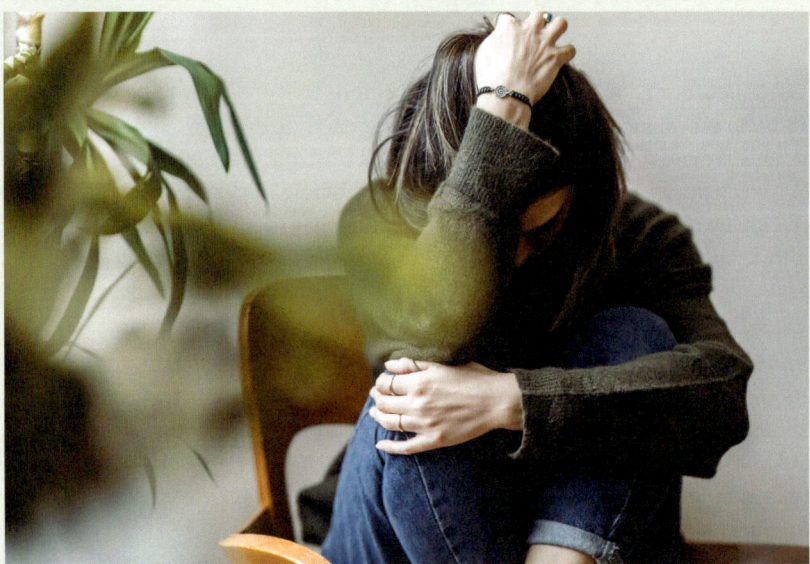

Figure 7.7   Ella's depression

Source: © Liza Summer/Pexels

Ella was diagnosed with depression at the age of 16. Her account reflects a biopsychosocial model of psychiatric disorder: she believes that her depression was caused by a combination of a chemical imbalance and learned behaviours. Various childhood events may have resulted in her depression. She became very introverted after her parents separated and her best friend moved away. During adolescence, Ella also began to have trouble sleeping and lacked energy. She feels unlucky that the doctors she saw were not attentive to her psychological symptoms.

When Ella was diagnosed, she began taking antidepressant medication. The initial side effects were unpleasant and included disrupted sleep and weight gain. However, these gradually reduced, and she felt like she was 'given my life back'. Ella feels that she can 'now be a normal person'. Diagnosis and treatment had other psychological benefits for Ella. The acknowledgement that her depression was a result of serotonin activity in her brain was a counter to people simply saying 'Cheer up! Why are you so miserable?', and implying that depression was somehow her fault.

However, Ella realised that although antidepressant medication had 'sorted out my brain chemistry', she was also aware that her depression was influenced by psychological factors: 'You have learnt all these negative ways of looking at things, and doing things … from your parents at times.' This realisation meant that Ella saw a need for psychotherapy to help her to learn better ways of dealing with events in her life and trying to change her 'total inferiority complex'. Her experiences of therapy helped her to develop a more positive approach to herself and her social interactions.

(Adapted from www.healthtalk.org © Dipex)

Anxiety Disorders

Anxiety disorder is an umbrella term that incorporates various forms of abnormal and pathological fear and anxiety. An anxiety disorder may have a specific limited focus, or it may be more diffuse.

Generalised Anxiety Disorder (GAD) is characterised by excessive fearful anticipation and worrying thoughts. Physical symptoms include agitation in the gastrointestinal, respiratory, cardiovascular, urinary, and muscular systems. Because GAD is not related to individual events or circumstances, it is separate from episodic anxiety such as phobia or panic disorder.

Phobias are anxious reactions to particular situations or objects. Unpleasant physical and psychological experiences of severe anxiety accompany phobias, so people may try to avoid the situations or objects which they fear. **Panic disorder** is diagnosed when panic attacks occur unexpectedly and in the absence of a single identifiable trigger for an anxious response. In panic attacks, the symptoms of anxiety rapidly escalate and catastrophic thoughts, such as 'I'm going to die', are common.

Anxiety disorders may have a genetic component (Ask et al., 2021). Neurochemical and brain imaging studies indicate abnormal activity in the amygdala, hippocampus, and prefrontal cortex and dysfunction in serotonin, noradrenaline, and dopamine systems (Liu et al., 2018). Experiences are often important for the development of phobias. The aetiology of panic disorder is less clear, but it may result from a combination of abnormal neural activity, excessive ANS responses to stress, and excessive fearful responses to the resulting autonomic arousal (Kim & Yoon, 2018).

Medical treatments for anxiety disorders include anxiolytics (for short-term use) and antidepressants for people with GAD or phobias involving depression. Psychological therapies include relaxation training, self-help methods, and CBT (van Dis et al., 2020). Combinations of psychotherapy and pharmacotherapy are often more effective than either single treatment.

Schizophrenia

Schizophrenia is characterised by disorders of thought, mood, and anxiety. The key features of **schizophrenia** are psychotic symptoms such as delusions and hallucinations. These **positive symptoms** are additions to usual pre-existing functioning (e.g. hallucinations). The **negative symptoms** of schizophrenia include a blunting of feeling, reduced capacity to express emotions, and incongruous emotions (e.g. laughing at sad news). Reductions in attention and memory may be present. Poverty of speech, depressed mood, and low motivation may combine with these emotional changes and lead to a withdrawal from normal social interactions.

Schizophrenia results from the interaction of genetic, physiological, and experiential factors. Twin studies indicate a genetic predisposition, and evidence of differences in neurotransmitter activity (McKnight et al., 2019). Complications during pregnancy, adverse childhood experiences, such as neglect or abuse, and early or prolonged cannabis use increase the risk of schizophrenia (Belbasis et al., 2018; D'Souza et al., 2022). Schizophrenia has been described as 'a classic battleground' for nature–nurture debates (St Clair & Lang, 2021).

Antipsychotic medications can be effective for treating positive symptoms, but do not affect the negative symptoms. Lack of adherence to schizophrenia medication is often a problem, and may be influenced by side effects, including weight gain (Yaegashi et al., 2020). However, various educational, technological, and social support interventions have been shown to improve adherence (Loots et al., 2021). Psychotherapy can be a useful adjunct to medication, but more robust research evidence is needed to identify the most effective approaches (Guaiana et al., 2022).

Personality Disorders

Personality disorders consist of inflexible patterns of behaviour that deviate from social expectations and cause distress, suffering, or harm to the individual or other people. These disorders may result from a combination of a genetic predisposition and experiential factors, such as brain injury during a complicated birth, difficult parent–child interactions, or traumatic experiences.

People with personality disorders are more likely than others to have physical or psychological conditions, and unhealthy patterns of alcohol and drug use, and they also have shorter life expectancy (J.K.N. Chan et al., 2023; Dokucu & Cloninger, 2019). Effective interventions are needed to address both the personality disorder and any comorbid conditions.

Because personality is relatively stable, personality disorders tend not to be very responsive to treatment. Furthermore, there are no drugs available specifically for treatment of personality disorders: instead, drugs may be used to treat anxiety, psychosis, or depression (Stoffers-Winterling et al., 2022). Psychosocial treatment often involves identifying ways to manage the person's behaviour in different social contexts. There is a need for more evidence of the efficacy of specific psychosocial interventions (Storebø et al., 2020).

Summary 7.3

- Psychiatric disorders result from the interaction and combination of four Ps: predisposing, precipitating, perpetuating, and protective factors.
- Biomedical and psychosocial factors can constitute predisposing, precipitating, and perpetuating factors.
- The two major systems for classifying psychiatric disorders are the DSM and the ICD.
- Psychiatric disorders differ from each other in terms of the presence, nature, and intensity of disorders of thought, mood, and anxiety.

7.3.3 Psychiatric Assessment

As noted earlier, many psychiatric disorders are syndromes of symptoms that may be aspects of different disorders (Krueger & Eaton, 2015). Furthermore, symptoms of depression and anxiety are commonly part of psychological and physical conditions. It is therefore important to conduct a thorough examination and assessment to evaluate differential diagnoses. The nature of many psychiatric disorders may make the psychiatric interview more difficult than a standard clinical interview (see Chapter 13) because people may be apathetic, anxious, angry, deluded, or aggressive.

The psychiatric history should first attend to the presenting complaint and its history, including the person's reports of the believed causes of the problem and their subjective experiences. It is also important to gain information about the person's pre-morbid history. There may be a need to corroborate reports provided by a person experiencing delusions or psychosis. The history should also gather information about the person's psychiatric and medical history, including details of any medications and other treatments. Information relating to the person's family history should identify the presence of any psychiatric disorders.

The **Mental State Examination** (Trzepacz & Baker, 1993) can aid psychiatric diagnoses. It provides a structured way of both observing and describing several aspects of psychological functioning:

- *Behaviour and appearance*: The focus here includes the visible signs of physical health or injury and psychological wellbeing.
- *Mood*: In addition to seeking the person's self-assessment of their mood, healthcare professionals should make their own assessment of the person's mood.
- *Affect*: In psychiatric disorders, affect may be blunted, irritable, suspicious, perplexed, or incongruous (i.e., not appropriate for the context).
- *Perception*: Note any illusions, such as mistaking one real object for another, as well as hallucinations.
- *Insight*: The focus here is on whether the person thinks that they have a psychiatric disorder or need treatment.
- *Speech and thought form*: The tone, speed, and volume of speech may vary in different disorders. Thoughts may be disjointed, illogical, or repetitive.

- *Thought content*: Pay attention to expressions of guilt, hopelessness, depression, anxiety, and depersonalisation (e.g. feeling unreal or detached).
- *Cognition*: Note deficits in memory and problem solving. The 'Mini-Mental State Examination' may help (Folstein et al., 1975; and see section 7.4.1).

─Clinical Notes 7.3─

Psychiatric Assessments

- Many psychiatric disorders present combinations of similar symptoms, so it is helpful to think of them as syndromes rather than simple discrete illnesses.
- The Mental State Examination can help you to detect possible psychiatric morbidity in people not presenting with psychiatric complaints.
- Be aware of how predisposing, precipitating, perpetuating, and protective factors influence the onset and maintenance of symptoms.
- Be sensitive to how psychiatric morbidity may affect people's capacity to be involved in making decisions about their treatment.

7.3.4 Management and Treatment of Psychiatric Disorders

When treating any illness, it is important to agree on a treatment plan with the person and to monitor their adherence and progress. Treatment should be planned in relation to immediate needs, short-term goals, and long-term goals. It may involve medical, psychological, and/or social interventions.

Drug Therapy

The drugs used in psychiatry can be divided into different categories, but some drugs can have more than one application (e.g. benzodiazepines have anxiolytic and hypnotic effects). Many have marked side effects that may result in low adherence (Yaegashi et al., 2020). Great care must be taken when considering prescribing psychotropic drugs to certain groups, including pregnant or breastfeeding women, children, elderly people, and people with digestive or heart disorders (McKnight et al., 2019). Care must also be taken when withdrawing or changing medication.

Psychotherapy

Psychotherapy is an effective component of treatment for many psychiatric disorders. As noted in Chapter 14, there are various types of 'talking cures', but all share the belief that there is therapeutic value in helping people to understand their past and present situation, to manage their symptoms, and to develop more productive ways of thinking about themselves, their illness, and social interactions. There is substantial evidence of the efficacy of cognitive behavioural therapy (CBT) and mindfulness for depression, anxiety disorders, phobias, and obsessive-compulsive disorders (Öst et al., 2023; Zhang et al., 2019). In some cases of depression,

CBT may be more effective than antidepressant drugs (Breedvelt et al., 2021). There is also growing evidence that self-guided online interventions are effective for various psychological conditions (de Oliveira et al., 2023; Eilert et al., 2022). Psychodynamic and psychoanalytic therapies are effective for many psychiatric disorders (Leichsenring et al., 2023).

In many cases, better outcomes result from a combination of medication and counselling than from either approach in isolation (Guidi & Fava, 2021). For example, in anxiety disorders, anxiolytics may alleviate the immediate physical symptoms and thereby facilitate psychotherapy.

Electroconvulsive Therapy

Electroconvulsive therapy (ECT) involves passing an electric current across a person's brain to alter its activity. There is evidence of its efficacy for depression (Elias et al., 2018), but the therapy attracts controversy (Meechan et al., 2022). It may also be useful for schizophrenia or post-traumatic stress disorder (PTSD) (Ali et al., 2019; Youssef et al., 2017). ECT tends to be used for severe conditions that have not responded to medication or which threaten the wellbeing of the patient or other people (e.g., mothers with puerperal psychosis, people with a high suicide risk).

Medical Decision Making in Psychiatric Disorders

Impaired cognitive functioning associated with some psychiatric disorders may hinder people's capacities to be involved in decision making or to give informed consent to treatment. People who lack insight may not recognise that they are unwell and require treatment. The concept of 'capacity' for decision making is important, but there is debate as to how it should be defined and implemented in the context of psychiatric disorders, and what should be done if it is thought that a person may lack capacity (Calcedo-Barba, 2020). Many of these issues also apply in the neuropsychiatric disorders described in the next section (Jayes et al., 2020).

Summary 7.4

- A thorough psychiatric interview involves taking a psychiatric history and conducting a Mental State Examination.
- Many psychiatric disorders present as syndromes, and symptoms are shared between many of these syndromes. This makes differential diagnosis important.
- When developing a treatment plan, medical, psychological, and social interventions should be considered.
- Psychological therapies can be as effective as medication for many psychiatric disorders, in particular mood disorders.

7.4 Neurological Disorders

Degeneration or damage within the brain and nervous system can lead to a range of disorders. Their precise nature is determined by the location and extent of the impairment to normal functioning. Because different brain regions have different functions, damage or disorders that are localised in specific brain regions tend to have specific outcomes. This section outlines several common neurological disorders, their psychological aspects, and their treatment. It is followed by sections on neuropsychological assessment and rehabilitation.

Multiple sclerosis (MS) is characterised by the inflammation and demyelination of the central nervous system. It may result in a loss of sensation or function in the limbs, incontinence, fatigue, pain, cognitive impairments, and mood disorders. MS is believed to be an autoimmune disorder, but the exact processes involved are not known, and there is no cure. The unpredictable and variable nature of MS impair psychological wellbeing and cognition, but psychological comorbidities in MS are often under-diagnosed (Solaro et al., 2018). Although there is no cure for MS, psychological interventions can be effective for managing depression and helping people to cope with the physical limitations arising from the condition (Faraclas, 2023).

Motor Neurone Disease (also called Amyotrophic Lateral Sclerosis or ALS) is a rare and terminal disorder which involves the progressive degeneration of motor neurons and leads to progressive weakness in the skeletal muscles. Its cause is not known, nor is it known why the sensory nerves, which have a similar structure, are not affected. Mood disorders often occur, and quality of life tends to be worse if there is greater functional impairment (Rosa Silva et al., 2020). Impairment to overall quality of life appears to be smaller if social support is available.

Disorders of the basal ganglia, such as Parkinson's disease and Huntington's disease, cause severe motor deficits (see 7.1.3), but also have important cognitive and emotional aspects. The symptoms of basal ganglia disorders have been referred to as the three Ds: dyskinesia, dementia, and depression (McHugh, 1989). **Parkinson's disease** is a severe, incurable motor disorder characterised by muscle stiffness, slowness of movement, an unstable posture, and muscle tremors (see Case Study 7.1). It is a progressive degenerative disorder resulting from a severe reduction in dopamine activity in the basal ganglia. Standard pharmacological treatment is the dopamine precursor L-Dopa, but the use of deep brain stimulation has also progressed (Wolff et al., 2023). Cognitive deficits are common and include impairments to memory and information processing. Depression, anxiety, lethargy, sleep disturbances, and pain are more common among people with Parkinson's disease than in the general population (Weintraub et al., 2022). CBT and mindfulness-based therapies can reduce psychological distress in people with Parkinson's disease (Ghielen et al., 2019; Roper et al., 2024).

Huntington's disease is characterised by involuntary rapid, ceaseless movements or tics. Other symptoms include a loss of coordination and balance, slurred speech, and difficulties in swallowing. It is a genetically determined disorder caused by the progressive degeneration of specific neurons. There is no cure for Huntington's disease and death usually occurs 15–25 years after symptom onset. Cognitive deficits are common, and people with Huntington's disease have an elevated risk of mood disorders and suicidal behaviour (Clark et al., 2023). Treatment focuses on addressing the physical and psychological symptoms, preventing complications, and providing psychological support.

Dementia involves the progressive loss of cognitive function due to damage or disease in the brain. In high-income countries, dementia is now one of the most common causes of death. Dementia is not a single disorder but a syndrome, the symptoms of which vary between people, depending on the location and cause of the disorder. Vascular dementias result from multiple small strokes which, in accumulation, produce a sufficient loss of neurons and accompanying changes in behaviour and cognition.

Dementia of Alzheimer type (DAT or **Alzheimer's disease**) accounts for over half of all dementias. It involves the progressive loss of neurons and synapses in the cerebral cortex and particular subcortical regions. Loss of neurons in DAT may be caused by a combination of genetic factors and environmental influences. DAT is characterised by progressive impairments to memory, cognitive capacities, and social functioning, which are commonly accompanied by confusion, irritability, and mood swings. People with DAT are more likely than the general population to experience anxiety, irritability, depression, and apathy, and greater psychological symptoms may be predictive of further cognitive decline (Asmer et al., 2018; Y.Y. Huang et al., 2023).

It can be difficult to make a differential diagnosis between depression and the early stages of dementia because depressed people often experience impaired concentration and memory, and depression and apathy often co-occur with dementia (Gilmore-Bykovskyi et al., 2019; see also Case Study 7.3).

Drug therapies have a small but significant impact on cognitive functioning in Alzheimer's disease, and exercise therapy can also be effective (H.A. Fink et al., 2020; Hort et al., 2023; Moniruzzaman et al., 2021).

Case Study 7.3

Identifying the Early Stages of Dementia

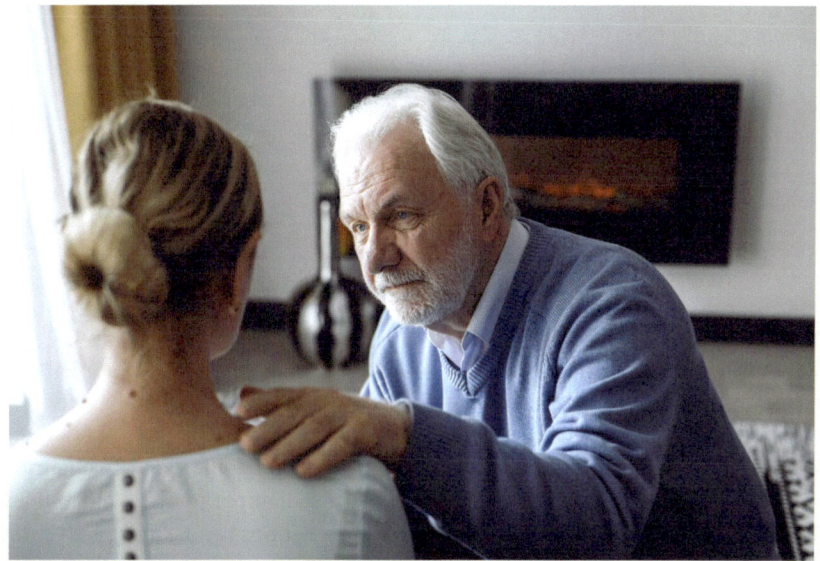

Figure 7.8 Signs of dementia in Andreas' wife Maria

Source: © Pavel Danilyuk/Pexels

As dementia develops, people may not have full awareness of changes in their behaviour or their own memory problems. Andreas visited his doctor on his own on what was supposed to be a joint visit with his wife Maria. He had become worried about changes in Maria's behaviour.

(Continued)

Andreas said that he did not notice the gradual changes occurring day to day, until it was pointed out to him by other people who had less frequent contact with her:

> One example was with my son. He lives overseas, so only visits now and then. He took Maria out shopping for a new coat, and when he came back said 'Why haven't you told me how down she is? She wasn't really interested in anything, and when we were having coffee, she was just in a world of her own'. When he told me how much she had changed since the summer it really shocked me.

> When he said that, I did wonder whether she might be depressed. But then there were other things, like forgetting to lock the house or the car – and she didn't like it when I pointed it out. I wasn't sure what was wrong, but it was starting to worry me. That worry must have grown because one time she said, 'Why are you always getting annoyed with me?' and I just said, 'It's because I'm so worried about you', and that made her really upset. So I suggested that we should see the doctor.

After a subsequent productive three-way discussion, the doctor was able to determine that Maria was displaying signs of dementia.

> Now that I have spoken to other people, I've realised that a lot of us went through the same kinds of things. At first, it's hard to notice that there is a series of unrelated and apparently insignificant things that you can only make sense of with hindsight and through talking to other people.

(Adapted from www.healthtalk.org © Dipex)

In a **stroke**, central nervous system neurons die because of disruptions to the blood flow to the brain (see Chapter 16). Neurological deficits often arise from a stroke. Post-stroke, people have elevated risks of depression and anxiety, and they are more likely to experience irritability, agitation, eating disturbances, and apathy (L. Liu et al., 2023; S. Zhang et al., 2020). There is, therefore, a need for physical, cognitive, and psychological rehabilitation. Psychiatric disorders after stroke are important in their own right, but they also hamper physical rehabilitation (Ahn et al., 2015). Evidence indicates that psychological interventions can be an effective way to treat mood disorders that arise after a stroke (Allida et al., 2023).

Acquired brain injury (ABI) is another cause of neurological impairment. Traumatic brain injuries commonly arise from blunt injuries to the head during 'closed head injuries', such as road traffic accidents, falls, assaults, or sporting injuries. In contrast, 'open head injuries' occur when a sharp object penetrates the skull and tend to result in more localised damage. Closed head injuries tend to result in a diffuse array of cognitive, behavioural, and emotional symptoms.

Because multiple mechanisms may be involved in ABIs, the resulting neural damage tends to be heterogeneous. Damage to the prefrontal cortex often leads to changes in personality and psychological adjustment, such as irritability, disinhibition, and aggression (Vaghela et al., 2023). Rates of depression and anxiety are elevated following ABIs. Overall quality of life tends to be impaired because of an interaction between biological factors such as the severity of the injury, psychological factors such as anxiety and depression, and social factors such as unemployment and reduced social participation (Mamman et al., 2024). Emotional support and psychosocial interventions may therefore play an important role in rehabilitation (see Research Box 7.2). ABIs can affect attention and working memory, and therefore impair people's capacity to be involved in medical decision making, but there is growing evidence of the value of some memory remediation strategies (Kohler et al., 2020; Lambez & Vakil, 2021).

Research Box 7.2

Improving Psychological Wellbeing after a Brain Injury

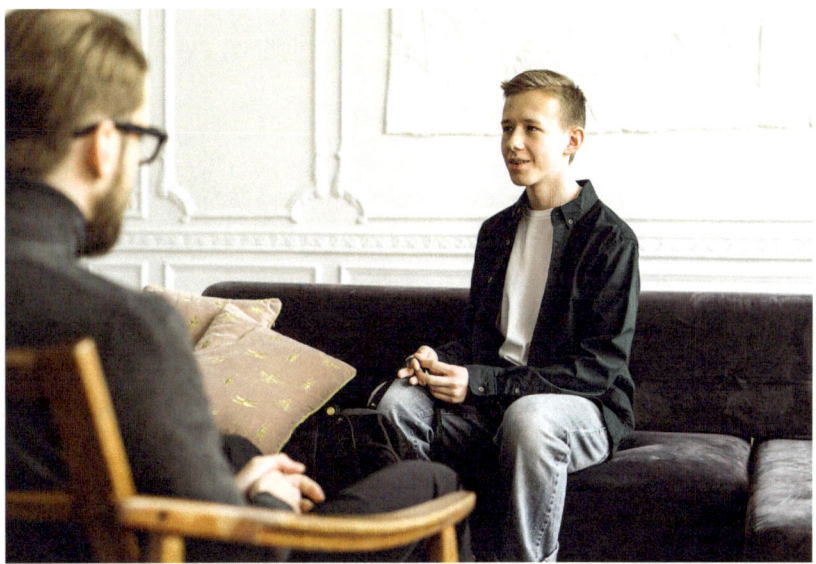

Figure 7.9   Adolescent in a CBT session

Source: © cottonbro studio/Pexels

Background

Rates of anxiety are elevated following acquired brain injury (ABI). Anxiety is bad in itself, but it can also limit educational and social activities, and this may explain elevated rates of depression. Adolescents are particularly susceptible to anxiety in social settings, so there is a need to find effective ways to reduce anxiety and enhance social rehabilitation following an ABI.

(Continued)

Method and Findings

This randomised controlled trial (RCT) evaluated an 11-session cognitive behavioural therapy (CBT) programme for anxiety that was adapted for adolescents post-ABI. Thirty-six Australian 12–19-year-olds with an ABI were randomly allocated to either the in-person CBT intervention or a wait-list control group. Anxiety, depression, and participation in daily activities were assessed before the intervention, immediately after the intervention, and then two and six months later.

The intervention resulted in reductions in anxiety and depression, which were not seen in the control group, and which persisted for the six-month follow-up period. There were no significant changes in participation in daily activities.

Significance

CBT can be an effective way to reduce anxiety and depression in adolescents with ABI. Further work could determine which specific components of the CBT led to change, how participation in daily activities can be enhanced, and whether online delivery could maintain effectiveness while also increasing accessibility.

Soo, C.A., Tate, R.L., Catroppa, C. et al. (2024) A randomized controlled trial of cognitive behavioural therapy for managing anxiety in adolescents with acquired brain injury. *Neuropsychological Rehabilitation*, 34(1): 74–102. doi:10.1080/09602011.2022.2154811.

Summary 7.5

- Neurological disorders may arise from progressive degenerative processes or acute events, such as a stroke or traumatic brain injuries.
- The severity and impact of neurological disorders depends on the location and extent of the neurological damage involved.
- Neurological disorders can cause impairments to physical functioning as well as changes in mood and personality.

7.4.1 Neuropsychological Assessment

Neuropsychological rehabilitation focuses on improving a person's physical, behavioural, and social functioning. An important part of rehabilitation programmes is a thorough neuropsychological assessment to establish the precise nature of any impairments, and to enable the individualisation of rehabilitation programmes (Luria, 1963 [1948]). Neuropsychological assessment may be conducted for various purposes: (1) describing and measuring cognitive deficits, (2) differential diagnosis (whether cognitive deficits are part of another psychiatric disorder), and (3) monitoring neuropsychological rehabilitation.

A complete neuropsychological assessment involves the examination of senses, as well as memory and problem solving. A useful tool is the **Mini-Mental State Examination** (MMSE), which provides a brief, standardised way of assessing someone's cognitive capacities (Folstein et al., 1975). The Montreal Cognitive Assessment and Addenbrooke's Cognitive Examination serve similar purposes (Bruno & Schurmann Vignaga, 2019; Patnode et al., 2020).

Physiological or neuroimaging assessments may also be made. Tests of cranial nerve function include assessments of movement and sense perception. Tests of motor nerve function include assessment of reflexes and observations of involuntary movements, weakness, or incoordination. Sensation of touch or temperature in the limbs can also be assessed. Further investigation may include computerised tomography (CT), magnetic resonance imaging (MRI), and functional MRI (fMRI). Analysis of cerebrospinal fluid can give information about infections and cancers.

7.4.2 Neuropsychological Rehabilitation

The prospects for recovery from neural damage are influenced by the size and location of any damage, the state of the brain before the injury, and the person's personality and coping styles (Luria, 1963[1948]; Wilson et al., 2017). Key tasks for rehabilitation include improving cognition, communication, mood, and behaviour. Prospects for rehabilitation following traumatic brain injury may be hampered if the brain injury means that the person is unaware of the need for rehabilitation, or has experienced changes in attention and personality that make it harder for them to engage with it.

Over recent decades, there has been a trend toward community-based neuropsychological rehabilitation. Such programmes are designed to enhance the development of independence (Wilson et al., 2017). They often involve the provision of appropriate support in the home and workplace. There has been increased use of technologies to aid memory, decision making, and the organisation of daily activities (Mura et al., 2018; D.S.M. Ong et al., 2021). Rather than being an exclusive relationship between patients and health professionals, rehabilitation has come to be seen as a partnership involving people's families. All parties in this partnership must work together to achieve optimal cognitive, physical, and social wellbeing (see Research Box 7.2).

Rehabilitation should be designed to achieve goals that are relevant to the person. This will make it more likely that the person and their family will remain involved in rehabilitation. The general principles of goal setting must apply here. Goals should be agreed with the person and should be SMART: **S**pecific, **M**easurable, **A**chievable, **R**ealistic, and have **T**imelines for achievement (see Clinical Notes 7.4).

Clinical Notes 7.4

Neuropsychological Rehabilitation and Goal Setting

- In designing rehabilitation for people with neuropsychiatric disorders, it is important to set goals and targets that are relevant for each person. This can increase their motivation and adherence. This general principle can be applied in other medical contexts.

(Continued)

- Goals should be SMART:

    o **S**pecific – stick to specific behaviours.
    o **M**easurable – behaviour must be measurable so progress can be recorded.
    o **A**chievable – within their capabilities. This often means you need to start with very small goals.
    o **R**ealistic – goals need to be easily carried out and attained within the context of the person's life.
    o **T**ime specific – give a time in which the goal must be achieved.

- An example of a SMART goal for a depressed and socially withdrawn person might be to walk to the local shops every day for a week.

Decisions about which approaches to use should be influenced by the nature of the goals to be reached and the capabilities of the person (Wilson et al., 2017). They may entail learning new ways of performing tasks or interacting with people and coming to terms with limitations. The techniques chosen should maximise the person's attention to the immediate tasks and longer-term goals. Rehabilitation must aim to improve not only cognitive functioning, but also mood and social functioning.

Summary 7.6

- Neuropsychological rehabilitation focuses on addressing the cognitive and emotional deficits arising from neural damage or degeneration.
- Neuropsychological assessment can be used as part of a diagnosis, for planning rehabilitation, and for monitoring progress. It focuses on cognitive capacity and may also involve physiological or neuroimaging assessments.
- The prospects for rehabilitation in neurological disorders are influenced by the characteristics of the neurological impairment (nature, size, location, etc.) as well as the characteristics of the person, such as their coping style.
- Neuropsychological rehabilitation should be designed to meet goals that are important to the person.

Conclusion

This chapter has given an introduction to a broad range of linked topics. The outline of healthy structure and function of the nervous system was followed by a section that highlighted the importance of sleep for cognitive functioning and wellbeing. The discussion of the role of predisposing, protective, precipitating, and perpetuating factors in psychological distress, psychiatric disorders, and neurological disorders highlighted the need to take a broad biopsychosocial approach to diagnosis and treatment.

Further Reading

Carlson, N.R. & Birkett, M.A. (2021) *Physiology of Behavior* (13th edition). Boston, MA: Allyn & Bacon. A standard textbook on neuropsychology and biological psychology, it contains detailed descriptions and illustrations of brain structures and functions.

McKnight, R., Price, J. & Geddes, J. (2019) *Psychiatry* (5th edition). Oxford: Oxford University Press. A comprehensive, clear, and authoritative overview of psychiatry. A major limitation is that it contains no references.

Stevens, L. & Rodin, I. (2024) *Psychiatry: An Illustrated Colour Text* (3rd edition). Edinburgh: Elsevier. Accessible, brief chapters on a range of topics. Each topic is covered in a two-page spread that gives a good introduction that can be supplemented by further reading.

Wilson, B.A., Winegardner, J., van Heugten, C. & Ownsworth, T. (eds) (2017) *Neuropsychological Rehabilitation: The International Handbook*. Abingdon: Routledge. Provides broad coverage of individual and group approaches to rehabilitation. It also includes numerous case examples, and considers approaches used in different countries.

Revision Questions

1. Describe the organisation of the nervous system (i.e. central, peripheral, autonomic divisions) and the functions of each division.
2. Explain why damage to the brain stem has different consequences than damage to the frontal lobes.
3. Discuss the accuracy of the statement: 'When a person is asleep, her/his body and brain are at rest'.
4. Describe how sleep deprivation may affect health professionals' competence.
5. Describe the 'three Ps' that are used to explain the onset and progression of psychiatric disorders. Why is it important to consider a 'fourth P'?
6. Why is combining drug therapy and psychotherapy often more effective for psychiatric disorders than either treatment in isolation?
7. Choose one neurological disorder. Outline its causes, physical and psychological symptoms, and prospects for treatment.
8. Why is a thorough neuropsychological assessment for rehabilitation necessary? What procedures are used in this assessment?
9. Outline the purposes and practices of neuropsychological rehabilitation.
10. Why may issues related to consent be more problematic in psychiatric and neurological disorders than in physical disorders?

8

PSYCHOSOCIAL DEVELOPMENT ACROSS THE LIFESPAN

—Learning Objectives—

This chapter is designed to enable you to:

- Describe the major psychosocial developmental changes that occur in childhood.
- Outline how language and thinking develop through childhood and adolescence.
- Describe the physical and psychological changes and challenges of adolescence.
- Discuss stability and change in physical and cognitive capacity during older adulthood.
- Appreciate how changes across the lifespan affect practitioner–patient communication.

Psychosocial development occurs across the lifespan. At different ages, we acquire different cognitive and social skills and enact different social roles (see Chapter 9). One way of thinking about these changes is by using Erikson's (1950) division of the lifespan into eight stages, each characterised by a particular developmental challenge that must be resolved for optimal psychosocial functioning (see Table 8.1).

Although these challenges are psychological in nature, health and illness can influence the extent to which people are able to resolve them. For example, physical disabilities may affect the development of autonomy in childhood. Similarly, people's health may be affected by their experience of each developmental conflict, such as adolescents engaging in risky behaviours as part of exploring their identities. Furthermore, health, health-related behaviour, and other experiences during childhood can affect morbidity and mortality during adulthood (Bjerregaard et al., 2020; Horesh et al., 2021; Nurius et al., 2015).

Erikson's (1950) model indicates that although childhood is important, development and change occur across the lifespan. This chapter, therefore, outlines a lifespan approach to development. Health professionals must be able to identify abnormal patterns of development and treat these appropriately to minimise disturbances to physical and psychological growth. We also need to be aware of people's capabilities at different ages to facilitate optimal practitioner–patient communication.

Table 8.1   Erikson's model of lifespan development

Age	Conflict	Outcomes
Infancy	Trust vs Mistrust	Children develop a sense of trust in other people when their carers provide reliable care and affection
Early childhood	Autonomy vs Shame/doubt	Children develop a sense of autonomy and independence derived from acquiring physical skills. Failure leads to shame and doubt
Preschool	Initiative vs Guilt	Children begin to assert control over their environment and develop a sense of purpose. Efforts to exert too much power result in disapproval and guilt
School age	Industry vs Inferiority	Children need to cope with new social and intellectual demands and develop feelings of competence
Adolescence	Identity vs Role confusion	Adolescents need to develop a strong personal identity. Failure leads to role confusion and a weak sense of self
Young adulthood	Intimacy vs Isolation	Adults need to form strong intimate relationships. Failure leads to loneliness
Middle adulthood	Generativity vs Stagnation	Adults need to create and nurture things that will outlast them (e.g. children or social changes) to provide feelings of accomplishment and usefulness
Maturity	Ego integrity vs Despair	Older adults need to feel fulfilled when they reflect on their lives. Failure leads to regret and despair

8.1 Childhood

Childhood is a time of astounding and rapid psychosocial development. It is important to understand typical patterns of psychosocial development so that deviations from these norms can be identified and addressed.

8.1.1 Attachment and Development

Attachment is a strong affectional tie felt for another. Children feel pleasure and joy when interacting with caregivers with whom they have a secure attachment, and comfort from being near them in times of stress. Unless infants have secure trusting attachments to their adult caregivers, normal cognitive, social, and emotional development may not occur.

Quality of Attachment

Various attachment styles have been identified. They can be broadly divided into secure attachment versus different types of insecure attachment. The original way in which attachment was measured is a research technique known as the 'strange situation' (Ainsworth et al., 1978). This is a situation in which a mother brings her child to a room with toys in it, leaves the child for a short while, and then returns. By observing how much exploration and play the child engages in, and how they respond to their mother's departure and return, children's attachments may be categorised into the attachment styles shown in Table 8.2. The most common type of attachment is the most adaptive one, with around 70% of children displaying secure attachment. These general patterns tend to be found in different 'western' cultures, but there may be some differences in other cultures (Agishtein & Brumbaugh, 2013; van Ijzendoorn & Kroonenberg, 1988).

Table 8.2 Attachment styles in the 'strange situation'

Attachment style	Child's behaviour when mother leaves	Mother's parenting style
Secure attachment	Child gets upset when mother leaves but calms down quickly when she returns, and explores the environment when she is there	Mother is quick to respond to physical and emotional needs of the child. Helps the child to cope with their stress
Avoidant attachment	Child explores the environment and does not respond when mother leaves or returns	Mother does not respond when child is upset: tries to stop child crying and encourages independence and exploration
Ambivalent attachment	Child gets upset when mother leaves but can be comforted by a stranger. When mother returns the child will act ambivalently and may resist contact or appear angry	Mother is inconsistent – varies between responding quickly and appropriately on some occasions and not responding on other occasions. Child is therefore preoccupied with whether mother is available before they can use her as a secure base
Disorganised attachment	Can be secure, ambivalent, or avoidant but also shows some difficulty coping when the mother returns, with behaviour such as rocking themselves or freezing	Mother's behaviour can be negative, withdrawn, inappropriate, roles not clearly defined, sometimes child maltreatment

The Importance of Secure Attachment

Secure attachments to carers are important because they develop feelings in children that they are worthy of love and care, and that others will be available to them in times of need. They establish children's 'internal working models' for all subsequent close relationships (Bowlby, 1973). The internal working models of children with less secure attachments do not include an expectation that they are worthy of love and care.

Secure attachment during childhood has broad and lasting influences on development. It promotes optimal development of the brain – especially the limbic system, which is crucially involved in emotional regulation (see Chapter 7). Insecure attachment resulting from neglect and a lack of stimulation can lead to serious underdevelopment in these brain regions (Lang et al., 2020; Ross et al., 2021). Secure attachment also results in better social competence and peer relations, better emotional competence and self-reliance, better cognitive function, and better physical and psychological health (Borowski et al., 2021; Park et al., 2023).

The importance of the interaction between genes and environment for neurological and cognitive development is an archetypal example of why 'nature versus nurture' debates have been replaced by an understanding of the interaction between genes and environment. The field of **epigenetics** focuses on how environmental factors – including social contextual factors – regulate the activity and expression of genes (Smeeth et al., 2021; Thumfart et al., 2022). Environmental influences such as a lack of nurturing in early childhood can lead to neurological and endocrine changes that can then be passed to the next generation (see section 1.5.2).

Given the importance of attachment, one might wonder whether all is lost if a secure attachment to parents does not develop or is not possible. Research has indicated that adopted children can develop secure attachments with their adoptive parents – especially those adopted at an earlier age (van den Dries et al., 2009). Most children also have a degree of resilience which will allow them to recover to some extent from earlier neglect or abuse.

How Does Attachment Develop?

Several different accounts for the development of secure attachments have been offered. Freud's **psychoanalytic theory** proposed that the mother becomes the primary love object in the baby's life because she satisfies the infant's need for food and oral pleasure. **Learning theory** argues that a positive perception of the mother is formed because the baby learns that breast-feeding satisfies hunger (and the mother learns that breastfeeding calms the baby).

Bowlby (1969) argued that Freud's psychoanalytic perspective fails to acknowledge attachment as a psychological bond in its own right rather than an instinct derived from feeding or sexuality. Bowlby's view concurred with Harlow's (1958) research with monkeys separated from their mothers, which showed that attachment is formed on the basis of comfort and protection rather than nourishment. In that research, baby monkeys separated from their mothers were found to prefer a fake surrogate 'mother' covered in soft fabric to a wire 'mother', even when the wire 'mother' provided milk.

Bowlby argued that humans have a set of in-built attachment behaviours that are designed to maintain close contact with a particular person who is perceived to be better able to cope with the world. In babies, the attachment behaviours include clinging to caregivers, crying for their attention, and smiling at their return. Even in the first week after their birth, babies prefer to look at faces that engage them in a mutual gaze, and assessment of neural activity in infants shows that they have enhanced neural processing of direct eye contact (Guellaï et al., 2020; Simion et al., 2011). Infants are very sensitive to attention from adults and to interpersonal interaction with adults, and they quickly notice when adults do not respond to them. For example, the image and the video referred to in Figure 8.1 show that when an adult who has been interacting

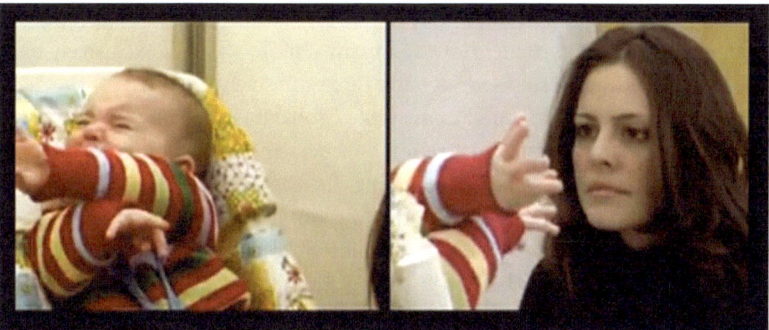

Figure 8.1   Still face study – infants become distressed if carers do not respond to them

Source: Still image taken from www.youtube.com/watch?v=YTTSXc6sARg&t=74s, reproduced with permission from University of Massachusetts

with an infant stops responding, the child quickly exhibits signs of discomfort and distress (Mesman et al., 2009).

Attachment develops in stages as infants develop greater skills for directing their attention and actions, such as the following and clinging behaviours assessed in the 'strange situation' with children aged from 12 to 18 months.

Parent–Infant Bonding

For an attachment to parents to occur, infants must know who their parents are. The process of **bonding** to carers begins before birth. In the first few days of life, babies use various senses to learn who their carers are. It is important, therefore, for parents to engage in behaviours which maximise this multisensory input for their children, as follows:

- *Physical contact*: mothers should be encouraged to keep babies in contact with them as much as possible to provide sensory input in the form of touch, warmth, smell, sound, and sight.
- *Smell*: babies quickly learn to associate their mother's smell with comfort, pleasure, and nourishment.
- *Sound*: from an early age, babies can distinguish between their mother's voice and the voices of other people, and will prefer their mother's voice to other similarly pitched female voices.
- *Sight*: even though their focal distance is only around 25 cm, three-day-old babies can visually distinguish between their mothers and other people.

Although most of the research has focused on mothers, bonding with fathers is important and the principles described above also apply. Parent–infant bonding in the first days sets an important foundation for subsequent parent–child interaction. However, all is not lost if there is less contact during the early period. Strong parent–child bonds can be formed with premature or sick babies who must spend time in incubators, and between parents and adopted children.

8.1.2 Breastfeeding and Development

Breastfeeding is an important mother–infant interaction. On the basis of solid empirical evidence of the health benefits, the World Health Organization (2013) advocates that infants be exclusively breastfed for the first six months of life. However, many children are not exclusively breastfed for six months. Globally, it is estimated that 48% of babies are exclusively breastfed for the first six months, and considerable change will be required to meet the Global Breastfeeding Collective's (2023) target to reach 70% by 2030. A review of breastfeeding practices in high-income countries revealed that although 91% of babies received some breastfeeding, the proportion breastfed until age six months was 45%, and the proportion exclusively breastfed was only 18% (Vaz et al., 2021).

A review of longitudinal studies that follow children from infancy into childhood found that those who were breastfed perform better on tests of intelligence, even after taking into account maternal intelligence and the home environment (McGowan & Bland, 2023). The optimal duration for breastfeeding appears to be around six to nine months, with lower test scores found for those not breastfed at all, breastfed for less than six months, or exclusively breastfed for more than nine months. Exclusive breastfeeding beyond nine months may produce nutritional deficiencies.

Several different factors may explain the links between breastfeeding and intelligence. First, nutrients in breast milk – especially long-chain fatty acids – may contribute to better neural development. Second, physical and psychological attention during breastfeeding may foster greater intelligence. Third, factors related to both breastfeeding *and* children's intelligence may be important. Chief among these are the characteristics of mothers who breastfeed, because better-educated and more intelligent mothers are more likely to commence and continue breastfeeding (Horta et al., 2015).

Meta-analyses of studies designed to follow children over time show that greater breastfeeding during infancy is associated with lower rates of childhood asthma, and may also protect against eczema and allergic rhinitis (Victora et al., 2016). Some of these positive effects may be due to the immunomodulatory qualities of breast milk and/or the avoidance of allergens. Longer breastfeeding also appears to reduce the risk of subsequent overweight/obesity, high blood pressure, and Type 2 diabetes (Victora et al., 2016).

Rates of early initiation of breastfeeding, exclusive breastfeeding, and continued breastfeeding can be improved when counselling and education are provided concurrently in home, community, and health systems settings (Chipojola et al., 2022; Tomori et al., 2022). An example is provided in Research Box 8.1. As in other domains, reviews of intervention efficacy highlight the importance of ensuring that they are composed of recognised psychosocial behaviour change techniques (Kassianos et al., 2019).

Research Box 8.1

Educating Fathers to Support Breastfeeding

Background

The World Health Organization (2013) advocates that infants be exclusively breastfed for the first six months of life. However, many children receive no breastfeeding, and very few are exclusively breastfed for six months. It is important, therefore, to identify effective ways to encourage and support mothers to breastfeed. Fathers are a potentially important, but under-used, resource.

Methods and Findings

In this Iranian study, 76 fathers were randomly allocated to either a control group or an intervention group, and were assessed for their own support for breastfeeding, and their partner's current level of breastfeeding. Men in the intervention group then received two individual in-person education and counselling sessions that outlined the benefits of breastfeeding and explained how to support their partner's breastfeeding. All men were followed up four months later. Comparisons between the two groups after four months revealed that the intervention was related to significant improvements in fathers' support for breastfeeding and increases in whether there was any breastfeeding or exclusive breastfeeding.

(Continued)

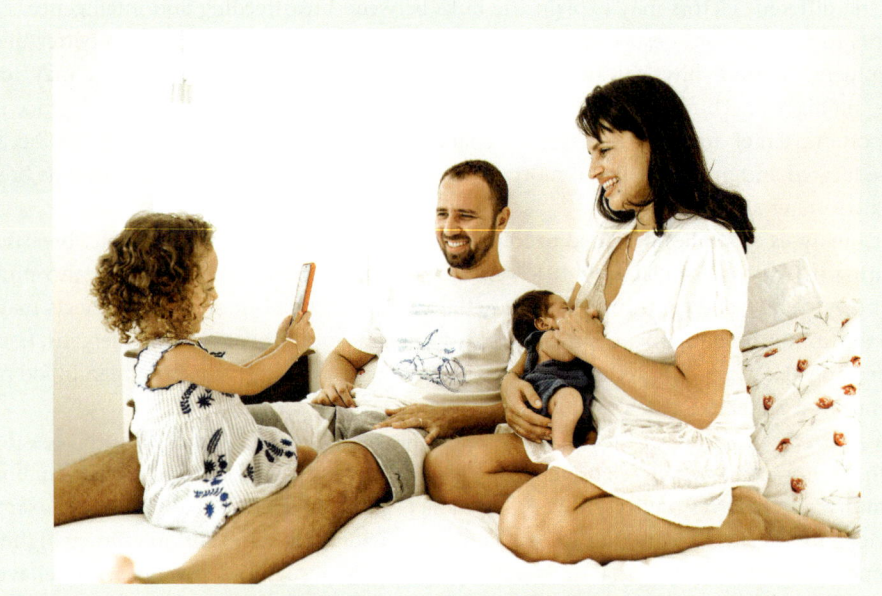

Figure 8.2   Fathers as social support for breastfeeding

Source: © Jonathan Borba/Unsplash

Significance

This study indicates that to promote breastfeeding, healthcare interventions should not only focus on mothers, but should also focus on fathers and other important sources of social support.

Panahi, F., Fakari, F.R., Nazarpour, S. et al. (2022) Educating fathers to improve exclusive breastfeeding practices: A randomized controlled trial. *BMC Health Services Research, 22*(1): 554. doi:10.1186/s12913-022-07966-8.

8.1.3 Language Development

Learning to use language is one of the most important intellectual capacities a child will ever develop. As well as being essential for communication in its own right, language is important for many other learning skills: imagine what school would have been like if you were not able to understand your teacher or ask questions! Various theories have been developed and applied to explain how children progress from nonsensical babbling at six months of age to grammatically sophisticated speech just a few years later.

Some researchers have emphasised the importance of **operant conditioning** and **observational learning** (Skinner, 1957; see Chapter 10). Such perspectives argue that children develop their capacity for language in response to encouragement and correction from parents and other people. They also argue that children's imitation of adult speech is important. Although children may learn the meanings of words in these ways, they cannot explain how children learn the complex rules of grammar – that is, rules about how words must be put together so as to make sense.

In contrast to behaviourism and social learning theories, **nativism** argues that children have an innate predisposition for language, that is, they have in-built capacities for making sense of language. Chomsky (1965) argued that humans are unique in having an innate biologically-based language acquisition device (LAD) which allows children who know a few words to generate grammatically correct statements and understand what others say. The argument that the LAD is a *unique* human feature has received support from studies of language learning in primates. Such research indicates that although primates can learn to use sign language or symbols to communicate, they possess no understanding of grammar. Although Chomsky's ideas have been influential, they have some limitations. In particular, although there are specialised language areas in the human brain (see Chapter 7), there is no evidence that the LAD is located in a specific brain region.

Interactionism appears to offer a bridge between the opposing perspectives of Skinner (1957) and Chomsky (1965). Interactionism argues that language learning is a combination of nature *and* nurture. Children learn language via the combination of an innate linguistic capacity, a strong desire to connect with others, a rich linguistic and social environment, and the reinforcement of their efforts.

Evidence for the interactionist perspective comes from the observation that adult–child communication is quite different from adult–adult communication. It involves closer physical proximity, more prolonged eye contact, exaggerated facial expressions and gestures, and the use of **motherese** or **parentese**. Parentese is an alternative name for adult–child speech, which is a simplified version of adult–adult speech. Table 8.3 shows that, compared to adult–adult speech, parentese is shorter, less complicated, and much slower.

Table 8.3 Comparison of 'parentese' and speech between adults

	Adult–child	Adult–adult
Utterance length	4 words	8 words
Utterances with conjunctions (e.g. because)	20%	70%
Utterances with a pause at the end	75%	51%
Speed (words/min)	70/min	132/min

These differences are significant changes, not slight adjustments. Other features of parentese are that it is more likely to be in present tense, is more likely to use proper names rather than pronouns (e.g. 'Daddy's nose is bleeding' rather than 'My nose is bleeding'), has more repetition, and features exaggerated intonation. Young children appear to prefer parentese – the intonation and rhythm can attract and hold their attention. These features mean that children's natural predisposition for language learning is nurtured through interactions with others (Ferjan Ramírez et al., 2024).

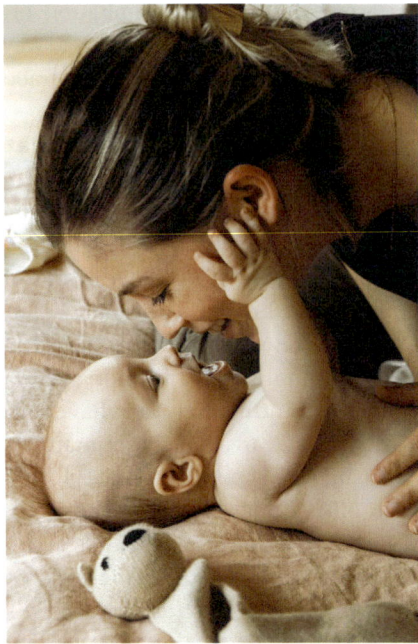

Figure 8.3 Mother–baby interaction and motherese

Source: © Febe Vanermen/Pexels

Stages of Language Development

Babies babble long before they speak their first real words. This is not a simple imitation of adult speech: it includes sounds that may not even be used in the language(s) spoken in a child's home. Babbling is a generalised system of vocalisations. Nature provides infants with the sounds they may need, and nurture gradually moulds the use of sounds that are appropriate for their language. It is important that parents show interest in babbling because this indicates to the child that they are part of the social system. Parents' communication with babies at this stage can also help them to learn that vocal sounds have meanings (e.g. people's names).

The mean age of babies saying their first word is 12 months (but the range is from eight to 18 months). By this age, infants begin to use sounds to convey meaning. However, the meaning of these single-word statements is not always clear: when an infant says 'ear', it may mean 'This is my ear', or 'My ear hurts', or something else entirely. Parents can help their children learn words by giving a 'running commentary' of what they are doing and using expressions and gestures to provide clues to meaning.

From around the age of two, children begin to use 'telegraph speech', which contains mainly nouns and verbs. Words are used to express desires (e.g. 'Feel tired'). From age three there is a rapid progression to complete sentences. In addition to using more words per sentence, children begin to use possessive pronouns ('mine', 'Daddy's'), negatives (e.g. 'can't' rather than 'no'), and modifiers (adjectives like 'big' and adverbs like 'quickly'). Language begins to be used to express thoughts and emotions. Some of these changes can be linked to developments in cognitive capacity. By age five, children have vocabularies of thousands of words and can understand quite complex sentences.

Implications for Practitioner–Child Communication

As in all contexts, communication will be best when there is a match between the demands of the situation and the capacities of the people involved. Medical consultations with children are affected by:

- *Children's language capacity*: very young children may not possess the precise vocabulary used by medical professionals (e.g. what does 'I have a tummy ache' really mean?).
- *Practitioners' communication skills*: health professionals should be sensitive to how a child's age may affect their ability to understand, and should make appropriate adjustments to their manner of speech.
- *Interaction between practitioner and child*: it is important to consider whether parents can be used as 'translators' for their children.

Health professionals need to be aware of how language capacity develops with age, and adjust their communication style as appropriate.

Summary 8.1

- All children have an innate capacity to learn language – the language acquisition device (LAD).
- The interactionist perspective argues that, in addition to the LAD, experience is important. For example, 'parentese' helps children to learn to use their innate capacity for language.
- Adults can help children to develop their language capacity by encouraging them and providing feedback.
- Health professionals should match their language to the capacities of children, for example, by using elements of 'parentese' in consultations with young children.

8.1.4 Intellectual Development

How does a child's mind grow? When and how do children begin to think symbolically, reason logically, and see things from another person's perspective? The following section attempts to provide answers to these questions and to discuss the implications for medicine and healthcare. It commences with the influential theory of Piaget, followed by a discussion of some criticisms of Piaget's theory and the insights offered by Vygotsky.

Piaget's Stage Theory

Central to Piaget's (1954) influential theory was the idea that a child's mind is not a miniature version of an adult's mind waiting to be filled with information: the child's mind develops into an adult mind through four discrete stages (see Figure 8.4). Although each stage can be broken into sub-stages, development always proceeds in the same order and the order of stages is universal. In this theory, the term 'operations' refers to the ways in which children work out problems. The stages in Piaget's theory are:

- **Sensorimotor stage**: Babies experience the world through their senses. They cannot 'think' because they live in the moment with no abstract concepts. However, they can exhibit intelligent behaviour (e.g. pulling a blanket to get a toy that is out of reach but resting on the blanket). Before eight months, infants do not understand object permanence, which is the awareness that things that are out of sight still exist.
- **Pre-operations**: Language acquisition brings a fundamental change to intellectual development because language is symbolic: words are symbols that refer to real things. Linked to this capacity for symbolic thought, a major change from the sensorimotor stage is the capacity to imagine things. This is reflected in play, where a stick can become a sword or a magic wand. In this stage, children are **egocentric**. They are unable to see things from another person's perspective or consider the point of view of others. For example, in hide-and-seek, children may think that if they cannot see you, then you cannot see them. In medical and healthcare contexts, children may not be aware that other people do not know what symptoms they are experiencing.
- **Concrete operations**: Children begin to learn to use logical processes. They can manipulate real (concrete) objects to solve problems, such as using their fingers or blocks to do addition and subtraction. In addition, children can learn the principle of conservation, that is, that moving, spreading out, or rearranging objects does not change them. In this stage, children develop the capacity to see things from another person's perspective.
- **Formal operations**: Children become able to reason not just on the basis of real physical objects, but also on the basis of hypotheses or propositions: for example, '$x^2 + 4 = 13$, what is the value of x?' During this stage, thinking becomes multidimensional: children become able to consider various possibilities rather than just the most obvious solution to a problem. Other important developments include metacognition (the capacity to think about thinking) and introspection (the capacity to think about emotions).

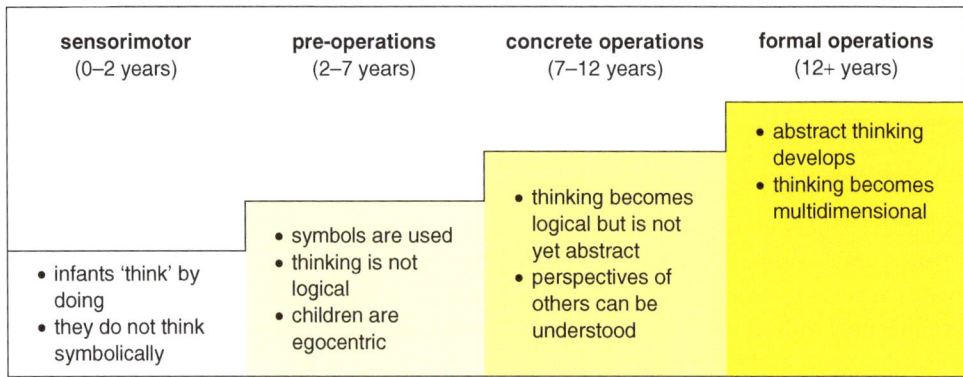

Figure 8.4 Piaget's stage model of intellectual development

Numerous studies have shown that development tends to follow Piaget's order. However, Piaget's ideas have been criticised (e.g. Lourenço, 2016). Development of intelligence is smoother and more gradual than Piaget's argument for step-like jumps between stages. Piaget also seems to have underestimated children's capacities and overestimated adults' capacities. For example, many adults do not always use formal operational reasoning. It has also been suggested that younger children's difficulty with reasoning tasks is strongly influenced by their inability to understand complex adult language. Furthermore, pre-operational children do have some capacity to consider others' perspectives.

Vygotsky's Theory of Social Development

A fundamental principle of Vygotsky's theory of social development is that full cognitive development requires social interaction (Daniels, 2017). Vygotsky emphasised the importance of culture for learning. At a broad level, culture teaches children both *what* to think and *how* to think. At the individual level, children learn through problem solving that is shared with someone else – a friend, a sibling, a parent, or a teacher. Compared with Piaget, Vygotsky gave greater emphasis to the importance of language in learning. Vygotsky argued that language is crucial for collaborative problem solving and that such collaborative problem solving is important for children's cognitive development.

Vygotsky argued that learning occurs in the 'zone of proximal development', which is the gap between what a child can do without help and what they can do with appropriate guidance or collaboration. With such help from adults or peers, children can perform tasks they would be incapable of completing on their own. Furthermore, teaching and learning will be more effective if there is a continual adjustment of the level of help given so that children become more independent at solving problems.

Understanding Others' Perspectives

As noted earlier, young children are egocentric: they cannot take on the perspective of others. Young children also lack a '**theory of mind**': they do not understand that other people have different thoughts, emotions, and perceptions. Autistic spectrum disorders are often characterised by impairments in theory of mind tasks.

Children aged two or three use words like 'want', which reflect the development of knowledge of an inner self. Over time, this understanding is applied to other people, and children come to understand that they can infer the mental states of other people. Thus, we may say that they possess a naïve theory of mind. Having a theory of mind allows us to empathise with others. However, it also allows us to deceive. For example, children who possess a theory of mind can understand what they need to do to feign illness to avoid school. Similarly, when poker players bluff, they are applying their theory of mind.

Healthcare consultations with young children clearly need to take into account the issues of egocentrism and an absence of a theory of mind. Young children may assume that others know what they are feeling and experiencing. Health professionals therefore need to encourage young children to explain all of their symptoms and concerns, even if these appear obvious to the child.

Children's Understanding of Illness

Children's understanding of illness and treatment varies with age (Lockhart & Keil, 2018; Toyama, 2016; see Research Box 8.2). Understanding of illness progresses from concrete, egocentric explanations to abstract, multidimensional explanations.

Although Table 8.4 suggests a stage-like development of understanding of illness, this is not strictly true: understanding illness is influenced by experience. Thus, young children with leukaemia may understand the disorder much better than other children of the same age. This suggests that explanations of illness and disease should build on prior experience and not be based simply on chronological age. Such findings also support Vygotsky's argument that children's understanding develops best if they receive appropriate help from considerate adults.

Table 8.4 Children's explanation of illness (Bibace & Walsh, 1980)

Age	Explanation of illness
2–4	Phenomenism – particular objects are believed to cause illness but there is no sense of the mechanisms involved
4–7	Contagion – illness is caused by proximity to ill people or to particular objects
7–9	Contamination – illness is caused by physical contact with an ill person and may be viewed as punishment for misbehaviour
9–11	Internalisation – illness is located within the body but may be caused by external factors, e.g. people get colds from being cold
11–16	Physiological – illness is caused by malfunctions in organs or systems which may be due to infections
16+	Psychophysiological – psychological factors like stress and fatigue can affect physiological processes, rather than only being an outcome

Children's understanding of illness can be enhanced by the use of developmentally appropriate interventions that break complex information into more easily digested pieces and present them in child-friendly ways (see Research Box 8.2). There is evidence that such interventions can alleviate children's fear of medical procedures, and that medical students who take part in such interventions subsequently feel more confident communicating with children about medical topics (Kis et al., 2022). Medical communication with young children – whether it is verbal consultation or information leaflets – should therefore avoid using abstract concepts. With all children, it is important to focus on their 'here and now' experiences and concerns.

Research Box 8.2

Child-Friendly Interventions Enhance Understanding of Illness

Background

The 'Teddy Bear Hospital' is a worldwide concept designed to reduce children's fear of hospitalisation and medical procedures, and to enhance their medical knowledge. Children bring their teddy bears to be treated by medical students playing the part of 'teddy docs'. Based on theories of child development and previous research, it was expected that taking part in a role-play situation suitable for children's developmental stage should enhance their knowledge of the body, health, and illness.

Method and Findings

The participants were 139 children aged four to five years attending kindergartens in Germany. Eight kindergartens were randomised to be intervention schools where the Teddy Bear Hospital was run, and eight kindergartens served as a control group. Children's understanding was assessed at the beginning and end of a two-week period. Children in the intervention group were assessed before and after visiting the Teddy Bear Hospital.

Results showed that children were able to learn effectively through role-play in the Teddy Bear Hospital. Children who visited the Teddy Bear Hospital had enhanced knowledge of the body, health, and disease at the second assessment. This was particularly clear in relation to their knowledge of internal organs.

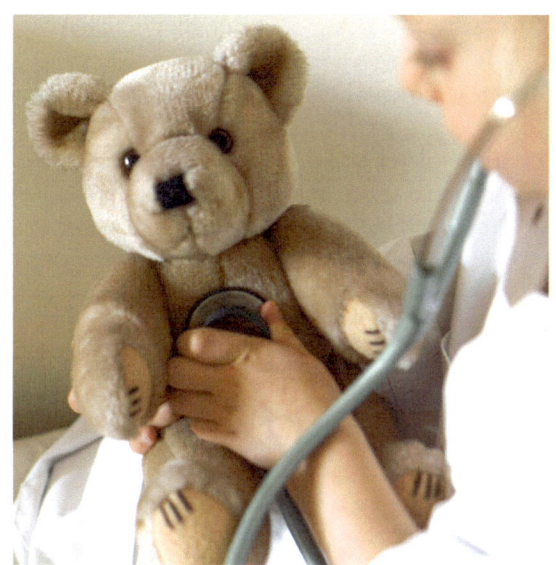

Figure 8.5　Role-play in the Teddy Bear Hospital

Source: © Derek Finch/Pexels

Significance

Children's understanding of illness can be enhanced by providing age-appropriate information in an appropriate format and context.

Leonhardt, C., Margraf-Stiksrud, J., Badners, L., Szerencsi, A. & Maier, R.F. (2014) Does the 'Teddy Bear Hospital' enhance preschool children's knowledge? A pilot study with a pre/post-case control design in Germany. *Journal of Health Psychology, 19*: 1250–1260.

Clinical Notes 8.1

Communicating with Children

- Adjust your consultation style to the capacities of children: pay attention to the language you use and the complexity of the ideas you are trying to convey.
- Younger children will not understand abstract concepts or internal bodily processes. However, be aware that some children can have very advanced knowledge of the illnesses they have been exposed to.
- Explain things to children in age-appropriate ways, such as using dolls or action figures to get their attention and help them to understand.
- Age-appropriate information booklets can increase children's understanding of illness, treatment, and recovery.
- If necessary, use parents or other adults to help you communicate with children.

Summary 8.2

- Young children's thought processes are fundamentally different from those of adults.
- Initial thought processes are based on real-world objects and an egocentric perspective.
- Before developing a 'theory of mind', children will not know that others do not share their thoughts/feelings and may not disclose pain/symptoms.
- Young children cannot understand abstract or unobservable concepts such as infection.
- Experience interacts with the developmental stage to produce an understanding of illness.
- Age-appropriate information increases children's understanding of illness and recovery.

8.2 Adolescence

Although adolescence is often equated with the physical changes of **puberty**, it is a biopsycho-social phenomenon that involves physical, cognitive, and social changes. The major psychological challenges of adolescence include adjusting to a changing body size and shape, coming to terms with sexuality, adjusting to new ways of thinking, and striving for emotional maturity and economic independence.

The average age of the onset of puberty is around 13 years, but there is a range of a few years around this average. Puberty begins one to two years earlier for girls than boys. It is the most rapid growth period after prenatal development and early infancy. During a period of around four years, adolescents grow an average of 25 cm/10 inches in height and gain 18 kg/40 lb in weight. There are also marked changes in hormone levels, especially testosterone and oestradiol (estradiol). The end point is sexual maturation and an adult physique.

In developed countries, the age of onset of puberty has fallen by three to four years over the last few hundred years due to improved standards of living, including better health and better nutrition. These factors are important because puberty's onset is associated with girls reaching a critical body mass (~48 kg/7.5 stone) and body fat proportion (~17%). These changes mean that it is now common to reach biological maturity at an age when cognitive and social maturity have not been reached.

8.2.1 Psychological Aspects of Puberty

Responses to puberty are different for boys and girls and are tied to different body shape ideals. In terms of body shape, girls tend to be less satisfied than boys (Alm & Låftman, 2018; Toselli et al., 2021). This is influenced by the fact that in high-income countries, the socially ideal body shape for women is often seen to be similar to that of pre- or early-adolescent girls (i.e. very thin), whereas the socially ideal body shape for men is adult (i.e. tall and muscular). However, it is important to note that during puberty both boys and girls feel worse about their bodies than before or after. There are also observed changes in mood. Boys tend to express more anger and irritability; girls tend to express more anger and depression. These alterations may be due to hormonal changes or responses to new life events and developmental challenges.

Puberty onset is earlier for girls than boys, and girls who mature early tend to dislike the experience. Boys may like maturing early because they are the first of their male peers to gain height and musculature. Many boys and girls express dissatisfaction with their body image during adolescence. Research indicates that although girls are more likely to express dissatisfaction with their bodies, levels of satisfaction often vary over adolescence (Lacroix et al., 2023). Such studies also show that many girls and boys feel under pressure to conform to the ideal body shapes of modern consumer culture and that peer criticism of appearance is an unavoidable part of adolescent life for both boys and girls. Concerns about appearance do not only apply to body shape; they are also influenced by cultural ideals of clear, blemish-free skin (Nguyen et al., 2016; Stamu-O'Brien et al., 2021). The importance of taking a biopsychosocial perspective (Chapter 1) is highlighted by the observation that in relation to both body image and skin, levels of satisfaction are influenced by psychosocial factors, such as the quality of relationships with family and peers, and academic performance.

Relationships with Parents and Other Adults

Important changes occur in parent–child relationships during adolescence. On one hand, adolescents separate their identity (individuate) from their parents, becoming more emotionally and behaviourally independent and autonomous. On the other hand, there is continued emotional connectedness, but changes to relationship quality (Arnett, 2004; Erikson, 1950, 1968; Soenens & Vansteenkiste, 2020).

One important domain of adolescent–adult interaction is medical consultations. Research indicates that many adolescents are dissatisfied with their interactions with health professionals. Some of this dissatisfaction stems from concerns about privacy and confidentiality; some arises from embarrassment from talking about sensitive issues such as body image, sexual behaviour, or illegal behaviours such as alcohol or drug use. It is therefore important to be sensitive to these concerns and to remind adolescents that information exchanged in consultations will be private and confidential. Such reassurance can make it more likely that adolescents will disclose sensitive health information (Baldridge & Symes, 2018; Kim & White, 2018). It is also important to encourage adolescents to develop their capacity to discuss their health concerns and to be involved appropriately in decision making during medical consultations (Grootens-Wiegers et al., 2017).

We often think of practitioner–patient communication as a two-way interaction. However, it must be acknowledged that parents may have legal rights and responsibilities relating to medical consultations involving children below the age of consent. It is therefore important to consider a triadic approach that addresses the complex interplay of adolescents, parents, and healthcare providers (Pampati et al., 2019). However, there is also a need to be aware that older adolescents may feel uncomfortable or dissatisfied with three-way communications involving themselves, health professionals, and their parents. This dissatisfaction may be more likely if they feel that they are being spoken about rather than spoken to. If parents insist on being involved in medical consultations involving their adolescent children, then it may be helpful to ensure that at least part of the consultation involves seeing the adolescent in a confidential context without their parents (Baldridge & Symes, 2018; Duncan et al., 2011).

—Clinical Notes 8.2—

Working with Adolescents

- Adjust your consultation style to the capacities and experiences of adolescents. Pay attention to the complexity of your explanation and check that they understand the terminology used.
- Be aware of adolescents' concerns about their appearance and body image.
- Be aware of people's embarrassment when talking about their health concerns. Respond in a non-judgemental way and reassure them that information will be treated confidentially.
- You may need to be tactful when negotiating with adolescents and their parents about the role of parents in consultations and decision making.

8.2.2 Cognition, Risk Taking, and Identity

Piaget's (1954) stage theory argued that formal operational thought develops during adolescence. The improved decision-making capacity of adolescents is supposed to make them better able to identify alternative courses of action, identify the consequences of each alternative, evaluate the desirability of each consequence, assess the likelihood of each consequence, and logically combine all of this information to make the best decisions about their behaviour. This should reduce the likelihood that they will make bad decisions. However, adolescents seem to be good at making bad decisions! This is reflected in the fact that accidents are the leading cause of death among young people (World Health Organization, 2024c), and in the high rates of unintended pregnancies (Ahinkorah, 2020; Kortsmit et al., 2023) and unhealthy behaviours (GBD 2019 Risk Factors Collaborators, 2020; Mokdad et al., 2016) among young people.

Although the development of metacognition (the capacity to think about thinking) and introspection (the capacity to think about emotions) should facilitate a better understanding of others, much of adolescents' thinking is directed toward themselves. Thus, adolescents may become self-absorbed and **egocentric**. However, this is different from the egocentrism that is characteristic of the pre-operational stage: pre-operational children cannot help their egocentrism, whereas adolescents can. The combination of metacognition, introspection, and egocentrism can lead to feelings of there being an imaginary audience observing our actions. Adolescents tend to have a heightened sense of self-consciousness and may feel that their behaviour and appearance are the focus of everyone else's concern and attention. In this stage, they may develop a 'personal fable' (Elkind, 1967). This is a belief that all of their experiences are novel and unique (e.g. 'nobody has ever felt love this strong'). The personal fable may be dangerous when it is applied to health-risk behaviour (e.g. 'I won't get pregnant' or 'I won't have a car crash'). Although young people may express unrealistic optimism about health risks, unrealistic optimism is not necessarily more common among adolescents than adults (Cohn et al., 1995; Knoll et al., 2015).

The term 'subjective expected utility' is used to explain the value people give to a particular outcome. Higher rates of risky or unhealthy behaviour may, however, reflect differences in beliefs about the subjective expected utility of different behaviours (Savage, 1954). Put another way, adolescents may not think the 'bad' outcomes of their risky behaviour are as likely or as bad as adults think they are.

A certain amount of risk taking is appropriate during adolescence. For example, Erikson's developmental theory highlights the importance of 'trying out' different identities and related behaviours during adolescence (Erikson, 1968; Fryt et al., 2022; Icenogle & Cauffman, 2021). Adolescents have increased access to a range of potentially risky behaviours, such as alcohol consumption, motor vehicle use, and sexual activity, and some of these behaviours are important aspects of their socialisation into adulthood. Furthermore, many health-risk behaviours are gendered, and adolescents may engage in risky behaviours as part of the development of their gender identities. Thus, many young men seek to test or display their masculinity by engaging in risky or unhealthy behaviours (de Visser & McDonnell, 2013).

Risky behaviour is also influenced by social contextual factors. For example, adolescents are more likely to take risks when they are with same-age peers but less likely to do so when alongside or with older adults (Centifanti et al., 2016; Knoll et al., 2017). Brain imaging studies suggest that activity in brain regions involved in affect, cognitive control, and social information processing varies according to the type of social context and the social actors who are present (e.g. adolescent peers evoke different effects than adults do; van Hoorn et al., 2019).

Summary 8.3

- Puberty onset is earlier today than 100 years ago. This has been influenced by improved standards of living and better diet.
- Responses to the process and outcomes of puberty are different for boys and girls.
- Major developmental tasks include adjusting to a new body size and shape, coming to terms with sexuality, using new cognitive capacities, and developing maturity and independence.
- Adolescents begin to disengage from family activities but one-on-one quality interactions with parents often stay the same.
- Adolescents' interactions with health professionals can be affected by embarrassment when talking about sensitive issues, concerns about confidentiality, and the presence of parents during consultations. It is important to be aware of, and responsive to, these concerns.
- Although adolescents have an improved decision-making capacity, their egocentrism may distort their perception of risk.

8.3 Adulthood

There is no clear line separating adolescence and adulthood. The differences between adolescence and adulthood have been blurred by the fact that in developed countries young people now take longer than previous generations to complete their education, gain their financial independence, establish their own households, form long-term relationships, and have children. It has therefore been suggested that the period from the late teens to the early twenties should be conceived of as 'emerging adulthood' (Arnett, 2004).

After rapid and profound changes in cognitive and psychological functioning during childhood and adolescence, 'established adulthood' is a time of relative calm (Mehta et al., 2020). However, it is during adulthood that patterns of behaviour and psychological states linked to the major causes of morbidity and mortality become established. There are many examples of these throughout this book, but particularly in the chapters on body systems (see Chapters 15 to 19).

Although adulthood is often thought of as a period of stability, there can be important changes. Many of these relate to changes in social roles and adjustment to major life events, such as having children, moving house, changing jobs, and experiencing the deaths of loved ones. Gaining, losing, or changing social roles can be stressful and may lead to depression (see Chapter 9). Furthermore, prolonged stress can have serious negative consequences for immune and endocrine function (see Chapters 3 and 15). Although stressful life events and negative role changes tend to be linked to poorer physical and psychological wellbeing, the impact of such events varies according to coping responses and social support. It is therefore important that adults develop and maintain effective individual coping skills and supportive social networks.

8.4 Old Age

Current life expectancy globally is 76 years for women and 71 years for men, but there are notable regional differences. For example, in Europe, life expectancy is 81 for women and 75 for men, and in Africa life expectancy is 67 for women and 62 for men (World Health Organization, 2024d). Life expectancy today is around 30 years longer than it was in 1900, and five years longer than it was in 2000. Although life expectancy has increased, birth rates have fallen, and, as a result, the proportion of the population who are elderly is increasing. It will be around 25% by 2050 (GBD 2021 Demographics Collaborators, 2021; GBD 2021 Fertility and Forecasting Collaborators, 2024).

Control of infectious diseases means that there is a lower burden of disease among young people and a concentration of illness and death among the elderly. This **compression of morbidity** has occurred because the age of onset of chronic disease has increased more rapidly than life expectancy – that is, people stay well for longer, but illness is compressed into the final phase of life (Fries et al., 1989; Newton, 2021). Combined with changes in population composition, it means that a greater proportion of medical consultations and expenditure will be concentrated on older people. So, unless you work in paediatrics or obstetrics, you are likely to encounter increasing numbers of elderly people.

8.4.1 Health Promotion among the Elderly

It is generally accepted that ageing involves reduced physical capacity. So, should older people resign themselves to physical decline? The answer to this question is a definite 'no'. Physical decline can be significantly reduced by encouraging older people to maintain or initiate healthy lifestyles. Research suggests that regular, moderate physical activity among older people can lead to significant improvements in some areas of immune function (Mathot et al., 2021). In addition, lung cancer and cardiovascular risk among smokers falls rapidly within a few years of quitting smoking (Caini et al., 2022; Tindle et al., 2018). Furthermore, even among older people, the likelihood of an earlier death is influenced by whether they continue or change unhealthy behaviours (Phan et al., 2022). However, behaviour change may be more difficult among older people than among younger people because their patterns of behaviour may have become more habitual.

─**Activity 8.1**─────────────────────────────

Beliefs about Ageing

- Stop for a moment and note the images that come to mind when you think about elderly people.
- Are the images that come to mind mostly positive or negative? Is there a mixture?

8.4.2 Ageing and Psychological Wellbeing

Stereotypes of elderly people are often contradictory. On the one hand, elderly people are seen as 'sages' with a lifetime's knowledge and experience. On the other hand, they are seen as 'senile' or 'demented'. In general, our society has a negative view of ageing, which is seen as the loss of youth and a decline in physical, cognitive, and social functioning.

As the proportion of older people in the population increases, so too will the number of people with dementia, and although the prevalence of **dementia** does increase with age, it is a myth that *all* old people suffer from fundamental intellectual decline (see Case Study 8.1) (GBD 2019 Dementia Forecasting Collaborators, 2022). Furthermore, there appear to be various effective ways to limit cognitive decline. Dementia is present in less than 5% of adults aged 60–69, less than 10% of those aged 70–79, and less than 25% of those aged 80–89 (Prince et al., 2015).

When discussing the intellectual capacities of the elderly, we must distinguish between 'crystalline intelligence', which reflects experience and long-term memory, and 'fluid intelligence', which reflects processing speed and short-term memory. Tests of fluid intelligence (e.g. IQ tests) suggest that many older people are 'mentally disadvantaged'. However, their behaviour does not match this description. One reason for this is that crystalline intelligence may compensate for declines in fluid intelligence. In addition, IQ tests may not assess real-world skills. 'Brain training' activities are often marketed as a solution to cognitive decline, but research shows that the gains tend to be limited to the specific tasks involved in the brain-training game (McPhee et al., 2019; Simons et al., 2016). So, practising anagram puzzles may make a person better at that task, but not better at managing changes to their household budget. To preserve broad cognitive functioning, people should engage in a broad range of cognitive activities, and these activities should ideally be tailored to the specific capacities and needs of the individual (Turnbull et al., 2022).

Age-related declines in fluid intelligence may be associated with physical health and organic change in the central nervous system. Reviews of research evidence indicate that increasing levels of physical activity among older adults may improve their cognitive function, regardless of their initial cognitive status (F.T. Chen et al., 2020), and that such benefits are also observed among the subsample of older adults with dementia (Zeng et al., 2023). This is in addition to the improvements in immune function noted earlier (Mathot et al., 2021).

Case Study 8.1

Successful Ageing

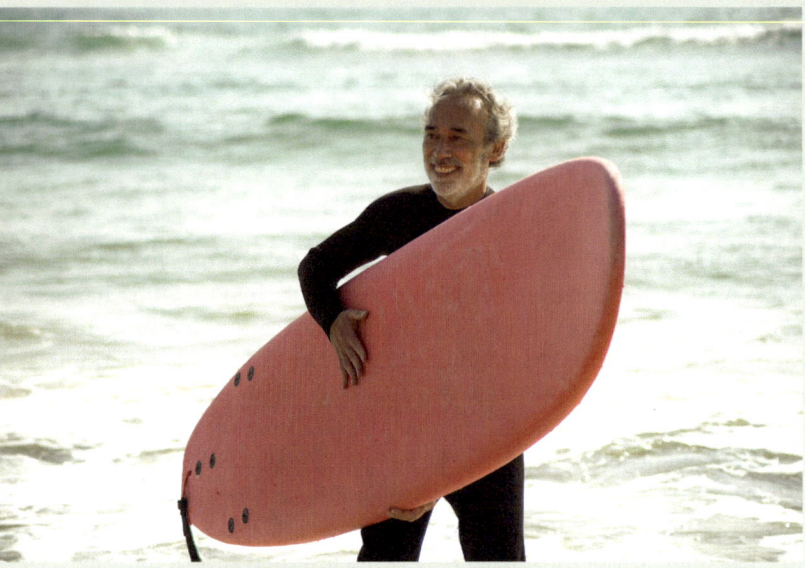

Figure 8.6   Staying active in older age

Source: © Kampus Production/Pexels

It is a myth that all old people suffer from a fundamental intellectual decline and restriction of their lifestyle. When Fred Hale Senior died in November 2004 at the age of 113, he was documented as the world's oldest man. Although few people achieve such old age, his experiences show that many elderly people maintain fully active lives:

- At 95 he tried boogie-boarding while visiting Hawaii.
- He participated in his last deer hunt at age 100.
- At 103 he was still living independently, shovelling the snow off his rooftop.
- His driving licence was renewed at age 104, but he gave up driving at 108, because slow drivers annoyed him.
- He maintained an active interest in sport and bee-keeping.

Although his longevity may have been influenced by genetic factors, his lifestyle was also important. He attributed it to eating three full meals at the same time each day, never smoking, rarely drinking alcohol, and eating at least a teaspoonful of honey and bee pollen every day.

Depression in Older Age

The prevalence of depression tends to increase with age. Depression tends to be associated with declines or losses in other areas, including functional disability, cognitive impairment, and social deprivation (Aziz & Steffens, 2013; Maier et al., 2021). As in earlier phases of life, depression is more common among elderly women than men. Psychosocial influences on increased rates of depression include role loss (see Chapter 9) – particularly among men for whom work was an important component of identity – and negative life events. Bereavement has an important impact on rates of depression. Older people are more likely than younger people to experience the death of their spouse and friends. Given that average life expectancy is longer for women, in each age band there is a greater proportion of widows than widowers. This may help to explain higher rates of depression among older women than men.

Clinical Notes 8.3

Working with Elderly People

- Be aware of your own stereotypes and prejudices related to ageing and the elderly. Do not let these lead to poorer care for older people.
- Adjust your consultation style to the capacities of older people.
- Do not assume elderly people are frail or senile – difficulty with hearing or talking does not mean they are stupid!

8.4.3 Healthcare of Older People

As older people are an increasing proportion of the population, there are concerns that increased demands for health and social care will have to be met by a smaller proportion of tax payers of working age, or an increased reliance on informal or voluntary carers, many of whom may themselves be managing the impacts of ageing (Morgan et al., 2020; Robine et al., 2007).

Negative stereotypes about ageing can lead to the stigmatisation of older people and a neglect of issues concerning them. It is often assumed that older people are physically frail, cognitively impaired, and have diminished social engagement. These stereotypes and prejudices then affect the quality of service provision: many elderly people are not treated with the respect and dignity to which all people are entitled (Liu et al., 2012; Rush et al., 2017). Mistreatment of older people in health and social care settings is not purely due to a lack of resources, but also reflects negative attitudes (Care Quality Commission, 2013; Yaghmour, 2022).

Although some elderly people experience substantial declines in cognitive function with age, most do not. It is therefore important for health professionals to check their patients' cognitive function and adjust their consultation skills accordingly. During consultations with older people who have clear declines in fluid memory, allow more time for information to be considered before asking further questions. It is important not to fill silences with more questions, as this can lead to a communication breakdown.

It is also important to consider people's expectations of consultations. Although younger people may expect and appreciate a more patient-centred approach to consultations, older people may be more comfortable with a patriarchal approach, wherein the practitioner is the expert who is expected to provide solutions and make decisions. At any age, it is important to tailor consultation styles to people's capacities and preferences: among older people, effective verbal and nonverbal communication strategies can have a positive impact on various patient-focused outcomes (Sharkiya, 2023).

Summary 8.4

- Compression of morbidity means that people stay healthier for longer, but have a concentration of illness and/or disability at the end of their lives.
- Even in old age, changes in health-related behaviour are beneficial to physical and psychological wellbeing.
- Ageing is linked to declines in fluid intelligence (i.e. cognitive processing speed), but not crystalline intelligence.
- Depression is common in old age, particularly in women.

Conclusion

This chapter has given an overview of the significant and widespread components of psychosocial development that occur across the lifespan. Many of these key changes occur alongside the physical developments of childhood and adolescence. However, it must be noted that across the lifespan, changes in psychological and social functioning are often closely linked to physical wellbeing.

—Further Reading—

The three textbooks below have been prepared for psychology students. They provide a lot of detail, but little attention is given to medical applications.

Bee, H. & Boyd, D. (2013) *The Developing Child* (13th edition). Boston, MA: Allyn & Bacon. A standard text on development during childhood and adolescence, it is very reader-friendly and has a range of illustrations of the major points.

Berk, L. (2015) *Child Development* (9th edition). Boston, MA: Allyn & Bacon. Also a standard text on child and adolescent development, it has reader-friendly images and text boxes to help you understand the key points.

Santrock, J. (2021) *Life-span Development* (18th edition). Columbus, OH: McGraw-Hill Education. Includes the whole lifespan, and while much of it covers childhood, it has a broader focus than the first two books listed here. Neverthelesss, it still provides information on childhood development.

—Revision Questions—

1   Why is infant–adult attachment important for children's development?
2   Describe the link between breastfeeding and intelligence.
3   How does the interactionist approach to language learning differ from the nativist (LAD) approach?
4   What should practitioners do to promote effective practitioner–child communication?
5   Describe the central features of Piaget's theory of cognitive development.
6   Explain why 'theory of mind' is important for medical consultations with young children.
7   Adolescents are supposed to have adult-like capacities for risk assessment, so why are they more likely to take risks?
8   What is meant by the compression of morbidity? How does this affect the number of medical consultations with older people?
9   Summarise the major changes in cognitive capacity observed in old age.
10 What factors need to be considered during consultations with older people?

9

SOCIAL PSYCHOLOGY

─Learning Objectives─

This chapter is designed to enable you to:

- Discuss the links between attitudes and behaviour, and the importance of attitude change in encouraging healthy behaviour.
- Describe how self-perceptions influence a range of health behaviours.
- Discuss the importance of group membership to individuals and how group membership can influence individual behaviour.
- Outline the different explanations of aggressive behaviour.
- Identify the factors that can increase the likelihood of prosocial behaviour.

Social psychology helps us to consider such issues as how we present ourselves to others, our health behaviour, how a group makes decisions, and even whether we are able to challenge senior doctors if we believe they are wrong. For example, in 2003 one junior doctor was ordered by a senior doctor to administer a combination of two drugs to a man with leukaemia. The combination was lethal. The junior doctor asked the senior doctor twice if this was correct, but was told to go ahead, with devastating consequences (Ferner & McDowell, 2006). Social psychology examines why we carry out such actions and which social forces contribute to them. In this chapter we consider how people's attitudes and beliefs about themselves can influence their behaviour, including their health-related behaviour. We then address the issues of conformity, aggression, and how individuals behave as members or leaders of groups.

9.1 Attitudes

In social psychology and health promotion, a great deal of attention is given to attitudes. **Attitudes** can be defined as a measure of people's like or dislike of an object. The 'object' may be a real object, a person, or a behaviour such as 'healthy eating'. The expectancy-value model suggests that attitudes are the product of expectancy about an object and the value given to that object (see Chapter 5). For example, attitudes toward condom use will be shaped by expectancies (e.g. condoms reduce sexual pleasure) and the value of the expectancies (e.g. sexual pleasure is important). Thus, two people with the same expectancy may have different attitudes because they give different values to this expectancy.

Attitudes reflect what we think about something, how we feel about it, and how we plan to behave (Eagley & Chaiken, 1993). Ideally, the thinking, feeling, and behaving components of attitudes will be consistent with each other. When we hold inconsistent beliefs or when our behaviour does not match our beliefs, it leads to unpleasant cognitive dissonance, which we will be motivated to reduce (Festinger, 1957). People may seek to reduce cognitive dissonance by changing either their attitudes or their behaviour. Thus, an overweight person who knows this is unhealthy may either decide to lose weight or change their beliefs about their weight.

9.1.1 Attitudes and Behaviour

Attitudes measured at one time can often be used to predict behaviour at a later time. Attitudes are therefore central to many models of health behaviour (see Chapter 5). However, it is important to note that other beliefs (e.g. normative beliefs) and social factors influence whether attitudes are acted upon.

Changing Attitudes and Changing Behaviour

Because attitudes predict subsequent behaviour, it is generally accepted that attitude change should be a productive way to change behaviour. The enormous sums of money spent on advertisements for cars, soft drinks, cosmetics, and so on reflect the belief that people's purchasing behaviour will change if their attitudes toward products are changed. For example, in the last decade, fast-food chains have changed their advertising to counter concerns that their meals are unhealthy in an effort to retain their market share. Mass media health promotion campaigns also try to encourage behaviour changes by changing people's attitudes toward healthy and unhealthy behaviours.

These efforts are based on the hypothesis that there is generally agreement between people's behaviour and the affective, cognitive, and behavioural components of attitudes (Eagley & Chaiken, 1993). According to the theory of cognitive dissonance, if we change people's attitudes toward their current unhealthy behaviours, this will set up dissonance between their new attitude and their established behaviours. They should then change their behaviour to reduce the dissonance between their attitudes and behaviour.

'Foot-in-the-door' techniques are an interesting illustration of how our desire to behave consistently with our attitudes can be manipulated (Burger, 1999). These techniques involve asking people to agree to a simple request, which they are likely to comply with. Later, the same person is asked to agree to a substantially more demanding request, which is the actual target behaviour. For example, one study of French university students found that smokers who had previously agreed to a request to stop smoking for two hours were significantly more likely than other smokers to agree to a request to stop smoking for 24 hours (Guéguen et al., 2016). 'Foot-in-the-door' techniques produce better responses to requests for the target behaviour because once a person has agreed to the small initial request, they have demonstrated to themselves and others that their attitudes toward the cause are favourable and that they are committed to the behaviour. Similar principles underlie campaigns such as 'Meat-free Monday' (www.meatfreemondays.com), which aim to encourage larger-scale dietary change by encouraging people not to eat meat on one day per week. People who engage more with the campaign are more likely to completely eliminate meat from their diets (de Visser et al., 2021). Other techniques for encouraging behaviour change through attitude change are addressed below.

Persuasive Messages

If we wish to change health-related behaviour by changing attitudes, then we must be sure about the most effective ways to do so. A message is most likely to change people's attitudes if it:

- Reaches its recipient – different approaches can be used, including discussion during consultations, leaflets, or the use of mass media.
- Is attention-grabbing.
- Is understood by the recipient – it must be couched in the appropriate language and 'pitched' at the appropriate level of complexity.
- Is seen by the recipient as relevant and important.
- Is remembered by the recipient, translated into an intention to change behaviour, and acted upon.

The characteristics of the sender of the message – be they individual health professionals or organisations such as Departments of Health – influence whether the message will be persuasive. We are more likely to be persuaded if the sender of the message is:

- *Credible*: the qualifications and occupational status of health professionals may increase their persuasive power.
- *Trustworthy*: the perceived objectivity of health professionals may increase their ability to encourage an attitude and behaviour change.
- *Appealing*: health professionals should aim for appealing personal presentation.

Inducing a certain amount of fear – for example, by using graphic images of illness or injury – may motivate people to change their behaviour, but fear campaigns can be counterproductive. If fear-based campaigns do not also include sufficient information about what people can do to avoid a feared outcome, and do not boost self-efficacy for self-protective responses to the feared outcome, then people may simply avoid the issue rather than focusing on the issue and their behaviour (Kok et al., 2018).

Clinical Notes 9.1

Persuading People to Change their Behaviour

If you wish to change people's attitudes to their health-related behaviour:

- Make sure the message is clear, relevant to them, and easy to remember.
- Think of whether it is better to emphasise the gains or losses associated with current and desired behaviour.
- Pay attention to your own persuasive power based on your qualifications, occupational status, and credibility.
- Be aware that how you present yourself can influence people's perceptions of your status and credibility.

Framing effects can also be important (Rothman & Salovey, 1997). They refer to whether a message emphasises the benefits of a certain behaviour or the losses associated with that behaviour. Theories of message framing argue that when we want people to take up behaviours aimed at detecting health problems or illness (e.g. breast self-examination or HIV testing), loss-framed messages may be more effective. When we want people to take up behaviours aimed at promoting prevention behaviours (e.g. using sunscreen or using condoms), gain-framed messages may be more effective. Whereas there is a lack of clear evidence that framing *per se* makes much difference to behaviour change (Ainiwaer et al., 2021), it is also important to consider the types of gains or losses that may be most motivating for people. One review led to the conclusion that, where possible, messages should be tailored to people's stage of change (see Chapter 5) and framed to focus on self-determined motives and goals (Pope et al., 2018).

Ambivalence

For many attitudinal objects we do not have simple positive or negative attitudes. Instead, our feelings are often mixed (Miller & Rollnick, 2002). For example, we may have positive attitudes toward certain aspects of drinking less alcohol (saving money, feeling safer, being more in control, avoiding hangovers, etc.), but negative attitudes toward other aspects of drinking less (feeling more socially inhibited, fear of missing out, etc.). This ambivalence can influence efforts to change health behaviours because ambivalent attitudes tend to be worse predictors of behaviour than homogeneous attitudes (Conner et al., 2003; Conner et al., 2021). Furthermore, studies of adolescents highlight interactions between peer norms and personal ambivalence related to the use of tobacco and marijuana (Hohman et al., 2014; Hohman et al., 2016). The findings suggest that one way to reduce use of tobacco or marijuana may be to highlight to young people their own ambivalence toward these behaviours.

Summary 9.1

- People are motivated to keep their attitudes consistent with their behaviour. Thus, efforts to change health behaviour will often focus on changing attitudes.
- Attitude change messages should be tailored to maximise their persuasiveness. This means paying attention to the content of the message, the style of delivery, and the characteristics of the person delivering the message.

9.2 Self Psychology

One important focus of our attitudes is ourselves. A person's self-image is important for their health and wellbeing. We naïvely tend to assume that our selves are singular, continuous, and consistent: I think that when I woke up this morning I was more or less exactly the same person I was yesterday and will be when I wake up tomorrow. People with some psychiatric conditions may not always have this sense of unity (see Chapter 7).

Despite feeling that we have a singular self, it is possible to think of different definitions or different components of our selves. One key distinction is the difference between a personal self (how I perceive myself) and a social self (how others perceive me). These two selves may not always be in agreement. For example, someone may be perceived as calm and confident when talking in public while actually being a bundle of nerves. A distinction can also be made between personal identity, which consists of everything that makes someone a unique person, and social identity, which consists of the things someone shares with members of groups that are important to them (e.g. family resemblance, national identity, occupation). Processes of group affiliation and conformity will be addressed later in this chapter. For now, we will focus on ideas of the self.

9.2.1 Self-Esteem and Self-Image

Self-esteem has important links to behaviour and health. Self-esteem consists of feelings and evaluations about ourselves. It is often thought that low self-esteem is unhealthy, but research suggests that this assumption may be simplistic (Arsandaux et al., 2020; Baumeister et al., 2003). For example, young people with higher self-esteem may be more likely to experiment with cigarettes, alcohol, or other drugs rather than avoiding such behaviours (Maas & Lefkowitz, 2015). One area in which there are clear links between low self-esteem and ill-health is in relation to eating disorders: low self-esteem is a significant predictor of disordered eating (Krauss et al., 2023). Self-esteem can also be lowered in certain illnesses, especially in chronic conditions, whether they are physical or psychological (Liu et al., 2019; Pinquart, 2013;). Positive self-esteem is reflected in the promotion of a positive self-image to oneself and other people.

Most of us put a lot of effort into developing and promoting a favourable self-image. A key part of self-image is our appearance. Goffman (1959) used the analogy of acting in a play to explain how and why we modify our appearance and behaviour depending on where we are (the scene) and who we are with (our audience). For example, the clothes we wear and the amount of time we spend on our appearance will probably vary depending on whether we are at home studying, going to a party, or attending a formal meeting (see Activity 9.1). Appearance can also be a marker of group membership (Figure 9.1).

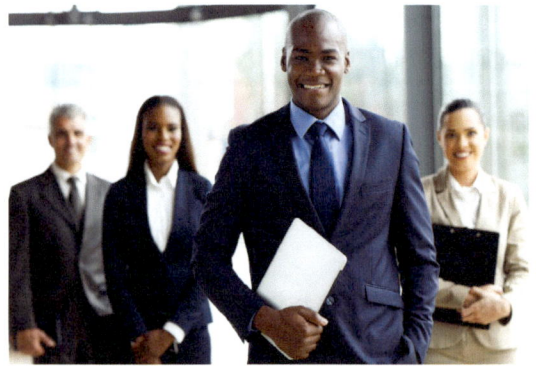 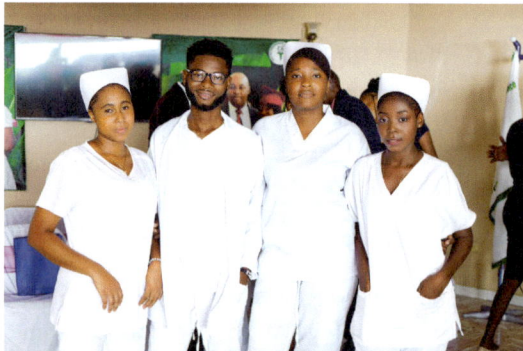

Figure 9.1   Group membership and dress

Source: © michaeljung/Adobe Stock; © Haguy Paulemon/Pexels

—**Activity 9.1**—

Self-Presentation and Clothing

Compare the following three settings:

1   The last time you were studying.
2   The last time you went out on a first date with someone.
3   The last time you had a formal interview.

In each of these situations:

- How much time did you spend planning what you would wear and getting ready?
- Did you do your hair and use cosmetics/shave?
- How did the clothes you chose reflect the self-image you were trying to project?

People also use appearance as a shorthand way of evaluating others. However, looks can be deceiving. In some cases, this can have implications for health. For example, we often assume that if a person looks healthy, they are healthy. This assumption can prove costly in the case of serious illnesses such as COVID-19 and HIV/AIDS, where there may be no visible signs of illness.

Hippocrates stated that physicians should be 'clean in person, well-dressed, and anointed with sweet-smelling unguents'. Research suggests that how physicians present themselves through their clothing and accessories influences people's trust and confidence in them (Petrilli et al., 2015). In general, people feel less positive about health professionals wearing casual clothes or jeans. However, preferences do vary between cultures and contexts: formal attire and white coats are generally preferred by older people, and preferences for attire are less obvious in intensive care or emergency settings.

How we behave in social situations is a component of maintaining a positive self-image. Most of us try to obey social conventions about appropriate and inappropriate behaviour in order to be perceived favourably. It is also important for our self-esteem to affirm positive aspects of ourselves when we are criticised. This can be done in various ways. The example in Highlight Box 9.1 shows that when we are criticised, we often try to publicly affirm positive aspects of our selves and/or denigrate the person who has criticised us.

One way to boost our self-image is to make social comparisons. One approach is to make downward comparisons with people whose problems or situation are worse than our own. For example, a person who has had a leg amputated following a car accident may feel better off than someone who has been made quadriplegic in a car accident. Another example is the responses of some drug addicts to criticism of their behaviour: 'functional' heroin addicts may compare themselves favourably to 'junkies' who engage in crime to support their drug use. In contrast, upward identification occurs when people highlight the similarities between themselves and others who are deemed socially superior so as to make their self-image more positive (Suls et al., 2002). People's upward identifications and/or downward comparisons have been found to lead to changes in anxiety and mood in people with severe challenges to their health (Petersen et al., 2012).

—Highlight Box 9.1—

Self-Affirmation

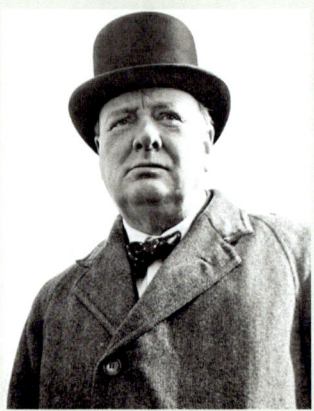

Figure 9.2 Photograph of Winston Churchill

The following exchange is reputed to have occurred between Labour MP Bessie Braddock and Conservative Prime Minister Winston Churchill:

Braddock: Mr. Churchill, you are drunk.

Churchill: And you, madam, are ugly. But in the morning, I shall be sober.

Churchill's response protected his self-image and self-esteem by highlighting the fact that his undesirable behaviour was temporary (and therefore not a fundamental part of him), whereas his critic's undesirable appearance was permanent.

Quote copyright © Winston S. Churchill

9.2.2 Attributions

Our efforts to create and maintain a positive self-image are also influenced by the attributions we assign to our own and others' behaviour. Internal attributions are based on the belief that a person's behaviour is internally motivated – that it is voluntary and reflects the person's attitudes. In contrast, external attributions are the beliefs that a person's behaviour is due to external factors such as luck, chance, or someone else demanding it.

In terms of our own behaviour, we tend to prefer internal attributions for our successes (e.g. 'I got an A for the exam because I studied really hard') and external attributions for our failures (e.g. 'I failed the exam because the lecturers set difficult questions'). In contrast, we tend to attribute others' behaviour to internal or dispositional causes rather than external or situational causes. This is known as the fundamental attribution error (Ross, 1977). This error means that we are more likely to attribute negative facts about other people (e.g. being unwell, anxious, or depressed) to their own behaviour or characteristics rather than to the broader social context. Examples of internal and external attributions for health are given in Table 9.1.

Table 9.1 Attribution errors and illness

	Internal attribution	External attribution
Obesity	They are lazy and greedy	There are not the right facilities or incentives to encourage activity and healthy eating
Depression	They are weak and unable to cope	They have experienced severely stressful life events

From this, it should be clear that attribution errors can have wide-ranging repercussions on clinical care through their impact on the doctor–patient relationship and understanding of the person's illness, and therefore treatment. In healthcare practice, we must be aware of making this error and ensure that we consider external and situational factors such as life circumstances and competing demands.

One application of attribution concepts within healthcare settings is the health locus of control (Wallston et al., 1978). An individual's locus of control reflects the extent to which they believe that they have control over their health. It can be divided into three components:

- *Internal*: the belief that what they do will affect their health. These people are more likely to seek information and to initiate and persist with changes in health behaviour.
- *Powerful others*: the belief that the most important influence on their health is other people, such as medical and health professionals, who possess knowledge and skills. These people may be more likely to seek and follow professional advice, but they are less likely to initiate changes in health behaviours.
- *External*: the belief that the maintenance of health and the onset of illness are due to fate, chance, or luck. These people are unlikely to take action to protect or promote their health.

The significance of attributions of control over health and illness is clear from longitudinal research which shows that children with a stronger internal locus of control have a reduced risk of obesity, hypertension, and poor physical or psychological wellbeing during adulthood (Gale et al., 2008), and that teenagers with a stronger external locus of control have a greater risk of obesity or harmful alcohol intake as adults (Cheng & Furnham, 2019). Furthermore, a more external locus of control has been found to be associated with lower psychological wellbeing (Hovenkamp-Hermelink et al., 2019; Kesavayuth et al., 2022). However, it should be noted that when people do not have any actual control over their situation, an internal locus of control may be detrimental. For example, the authors of a study of over 5,000 people with multiple sclerosis concluded that among people with that incurable terminal condition, having an external health locus of control was associated with better quality of life (Rothman et al., 2023).

9.2.3 Ideal Self and Actual Self

To varying degrees, most of us have biased appraisals of ourselves. Most of us probably think that we are more generous, helpful, and caring than others think we are. There may also be a discrepancy between our *actual* self (how we currently are) and our *ideal* self (how we would like to be) (Higgins, 1987). Perceived gaps between our ideal and actual selves can motivate a behaviour change. For example, a man may be motivated to take up regular exercise because when he looks in a mirror, he does not see the ideal athletic physique he desires.

Sometimes, the discrepancy between the ideal self and actual self can be distorted, with important consequences for our physical and psychological wellbeing. This is often observed among people with eating disorders such as anorexia nervosa and bulimia (Paterna et al., 2021; Walker et al., 2018). Influenced by cultural preferences and media images, many young women (and increasingly men) with eating disorders desire an ideal body image that is unrealistically thin and unhealthy (Mitchison & Mond, 2015; see Case Study 17.1). Men may also be affected and strive to attain an ideal physique which is unrealistically muscular (Badenes-Ribera et al., 2019; see Case Study 9.1). Research Box 9.1 describes the impact of a media literacy intervention designed to counter the impact of unrealistic media images (Kurz et al., 2022).

Research Box 9.1

Media Literacy Training to Counter the Impact of Unrealistic Body Images

Background

Media images influence many young women to internalise an ideal, thin body image that is unrealistic and unhealthy. This study investigated the impact of 'SoMe', a social media literacy programme for body image, dieting, and wellbeing for adolescents.

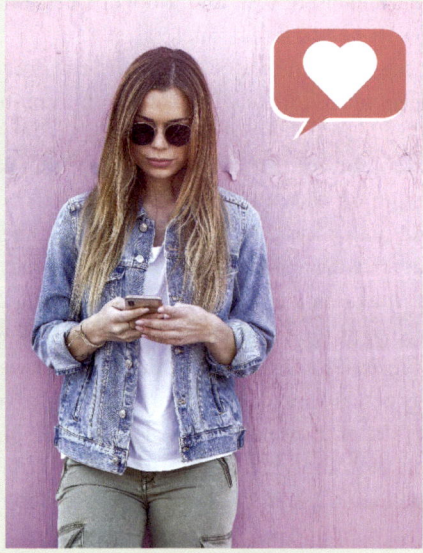

Figure 9.3 A secondary school student on social media

Source: © CDPiC/Adobe Stock

Method and Findings

Participants were 892 Australian secondary school students aged 11–15 years. The 483 students in the intervention schools received four weekly SoMe classroom sessions, and the 409 students in the control schools received lessons as usual. All completed a survey at the start of the study, after one week of the intervention period, and then six and 12 months later. The results revealed that girls in the intervention schools were less likely to report dietary restraint or depressive symptoms at six-month follow-up. No intervention effects were found among the boys.

Significance

Previous studies indicated that social media literacy training can affect what adolescents think about social media images, their own bodies, and their eating behaviour. The findings of this trial suggest a need to refine the intervention to maximise its existing impact, and a need to identify the young people who would benefit most from it.

Gordon, C.S., Jarman, H.K., Rodgers, R.F., et al. (2021) Outcomes of a cluster randomized controlled trial of the SoMe social media literacy program for improving body image-related outcomes in adolescent boys and girls. *Nutrients, 13*(11): 3825. doi:10.3390/nu13113825.

─Case Study 9.1─

Self-Image and Body Building

Sometimes the discrepancy between the ideal self and the actual self can be distorted, with significant consequences for physical and psychological wellbeing. Muscle dysmorphia is a form of body dysmorphic disorder in which men who are already more muscular than most men become preoccupied with the desire to be more muscular than they are.

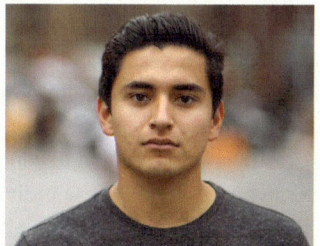

Figure 9.4 Tony's muscle dysphoria

Source: © blvdone/Adobe Stock

   Tony initially became interested in weight training when he was in high school. He had always felt small and was impressed by a friend's change in physique after he started weight training. Tony quickly became 'hooked' on training. He began spending increasing amounts of time at the gym and less time with friends. He found himself constantly thinking about his body and comparing it to those of other men at the gym. Although he had developed an extremely muscular physique according to any objective standard, he felt ashamed of his lack of musculature, and when he was not at the gym, he would wear baggy trousers and loose t-shirts to hide his body.

> No matter how big I got, or how much bigger I was than other guys, it didn't matter – I had to be even bigger. I started using supplements, but I wasn't getting bigger fast enough … so last year I started using steroids.

(Continued)

The steroids have produced some benefits, but they also have unwanted side effects. For someone so concerned about his appearance, the development of acne has been hard to bear. Tony's desire to be bigger has also led him to suffer in other ways:

> I started pushing myself too hard and was getting all these injuries … but that only made me want to train harder when I recovered to make up for the lost time. My shoulders and knees are shot from pushing weights that are too heavy.

Summary 9.2

- Our beliefs about who we are and who we want to be can have strong influences on our behaviour.
- We tend to attribute our successes to our efforts and our failures to external factors.
- The fundamental attribution error is our tendency to attribute other people's poor health or lack of success to their disposition or character rather than to the broader social context.
- Our beliefs about what influences our health (our efforts, other people, or fate) can influence the likelihood of initiating and maintaining healthy behaviours.

9.3 Individuals and Groups

Humans have a basic need for the company of others to avoid loneliness, to gain attention from other people, to bolster their self-image, and to reduce anxiety. Some people do prefer to live in isolation, but they are exceptions to a very strong social norm. For most people, group membership and group identity are important components of individual identity. Having a strong positive group identity can benefit our psychological and social wellbeing. However, group membership may restrict our individual freedom due to pressures to conform to group norms, and membership of some groups may expose individuals to prejudice, stigmatisation, and victimisation.

When you start working as a health professional you will acquire various identities, from the broad group of 'health professionals' down to the specific group forming the discipline or team in which you work. Social identity theory (Tajfel & Turner, 1986) proposes that a sense of belonging to valued groups is an important component of maintaining a positive self-image. Our membership of groups may be based on things we cannot change, including obvious physical characteristics such as ethnicity, sex, and age. However, our membership of other groups reflects the choices we make, such as our occupation, sporting team, or subcultural group (e.g. skaters, hipsters). Important markers of group identity include styles of dress and the kind of language used (vocabulary, accent, slang, etc.).

9.3.1 Social Roles

Most everyday interactions run smoothly because of shared beliefs and assumptions about how people should behave. Many social interactions are quite complex, and most of us behave in ways that indicate our awareness of what is appropriate and inappropriate behaviour. It is usually only when someone 'breaks the rules' that we will become conscious of them.

Goffman's (1959) dramaturgical theory suggests that social interactions can be thought of as being like a play in which interactions between people inhabiting different **social roles** are guided by shared assumptions about normal or appropriate behaviour. Social roles can be ascribed or acquired. Ascribed roles are those that are given to us independently of what we do (e.g. daughter/son). Acquired roles are those we attain through experience and social recognition (e.g. midwife). Each social role entails certain rights and responsibilities. Different social roles also allow us to behave in certain ways. To be recognised as socially competent, we must behave in ways that are appropriate to our social roles.

Changes in social roles can be stressful because of the links between social roles, identity, and social recognition. Gaining new roles can also be stressful because we need to learn new patterns of behaviour and prove that we are competent (e.g. getting a job promotion, becoming a parent). Feelings of failure or incapacity in social roles can lead to depression. Role loss can also be stressful (e.g. someone who has retired after 45 years working for the same employer). Role conflict (e.g. people trying to balance the new role of 'parent' with the established role of 'professional') can be another source of stress.

The concept of social roles is important in medicine and healthcare (Parsons, 1975). A person inhabiting the sick role has the right to relinquish other obligations – they can take time off work/school and avoid having to do daily activities, such as washing the dishes or taking out the rubbish. However, the sick role also entails obligations, such as the obligation to strive to get better, to follow medical advice, and not to engage in activities that may hinder recovery. Another important aspect of the sick role (as an ascribed role) is that it must be formally acknowledged. Because health professionals usually have to certify sick leave, they can be thought of as gatekeepers of the sick role. The social role of doctors bestows certain rights on them, such as the right to ask personal questions and conduct physical examinations. However, it also entails responsibilities, such as upholding professional standards and maintaining patient confidentiality.

9.3.2 Conformity

People generally have strong tendencies for conformity to the expectations of the groups to which they belong. The more we want to belong to a group, the more important it is for us to conform. Research has shown that people tend to go along with what others think – sometimes going against their own better judgement (Asch, 1956). When other group members have expressed a unanimous opinion, many people may find it hard to speak out against it.

Activity 9.2

Conformity

Imagine you are on your first day as a junior doctor. On ward rounds a senior consultant suggests a treatment that you believe is wrong. Several of the other group members seem to agree with the senior consultant.

- How easy would it be to say what you think rather than conforming to the group?
- What would you do?

Conforming to group norms can help to maintain distinctions between groups. One way to protect or improve our self-image is to make favourable comparisons between the groups to which we belong (the ingroup) and other groups (outgroups). For example, if the team I support wins an important match, I will feel good about myself and happy to be part of my ingroup rather than the outgroup (i.e. not part of a losing team). However, making favourable comparisons often means relying on and reinforcing prejudices and stereotypes about outgroups.

Groups can also have powerful effects on decision making. With group decision making it is not always the case that 'the whole is greater than the sum of its parts' (Levine, 2018). This seems to be because of the influence of social motives. The urge to conform can sometimes stifle creative thinking, and this may be particularly so for new members of groups. For example, junior doctors or medical students may have fresh insights but find it difficult to question the professional opinions of other members of the team.

Group decisions are often narrower than the decisions of individual group members. The phenomenon of polarisation means that through group discussion, agreement within a group tends to intensify so that each individual's attitude becomes stronger. For example, imagine we have six individuals who have moderately positive attitudes toward euthanasia. Following a group discussion there will tend to be a concentration and polarisation of attitudes: the group will become more positive toward euthanasia. If individuals were moderately opposed to euthanasia before the group discussion, the group attitude would be more extremely opposed following group discussion. Three explanations have been given for why this polarisation occurs (Hogg & Vaughan, 2008):

- *Persuasive arguments*: people in groups of like-minded people will hear arguments that they already agree with as well as new arguments supporting their original beliefs. These arguments will galvanise the initial attitude. In addition, making public commitments to our own beliefs via statements to other people may strengthen our initial attitudes.
- *Social comparison*: to prove they really belong to the group and to seek approval, individuals will make more intense statements of their initial belief.
- *Self-categorisation*: people will develop stereotypes of group members and be aware of what distinguishes the ingroup prototype from stereotypical outgroup members. Therefore, for individual and group identity reasons, people's opinions will move toward the ingroup prototype.

Another example of how group decision making may be worse than individual decision making is called **groupthink** (Janis & Mann, 1977). Groupthink occurs when the desire for group unanimity overrides rational decisions. It is more likely to happen when a group is already homogeneous and cohesive. However, groupthink also depends on the characteristics of the situation, such as if a decision has to be made in stressful or rushed situations or when the group is isolated from external sources of information. Thus, groupthink may be most likely to occur when cohesive groups are placed in stressful situations. Given the urgency of many healthcare situations, it is vitally important that teams are aware of how groupthink can lead to erroneous or poor decision making.

9.3.3 Obedience, Power, and Leadership

The processes of conformity just described refer to situations in which people think or behave in certain ways because of a perceived pressure to do so. Of course, there are many situations in which we behave in certain ways because of a need to be obedient to people who have power or authority.

Obedience

The powerful effects of obedience to authority have been observed in many settings, including those directly relevant to medicine and healthcare practice. In a classic study of obedience, study participants were told by a researcher in a white coat to give increasingly strong electric shocks to 'learners' who made mistakes in a word memory task (Milgram, 1974). No shocks were actually given, but the 'voltage generator' included descriptions of increasing voltage levels – 375 volts was labelled 'Danger: Severe Shock', and 435 volts was labelled 'XXX'. If participants hesitated or asked to stop, the researcher urged them to go on, informing them to treat silence or non-responses as errors and to administer another shock. Although it was predicted that fewer than 10% of participants would administer shocks greater than 195 volts (labelled 'Very Strong Shock'), all of the participants went beyond this. In fact, 63% went all the way to 450 volts. Subsequent analyses have indicated that key influences on obedience in this study included how legitimate the researcher was perceived to be, and how directive and consistent they were, as well as the proximity of the participant and the 'learner' (Haslam et al., 2014).

The impact of obedience to authority has also been observed in healthcare contexts. Hierarchies of power and influence mean that junior doctors, nurses, or other health professionals may feel unable or unwilling to question the decisions of senior physicians. Research indicates that in some cases nurses would be prepared to act in ways that go against their professional standards or established procedures, if requested by a senior physician (Hofling et al., 1966; Rank & Jacobson, 1977). Fortunately, procedures, systems, and technology can be established to counter these tendencies in various health professions (Naseralallah et al., 2022).

Leadership and Influence

Effective leadership involves the appropriate use of authority and influence to ensure the efficient management of people and resources to achieve group aims. Good leadership involves more than simply 'getting the job done'. Good leaders will aim to develop and maintain good team relationships and provide appropriate opportunities for individual input.

Leadership styles can be grouped into three broad categories. Autocratic leaders assume total responsibility for making all decisions and managing team members. This style characterises dictators, who do not tolerate the views and decisions of ingroup or outgroup members. Democratic leaders are consultative, allowing group members to be involved in decision making, planning, and the monitoring of performance if they possess the appropriate knowledge and skills. Laissez-faire leaders do not impose their leadership, but allow group members to decide on goals and strategies. In most professional settings, it is rare to find purely autocratic or laissez-faire leaders. However, democratic leaders may tend more toward autocratic or laissez-faire styles: the context may determine the extent to which they do so.

Leaders often vary in terms of how they try to encourage or enforce compliance with their decisions (Raven, 1965). One common strategy is to apply the principles of operant conditioning (see Chapter 10). According to this approach, good performance may be recognised via bonuses or other material rewards. One example is performance-related pay. In contrast, coercive leadership is based on a leader threatening to remove privileges or administer punishments if their instructions are not obeyed.

It is also possible to identify different sources of authority or reasons for leadership. One basis for power is recognised hierarchies of power. These are often based on the leader possessing superior knowledge, experience, or expertise. Thus, a consultant is in a superior position relative to a junior doctor. However, this is not always the case. For example, in the military a newly-commissioned officer has a higher leadership position than a senior non-commissioned officer with 40 years of experience. It is also important to note that people sometimes become leaders not because of their expertise or experience, but because of their charisma, charm, or connections to powerful people.

Clinical Notes 9.2

Hierarchy and Leadership in Medicine

- Being a doctor entails certain rights and responsibilities. Your reputation will be damaged if you disregard these responsibilities or abuse these rights.
- Pay attention to the different leadership skills people use. Use good leaders as role models and avoid following the examples set by bad leaders.
- Be aware of your own tendency to conform to authority. Ask yourself whether it is always in patients' best interests to do what your superiors suggest.
- Be brave enough to challenge your superiors if you think they have made a decision that will not result in the best care for patients.

9.3.4 Stereotypes and Prejudice

Another aspect of the study of individuals and groups to consider is stereotypes and prejudice. **Stereotypes** are generalisations that we make about specific social groups and members of those groups. They are 'rules of thumb' which are broadly correct, but may sometimes be erroneous (Tversky & Kahneman, 1974). The social groups for which people have stereotypes are various and include nationality, occupation, and religion. However, they can be more specific.

Stereotypes form the basis of many jokes in which a dominant ingroup denigrates an outgroup that is perceived as being inferior. For example, Australians make jokes about New Zealanders. You may also be aware of jokes based on stereotypes of different medical specialisations (e.g. orthopaedic surgeons, anaesthetists, psychiatrists). Although many of these jokes may appear harmless, it is important to note that incorrect or inaccurate stereotypes can lead to undesirable social behaviour.

Prejudice toward particular social groups is commonly based on inaccurate stereotypes. Taken literally, prejudice means to judge prior to having the relevant facts. History is replete with clashes between groups based on erroneous assumptions about differences due to nationality, ethnicity, or religion.

Activity 9.3

Stereotypes of Patients

Take two minutes to write down words that describe people with HIV/AIDS, people with chronic fatigue syndrome, and people with cancer.

- How did you acquire these beliefs?
- How were your interactions with people with these conditions shaped by your initial beliefs?
- How have your initial beliefs been changed by your interactions with people with these conditions?

Stereotypes and prejudice can also affect healthcare. Stereotypes and prejudices about people with certain health conditions, ethnic minorities, or the elderly (Stone et al., 2019; see Case Study 8.1) matter because of the known links between attitudes and behaviour noted earlier. Health professionals should not let people's personal characteristics or backgrounds influence their clinical decisions or the quality of care that they provide. However, prejudice and stereotyping can lead to poorer healthcare and worse health outcomes (Akinade et al., 2023; Hall et al., 2015). Prejudices about mental illness can result in poorer care for some people. For example, studies of both practising primary care physicians and medical students reveal that they tend to have prejudices against people with mental illness that result in reduced access to healthcare (Dixon et al., 2008; Lawrie et al., 1998). Research Box 9.2 provides an example of studies designed to determine when and how to intervene to address prejudicial attitudes.

When discussing stereotypes and prejudice, it is important to address both explicit stereotypes – that is, beliefs that we are consciously aware of and accept – and implicit or unconscious biases. Unconscious biases can be activated quickly and unknowingly by characteristics such as a person's gender, accent, or weight. Even if we do not hold explicit stereotypes related to these characteristics, we seem to soak up general social prejudices from the world around us. We are all susceptible to unconscious biases, and health professionals' unconscious biases can affect patient care (Antonopoulos et al., 2023; FitzGerald & Hurst, 2017; Groves et al., 2021; Vela et al., 2022). There is some evidence that training in biases, stereotyping, and prejudice can change beliefs and behaviours (Heim et al., 2020; Ricks et al., 2022). However, there is also a need to address systemic racism and sexism within healthcare systems, because it has been argued that implicit biases reflect systemic biases (Payne & Hannay, 2021), and that addressing biases in individuals will be ineffective if the systems within which they live and work do not also change (Vela et al., 2022).

Stereotyping in healthcare is not restricted to health professionals. Patients' stereotyped beliefs about health professionals also matter. One study found that people who expressed more negative stereotypes about doctors were less likely to seek healthcare when they became ill, were less satisfied with the care that they did obtain, and were less likely to adhere to the treatment prescribed by their doctor (Bogart et al., 2004). Identifying the reasons for people's negative stereotypes in an attempt to change these attitudes may help to improve the health of the population. It may also be important for health professionals to try to change their behaviour so that they do not reinforce unhelpful stereotypes.

Research Box 9.2

Health Professionals' Attitudes Toward Mental Illness

Background

Many health professionals have negative stigmatising attitudes toward people with mental illnesses. However, it is not always known what training should be given to those learning to be health professionals, and whether the issues are more or less prominent in different professions.

(Continued)

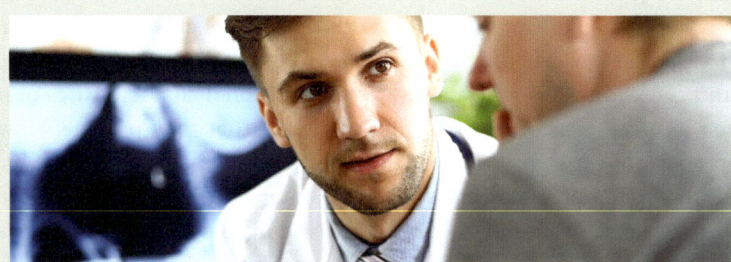

Figure 9.5   Health professionals' stigmatising attitudes

Source: © H_Ko/Adobe Stock

Method and Findings

This study was designed to compare the attitudes of students in nursing, medicine, occupational therapy (OT), and psychology. Measures of attitudes were completed by 927 final-year students at six universities in Chile and Spain. The results indicated that, compared to students of psychology and OT, medical and nursing students had more stigmatised views of psychiatric conditions. They had more negative attitudes about the dangerousness and recovery prospects of patients with psychiatric conditions, and they were also less likely to disclose their own mental health problems.

Significance

The authors concluded that there is a need for education and other interventions to counter stigmatising views of psychiatric conditions among all health science students, but especially in nursing and medicine programmes. They suggested that one way to do this could be through social contact with people who have been successfully treated.

Masedo, A., Grandón, P., Saldivia, S., et al. (2021) A multicentric study on stigma towards people with mental illness in health sciences students. *BMC Medical Education, 21*(1): 324. doi:10.1186/s12909-021-02695-8.

Clinical Notes 9.3

Avoiding Prejudice and Careless Assumptions in Healthcare

- Be aware of your attitudes toward different groups of people, whether they are ethnic groups, particular types of patients, or particular professions in healthcare.
- Ensure that your attitudes do not affect your treatment of different patients.
- The fundamental attribution error means that we are prone to assume that people's behaviour is due to them and not their circumstances.
- Remember that people's behaviour is often strongly influenced by their history or current social circumstances, so do not assume that people are intrinsically difficult or badly motivated.

Summary 9.3

- Group membership is an important part of individual identity.
- Different social roles entail different rights and obligations. In medicine, social roles influence the behaviour of doctors and patients (e.g. the sick role).
- People tend to conform to the expectations of the groups to which they belong.
- People often obey leaders without questioning them, sometimes even when what they are being asked to do is harmful to others.
- Group decision making can be impaired by the tendency toward conformity and because alternative positions are not considered.
- Effective leadership involves the appropriate use of authority and the best use of the skills and capacities of group members.
- Stereotypes are cognitive short-cuts which are a core aspect of prejudices. They can exert important influences on behaviour, including health-related behaviour.

9.4 Antisocial and Prosocial Behaviour

We finish this chapter by considering two contrasting types of interpersonal behavious that are important in medicine and healthcare – antisocial behaviours such as aggression, and prosocial behaviours such as helping and donating.

9.4.1 Aggression

Aggression involves behaviours that are enacted to cause physical or psychological harm or pain to another person. Aggression can be actual (e.g. physical attacks) or symbolic (e.g. burning flags). Different explanations of aggression are outlined below. Strategies for dealing with angry or aggressive people are covered in Chapter 13.

The frustration-aggression hypothesis (Berkowitz, 1989) argues that when we are prevented from achieving our goals, we become frustrated, and this can lead to aggression. Although frustration may be a significant factor in the lead-up to aggression, it cannot be the sole cause. For example, if someone is frustrated because a library book they want has not been returned, they do not automatically become violent, because they know that the library is not an appropriate place for aggressive behaviour. The cue-arousal theory of aggression therefore argues that frustration is more likely to lead to aggression if there are situational cues that aggression is an appropriate response (Geen & O'Neal, 1969). In healthcare contexts, such situational cues may include rude or aggressive behaviour that is exhibited by other patients or health professionals. Other situational influences include the effects of alcohol and other drugs, which may impair cognition or reduce inhibitions against violent behaviour.

Patient aggression and violence are prominent occupational hazards for health professionals. A review of over 100 studies from 30 countries revealed that around one-sixth (17%) had experienced physical violence perpetrated by patients or visitors, and that almost half (47%) had experienced physical violence or abuse (Wu et al., 2024). Furthermore, a review of 30 studies involving over 10,000 nursing students indicated that just over half (55%) had experienced workplace violence (Mohamed et al., 2024). These assaults can have a serious negative impact on staff wellbeing (Lanctôt & Guay, 2014). Aggression and violence may be more common in particular settings, such as emergency departments and psychiatric departments, and younger staff may be more vulnerable to assault. Violent or aggressive behaviour appears to be more likely if patients are anxious, in pain, or are concerned about the financial aspects of their treatment: when these features are present, patients may be more attentive to threatening stimuli, and aggression may be a response to increased feelings of threat.

The likelihood of aggressive behaviour appears to be influenced by organisational and situational influences such as prolonged waiting times and crowded waiting areas (which can increase patient frustration) and by medical procedures that induce pain or anxiety (Wu et al., 2024). Training staff to deal better with aggressive or violent people may reduce the risk that they will experience verbal or physical assaults, and it can reduce the negative emotional impact of assaults that do occur (Schablon et al., 2012), but there is a need for more robust evidence about how best to prepare people and healthcare settings to reduce the risk of violence and to reduce its impact when it does occur (Spelten et al., 2020).

People with certain conditions may be more likely to become aggressive. This can be particularly likely in dementia or psychiatric conditions characterised by cognitive impairments, delusions, or disinhibition (see Chapter 7). However, situational factors matter because not all people with such conditions will become aggressive or violent: this is recognised by health professionals, who cite staffing, policies, and resource limitations as contributory factors (Fletcher et al., 2021). However, attribution errors (referred to earlier) are also evident, in that health professionals tend to attribute aggressive behaviour among people with psychiatric diagnoses to internal characteristics, whereas users of mental health services tend to attribute their aggressive behaviour to external or situational factors, such as being provoked, belittled, or annoyed by staff (Fletcher et al., 2021). Patients and healthcare professionals tend to be in agreement that a good therapeutic relationship protects against aggression (Fletcher et al., 2021).

9.4.2 Prosocial Behaviour

Although social psychology often focuses on why people engage in undesirable behaviours such as aggression and prejudice, many researchers focus on positive social behaviours, such as helping and altruism. Such prosocial behaviours include the activities of health professionals and other healthcare workers, although people may not engage in such behaviours for purely altruistic reasons.

Altruistic behaviours are prosocial behaviours that we engage in without expecting to be rewarded, even though the feeling of 'doing good' that arises from altruistic behaviours may be a form of reward in itself. Some people argue that our capacity for empathy explains why we help others: we can imagine what it would be like to be in their position, so we try to help them (Persson & Kajionus, 2016). Others argue that we choose to help others to relieve our own distress at seeing someone in need of help (Cialdini et al., 1987). It is also possible that people engage in seemingly altruistic behaviours because they expect a reward or recognition in the future (e.g. we may do voluntary work because we think it will look good on our CV). Consenting to donate one's organs can be seen to be a purely altruistic act because there is no possibility of a reward for such behaviour. However, the knowledge that we will be helping others after we die can also be construed as a reward.

In more mundane everyday circumstances, the likelihood that we will help others is influenced by our perceptions of the costs and benefits of helping. We are more likely to help others if we perceive that doing so will not be too taxing for us in terms of time, effort, and emotion (Piliavin et al., 1969). For example, we are less likely to help someone get their cat out of a tree if we are rushing to a job interview. This principle helps to explain mobile blood donation services. Such services eliminate some of the time and money costs associated with donation, thereby increasing the attractiveness of this behaviour.

In addition to being influenced by perceived personal costs and benefits, the likelihood of helping others is influenced by our perceptions of whether other people are helping. Social learning and modelling concepts (see Chapter 10) suggest that we are more likely to help if we can see others doing so, and less likely to help if we see others not getting involved. In situations where nobody helps, this can be because of a diffusion of responsibility. Each individual assumes that somebody else will take responsibility for helping, with the net result that nobody does so (Latané & Darley, 1970). This phenomenon can be illustrated by the fact that people are more likely to help when they are not in groups. For example, if a person has an epileptic seizure, people are more likely to help if they are the only bystander, but the likelihood of helping decreases as the number of inactive bystanders increases. Reviews of published research provide evidence for the bystander effect, but also find that the effect is weaker in dangerous emergency situations or when there are stronger social norms for helping (Fischer et al., 2011; Mainwaring et al., 2023).

Social cues to helping can be used to encourage prosocial behaviour (just as social cues may encourage aggression). Examples include the coloured badges, ribbons, and wristbands worn to demonstrate support for various charities. These are in some part symbolic of a material exchange (e.g. you donate money so you get a reward). They are also a public demonstration of commitment and a signal to others that they should also consider supporting the cause.

Summary 9.4

- Several different theories of aggression have been put forward. Although there is support for most theories, no single theory explains all acts of aggression.
- Aggressive behaviour appears to be a combination of individual tendencies toward aggression, the psychological state of the individual at a particular time, and situational cues or stressors.
- Altruistic behaviours are helping or prosocial behaviours that people do for others with no expectation of a personal reward.
- The likelihood of helping appears to be influenced by the personal costs and benefits of helping.
- The behaviour of others is also a cue for helping behaviour. We are more likely to help if we can see others helping, or if there are no other people available to offer help.

Conclusion

This chapter has given an overview of some key components of social psychology that are applicable to health and healthcare. The material presented here illustrates how our beliefs about ourselves and other people influence healthy and unhealthy behaviour, antisocial behaviour, and prosocial behaviours.

—Further Reading—

Hogg, M.A. & Vaughan, G.M. (2022) *Social Psychology* (9th edition). Harlow: Pearson Prentice Hall. A good introduction to a wide range of social psychology topics. However, this book is designed for psychology students, so it lacks a specific focus on the application of key concepts to health contexts.

Stroebe, W. (2011) *Social Psychology and Health* (3rd edition). London: McGraw-Hill Education. Discusses health and related interventions from a social psychological perspective.

—Revision Questions—

1   What is meant by the term 'cognitive dissonance'? How can it be used to encourage healthy behaviour?
2   Outline the characteristics of messages and messengers that will increase the likelihood that people will respond to them in positive ways.
3   How does the clothing doctors wear affect people's perceptions of them? Why is this the case?
4   How can perceived discrepancies between people's actual and ideal selves prompt behaviour change? Give one healthy example and one unhealthy example.
5   What is meant by the 'fundamental attribution error'? Give two health-related examples of this phenomenon.
6   What is meant by the term 'sick role'? What does it mean to say that doctors are 'gatekeepers' of the sick role?
7   How well does the proverb 'Many hands make light work' apply to medical decision making? Discuss with reference to the concepts of conformity and groupthink.
8   What is a stereotype? What is the link between stereotypes and prejudice?
9   Why is the cue-arousal theory likely to be a better explanation of aggression than the frustration-aggression hypothesis?
10   Describe the characteristics of situations that make it more likely that people will help others.

10

COGNITIVE PSYCHOLOGY

---Learning Objectives---

This chapter is designed to enable you to:

- Describe perceptual processes and give examples of how they are relevant to medical settings.
- Understand the processes of attention and how they contribute to medical errors.
- Describe classical and operant conditioning and discuss how they can be used in clinical practice.
- Understand the characteristics of short- and long-term memory.
- Use this information to help devise effective ways to revise for exams.

Learning to be a health professional involves the accumulation of knowledge, clinical, and technical skills, all of which are driven by cognitive processes of perception, attention, learning, and memory. Understanding how these processes work can help us in various ways. We can find better ways to learn, to be more aware of the conditions under which medical errors might occur, and to help people to change behaviours (e.g. helping children with eczema to stop scratching). In this chapter we look at perception, attention, learning, and memory, with examples of how they are relevant to healthcare.

10.1 Perception

Perception involves the way information from our environment is transformed via our senses (sight, hearing, smell, touch, and taste) into experience. It is helpful to clarify the difference between perception and attention, which we look at in the next section. **Attention** refers to those aspects of our environment we focus on and process.

Let us start with visual perception because, on the surface at least, it appears quite straightforward. Light from the environment is projected onto our retina and transformed into electrical impulses by the rods, cones, and ganglion cells of the retina. These impulses are transmitted via the optic nerve to the visual cortex where we 'see' the image. However, the mind has a strong influence on how we interpret stimuli. Activity 10.1 provides an example.

—Activity 10.1—

Visual Perception

- How many F and T letters are there in this sentence?

'INFERTILITY TREATMENT IS THE RESULT OF YEARS OF SCIENTIFIC STUDY COMBINED WITH THE EXPERTISE OF CLINICIANS'

Many get the task in Activity 10.1 wrong because we tend to process small and frequently used words, such as 'the' and 'of', as single units. It makes it much harder to 'see' the individual letters in these words. Visual perception is therefore a combination of visual stimuli (bottom-up processing) and our existing knowledge (top-down processing).

Other examples of top-down processing are size and shape constancy and depth perception. Size and shape constancy means that an object is perceived as remaining the same despite the fact that it appears larger as we move toward it, and changes shape depending on the angle from which we see it from. Our mind knows that most objects do not change shape, so therefore concludes that we are moving and seeing it from different perspectives. This knowledge is used in the perception of depth. For example, we know that people are approximately similar in size. In Figure 10.1a we can therefore see that the person in the background is further away from the camera. In this instance, our previous knowledge about people's size gives us clues about depth. Our interpretation of it happens very rapidly at an unconscious level. This effect is so strong it can even override our conscious perceptual processes. Compare the size of the image of the person in the background with the image of the person in the foreground. How much smaller would you say the person in the background is compared to the person in the foreground? Now look at Figure 10.1b, in which the image is actually brought forward in the picture. Most people would not have judged the image to be this small because size constancy and depth perception automatically bias our judgement.

The study of perception has established that not only are we unable to realise the extent of some true differences (such as the difference in size between the two people in Figure 10.1), but that we are also quite selective and biased in what we perceive. The underlying concept here is that of **perceptual sets**, where the influence of attention, previous experience, and motivation are combined so we perceive information that is relevant to us, both as humans and individuals. A perceptual set is influenced by the factors summarised in Highlight Box 10.1. Threshold for perception is where one stimulus has a lower or higher threshold for perception than others. If someone shouts 'Fire', it is more likely to get your attention than if they shout 'Air'. Similarly, in a noisy environment where lots of people are talking, you might suddenly become aware that someone across the room has said your name. This is because you have a lower threshold for 'hearing' your name.

a

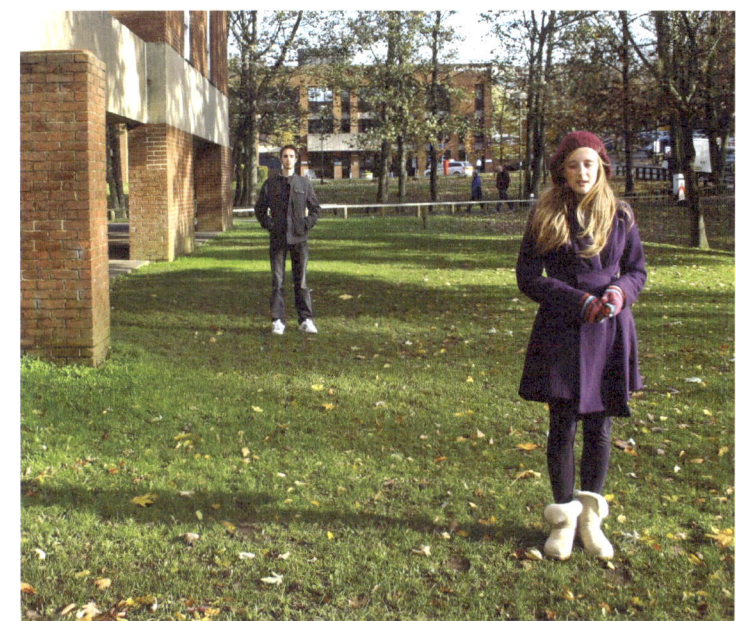

b

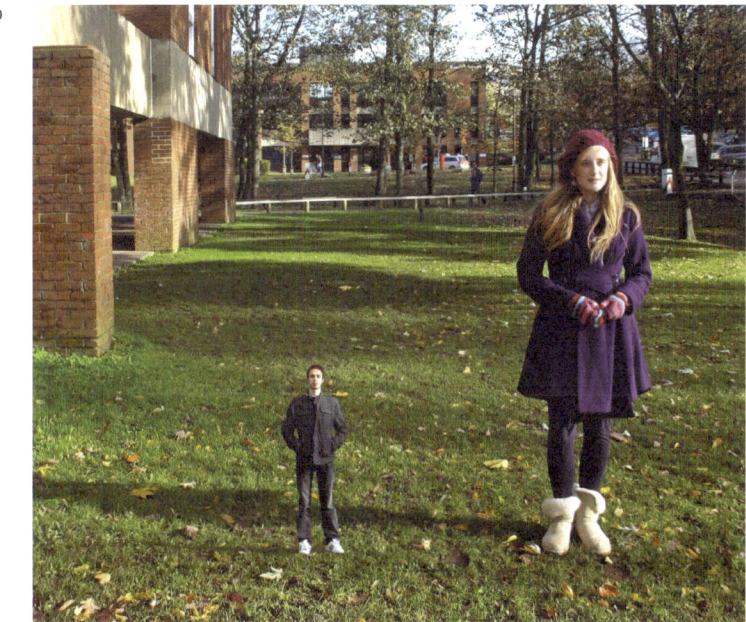

Figure 10.1 Size constancy and depth perception

The influence of experience is evident through the effects of size constancy and depth perception. Experience, expectations, and individual values combine to influence perception in more subtle ways as well. For example, poor children and adults overestimate the size of coins compared to more affluent people (Hitchcock et al., 1976). In healthcare contexts, studies of symptom perception show that just telling people that a stimulus might be painful makes them more likely to report pain in response to it. Furthermore, observing others experiencing pain or pain relief can affect our own experiences of pain (Meeuwis et al., 2023). The placebo and nocebo effects provide classic examples of the role of expectations and learning in the perception of symptoms (see Chapter 4). Research also indicates that expectancies influence pain intensity processing in the central nervous system (Atlas, 2023).

Our physical and psychological state affects what we perceive in several ways. First, our level of arousal determines how much attention we pay to our environment. When we are sleeping, we do not consciously perceive much, if anything, of our external environment unless there is a large change, such as a loud noise or a change in temperature. The processes through which people perceive stimuli when in a low level of consciousness are important in anaesthesia. Anaesthesia aims to remove conscious awareness, yet approximately 1% of people report some perception during surgery, and this experience can have adverse effects on wellbeing (see Research Box 10.1) (Kim et al., 2021; Tasbihgou et al., 2018). Second, our motivational state also influences what we pay attention to in our environment. For example, when we are hungry, we are more likely to notice food-related stimuli (Juvonen et al., 2020).

─Highlight Box 10.1─

Factors That Influence Perceptual Sets

- Threshold for perception
- Past experience
- Current drive state
- Emotions
- Individual values
- Environment
- Cultural background and experience

─Research Box 10.1─

Awareness and Memory during Obstetric Anaesthesia

Background

Awareness during anaesthesia (ADA) may be more common in obstetrics contexts than in other contexts because of several risk factors: the almost universal use of neuromuscular blocker drugs, rapid sequence induction, a high incidence of difficult airway management, and emergency or out-of-hours surgery.

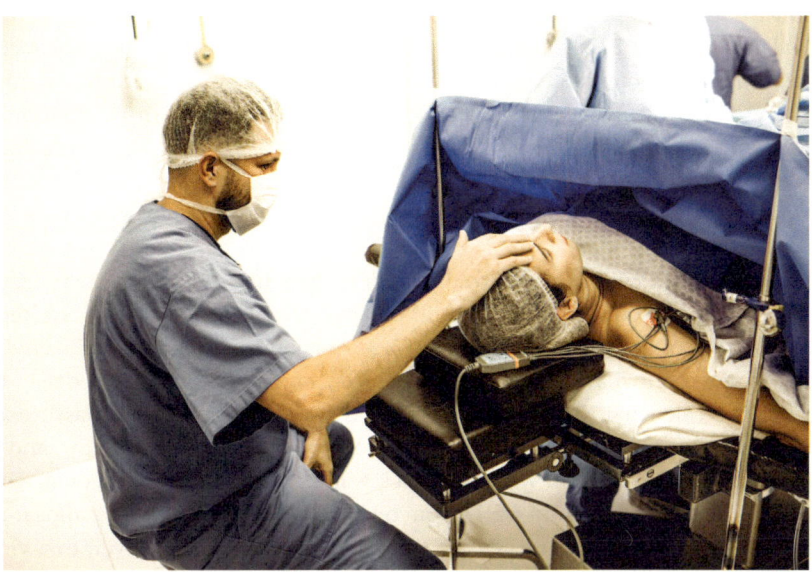

Figure 10.2   A woman under anaesthesia

Source: Jonathan Borba/Pexels

Method and Findings

This study included 3,115 women recruited from 72 hospitals in England. The study design included screening for ADA three times following surgery: within the first 24 hours, after 24–48 hours, and after 30 days. This procedure has been found to optimise accurate recall. All women who reported ADA were followed-up for 12 months using interviews and self-report checklists of symptoms for post-traumatic stress disorder (PTSD).

Twelve patients (0.4%) had certain or probable ADA, most of whom described distressing experiences involving pain or paralysis. Four of the 12 women screened positive for PTSD, with another marginally not meeting diagnostic criteria. PTSD is significantly more likely among women who reported ADA. Five of the 12 women with ADA had moderate to severe anxiety about future anaesthesia or related healthcare.

Significance

The high incidence of ADA and its strong links to psychological harm indicate a need to ensure appropriate follow-up for patients and staff. Generic psychological support pathways for ADA may be helpful, but the authors suggested that these may need to be refined for the obstetric setting.

Odor, P.M., Bampoe, S., Lucas, D.N., Moonesinghe, S.R. et al. (2021) Incidence of accidental awareness during general anaesthesia in obstetrics: A multicentre, prospective cohort study. *Anaesthesia, 76*(6): 759–776. doi:10.1111/anae.15385.

Emotions affect what we attend to and perceive. It has been well established that anxiety is associated with increased perception of threat and a narrowing of attention onto threatening stimuli (Valadez et al., 2022). This general pattern is also observed in the specific context of healthcare: illness-related anxiety is related to biased processing of health-threatening information (Du et al., 2023). Perceptual changes can also be seen for positive emotions. Classic studies of young children's perception found that before Christmas, children's drawings of Santa Claus were much larger and more elaborate than after Christmas, suggesting that children's emotional state influenced their perception and representation of Santa Claus (Sechrest & Wallace, 1964).

The environment provides the external stimuli that we interpret into experience. In spite of the influence of top-down influences and our perceptual set, most of us are remarkably accurate in what we see. This is partly because our previous experiences of the environment can help us to interpret what is happening. However, sometimes our knowledge of the environment can override what we see and result in a distorted perception. A classic example of this is the Ames room – a specially constructed room where the walls, window, and floor are faked to look like a square room when the back wall is in fact on the diagonal. The design means that if a person in the room walks from one corner to the other, they appear to shrink or grow. In reality, this is because they are walking further away. However, to a viewer, the perceptual cues that the room is square can override this, so they 'see' the impossible, that is, that the person shrinks or grows as they walk (there are many examples of the Ames illusion online).

Cultural factors influence perception less than might be expected. Many aspects of visual perception are consistent across cultures. One of the strongest effects of culture on perception is that we are quicker and better at recognising people of our own ethnic group compared to people of another ethnic group (Meissner & Brigham, 2001). This can influence how health professionals interact with people of different ethnicity. Reviews of cultural influences on practitioner–patient communication show that consultations with people from ethnic minorities involve less emotional expression by the doctor and patient, and less verbal expression by patients (Schouten & Meeuwesen, 2006; Zhao, 2023). It has been suggested that perceptual biases contribute to culture-related communication difficulties in healthcare consultations. There is increasing awareness of the need to address unconscious biases in healthcare and other contexts (Vela et al., 2022) (see also Chapter 9, section 9.3.4, and Chapter 10, section 10.5).

So far, we have discussed the influence of perceptual sets on normal visual perception. However, we also need to understand abnormal perceptual processes, which are relevant to many disorders, including autism and schizophrenia. For example, people with autism and people with antisocial characteristics tend to have poorer perception of expressions of emotion (Díaz-Vázquez et al., 2022; Marsh & Blair, 2008). Schizophrenia and other psychotic experiences are particularly interesting because they involve the perception of illusory events as real. Research suggests that psychotic-type thinking is more likely when people with schizotypal characteristics are put in situations of perceptual ambiguity and overload (Grave et al., 2017), and that the ability to process emotions is most impaired when people are experiencing negative symptoms or are in an acute illness state (Mandal et al., 2023). Better understanding of how perceptual capacity is affected by situational factors could inform better management and treatment of schizophrenia.

Summary 10.1

- Perception is the way information from our environment is transformed and interpreted into experience.
- Perception is the combination of environmental stimuli (bottom-up processing) and existing knowledge (top-down processing).
- A perceptual set is where attention, previous experience, and motivation determine the information each person perceives.
- Perceptual sets can be influenced by thresholds for perception, past experience, individual values, current drive state, emotions, environment, and culture.

10.2 Attention

Attention is the ability to select information in the environment to attend to and process. Attention is therefore an important part of perception, learning, and performance – particularly in situations where we need to multitask (i.e. divide our attention between different tasks). What we attend to and how much attention we pay to it is influenced by our physical arousal, motivation, and emotion. Attention can also be biased by these factors. Knowledge of how attention works can therefore help us to understand errors in healthcare, such as giving wrong drug dosages or making surgical errors.

Attention involves many different mental processes, and it would be wrong to think in terms of a single attentional system. For example, studies of people with brain injuries show that they often have problems with some aspects of attention, but not all. Attention can be voluntary, such as when we concentrate on learning or doing a task, or involuntary, such as when a loud noise or sudden movement grabs our attention. Attention has been likened to a spotlight or filter that can have either a broad or narrow focus. When attention is focused, central information is processed in detail, but peripheral information may be ignored or lost. To be able to function well in various situations, we need to be able to:

- Focus our attention on a particular stimulus.
- Remove or disengage our attention from a stimulus.
- Shift attention between different stimuli.

Attention is intertwined with cognitive processes of perception and memory (see Figure 10.3). **Sensory buffers** are short-term stores of incoming information that can be used to select which

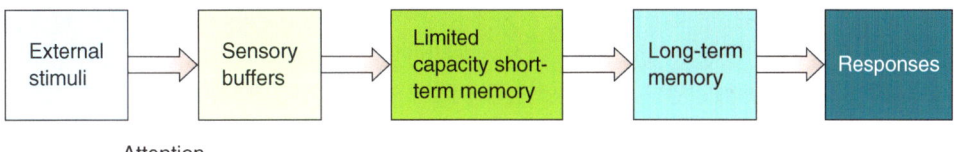

Figure 10.3 Cognitive processes

information to attend to consciously. Auditory sensory buffers register all incoming sounds for a few seconds, so this information is potentially recoverable during this time. A good example of this is when we 'tune out' of a conversation for a few seconds but can then replay what was just said in our head. This ability is especially useful if we are accused of not listening to what someone has just said!

Many theories of attention propose that we have a **limited capacity processor** that restricts the amount of information we can consciously attend to. Research has broadly confirmed this theory, but there is evidence that we can still unconsciously perceive information not attended to, and that our capacity to process information or to multitask increases as tasks become more practised or automatic and hence demand less conscious attention. For example, neuroimaging research indicates that even when we do not consciously attend to stimuli, there is similar but weaker neurological activation in the same parts of the brain that are activated during conscious attention (MacLean et al., 2023; Talsma et al., 2010).

10.2.1 Attention and Clinical Skills

Clinical skills are essential for medical practice. During your training you will learn skills such as clinical interviewing, physical examinations, and medical procedures. Skill acquisition draws on the processes illustrated in Figure 10.3. Learning a new skill demands our concentrated attention, short-term memory, cognitive motor processes, and effortful responses. Initially, attention is needed for both perception and response stages. As we learn and practise a skill, it gradually becomes easier and requires less of our attention or concentration. There are three broad stages in skill acquisition (Adams, 1971):

1   *Cognitive stage*: development of a mental representation of the skill and how to perform it. At this stage, learning usually relies on explicit instruction through teaching from an expert, demonstration, and self-observation (e.g. relying on a senior colleague to tell you what to do when taking blood).
2   *Associative stage*: development of an effective motor programme such that the person is able to carry out the broad skill but lacks the ability to perform finer subtasks with fluency. Development is guided by knowledge or feedback (e.g. being able to drive but being consciously aware of actions such as turning the wheel and changing gear).
3   *Autonomous stage*: the skill is largely automatic and relies on implicit knowledge and motor coordination, rather than explicit instruction (e.g. being able to drive without conscious effort).

Studies of skill acquisition show that practice may be more important than aptitude (Ericsson, 2020). However, practice has to be deliberate and focused, with adequate monitoring of performance and outcomes. If learning or practice is spaced out over time, it also improves learning (see section 10.4 on Memory). In the healthcare context, similar principles appear to apply – practice, with appropriate supervision and feedback, is crucial to developing expertise (Ericsson, 2015).

Multitasking is easiest when the skills have been developed to the autonomous stage, and the tasks are not too similar or complex (e.g. talking to someone while driving a car). However, even under easy conditions, multitasking entails competing processes which influence how each task is carried out. For example, using a phone while driving results in slower response times, a reduced ability to notice when the car in front slows down, and less attention to sensory inputs. This effect on driving appears to occur regardless of whether the phone is hands-free (Lipovac et al., 2017). Studies of attention have shown that incorrect actions or mistakes are most likely:

- When the correct response is not the strongest or most habitual.
- When our full attention is not given to the task.
- Under conditions of stress and anxiety.

The advantage of developing a skill to the autonomous stage is that it frees up some of our attention for multitasking (although other tasks will still impinge on the autonomous one). The disadvantage is that autonomous behaviour is no longer consciously controlled, so it is possible to make mistakes. This is particularly relevant to healthcare: it is estimated that in the USA alone over 200,000 patients die every year from preventable mistakes (Ferner & McDowell, 2006). The majority of cases arise from errors in administering or prescribing medication, wrong treatment, inaccurate diagnosis, and surgical errors (see Research Box 10.2).

─Research Box 10.2─

Medical Mistakes and Manslaughter

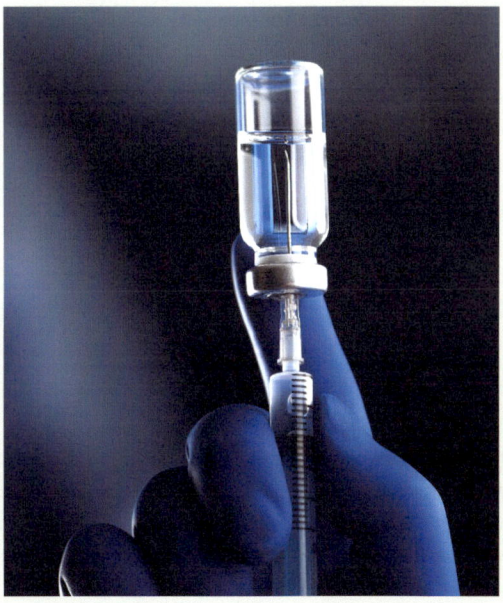

Figure 10.4   Medical errors

Source: © Alernon77/Adobe Stock

(Continued)

Background

Medical errors sometimes lead to people dying. It is therefore important to identify the causes of medical errors and to find ways to prevent them from happening.

Method and Findings

Newspapers and journal archives in the UK were searched to identify legal cases where doctors were charged with manslaughter to examine the causes of death. Between 1795 and 2005, 85 doctors were charged with manslaughter, with a large increase in prosecutions since 1990. The majority of doctors were acquitted, and only 29% were convicted or pleaded guilty. The main causes of manslaughter (with examples) were as follows.

Mistakes (44%): Errors in Planning

A 20-year-old man with muscular dystrophy died after circumcision. The surgeon guessed the man's weight and inadvertently gave three times the recommended dose of lidocaine. He was charged with manslaughter but acquitted.

Slips (20%): Errors Due to Distraction or a Failure of Concentration

A six-week-old boy died after cardiac arrest during surgery for pyloric stenosis (a narrowing of the opening from the stomach to the small intestine). The anaesthetist injected air into the bloodstream instead of the nasogastric tube. The anaesthetist was charged with manslaughter but acquitted.

Violations (19%): Deliberate Violation of Medical Practice

A two-year-old boy died from hypoxia that occurred during a hernia operation. The anaesthetist had deliberately inhaled anaesthetic before and during the operation. He was charged with manslaughter and found guilty.

Technical Errors (4%): Failure to Carry Out an Appropriate Action

A 16-year-old girl being treated for leukaemia died after an attempt to insert a Hickman line (central venous catheter) caused cardiac rupture. The surgeon was charged with manslaughter but acquitted.

Significance

Nearly two-thirds of patient deaths brought to prosecution are due to unconscious errors (mistakes or slips) that could be a direct consequence of automatic behaviour. The authors of this review of medical manslaughter cases argue that the prosecution of individual doctors would not improve patient safety as much as changing healthcare systems to incorporate checks to reduce unconscious errors.

Ferner, R.E. & McDowell, S.E. (2006) Doctors charged with manslaughter in the course of medical practice, 1795–2005: A literature review. *Journal of the Royal Society of Medicine, 99*: 309–314.

Skilled surgeons can carry out surgery relatively autonomously at the same time as doing other things, such as talking to colleagues about unrelated issues. Many surgeons listen to music while operating. Although music can be quite calming emotionally and physically, research into attention suggests that if something goes wrong and quick decisions or actions are required, music can interfere with our ability to focus attention on the emergency situation and responses. Research suggests that this is particularly the case for novice surgeons, possibly because of the effects of practice and automaticity. Furthermore, preferred and non-preferred music may have different effects, with non-preferred music impairing performance in similar ways to other distractions (El Boghdady & Ewalds-Kvist, 2020; Gil et al., 2020; see also Figure 10.5).

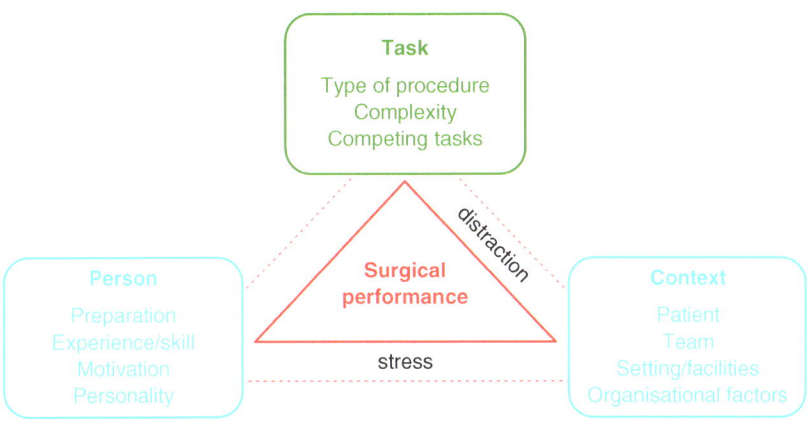

Figure 10.5   Influences on surgical skill (adapted from Schout et al., 2010)

Source: Adapted by permission from Springer. Schout, B.M.A., Hendrikx, A.J.M., Scheele, F., Bemelmans, B.M.H. & Scherpbier, A.J.J.A. (2010) Validation and implementation of surgical simulators: A critical review of present, past, and future. *Surgery & Endoscopy, 24*(3): 536–546

10.2.2 Biased Attention

As with perception, attention is biased toward certain stimuli. Normal and abnormal biases have been found. Normal biases include being more likely to attend to faces and emotional stimuli. For example, infants spend more time looking at faces or face-shaped stimuli than other shapes, and seem to have an innate preference for them (Dannemiller & Stephens, 1988; Wilkinson et al., 2014). Studies of reaction times to different objects indicate that we are quicker to pay attention to emotional items and take longer to disengage from them. Neuropsychological research shows that emotional stimuli produce stronger neurological responses than neutral stimuli and can affect working memory (Schweizer et al., 2019; Vuilleumier & Huang, 2009). These are specific examples of attention tending to be biased when we are overloaded by other stimuli or stressed.

Attention is biased – or abnormal – in some psychological disorders. People with eating disorders are more likely to attend to stimuli that are food-, body-, or weight-related (Stott et al., 2021). Anxious people are more likely to attend to threat-related stimuli and may be hypervigilant for particular stimuli (Bar-Haim et al., 2007; see also section 4.1.1). This is the case in generalised anxiety disorder, obsessive-compulsive disorder, post-traumatic stress disorder

(PTSD), and phobias. For example, a person with a blood phobia will continually scan the environment for signs of blood, and this takes up cognitive processing and attentional resources. More generally, attentional bias toward health-related threats may contribute to the development and maintenance of health anxiety (Shi et al., 2022). In other psychological disorders, normal biases may be disrupted. For example, a review of studies of pregnant women and new mothers revealed that, compared to non-depressed women, mothers with depression or anxiety are more likely to identify negative emotions such as sadness in infants' faces, and less accurate at identifying positive emotions such as happiness (Webb & Ayers, 2015).

Emotions are also important in how attention is directed and focused. Positive emotions are associated with a broadening of attention and negative emotions with a narrowing of attention onto particular stimuli (Schweizer et al., 2019; Vuilleumier & Huang, 2009). This can have various repercussions. On one hand, narrowing our attention in emergency situations is useful because it helps us to focus on the problem and what actions are needed to resolve it. On the other hand, this narrow focus means subsidiary or peripheral information is potentially ignored or less likely to be picked up. Knowledge of attention processes shows that, to a certain extent, slips and mistakes are inevitable parts of being human. It is therefore important to recognise the role of systems and organisations in such circumstances. If adequate systems of checking and monitoring are in place, then individual errors are more likely to be caught and corrected before they have severe consequences. The World Health Organization has produced such a 19-item checklist for surgical safety (WHO, 2009).

Summary 10.2

- Attention concerns the ability to select information in the environment to attend to and process.
- Attention influences the way in which we perceive, process, and respond to stimuli.
- Learning new skills involves concentrated attention, short-term memory, cognitive motor processes, and effortful responses.
- There are three stages involved in learning skills: cognitive, associative, and autonomous.
- At the autonomous stage, skilled behaviour can be carried out without conscious or effortful control.
- Multitasking requires divided attention and is easiest when one or both tasks are practised and autonomous.
- Mistakes are most likely to occur when the correct response is not strongest or habitual, when our full attention is not given to the task, and in conditions of stress or anxiety.
- Attentional biases include a bias toward emotional expressions and voices and the influence of emotions on the breadth of attentional focus.
- Abnormal biases are found in some psychological disorders.

10.3 Learning

Learning can be defined as the acquisition of knowledge or skills through experience, observing, studying, or being taught. **Associative learning** is how we learn the relationship between two events that occur together. For example, if one event occurs at the same time as another, it indicates a temporal relationship; if one event always follows another, it indicates a causal (and temporal) relationship. Different learning processes have a range of implications for healthcare, both in terms of your own learning and helping patients to recover and change their behaviour. Key learning processes include classical conditioning, operant conditioning, modelling, and imitation. Conditioning processes are particularly useful when working with young children or people with cognitive impairments who are less likely to change their behaviour in response to verbal reasoning.

10.3.1 Classical Conditioning

Classical conditioning is best known and illustrated by the work of Pavlov and his dogs. Dogs have a normal reflex to salivate when food is presented. Food is therefore an unconditioned stimulus and salivation is an unconditioned response because it occurs naturally without learning. Pavlov noticed that his dogs began to salivate at other times, such as when he entered the room, because they had learned that he was associated with being fed. Pavlov formally demonstrated classical conditioning by ringing a bell just before feeding the dogs. The bell was initially a neutral stimulus because it was not associated with food and did not produce salivation. However, after a short while, the dogs began to salivate when they heard the bell. The bell had therefore become a conditioned stimulus and salivation to the bell a conditioned response, because the dogs had learned the association between the bell and food.

Many other characteristics of classical conditioning have been identified. For example, the *nature of the stimulus* is important, as some stimuli are more easily conditioned than others. Novel foods or drinks are more readily associated with physical symptoms such as nausea. This is probably due to biological mechanisms that encourage learning in situations that may be dangerous – in this case, to prevent us eating poisonous foods. Therefore, if a novel food or drink is associated with illness or vomiting, most of us will develop an aversion to that food.

Activity 10.2

Learning not to Like

- Is there a food that you particularly dislike and will not eat? What learning processes do you think this dislike may be due to?

The *order and timing of the stimulus* will also determine whether conditioning takes place. The neutral stimulus (e.g. a bell) must be presented very shortly (e.g. half a second) before the unconditioned stimulus (e.g. the food) for conditioning to occur. If it is presented afterwards, very little or no conditioning will take place.

Finally, conditioning can be blocked or unlearned. Once classical conditioning has occurred, then attempts to condition a third stimulus can be blocked. In other words, once dogs learn that the bell predicts food, they will not always respond if a third stimulus, such as a flashing light, is introduced, but they may continue to rely on the bell. Conditioning can be *extinguished* or undone by presenting the conditioned stimulus (e.g. the bell) repeatedly without the unconditioned stimulus (e.g. the food).

Classical Conditioning and Physical Symptoms

Many physical responses can be classically conditioned, including immune and neuroendocrine responses (Figure 10.6), allergy symptoms, and nausea. Classical conditioning is therefore highly

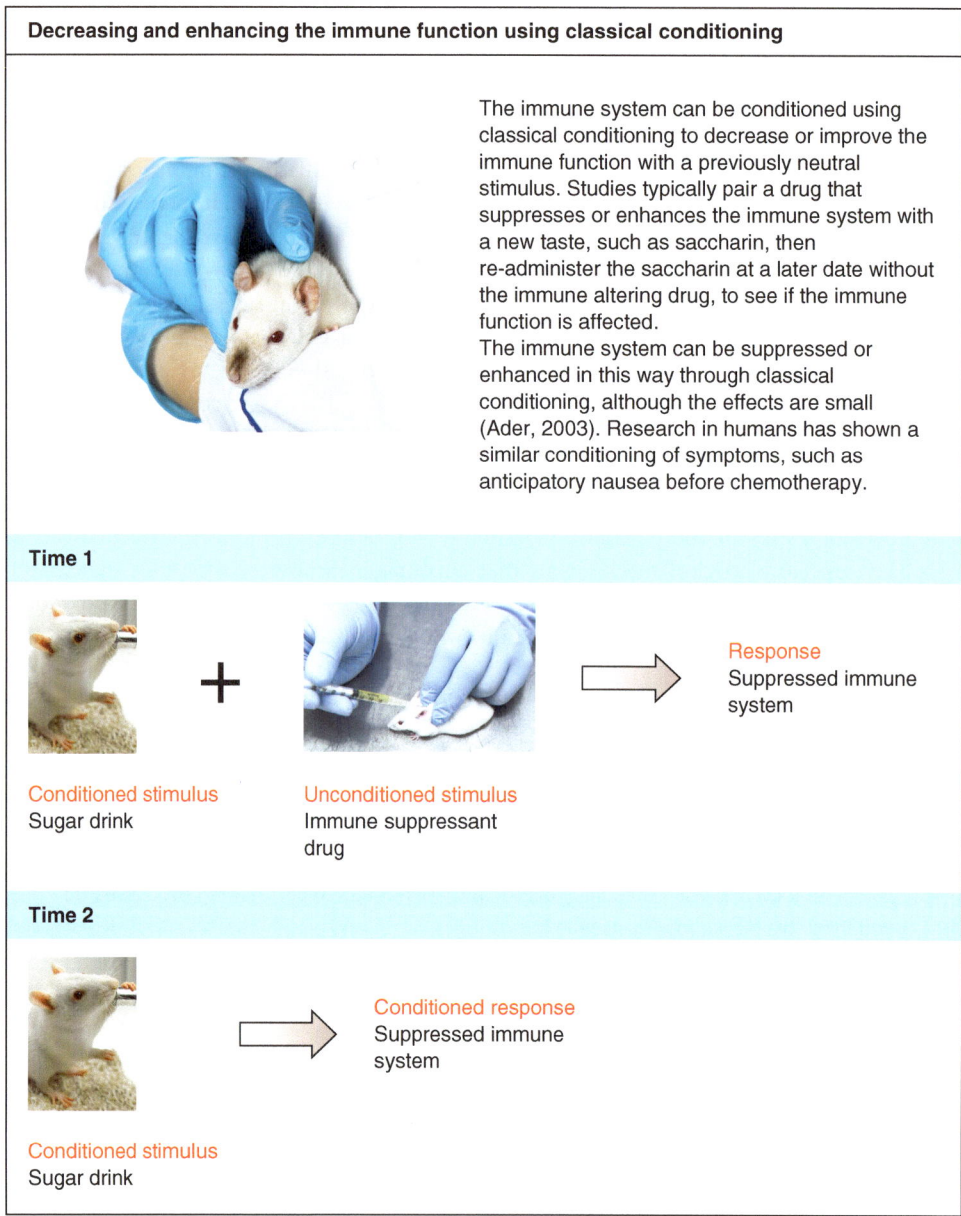

Decreasing and enhancing the immune function using classical conditioning

The immune system can be conditioned using classical conditioning to decrease or improve the immune function with a previously neutral stimulus. Studies typically pair a drug that suppresses or enhances the immune system with a new taste, such as saccharin, then re-administer the saccharin at a later date without the immune altering drug, to see if the immune function is affected.

The immune system can be suppressed or enhanced in this way through classical conditioning, although the effects are small (Ader, 2003). Research in humans has shown a similar conditioning of symptoms, such as anticipatory nausea before chemotherapy.

Time 1

+

Response
Suppressed immune system

Conditioned stimulus
Sugar drink

Unconditioned stimulus
Immune suppressant drug

Time 2

Conditioned response
Suppressed immune system

Conditioned stimulus
Sugar drink

Figure 10.6   Classical conditioning and placebo

Sources: Hands in medical gloves hold a rat © Olexandr/Adobe Stock; photograph of rat drinking reproduced courtesy of © Edstrom; researcher administered drug into the mice by subcutaneous injection © Hyung Keun/Adobe Stock

relevant to healthcare and occurs in many clinical situations, especially where illness or treatment involves pain or other adverse symptoms. The sights, sounds, or smells associated with hospitals may induce physical and emotional responses, such as anxiety or nausea. A good example of classical conditioning involves chemotherapy. Cytotoxic drugs can often have strong side effects such as nausea and vomiting, and up to 30% of people undergoing chemotherapy will experience anticipatory nausea and vomiting by the fourth session of chemotherapy (Kamen et al., 2014). This is because some aspects of the hospital environment become associated with symptoms of nausea and vomiting through classical conditioning. Thus, when people are re-exposed to the hospital stimulus associated with chemotherapy, they will feel nauseous or vomit even before they receive the chemotherapy.

Our understanding of classical conditioning can be used to reduce symptoms or induce positive physical responses. For example, we know that physical symptoms are more easily conditioned in response to novel food or liquid. We also know that once conditioning has occurred, it can block a third stimulus becoming conditioned. For example, giving people a novel drink before each chemotherapy infusion can prevent anticipatory nausea or shortens the time that nausea is experienced during chemotherapy because the nausea becomes associated with the drink and not the hospital context (Stockhorst et al., 1998). This association has also been demonstrated with allergy symptoms. If people are given a novel drink just before taking antihistamine drugs for five days, the drink alone will start to trigger the same drop in basophil activity and improvement in symptoms as the antihistamine drug (Goebel et al., 2008). Classical conditioning therefore plays an important role in placebo effects (see Chapter 4) and may underpin many of the effects of complementary and alternative therapies.

Classical Conditioning and Psychological Problems

Classical conditioning can be involved in the development of psychological problems such as phobias. A traumatic experience can lead to a particular object becoming associated with severe anxiety and fear. Subsequent exposure to this object can then trigger severe anxiety and, if the person subsequently avoids the object, a phobia may develop. An example of this is needle phobia, which can develop following a negative experience of an injection or blood test. To treat phobias, we need to extinguish the learned association by exposing the person to the object while reducing or minimising the conditioned response. This is usually done through flooding or systematic desensitisation, which are based on the fact that strong anxiety responses cannot be sustained indefinitely. Flooding involves exposing a person to the feared stimulus for a long enough time so that their anxiety reduces and the association between the stimulus and anxiety is extinguished. However, this is very hard for people with phobias to accomplish because it is an extreme way to face their fear.

Systematic desensitisation is a more gradual procedure where people are taught relaxation techniques and gradually exposed to stronger versions of the feared object or situation. For example, a person with a needle phobia might be asked to imagine a needle and immediately initiate the relaxation technique. Once they are relaxed in this situation, they might repeat it while looking at a picture of a needle, then a real needle, then perhaps a nurse giving someone else an injection. Thus, they can learn to relax when exposed to the feared stimulus and the association is gradually extinguished. Research shows that both flooding and systematic desensitisation are highly effective treatments for phobias (Böhnlein et al., 2020; Odgers et al., 2022). Advances in technology mean that information technology can be used to deliver systematic desensitisation programmes for anxiety and various phobias, including those specifically related to healthcare (Jiang et al., 2020; Schröder et al., 2023).

10.3.2 Operant Conditioning

Operant conditioning is learning from the consequences of our behaviour and reinforcement. In operant conditioning, behaviour is shaped by its consequences. Reinforcement increases the behaviour of interest:

- Positive reinforcement encourages a desired behaviour by linking it to positive consequences (e.g. continuing to go to the gym because people compliment your changed appearance).
- Negative reinforcement encourages a desired behaviour by removing unwanted experiences (e.g. continuing to take medication because it reduces unpleasant symptoms and pain). This kind of reinforcement is highly relevant to avoidance or escape behaviours, where people learn to avoid situations that harm them or make them anxious.

In contrast, punishment decreases the likelihood of the behaviour of interest:

- Positive punishment discourages an undesirable behaviour by linking it to an unwanted experience (e.g. stopping running because it leads to knee pain, or stopping drinking after experiencing terrible hangovers).
- Negative punishment discourages an undesirable behaviour by linking it to the removal of something that is wanted (e.g. no longer being rude to parents because doing so results in the removal of screen time).

Behaviour is very quickly learned if it is followed by positive reinforcement, such as food or praise. Primary reinforcers are those needed for survival, such as water, food, sleep, and sex. Secondary reinforcers are those that acquire value through experience, such as money, praise, and attention. People's behaviour can therefore be 'shaped' by reinforcement. Different patterns of reinforcement are given in Highlight Box 10.2 and vary in effectiveness. Variable ratio patterns of reinforcement usually lead to the strongest responses and are hardest to extinguish. This may partly explain why gamblers often find it hard to stop. It also has repercussions for drug abuse treatment. For example, methadone blocks the positive effects of heroin, but if it is used intermittently and the drug user gets occasional highs from heroin, they are on a variable ratio pattern of reinforcement and may find it even harder to stop.

—Highlight Box 10.2—

Patterns of Reinforcement

- Fixed ratio: behaviour is always rewarded after a fixed number of times (e.g. bonuses when you reach a target).
- Variable ratio: behaviour is usually rewarded after an average number of times, but it varies (e.g. slot machines or fixed-odds betting terminals).
- Fixed interval: behaviour is rewarded after a fixed time interval (e.g. once a week).
- Variable interval: behaviour is rewarded at varying time intervals.

Research has shown that punishment is much weaker than positive reinforcers, and that any effect of punishment is short-lived. In fact, it has been argued that punishment only suppresses a response, rather than leading to new learning. It may explain why a hangover is not enough to stop people drinking again! Given this knowledge, it does seem odd that our society places so much emphasis on punishment, from disciplining children to our penal system (Eysenck, 2000).

Operant Conditioning and Healthcare

Operant conditioning shows that to learn and improve at any task, including healthcare, we need feedback on our performance – preferably immediately – and that such feedback is most powerful if it is positive. Operant conditioning can be used by health professionals to encourage adaptive behaviours and is particularly useful with children or people with cognitive impairments (see Case Study 10.1). Research with people with severe learning disabilities shows that behaviours such as destructive out-bursts or refusing to eat can be changed very effectively by positively reinforcing an alternative behaviour (Petscher et al., 2009). Operant conditioning can also be useful for families caring for ill relatives. For example, chronic pain behaviours can be reinforced if families are overly sympathetic, or urge the person to lie down or rest and then do everything for them. Although the family may believe they are doing the right thing, in the long term it will lead to more pain behaviour. Hence, families need to learn to ignore pain behaviour and respond positively to non-pain behaviour.

Case Study 10.1

Conditioning and Paediatric Pain

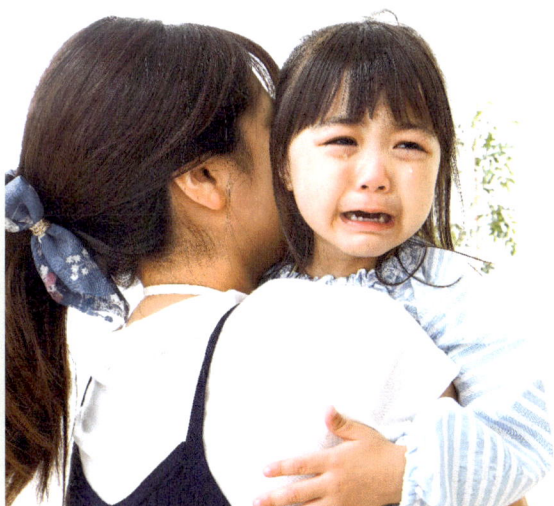

Figure 10.7   Akiko's paediatric pain

Source: © maroke/Adobe Stock

(Continued)

Akiko has third-degree burns to her legs. She needs physiotherapy and must wear uncomfortable splints on her legs. Treatment is not progressing because Akiko becomes increasingly
upset until therapy is stopped. Her mother tries to comfort her but finds it very difficult and is
starting to question whether therapy is really necessary.

The physiotherapist sometimes tries offering Akiko sweets to pacify her, but Akiko seems to be
getting worse rather than better. When Akiko is put into bed, she struggles until she has removed
the splints. If she can't get them off, her crying intensifies to the point of screaming, and she
remains sobbing well into her sleeping time until she falls asleep, or staff come and distract her.

Akiko has learned that the more she cries and struggles the more likely it is that:

- Her mother will cuddle her.
- She will be offered sweets.
- The splints will be removed.
- The physiotherapy will stop.
- Staff will come and distract her.

Some of these reinforcements are occasional, so they may be a variable ratio pattern of reinforcement
which leads to the strongest responses and is hard to extinguish.

How could you use Conditioning to help?

To help Akiko we need to minimise the punishment (pain and discomfort) associated with
physiotherapy, stop reinforcing the negative behaviour, and positively reinforce the behaviour
that helps her to recover. Measures could include:

- Ensuring Akiko has adequate pain relief and perhaps reducing the length of physiotherapy
  initially to help her cope with it.
- Star charts, praise, and treats to reward her when she keeps her splint on for a period of
  time, does physiotherapy exercises, etc.
- Preventing distress by using distraction and encouragement at critical times (e.g. the
  beginning of physiotherapy and bedtime) can also help.
- Teaching her ways to relax or cope during physiotherapy or when in bed that may reduce
  the pain felt.
- Using a decreasing schedule of contact. For example, when she first cries in bed a staff
  member checks her and with minimal words or contact tells her it is OK and she must
  keep the splint on. Akiko can then be left for increasingly longer intervals with minimal or
  decreasing interaction at each point. The splints must be put back on if she removes them.
- Physiotherapy should not be ended because of Akiko's distress. However, her distress
  needs to be managed sensitively.

10.3.3 Modelling and Imitation

Social learning theory has shown that we also learn by observing and imitating others. In a series
of famous experiments, Bandura showed that when children observed an adult being aggressive
toward a life-size doll, they were more likely to do the same when playing with the doll (Bandura

et al., 1961). A meta-analysis of research conducted using various experimental designs found that whereas playing violent video games increases aggression and aggression-related variables, playing prosocial video games has the opposite effect, and can be used in interventions to improve social relationships (Greitemeyer, 2022). However, social learning cannot account for all of our behaviour, because we do not imitate the behaviour of everyone we encounter. Social learning is more likely to take place if the person who is seen to be rewarded is high-status (e.g. a teacher, a medical consultant), is similar to us (e.g. colleagues, family), or friendly (e.g. friends).

Modelling and imitation are integral parts of health professionals' education. Students learn from observing and (selectively) imitating the behaviour of senior staff. Positive role models can be used in other settings to promote positive behaviours, such as health promotion campaigns, patient support groups, and helping people to prepare for surgery. The importance in health promotion of using models that are perceived as similar or relevant is illustrated by the health promotion campaign in Chapter 14 (see Figure 14.5).

Summary 10.3

- Associative learning occurs when we learn the relationship between two events that happen together.
- Classical conditioning occurs where a neutral stimulus (e.g. a bell) is paired with an unconditioned stimulus (e.g. food) to produce a conditioned response (e.g. salivation to the bell).
- Physical responses can be classically conditioned, including immune and neuroendocrine responses, allergy symptoms, and nausea.
- Classical conditioning can be used to create placebo effects and may underpin some of the effects of alternative therapies.
- Phobias can be a result of classical conditioning and are treated using extinguishing methods, such as flooding or systematic desensitisation.
- Operant conditioning occurs when we learn through the consequences of our behaviour – namely, positive or negative reinforcement, or punishment.
- Positive reinforcement is an effective way to encourage adaptive behaviour.
- Modelling and imitation can also influence behaviour, but people are selective in whose and what behaviour they imitate.

10.4 Memory

How and why we remember things affects every aspect of our lives – from day-to-day functioning to exam performance. The importance of memory is most apparent in the devastating impact of disorders such as dementia and amnesia. Understanding memory processes can help us to improve our own memory, and also the way we give information to patients so that they are more likely to remember it. Research suggests that people immediately forget around 50% of information they are told in consultations (Kessels, 2003; Richard et al., 2017). Furthermore, the greater the amount of information that is given, the worse recall is (Selic et al., 2011). This section addresses the basic organisation and characteristics of memory and its relevance to healthcare – namely, effective revision techniques and clinical applications.

10.4.1 Organisation and Characteristics of Memory

Learning and memory involve three stages of encoding, storage, and retrieval. Encoding takes place when the stimuli are presented and memory traces are created. Storage involves organising and storing information. Retrieval involves how we access and recall stored information. Memory problems can occur at any of these stages – information can be encoded wrongly (or not at all), storage may be partial, or retrieval may fail.

Memory is thought to be broadly structured as shown in Figure 10.3. Initially, information is held in sensory buffers. Some of this information is then processed by our short-term memory and the relevant or learned information will go on to be stored in our long-term memory.

The short-term or working memory is used to manipulate and temporarily hold incoming information. Examples of using our working memory are when we first learn a person's medical history, make a diagnosis, or calculate drug dosages. The working memory has visual and auditory components, both with a limited capacity. For example, the auditory loop will usually only hold as many words as we can read aloud in two seconds. This is consistent with early research that established that the average short-term memory span is 7+2 pieces of information (Miller, 1956). However, if the information has meaning or is chunked together, then our memory span can be significantly increased. An everyday example is chunking telephone numbers. It is much easier to remember 0141 337 4501 than 0-1-4-1-3-3-7-4-5-0-1.

Other characteristics of working memory are primacy and recency effects. The recency effect means people are most likely to remember information that has been most recently presented, such as the last few words on a list. It is probably because this information is most accessible in our working memory. The primacy effect means people are more likely to remember items at the beginning of a list compared to the middle. This is probably because of the extra time they have

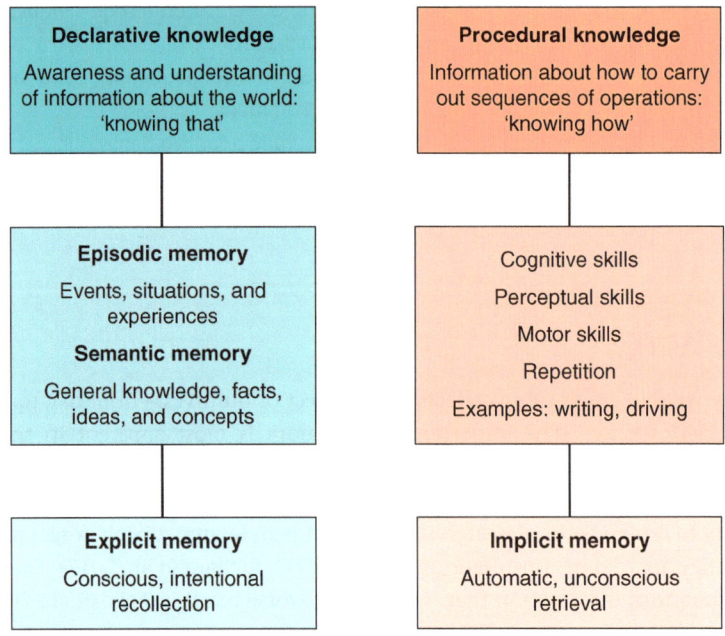

Figure 10.8 Long-term memory stores (adapted from Eysenck, 2000)

had to rehearse these items. Thus, when giving information, we need to present the most important information first and last, and chunk information so that more is remembered.

The long-term memory holds information for future retrieval and is dependent upon the formation of associations between nodes when information is active in our working memory. Repetition of material is important for consolidating long-term memory. Different types of long-term memory are shown in Figure 10.8 and many theories have been put forward about how long-term memory stores work. The known characteristics of our long-term memory are shown in Highlight Box 10.3.

─Highlight Box 10.3─

Characteristics of Memory

- Distinctiveness: distinctive or unique information is more likely to be remembered.
- Elaboration and processing: if information is elaborated in terms of meaning it will be processed more deeply and remembered better.
- Categorisation: information is stored in semantic categories (e.g. animals, food, people), which influences how quickly new information is processed and recognised.
- Spacing and chunking: chunking information increases the amount that can be learned and spacing out learning over time improves memory and retrieval.
- Construction of memories: memories are actively constructed and can be influenced by subsequent events (e.g. eyewitnesses' memory is notoriously subject to distortion).
- Context dependent: memories are associated with the context in which they were encoded, which includes environment and mood. Retrieval is therefore better in the context in which it was first encoded.
- Power of retrieval: the more frequently information is retrieved the better it is remembered – probably because the neural trace is strengthened.

10.4.2 Memory and Studying a Health Profession

Given what we know about memory, it is peculiar that many students do not revise effectively. With a few rare exceptions, studies of people with an outstanding memory have shown that it is down to practice and using strategies, such as mnemonics, rather than being innately gifted. Memory is improved through (Chase & Ericsson, 1982):

- Meaningful encoding (e.g. relating information to knowledge you already have).
- Structured retrieval (e.g. adding as many different cues as possible to the information to help retrieval).
- Practice and repetition (e.g. to make memory processing quick and automatic).

Successful encoding of information involves understanding the meaning rather than learning things by rote. Elaborating and organising information means that it is processed more deeply and integrated into existing knowledge. Effective revision strategies include summarising notes and reorganising the information into different categories, thinking about connections between new information and the things you already know, finding personal relevance or a connection, adding visual images or drawing diagrams or mind maps. Encoding is better if it is spaced out rather than crammed into one long session. Research clearly shows that spacing learning over time results in better memory and retrieval (Groome & Eysenck, 2016). The most effective strategy entails gradually increasing the time between each session.

Using visual imagery can increase our learning because it means both the auditory and visual aspects of our working memory are being used, and it adds further associations in the long-term memory. Visual imagery has been shown to increase memory performance, particularly if objects are pictured together (Groome & Eysenck, 2016). For example, if you have to remember to get a suture kit, a sandwich, and patient records for Ms Alade, you might visualise Ms Alade with a sandwich that has been sutured up balancing on her head. This is a visual mnemonic. Mnemonics are strategies that can help you to remember lists of information that have little connection or meaning. Mnemonics are effective memory aids, and are widely used in medical education for things such as how to perform examinations for pain (e.g. SOCRATES = Site, Onset, Character, Radiation, Associations, Time course, Exacerbating/relieving factors, Severity).

Research has shown that students who use strategies like these to improve their revision and memory do better in exams (Zhou et al., 2016). In particular, summarising notes and drawing mind maps are very effective. If you want to find out more about how to improve your revision techniques, see the Further Reading at the end of this chapter.

The increasing availability of information technology means that in many cases recording of lectures and other learning sessions are available. Watching recordings of learning sessions you have attended can be a useful way to consolidate learning (via repetition). In this context, it is notable that watching a recording twice at double speed may be more effective than watching it once at normal speed (Murphy et al., 2022). However, actively watching by taking notes appears to be more effective than simply passively watching (A. Chen et al., 2024).

─Research Box 10.3─

Using Repetition of Lectures to Boost Memory

Background

Recent research has indicated that watching recordings of lectures at up to double speed does not impair memory. Learning theories support the idea that watching lectures twice at double speed may lead to better memory than watching them once: it can make learning more efficient. However, it is not known whether watching lectures at double speed impairs note-taking, and whether speed or note-taking has a greater impact on learning.

Method and Findings

Researchers conducted two experiments: the first included 201 students and the second 133 students. Participants watched the lecture at normal speed or double speed and either took no

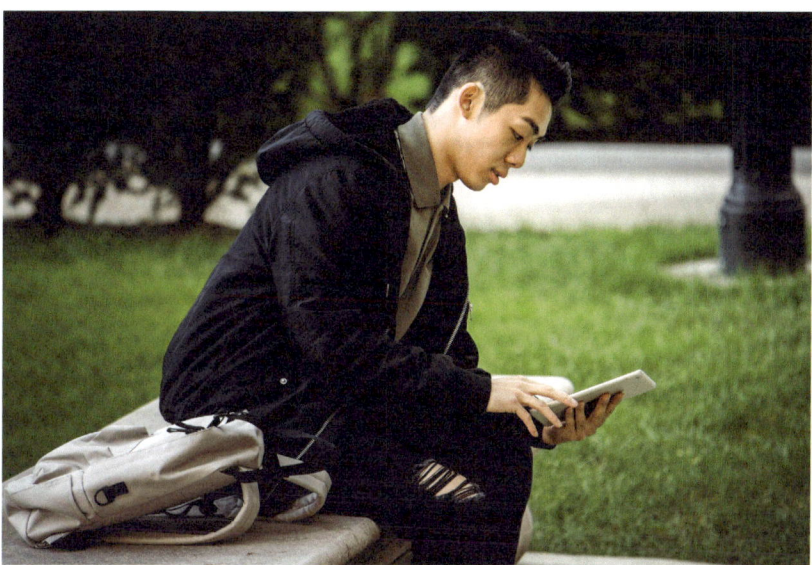

Figure 10.9 A student watching a recorded lecture

Source: © Armin Rimoldi/Pexels

notes, made written notes, or made notes on a laptop. The analyses revealed no significant differences in performance between individuals who took notes from a double-speed recording and those who took no notes at normal speed. Overall, it was also found that note-taking enhanced memory regardless of the speed of lecture play-back, and hand-written note-taking was linked to the best outcomes. Note-taking in written format or on a laptop helped individuals to stay focused and engaged during the lecture, and appeared to help them to process and retain information presented during lectures.

Significance

The authors concluded that if students choose to watch lecture videos at accelerated speed, then they should take notes while doing so. This is because such active learning can support memory for lecture content.

Lameris, A.I., Hoenderop, J.G., Bindels, R.J. & Eijsvogels, T.M. (2015) The impact of formative testing on study behaviour and study performance of (bio)medical students: A smartphone application intervention study. *BMC Medical Education, 15*: 72.

Chen, A., Murphy, D.H., Brabec, J.A. & Bjork, R.A. (2024) The effects of lecture speed and note-taking on memory for educational material. *Applied Cognitive Psychology, 38*(1): e4166. doi:10.1002/acp.4166.

Retrieval in exams can be improved using the characteristics of memory previously outlined (see Highlight Box 10.3). First, the more times you retrieve a piece of information the more you will remember it. Therefore, doing practice exams, testing yourself and others, or talking about topics are all good strategies to help you to remember information better. Smartphone applications for testing knowledge are an accessible and effective way to improve knowledge (see Research Box 10.3) (Lameris et al., 2015; O'Connor and Andrews, 2018). Second, memory is context-dependent. In other words, you are more likely to remember information if the context in which you learned it and then recall it remains the same. Therefore, try to revise under exam conditions. If you get writer's block in an exam, try to imagine yourself in the lecture theatre or the place where you revised. Focus on cues such as what was around you, the PowerPoint slides, the paper you wrote on, books, etc. Such methods can help you to retrieve the information you need.

Clinical Notes 10.1

How to Revise Effectively for Exams

- Summarise lecture notes and draw diagrams or mind maps.
- Concentrate on the meaning of the information rather than rote learning.
- Elaborate information as much as possible. How does it fit with what you already know? How does it relate to your personal experience? How can you use it clinically?
- Chunk information into meaningful groups or categories.
- Use mnemonics to remember lists – distinctive mnemonics are more easily remembered.
- Space out your learning – do not cram revision into one long session.
- Recall information regularly through testing yourself and doing mock exam papers.
- Work with other people in revision groups where you can explain or discuss different topics.
- If you are stuck in exams, think back to the context in which you learned the information.
- Use websites and smartphone apps to help you to revise.

10.4.3 Clinical Applications

There are many clinical applications of understanding memory, not least in trying to treat memory disorders such as Alzheimer's disease, or understanding why most of us have no memories of the first years of our lives.

Particularly vivid 'flashbulb' memories are commonly reported by people after shocking or traumatic events that evoke strong emotions, such as car accidents or myocardial infarction (Catarino, 2015; Tedstone & Tarrier, 2003). Re-experiencing these memories through flashbacks can be a symptom of PTSD. Research has shown that in situations of strong emotion people tend to remember emotions at the expense of facts. For example, if a doctor appears worried, their patient may think the situation is more severe, will focus on the doctor's worries, may become more anxious themselves, and will remember fewer facts from the consultation (Shapiro et al., 1992). However, doctors' use of affective communication – by being empathic, reassuring, and supportive – can reduce people's physiological arousal and result in better recall of information (Visser et al., 2017).

The most common clinical situation where memory is important is giving information to patients. Figure 10.10 and Clinical Notes 10.2 draw together several topics covered in this chapter and apply them to medical consultations (Dommershuijsen et al., 2019; Watson & McKinstry, 2009). Patient satisfaction is influenced by better understanding and recall of information, and patients who are more satisfied and who recall more information have better adherence to treatment. This in turn leads to better outcomes. An important initial task is to avoid or remove distractions, and to capture the person's attention. If a person is upset or distressed, then they may be unable to attend fully to factual information. If this is the case, then it may be best to address their emotional wellbeing first and to consider finding another time to communicate factual information. When you do have a person's attention, it is important to ensure that they understand what you are trying to convey. You can use written and visual information aids to help explain concepts (Sharko et al., 2022; Sletvold et al., 2020). Asking people to say in their own words what they have been told is a good way of checking their comprehension, and it allows you to correct any inaccuracies: there is evidence that this 'teach back' technique is effective for improving patients' knowledge (Talevski et al., 2020). Given that people forget so much information, it is sensible not to rely solely on a person's memory. It may be useful to provide them with records of the information you have conveyed. These could be printed notes, recordings of consultations, links to online resources, or the use of apps for smartphones or tablets (Timmers et al., 2020).

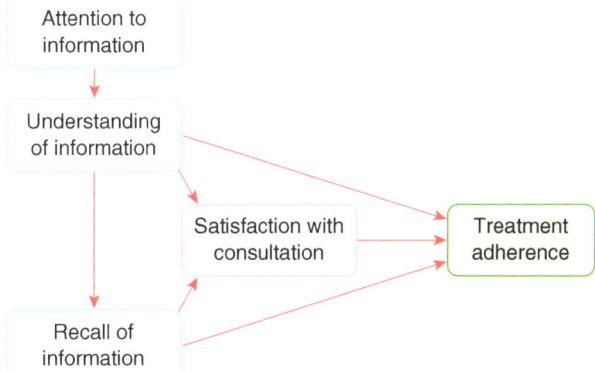

Figure 10.10   The importance of attention and memory in medical consultations (adapted from Kessels, 2003)

Clinical Note 10.2

Giving Information in Consultations

- Remove distractions and ensure that the person is able to focus on the information exchange.
- Put important information first and last.

(Continued)

- Emphasise the information that is important.
- Chunk information into meaningful groups or categories.
- Make the categorisation explicit (e.g. 'now I am going to tell you what is wrong with you, what tests are needed, and what you must do').
- Use repetition.
- Make the information salient to the person.
- Use simple words and short sentences.
- Be specific.
- Avoid overloading people by giving them too much information.

10.5 Cognitive Biases in Healthcare

The material presented thus far in this chapter indicates that perception, attention, and memory are not simply neutral and objective. To some extent, we perceive what we expect to perceive, and we pay more attention to what we expect to be important. In many predictable contexts this process is adaptive, because it frees up some of the limited cognitive capacity we have to manage complex situations. However, these biases may not always be correct, and they may interfere with the accurate interpretation of novel information that we receive. As noted above (section 10.2.2), we may be particularly vulnerable to biased perception and attention when we are overworked or overloaded with other stimuli. Increasingly, cognitive biases are recognised as an important reason for errors in diagnosis, treatment, and healthcare (Fiscella et al., 2021; O'Sullivan & Schofield, 2018). Table 10.1 summarises some of these biases, and the methods we can use to avoid them when making clinical decisions are presented in Clinical Notes 10.3 (O'Sullivan & Schofield, 2018).

Table 10.1 Decision-related biases in healthcare (O'Sullivan & Schofield, 2018)

Availability bias	A tendency to pay more attention and give more importance to information that is more readily available to us
Framing effect	We respond differently to the same information if it is presented with different reference points, e.g. a 97% survival rate may be perceived more favourably than a 3% death rate
Confirmation bias	A tendency to interpret information gained during a consultation in ways that fit our preconceived diagnosis, rather than making a diagnosis purely based on the information provided
Search satisfying	A tendency to stop looking for further information or alternative answers once the first plausible solution has been found, e.g. as noted in many chapters in this book, differential diagnosis is important to determine whether presenting symptoms of anxiety or depression are primary ailments or symptoms of other conditions
Diagnostic momentum	A tendency to continue a course of action instigated by other health professionals rather than considering the available information and changing the plan. Given what we know about obedience (Chapter 9), this may be especially likely if the earlier decisions were made by more senior colleagues
Base rate neglect	A tendency to ignore the base rate incidence of conditions if the person does not fit the risk profile, e.g. a teenager with heart issues
Overconfidence	Inflated beliefs about our diagnostic ability can lead to increased errors. Confidence in our judgements is not an indicator of the accuracy of these judgements

Furthermore, the biases we have mean that we may treat others unequally and unfairly. The material in Chapter 9 showed how stereotypes and prejudice can influence various social interactions, including the provision of healthcare. There is also ample evidence that even if we consciously feel that we are not biased or prejudiced, implicit or unconscious biases affect our interactions with other people. The behaviour of health professionals is influenced by unconscious biases related to gender, ethnicity, and other patient characteristics, such as weight (Fitzgerald et al., 2022; Hall et al., 2015; Maina et al., 2018). Unconscious biases related to gender, ethnicity, and even things like a person's accent can also affect health professionals' initial selection onto degree programmes and subsequent career progression (Capers et al., 2017; Noone & Najjar, 2021; Roessel et al., 2019). In general, these biases lead to worse experiences and outcomes for women, ethnic minorities, and people with other non-normative, marginalised, or stigmatised characteristics. There is, therefore, a need for individuals to be aware of their unconscious biases or implicit assumptions, and for these to be addressed in health professionals' training and continuing professional education (Gleicher et al., 2022; Mavis et al., 2022).

—Clinical Note 10.3—

Reducing Bias in Clinical Decisions

- Slow down when making decisions about diagnoses and treatment.
- Be aware of base rates for your diagnosis and differential diagnoses.
- Actively look for alternative explanations or diagnoses.
- Ask questions to disprove your working diagnosis.
- Remember that you might be wrong, and consider the implications.

Summary 10.4

- Learning and memory involve three stages of encoding, storage, and retrieval.
- Memory involves sensory buffers, the short-term or working memory, and long-term memory stores.
- Short-term or working memory manipulates and temporarily holds incoming information.
- Long-term memory stores hold information for future retrieval.
- Memory is improved through meaningful encoding, structured retrieval, and practice.
- Characteristics of memory can be used to improve revision techniques and memory performance.
- Memory is context-dependent, which includes the physical and emotional context.
- We can use our understanding of memory to give information to people in ways that make it more likely they will remember it.

Conclusion

An understanding of perception, attention, and memory is important for students of medicine and healthcare as it can make learning more effective. The principles and processes described in this chapter are also important for interactions with patients. The case studies, highlight boxes, research boxes, and clinical notes presented in this chapter highlight the practical implications of better understanding of perception, attention, and memory processes.

—Further Reading—

Llewellyn, C.D. et al. (eds) (2019) *The Cambridge Handbook of Psychology, Health and Medicine* (3rd edition). Cambridge: Cambridge University Press. Includes short chapters on cognitive dysfunction in intellectual and developmental disability, dementias, amnesia, aphasia, head injury, and stroke.

Cottrell, S. (2019) *The Study Skills Handbook* (5th edition). London: Red Globe. A useful guide to study skills that is very action-orientated, providing plenty of activities based on the principles discussed above. It has a useful companion website.

Groome, D. & Eysenck, M. (2016) *An Introduction to Applied Cognitive Psychology* (2nd edition). Hove: Psychology Press. An introduction to how cognitive theory and evidence relate to things like everyday memory, biological cycles, performance, and decision making.

—Revision Questions—

1   What is a perceptual set? Discuss the evidence for three factors that influence our perceptual set.
2   How do we learn skills? Outline the three stages involved in learning skills.
3   Discuss the conditions under which people can multitask. What is the relevance of multitasking for clinical practice?
4   Discuss two biases of attention and their implications for clinical practice.
5   What is classical conditioning? How can it be used to create a placebo effect?
6   Describe operant conditioning. What are the most effective forms of reinforcement?
7   Describe modelling and imitation and the three characteristics that make it more likely that children will imitate someone's behaviour.
8   What are (1) short-term memory and (2) long-term memory? What characteristics do they possess?
9   From your understanding of memory, discuss five techniques that can be used when giving information in consultations.
10 How can our understanding of memory help to improve revision techniques and memory performance?

SECTION III
HEALTHCARE PRACTICE

11

DIVERSITY, INCLUSIVITY, AND EQUALITY IN MEDICINE AND HEALTHCARE

Learning Objectives

This chapter is designed to enable you to:

- Outline the key social determinants of health and health inequalities.
- Explain what cultural adaptation of healthcare interventions entails, and why it is important.
- Understand the concept of intersectionality and how it affects health and health outcomes.
- Appreciate why it is important that the healthcare workforce reflects population diversity.

Psychological approaches to health and illness, including psychological interventions, tend to focus on the knowledge, beliefs, and behaviours of individuals. However, it is important to acknowledge that health and illness are also affected by the social contexts in which individuals live. Health status is more than simply a consequence of biological, physiological, or genetic factors; it is also affected by much broader economic, social, cultural, and environmental elements.

11.1 Social Determinants of Health Inequalities

The conditions in which people are born, grow up, live, and work influence their health (World Health Organization, 2008). **Social determinants** frameworks focus on how the circumstances in which people live shape their health, use of health services, and life expectancy (Marmot, 2005).

There is considerable evidence of social gradients in health: people from minority groups and people of lower social status have greater health risks, less access to health services, poorer health, and lower life expectancy than those with higher status. For example, life expectancy for Indigenous Australians is eight years shorter than life expectancy for the non-Indigenous population (Australian Bureau of Statistics, 2023) and similar patterns are observed in other countries with histories of colonisation (Figure 11.1). Social gradients affect not only physical wellbeing, but also the risk of mental illness, access to psychological services, and the outcomes of psychological treatment (Allen et al., 2014; Marmot & Wilkinson, 2006). The observed differences derive from an unequal distribution of resources and a failure to tailor services to the broad spectrum of society.

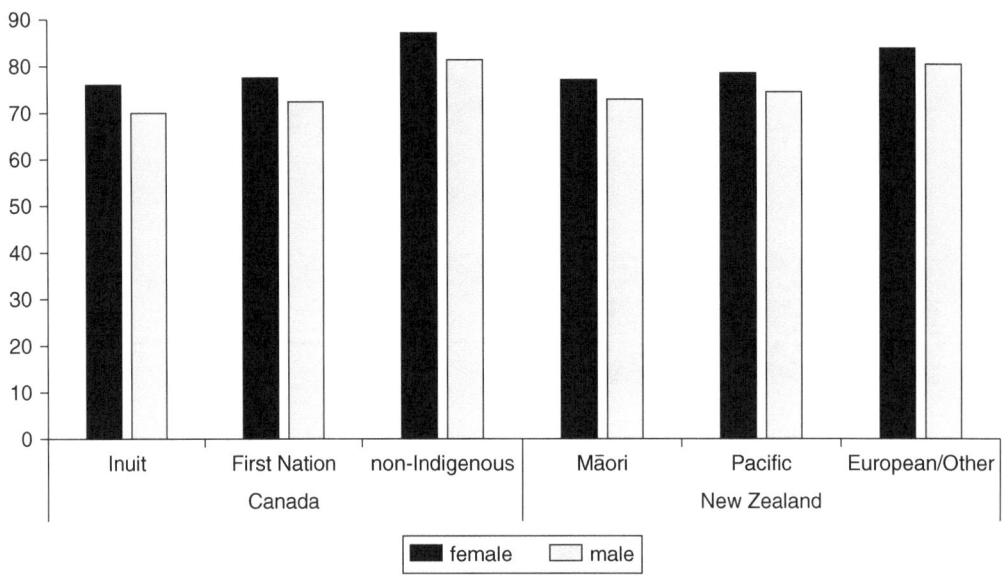

Figure 11.1   Life expectancy is shorter for Indigenous populations than for the ethnic majority (data from New Zealand Ministry of Social Development, 2016; Tjepkema et al., 2019)

Social gradients are linked to **health inequalities**, which the World Health Organization (2024e) defines as 'unfair and avoidable' differences in health between and within countries. Social determinants can have a greater influence on health than lifestyle or healthcare, and it has been estimated that they may explain at least one-third of the observed variation in health outcomes (World Health Organization, 2024e). Key social determinants of worse health and worse health outcomes include adverse childhood experiences, such as abuse or neglect, lower levels of education, lower incomes, unemployment and job insecurity, less stable housing and food access, and social exclusion and discrimination. Some of these are outlined in the remainder of this section and are addressed in greater detail elsewhere (Marmot & Wilkinson, 2006).

Disabilities can have their own impacts on health and wellbeing, and may also magnify the impacts of other health conditions. People with disabilities are more likely than others to have comorbid conditions (World Health Organization, 2024f). Furthermore, disabilities may affect people's engagement with, and experiences of, healthcare and health promotion activities. The broad array of disabilities is too great to address here – they may be cognitive and/or physical and may be congenital or acquired – but many of these issues are addressed elsewhere (Soorenian & Olsen, 2024).

11.1.1 Socioeconomic Status

One of the most important social determinants of health is **socioeconomic status** (**SES**), which is sometimes referred to as social class. SES is not a single characteristic, but instead reflects a combination of an individual's (or their family's) access to economic resources and their social position in relation to other people. Poor health and poverty go hand in hand. People with lower levels of education and/or income tend to have less healthy patterns of behaviour, poorer physical and psychological wellbeing, less access to healthcare, and shorter life expectancy (Braveman & Gottlieb, 2014; Kino et al., 2017; Walker & Druss, 2017).

It is known that life expectancy tends to be longer in richer countries (Jetter et al., 2019), but regardless of how wealthy a country is, wealthy people in any country tend to have better health and longer life expectancy than less wealthy people. Countries with greater income inequality (i.e. a greater difference in wealth between the richest and poorest people) have larger health disparities (Marmot & Wilkinson, 2006) and higher rates of psychological distress (Patel et al., 2018). It is clear that health is affected by both absolute wealth and relative wealth.

Education and income are key social determinants of health and health outcomes. For example, large-scale population-level studies conducted in Australia (Welsh et al., 2021) and across Europe (Mackenbach et al., 2019) reveal that those who are less well-off have significantly shorter life expectancies. The data in Figure 11.2 show clear step-wise social gradients in health markers and health outcomes: in all cases, social advantage is associated with better health.

Notably, links between SES and health are found for both objective measures of SES, such as income or education, and subjective measures of SES, such as where people see themselves on a 'ladder' relative to other people, or to which social class they think they belong (Präg, 2020). Furthermore, perceived SES has an effect on health over and above actual SES. For example, data from nearly 20,000 people in the English Longitudinal Study of Aging indicate that subjective SES has a significant impact on self-rated health even after taking into account objective measures of wealth, income, education, and employment status (Coustaury et al., 2023).

The social gradient applies not only to class or social status, but is observed along many other dimensions in which there is a favoured or powerful majority group and one or more minoritised groups or minorities. Some of these differences are outlined in the remainder of this section.

11.1.2 Sex/Gender

Sex and **gender** have a strong influence on health and health outcomes. Statistics reveal some stark differences between women's health and men's health. In nearly every country, life expectancy is several years shorter for men than for women. This difference is strongly influenced by the observation that women are more likely to engage in health-protective behaviours, such as vaccination and sunscreen use, and less likely to engage in harmful behaviours, such as excessive alcohol use (QuickStats, 2021, 2022; World Health Organization, 2018). In addition, women are more likely than men to engage in screening behaviours or to consult health professionals for psychological or physical concerns (Ballering et al., 2023; Höhn et al., 2020; Pei et al., 2024). Such sex differences should not simply be interpreted as the result of biological differences. The health of men living in different countries can vary greatly, and the health of women within the same country (e.g. women of different ethnicity) can also vary greatly. In addition, average male life expectancy in some countries is longer than average female life expectancy in other countries (World Health Organization, 2024d).

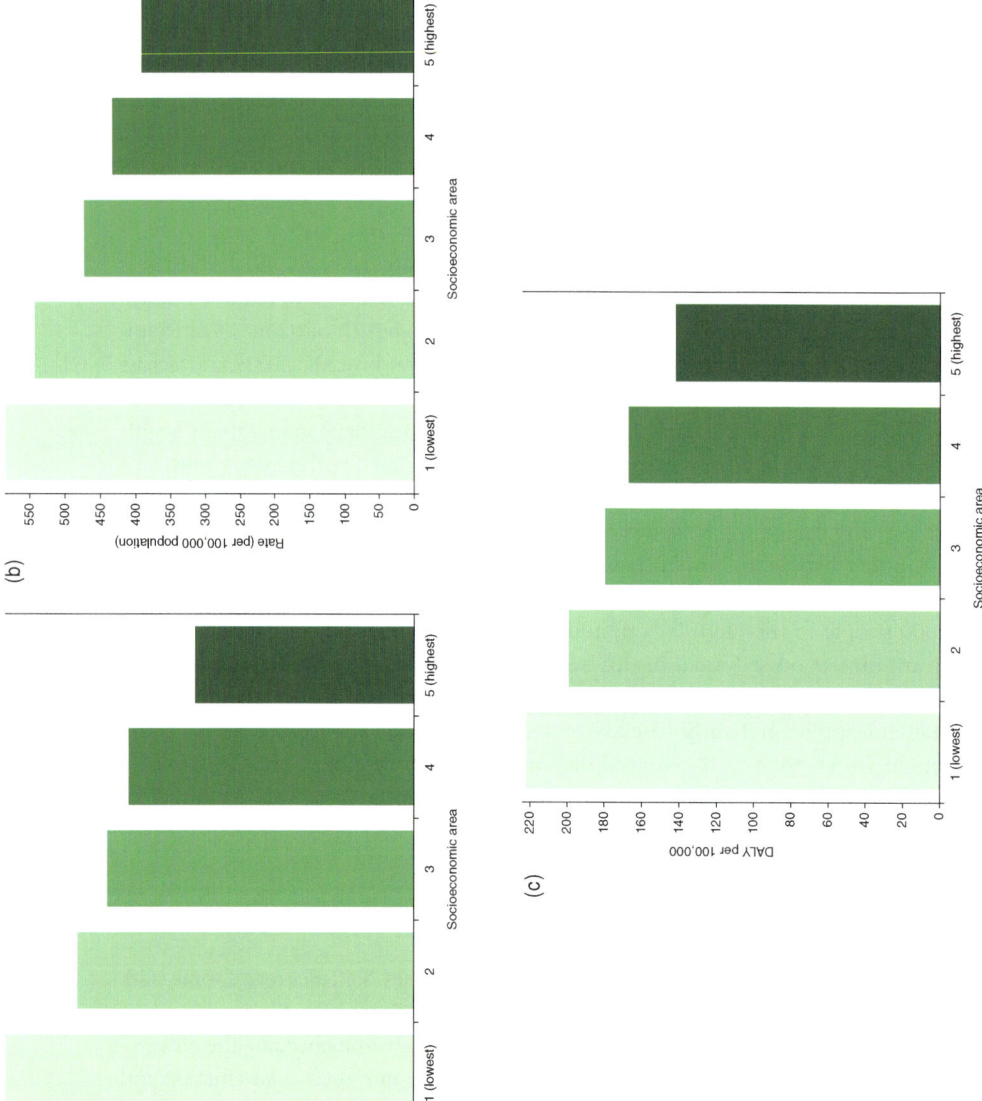

Figure 11.2 Health across socioeconomic groups in Australia: (a) Prevalence of diabetes by socioeconomic area, 2020; (b) All-cause mortality rate, by socioeconomic area, 2020; (c) Total burden of disease, by socioeconomic area, 2018 (adapted from Australian Institute of Health and Welfare, 2024)

People often use the terms 'sex' and 'gender' interchangeably, but they have quite distinct meanings. Sex and sex differences are biologically based: they refer to comparisons between people who are biologically female and people who are biologically male. Gender refers to the social construction of femininities and masculinities through 'feminine' and 'masculine' behaviours. Of course, there are some basic biological characteristics that distinguish all men from all women, but femininity is not a single thing – compare Margaret Thatcher and Marilyn Monroe – and nor is masculinity a single thing – compare Genghis Khan and Freddie Mercury. Some have argued that gender is better conceptualised as a verb than a noun: femininity is not something that women *have*, but something that they *do* (West & Zimmerman, 1987). Many social behaviours, including types of jobs, expressions of emotion, and competitiveness, have clear links to traditional definitions of gender.

Furthermore, many behaviours have gender stereotypes: boys and men are encouraged to take risks and not to show weakness, whereas women are often expected to take care of themselves and others (Courtenay, 2000). This helps to explain within-sex differences in health that cannot be explained by biological differences. For example, men who believe more in 'traditional' definitions of masculinity are more likely to engage in unhealthy 'masculine' behaviours, such as excessive alcohol consumption, and are less likely to engage in healthy 'feminine' behaviours, such as consulting health professionals about physical or psychological wellbeing. However, there is some evidence of generational shifts from these traditional patterns (de Visser & McDonnell, 2013; Lacasse & Jackson, 2020; McCreary et al., 2020; McGraw et al., 2021; Seidler et al., 2016). Furthermore, health professionals' beliefs about masculinity and femininity can influence how they respond to men's and women's psychological and physical symptoms (Möller-Leimkuhler, 2002; Samulowitz et al., 2018). For example, a review of studies of pain revealed that although women experience more pain, their reports of pain are taken less seriously than men's, are more likely to be considered to be psychological, and are less likely to be treated appropriately. In contrast, when 'stoic' men do express pain, it tends to be taken more seriously and treated more appropriately (Samulowitz et al., 2018).

The need to think beyond binaries of male and female is highlighted by increasing awareness of the proportions of people who have non-binary identities, and the observation that they often experience worse physical and psychological wellbeing than men and women whose gender identity matches their biological sex (Drabish & Theeke, 2022; Scheim et al., 2024). In this context, it is important that medical records and health research incorporate accurate gender data that reflect individual experiences and population diversity (Davison et al., 2021; Hay et al., 2019). Having said that, it is also important to note that in much of the research referred to throughout this book, little attention is given to gender diversity, and when analyses do address gender, results tend to be conceptualised in binary terms based on biological sex. In some contexts, the term '**cisgender**' is used to describe people whose biological sex corresponds with their gender identity, in contrast to '**transgender**' women and men whose gender identity does not correspond with their biological sex.

The healthcare experiences of transgender and gender-questioning people are of increasing relevance: barriers to access are widely reported (Safer et al., 2016). It is necessary for healthcare professionals to display an open and non-judgemental approach, to use correct terminology (e.g. using the pronouns preferred by each patient), and to be aware of relevant treatment and support services (Crowley et al., 2021). However, healthcare professionals, like people in other domains, often struggle to provide appropriate and sensitive care, which indicates a need for better knowledge and training (Brooks et al., 2018).

Gender-affirming healthcare focuses on transgender people's physical, psychological, and social wellbeing by affirming their gender identity, and validating transgender identity rather than treating it as a disorder. The underlying aim of gender-affirming care is to align a transgender person's physical traits with their gender identity. This may entail medical, surgical, psychological, and/or social interventions (Healthline, 2022).

—Highlight Box 11.1—

Terminology: 'Opposite' or 'Other'?

What is the opposite of male? Is there an opposite? What is the opposite of female?

Contrary to common parlance based on binaries, 'female' and 'male' are not opposites. They are no more opposite than apples and oranges are opposite types of fruit. Nor are 'feminine' and 'masculine' opposites.

Given the growing awareness of diversity in experiences and expressions of gender, it is preferable to use the term 'other' rather than 'opposite' when comparing sexes or genders.

11.1.3 Sexuality

Health behaviours and health outcomes also vary along the lines of **sexuality**. The term 'sexuality' reflects one or more of identity, attraction, and behaviour: the relative importance or relevance of these aspects may vary depending on what outcomes we are interested in. For example, if we are interested in the risk of STI transmission, then behaviour is key, and identity or attraction may be less relevant. Identity, attraction, and behaviour often overlap, but it is not necessary that they do (Richters et al., 2014). For example, a man may identify as heterosexual, feel attracted to women and men, but only have sex with men. Alternatively, a woman may be attracted to men, but not be sexually active, and identify as asexual.

People who identify as lesbian, gay, bisexual, or transgender (often abbreviated as **LGBT**) tend to have poorer psychological wellbeing and are more likely to attempt or complete suicide (O'Brien et al., 2016; Pitman et al., 2021). Heterosexual people have better psychological wellbeing than people of other sexualities. A meta-analysis of 12 UK population health surveys indicated that heterosexual people are significantly less likely to report anxiety and depression or other symptoms of low mental wellbeing than are lesbian women and gay men, bisexual women and men, or people with other sexualities (Semlyen et al., 2016; see Figure 11.3).

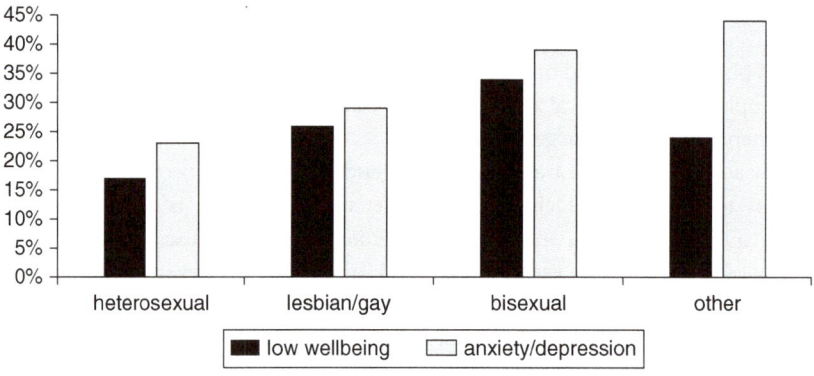

Figure 11.3   Higher prevalence of psychological difficulties among sexual minorities (data from Semlyen et al., 2016)

LGBT people are also more likely than heterosexual people to smoke tobacco, drink alcohol excessively, or use illicit drugs (Fish & Exten, 2020). Important reasons for poorer wellbeing and less healthy behaviour among LGBT people include minority stress arising from prejudice, discrimination, and violence (Fish & Exten, 2020; Hughes, 2016).

LGBT people are more likely to experience barriers to using health services (Frederiksen-Goldsen et al., 2023). Many LGBT people may avoid health services because health professionals do not understand their specific needs or because they feel marginalised by health professionals' heteronormative assumptions (i.e. unquestioningly assuming that heterosexuality is a given and is normal instead of being one of many possibilities). Furthermore, a large cross-sectional study of over 800,000 responses in the English General Practice Patient Survey dataset revealed that LGBT people were less likely than heterosexual people to feel confident in managing their health (H. Cross et al., 2023).

11.1.4 Ethnicity

Ethnicity is an important influence on health behaviours and health outcomes: people from ethnic minorities tend to have poorer health. Some of these differences may be due to biological differences between ethnic groups. For example, a 13-year follow-up study of nearly 60,000 Canadians revealed that the risk of diabetes was significantly higher among people of south Asian, Black, or Chinese ethnicity than among white adults (Chiu et al., 2011). Furthermore, the risk of diabetes for a white person with a Body Mass Index (BMI) of 30 (the lower boundary of the standard 'obese' category) was comparable to that of south Asian, Black, and Chinese people with much lower BMIs at the standard boundary between 'healthy' and 'overweight'. This highlights a need for ethnicity-specific BMI targets and prevention strategies.

There are also clear ethnic disparities in wellbeing: again, people from ethnic minority groups often have worse physical and psychological wellbeing (Australian Institute of Health and Welfare, 2023). For example, Figure 11.4 shows considerable variation in health markers across ethnic groups in the USA, and illustrates that different groups vary in relation to each other. However, instead of thinking only in terms of ethnicity-related physiological differences in disease onset and progression, we also need to consider whether health promotion activities, health

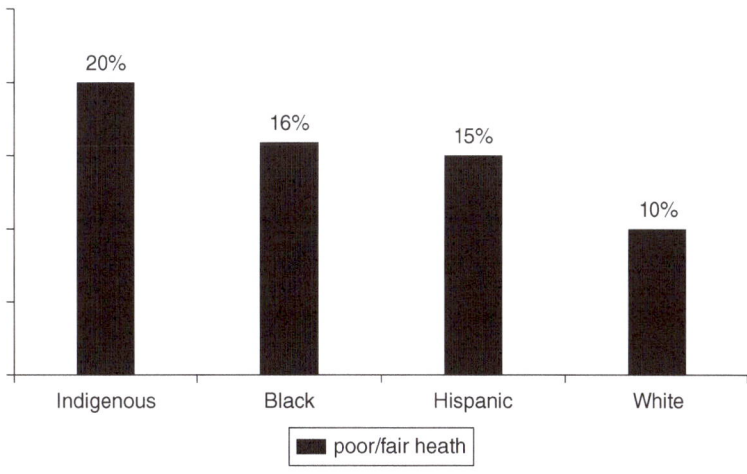

Figure 11.4   Variation in health markers across ethnic groups in the USA between 1991 and 2019.

Source: US Centers for Disease Control and Prevention. Respondent-assessed fair or poor health status, by selected characteristics: United States, selected years 1991–2019. Viewed on 21/10/2024 at: https://ftp.cdc.gov/pub/Health_Statistics/NCHS/Publications/Health_US/hus20-21tables/HStat.xlsx

services, and individual health professionals are aware of, and responsive to, cultural diversity (Memon, Taylor et al., 2016). Ethnicity-related health disparities may not be due to ethnicity *per se*, but rather due to the relative social standing of different ethnic groups within any country. To say that another way, the differences are not due to genetic differences between ethnic groups, but to the psychosocial experiences of members of ethnic groups.

Highlight Box 11.2

Terminology: 'Race', or 'Ethnicity', or Something Else?

In medicine and the health sciences, decisions and actions must be evidence-based. With this in mind, the concept of 'race' should be questioned. There is a shadowy history of pseudo-scientific studies that tried to prove the biological superiority of some population groups over others. However, it is now recognised that there is no biological basis to support 'race' as a biological reality: 'race' is a social construct. Nevertheless, even if 'race' does not exist, 'racism' does.

The term 'ethnicity' is also a social construct, but it is not based on (unsupported) biological claims. Instead, ethnic groups are defined by historical, cultural, and linguistic characteristics. The preferred or prevalent terminology varies between countries. Whereas 'ethnicity' is preferred in the UK, 'race' is widely used in the USA. Whereas many researchers refer to 'ethnic minorities', others prefer the term 'minoritised ethnicities' to reflect marginalisation compared to a dominant group. In other contexts, different terminology is preferred. For example, many Australian researchers refer to culturally- and linguistically-diverse (CALD) groups. You may also see the term 'global majority' used to refer to non-white people and populations.

A simple example of the importance of ethnicity in access to and use of health services comes from the domain of health promotion. If health promotion materials are only produced in the most common language or languages, then people who speak other languages will miss out on the information, which may mean that they are less likely to enact healthy behaviours and/or less likely to cease unhealthy activities. Thus, the language a person speaks, and their access to linguistically-appropriate information, can indirectly affect health. However, as noted in the next section, the translation of words may be only part of a broader need to adapt health promotion activities and health services to meet the needs of all ethnic groups.

Summary 11.1

- The social determinants framework focuses on how demographic and social factors affect people's health, use of health services, and health outcomes.
- Socioeconomic status is a key social determinant: people who are worse off in terms of education, income, or wealth tend to have poorer experiences of physical and psychological health.
- Social gradients are reflected in health inequalities: people who are marginalised, disempowered, or are members of minority groups tend to have worse healthcare experiences and worse health outcomes.

11.2 Addressing Social Determinants to Reduce Health Inequalities

The clear social gradients and health inequalities referred to in section 11.1 have prompted many to argue for, and work towards, developing health promotion and healthcare that is sensitive to, and responsive to, cultural differences. When discussing inequalities in healthcare, we need to consider various elements:

- Access to services: do all people have access to the same services, or to services of comparable quality? If not, why not?
- Engagement with services: do all people make use of the services that are available? If not, why not?
- Experiences of services: do all people have comparable, and good, experiences when they do engage with services? If not, why not?
- Outcomes of engaging with services: do all people experience comparable, and good, outcomes from engaging with services? If not, why not?

Evidence suggests that access, engagement experiences, and outcomes often vary greatly between population groups and in ways that tend to disadvantage minority groups (Caraballo et al., 2022; Eken & Powers, 2021; Fontil et al., 2022).

11.2.1 Cultural Competence

The benefits of **cultural competence**, which is sometimes referred to as **cultural sensitivity**, in approaches to mental health have been acknowledged for some time (e.g. Bernal et al., 1995; López et al., 1989; Rogler et al., 1987). Perhaps the most obvious example of a need for cultural adaptation is when an intervention developed in one country is transferred to another country. A logical first step would be to translate the materials from the original language to the language used in the new context – or, more appropriately, into the languages used in the new context.

However, simple translation may not always be possible because different languages may not have equivalent terms. For example, a language may use terms such as 'sadness' or 'low mood' to refer to the more complex phenomenon of 'depression'. Furthermore, within different cultural contexts the experiences that are described by specific words may have quite different meanings. For example, within secular contexts, hearing voices may be considered as an auditory hallucination that reflects some kind of disorder, whereas from a different perspective, hearing the voice of gods, angels, or demons could be understood as a religious experience (Cook, 2019). This suggests that translating words may be a necessary part of adapting materials and practices, but that other actions may also be needed as part of the cultural adaptation of healthcare (see section 11.2).

To properly address culture, it is necessary to ask what we mean by culture. Commonly-used definitions refer to culture as the general customs and beliefs that characterise the way of life of a particular group of people. Such definitions can be conceptualised at the national level and may be linked to stereotypes (e.g. the idea of Australian culture as being characterised by beaches, barbecues, and beer) (see Chapter 9, section 9.3, for more on stereotypes). However, the term 'culture' (or 'subculture') can also refer to the beliefs and social practices of ethnic or religious groups, or to other social subcultural groups.

It is important to note that much of the material covered in this chapter refers to the conscious awareness of perceived or actual differences between groups. However, as noted in Chapter 9, our thoughts and behaviour may also be affected by unconscious biases.

Activity 11.1

Is Diversity Visible?

As you read the text and the examples in this book, and others that you encounter during your education and training, consider how well diversity is addressed. Questions that you may wish to ask include:

- Are the experiences of diverse members of the population addressed?
- Do the examples that are given reflect population diversity?
- Have interventions been developed or adapted to reflect population diversity?

Also pay attention to who is present and who is absent as participants or researchers.

11.2.2 Cultural Adaptation

Cultural adaptation can be defined as the systematic modification of an evidence-based health intervention to acknowledge the influence of patients' linguistic, cultural, and social contextual background. It is a logical and ethical extension of an awareness of health disparities, and it can be used to address health disparities. Cultural adaptation involves identifying the core components of an intervention and the cultural factors that may affect the delivery of the intervention, and modifying the intervention to accommodate these cultural factors. The adaptation is to ensure that the intervention is suitable for the target population (Castro et al., 2010). The 'intervention' may be a specific treatment or therapy, or it could be conceptualised more broadly as a health system. Research Boxes 11.1 and 11.2 look at two studies on interventions that were culturally adapted to reach their target populations.

Various cultural adaptation frameworks and processes have been developed (e.g. Hwang, 2006, 2009; Naeem et al., 2019). Each describes a specific version of the general principles outlined above. For example, the Formative Method for Adapting Psychotherapy (FMAP: Hwang, 2009) is a five-step method for adapting psychotherapy. It is defined as being 'community-participatory' because it involves community members in the development of the intervention, and as being 'bottom-up' because it begins with an exploration of the needs of patients and other relevant people to ensure that it is grounded in the experiences of the specific target group. The five-step process is illustrated in Highlight Box 11.3.

Highlight Box 11.3

An Example of a Cultural Adaptation Framework

Applications of the Formative Method for Adapting Psychotherapy entail working through the following five stages:

1 Collaborating with stakeholders to generate knowledge.
2 Integrating information from step 1 with empirical and clinical knowledge.
3 Reviewing the initial adaptations with stakeholders and proposing further revisions.
4 Testing the acceptability and feasibility of the culturally-adapted intervention.
5 Finalising the intervention for broader delivery.

Research Box 11.1

Culturally Relevant Interventions

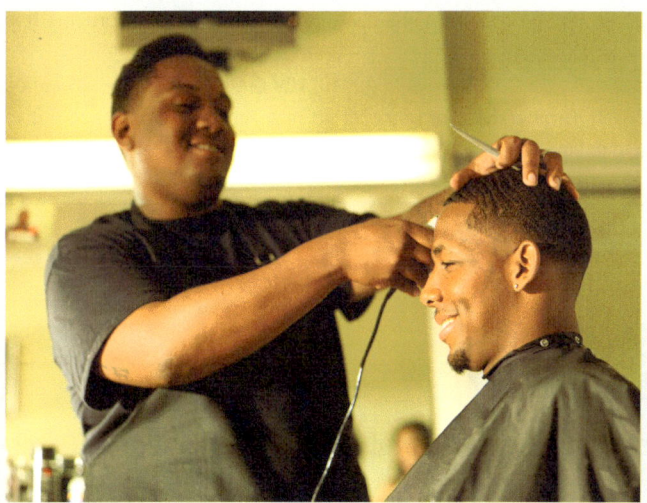

Figure 11.5   A barbershop in New York City

Source: © Joshua Resnick / Adobe Stock

(Continued)

Background

In the USA, Black heterosexual men are at greater risk of HIV infection, late diagnosis with HIV, and HIV mortality. HIV infection in this group is predominantly attributable to sexual behaviour, but there is a lack of effective condom-promotion interventions designed specifically for Black men. The aim of this study was to use the strong connections and frequent interactions that barbers have with this important, but overlooked population.

Methods and Findings

Twenty-four barbershops in New York City delivered the Barbershop Talk with Brothers (BTwB) intervention, which was a strength-based intervention designed to promote attitudes, social norms, self-efficacy, and communication skills supportive of condom use. A further 29 barbershops in the city served as the control group. Data were collected from 860 men who reported multiple sexual partners in the preceding six months, and at least one episode of sex without a condom. They completed surveys at baseline and at six-month follow-up. The two groups had comparable reports of condom use at baseline, but differed in relation to other demographic variables. After taking into account these baseline differences, it was found that men in the intervention group were significantly less likely to report unprotected sex at six-month follow-up.

Significance

The brief BTwB intervention was an effective way to embed a public health intervention within existing barbershop communities. The principles underlying the approach can be – and have been – used in other settings with different population segments to recruit trusted community members to deliver health promotion in settings that do not typically provide health services.

Wilson, T.E., Gousse, Y., Joseph, M.A. et al. (2019) HIV prevention for Black heterosexual men: The Barbershop Talk with Brothers cluster randomized trial. *American Journal of Public Health, 109*(8): 1131–1137. doi:10.2105/AJPH.2019.305121

—Research Box 11.2—

Cultural Adaptation of a Mental Health Intervention

Background

Better engagement with treatment for a first episode of psychosis leads to better outcomes. However, people often disengage from services, especially those from minoritised groups and/or those with diverse ethnic backgrounds. The Early Youth Engagement study (EYE-2) tested a new intervention that was designed to reduce disengagement. A key part of the development of the intervention was cultural adaptation to incorporate the needs of the diverse range of service users.

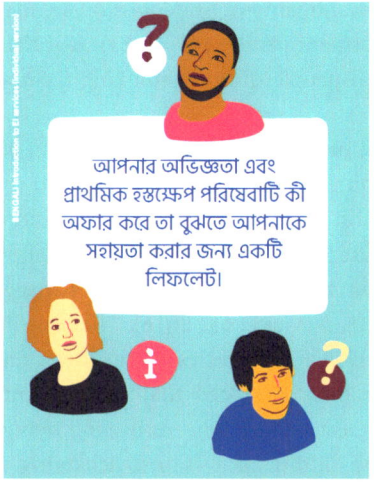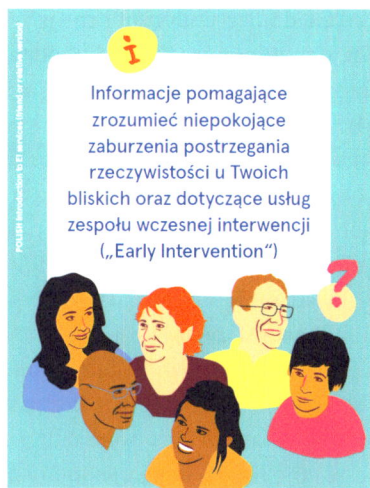

Figure 11.6 Cultural adaptations to address language barriers

Source: NHS, https://www.likemind.nhs.uk/

Methods and Findings

Twenty-one young adult service users completed semi-structured interviews about their perspectives on EYE-2 approaches and resources. Data were collected across three inner-city sites in England, and the sample was chosen to allow analysis of diversity across ethnicity, spirituality, and sexuality. Thematic analysis of the interviews highlighted that efforts to enhance engagement among minoritised groups must address language barriers. However, at a broader level, they must address culturally-specific differences in cognitions and beliefs about psychosis (e.g. how do religious or spiritual beliefs affect how people understand anomalous psychological experiences such as psychosis?). There is also a need to acknowledge the stigma and discrimination related to psychiatric conditions in general, and psychosis in particular. The analysis also highlighted the importance of trust in the therapeutic alliance and individual differences in therapeutic preferences. Furthermore, the findings highlighted the impact of intersectionality, such that greater stigma and discrimination may be experienced by people experiencing psychological distress who come from minoritised social groups.

Significance

The themes were mapped onto a cultural adaptation framework. This process highlighted that, as a first step, there is a clear need to make resources, services, and research more accessible for speakers of various languages. However, there is also a need for broader cultural adaptation that recognises how psychosis is experienced and understood in different cultural and social contexts.

Rathod, S., Phiri, P., de Visser, R.O. et al. (2023) Applying the cultural adaption framework to the Early Youth Engagement (EYE-2) approach to early intervention in psychosis. *British Journal of Clinical Psychology, 62*(3): 537–555. doi:10.1111/bjc.12423

The value of cultural adaptation in various contexts is highlighted in reviews which show that culturally adapted interventions for the psychosocial treatment of depression are more effective for reducing symptom burden than standard treatment (Anik et al., 2021), and that culturally adapted interventions are more likely to result in people quitting smoking (Leinberger-Jabari et al., 2024).

Cultural adaptation displays respect for the cultural diversity that exists within populations, improves communication by overcoming conceptual and linguistic barriers, and increases the participation of members of the target population by making interventions more engaging (Kreuter et al., 2004; Resnicow et al., 1999; see Case Study 11.1). For example, one study found that culturally adapting smoking cessation programmes led to higher levels of engagement and participation than a standard programme (Memon, Barber et al., 2016). That qualitative study used in-depth interviews with women from deprived communities in south-east England who had used stop smoking services in the past. Findings indicated that services could increase smoking cessation rates if they were tailored to meet women's needs by improving the continuity of care, providing more flexibility in the timing of sessions, delivering sessions in accessible locations, providing cost-free smoking cessation aids, and providing better and more appropriate peer support.

Case Study 11.1

Identity-First or Person-First Language?

It is important to pay attention to the language we use when describing people and their conditions.* Compare the following statements:

> I call myself a person living with HIV/AIDS, because I am a person who also happens to be HIV-positive. I was a person for 24 years, and I have been a person living with HIV/AIDS for 12 years. Calling someone an 'AIDS victim' or 'AIDS sufferer' makes them seem weak, when they are probably stronger than most people. (Ang)

> I am an autistic person. Autistic is in my personality, my imagination, and my soul. It is me: it cannot be separated from me… but please don't use 'autistic' as a noun: I am not an autistic; I am a person. (Lee)

The first is an example of '**person-first**' language; the second is an example of '**identity-first**' language. Some people and organisations oppose person-first language because they believe that identification of a specific trait in this way suggests that the trait is negative. In other contexts, people reclaim terms that were historically used in derogatory ways and thereby reduce their negative impact. Examples are terms such as crip and queer.

However, it is important to note that, within groups, there may be variety in preferred terminology. For example, many autistic people prefer other terms. To reduce the risk of errors, ask people what terms they prefer to be used.

* *Note*: we may also question whether 'patients' is always the preferred term, or whether 'service users' or simply 'people' may be a more appropriate term. Similarly, terms such as 'disease', 'illness', and 'disorder' are not simply interchangeable.

11.2.3 Cultural Congruence

One way of adapting the delivery of healthcare to the needs of a diverse population of patients is the practice of trying to match patients from minority groups with practitioners from the same minority groups. Most commonly, this has been achieved with a focus on ethnic matching, although many reports use the term 'racial matching' (Cabral & Smith, 2011). A meta-analysis of ethnic matching in mental health services suggested that it had positive, but variable, effects (Cabral & Smith, 2011). The results indicated that patients had a moderately strong preference for a therapist of their own ethnicity, and that they tended to perceive therapists of their own ethnicity more positively than other therapists. There was not strong evidence that matching led to better treatment outcomes. Of course, the ability to undertake ethnic matching is limited by the capacity of services to offer matching, and their motivation to do so. Research suggests that one or both of these aspects are commonly lacking. For example, a study of the perceived importance and prevalence of ethnic matching in substance use disorder treatment centres revealed that in just over half (58%) of the clinics there was the potential to match counsellors with ethnically similar clients, but that among these, 26% never ethnically matched clients and therapists and only 7% always did so (Steinfeldt et al., 2020).

Although some service users may prefer ethnic matching, not all people think that it is the most appropriate approach. Alternative approaches favoured by some service users include a focus on broader cultural appropriateness or a person-specific service (Olaniyan & Hayes, 2022). Matching can also be conducted according to other characteristics. For example, one study conducted in the context of primary care indicated that both male and female patients often prefer to see a same-gender primary care physician, but that this preference was stronger among men (M. Fink et al., 2020). Beyond demographic similarities or differences, other patient preferences could be considered as part of providing person-specific care (Olaniyan & Hayes, 2022). For example, one study explored the relative impact of physician gender and physician communication style, and found that their relative importance may vary for male and female patients (Schmid Mast et al., 2007).

11.2.4 Intersectionality

When cultural adaptation work is done, it tends to focus on single dimensions such as socioeconomic status *or* ethnicity *or* sexuality. However, people have a socioeconomic status *and* an ethnicity *and* a sexuality, and they may have a combination of minority and majority characteristics.

Thus, a middle-class woman in Northern Europe could possess the additional majority character-istics of white European ethnicity and heterosexual identity, and her experiences may be quite different from those of a middle-class white European lesbian woman, and both of these women may have different experiences from a middle-class lesbian woman from South-East Asia.

The concept of **intersectionality** draws attention to the ways in which inequalities related to SES, gender, sexuality, ethnicity, or other characteristics can combine to magnify inequalities in health behaviours and health outcomes (Mereish & Bradford, 2014). The concept was first introduced in the context of social justice to emphasise that minority characteristics often inter-sect to magnify social disparities, and that this fact is often overlooked (Crenshaw, 1991). However, it is clearly important for social studies of health and illness. When designing and providing health services, we must be responsive to diversity and intersectionality. If we are to understand (and address) health inequalities, then we must:

1   Acknowledge the existence of multiple intersecting identities.
2   Acknowledge how the experiences of people with multiple intersecting minority characteristics reflect structural inequalities (Bowleg, 2012).

Intersectionality is a way of understanding complex interactions of different forms of oppres-sion and privilege, including SES, gender, sexuality, ethnicity, and other social categories. The challenges of intersectionality in cultural adaptation arise when individuals face multiple and overlapping barriers that are linked to their intersecting social identities. For example, a Muslim woman who wears a hijab and lives in a non-Muslim, 'western' culture may face discrimination and exclusion based on both her religion and gender.

—Activity 11.2—

Privilege Walk

One way to think about how different aspects of experience and identity intersect is to under-take a 'Privilege Walk'. Depictions of this activity are available online (e.g. www.youtube.com/watch?v=hD5f8GuNuGQ).

The privilege walk begins with a group of people, such as students or work colleagues, lining up shoulder to shoulder along a starting line across the middle of the room. The session facilita-tor reads out various markers of privilege or advantage and in response, each member of the group takes one step forward or one step back depending on whether the characteristic applies to them. Statements may include:

- If you have ever been made fun of or bullied because of something you cannot change, take one step back.
- If you can show affection to your romantic partner in public without fear of negative reactions, take one step forward.
- If you have ever been diagnosed with a physical, psychological, or learning disability, take one step back.

- If you get time off work for your religious celebrations, take one step forward.
- If the primary language spoken in your childhood home was not English*, take one step back.
- If you can see a doctor whenever you feel the need, take one step forward.
  (* match to the official language(s) of the country in which people live)

By the end of the list, the group that had started shoulder to shoulder is dispersed along the length of the room, with the most privileged standing furthest toward the front. The more privileged people who have engaged in this task, including the authors of this textbook, are often surprised at the extent of their unacknowledged privilege.

Statistical analysis typically measures variation according to single variables. For example, research may explore the effects of gender differences, and separately explore the effects of ethnic differences, but not explore similarities and differences between men and women of different ethnicities. Although separate and simple categories such as gender or ethnicity have some explanatory power, it is limited (Bowleg, 2012). If we take an intersectional approach, then we must conceptualise and analyse health disparities in the complex and multidimensional ways that reflect people's identities and experiences, but this means that analysis becomes more numerous and more complicated. For example, if we create simple binary measures of SES (higher/lower), gender (woman/man), and ethnicity (majority/minority), then we end up with eight combinations and 28 comparisons between pairs. If we use more nuanced measures of SES, gender, and ethnicity than simple binaries, or if we add more demographic variables, then we end up with even more combinations and even more comparisons. This raises questions about the limited scope of ethnic matching (see above) because that practice privileges ethnicity as the most important variable. However, in some situations, other characteristics, such as gender, disability, or SES, may be more relevant to patients.

Although intersectionality is clearly important, it has also been noted that 'this framework complicates everything' (Hankivsky & Christoffersen, 2008: 279). Nevertheless, to ignore this complexity risks reinforcing multiply-determined health inequalities. The case studies and examples presented throughout this textbook have been chosen to include examples from a range of contexts. However, reflecting the state of the academic literature, participants tend to be WEIRD – that is, they tend to come from Western, Educated, Industrialised, Rich, and Democratic countries. As suggested in Activity 11.1, pay attention throughout your studies to who is present and who is absent – as participants, as researchers, and as educators.

Summary 11.2

- Cultural competence is reflected in an awareness that one-size-fits-all approaches to health promotion and healthcare may not meet the needs of all people.

(Continued)

- Cultural adaptation is the process of systematically modifying health promotion interventions or healthcare practices to acknowledge the diversity in patients' linguistic, cultural, and social backgrounds.
- The concept of intersectionality draws attention to how inequalities related to SES, gender, sexuality, ethnicity, and other characteristics combine in ways that intensify health inequalities.

11.3 Diversity in Healthcare Workforces and Healthcare Systems

Attention has been given thus far to patient experiences and patient preferences. Within that analysis, there has been some discussion of the characteristics of healthcare providers, particularly in relation to matching. For these reasons, it is important to have a healthcare workforce that represents the population that it serves (Stanford, 2020). However, the medical professions and wider healthcare workforce also need to reflect the diversity of the broader population (British Medical Association, 2019). All members of the population should have opportunities to undertake the education and training required to enter the health professions, and to progress along their career pathways. However, the experiences of staff and opportunities for development are not equal (British Medical Association, 2019). This is not only because it is good for individuals from minority groups, but also because environments that are diverse and inclusive have greater professional satisfaction and better outcomes for patients (British Medical Association, 2019).

Unfortunately, many healthcare professionals experience a lack of respect for diversity, and an absence of truly inclusive working cultures and contexts (British Medical Association, 2019). For example, one UK study of female Muslim health professionals and medical students revealed that the majority of participants experienced difficulties trying to wear a headscarf and conforming to 'bare below the elbow' dress codes in operating theatres (Malik et al., 2019). It was notable that many respondents felt that their career opportunities had been restricted by the medical profession's responses to their adherence to religious dress codes. For example, one woman reported: 'I decided not to go into surgery due to dress codes.' Another said that because surgery was her dream career, she 'just found a way around it', but also noted that 'some staff don't make it easy'. The different experiences of Muslim men and women in this context again highlight the need for intersectional approaches.

It could be argued that the safety of all patients needs to be balanced against the religious practices of some healthcare professionals. However, the specific and striking example of surgery is a marker of a broader phenomenon that may reflect an under-representation of ethnic minorities in senior roles. Studies in various countries reveal that although there have been increases in the proportions of people from ethnic minorities at the entry-point of education and training in the health professions, they are still strikingly under-represented at senior practitioner levels and in senior management (NHS England, 2022; Salsberg et al., 2021; Stanford, 2020). Increasing diversity and inclusivity at all levels of the health services is a vital step towards ensuring equality.

Conclusion

This chapter has outlined the key social determinants of health and health inequalities, and illustrated how people have poorer experiences of physical and psychological health and healthcare if they come from less privileged or more marginalised backgrounds. The existence of social gradients and related health inequalities highlights the need for the cultural adaptation of healthcare interventions so that they are suitable for all subgroups of the population. Cultural adaptation is a process of modifying health promotion interventions or healthcare practices to ensure that they reflect the linguistic, cultural, and social diversity in the population. At the same time as ensuring that all healthcare professionals understand the importance of addressing the healthcare needs of all members of the population, there is a need to ensure that all members of the population have the same opportunities for education and training as health professionals.

Further Reading

Marmot, M. & Wilkinson, R. (2006) *Social Determinants of Health* (2nd edition). Oxford: Oxford University Press. An update of a landmark book that provides a convincing overview of the important ways in which health is influenced by early life experiences, social circumstances, work and unemployment, ethnicity, and many other social factors.

Rose, P.R. (2020) *Health Equity, Diversity, and Inclusion: Context, Controversies, and Solutions* (2nd edition). Boston, MA: Jones & Bartlett. The second edition of an earlier book that expands the focus from exploring heath disparities to explaining how to work to promote health equity. There is an accompanying test bank that includes a collection of questions tailored to the book's content.

World Health Organization (2023) *Integrating the Social Determinants of Health into Health Workforce Education and Training*. Geneva: WHO. This PDF document is free to download and is a useful companion piece to the two other suggestions for further reading. It emphasises the need to ensure that health and care workers understand how social determinants affect health, and that they are helped to develop the skills needed to address health inequalities.

Revision Questions

1   What is meant by the term 'social gradients in health'? Explain using examples from published research.
2   Choose a dimension of social diversity (e.g. education, ethnicity, sexuality) and outline how it is related to health, access to health services, or experiences of healthcare.
3   Discuss the accuracy of the statement: 'Ethnic differences in health can be fully explained by biological differences.'

4   Explain the difference between the terms 'sex' and 'gender'. Give an example of a sex difference in health outcomes and a gender difference in health behaviour.

5   How might socioeconomic status affect access to, experiences of, and/or outcomes of engagement with health services?

6   Why is there a need to apply cultural adaptation frameworks in health promotion?

7   What are the benefits of cultural adaptation in health promotion?

8   Explain what is meant by 'intersectionality'. Why is intersectionality an important influence on health outcomes?

9   What challenges does intersectionality pose for cultural adaptation?

10   Why is it important that the demographic profile of the healthcare workforce reflects the diversity of the broader population?

12

EVIDENCE-BASED PRACTICE

Learning Objectives

This chapter is designed to enable you to:

- Define evidence-based practice.
- Identify the sources of information to be used in evidence-based practice.
- Describe the factors that influence people's adherence to prescribed treatment.
- Discuss the importance of effective communication between clinicians and patients.

Ideally, all decisions about treatment would be based on sound evidence. This ideal lies behind the promotion of evidence-based practice. But what is meant by 'evidence-based practice', and what counts as evidence? This chapter begins with a description of evidence-based practice. The second section focuses on evidence from research on adherence to treatment, and the third section describes research into practitioner–patient communication. Chapter 13 builds on the last section and outlines the communication skills to use in clinical consultations that can help improve patient outcomes.

12.1 Evidence-Based Practice

Evidence-based practice is widely accepted as fundamental to best practice. The formation of clinical guidelines and institutions such as the National Institute for Health and Care Excellence (NICE) in the UK are founded on the importance of evidence-based practice.

12.1.1 What is Evidence-Based Practice?

Evidence-based practice reflects the principle that 'decisions about healthcare are based on the best available, current, valid and relevant evidence. These decisions should be made by those receiving care, informed by the tacit and explicit knowledge of those providing care, within the context of available resources' (Dawes et al., 2005: 1). This and other definitions of evidence-based practice highlight the importance of integrating robust research evidence and clinical expertise, and acknowledge that patient choice is important. An important aspect of evidence-based practice is therefore taking into account the details of each person's predicaments, rights, and preferences. In a useful guide, Straus et al. (2018) state that for evidence-based practice we must:

1   Formulate an appropriate question. Questions must be phrased in a way that allows us to determine whether they have been answered. For example, if we want to know which of two possible treatments is better, then we need to define beforehand what we would consider to be a clinically significant difference – we will then have a criterion to apply to our answers.

2   Find the best evidence to answer this question. The different sources of evidence will be discussed in more detail below.

3   Evaluate and appraise the evidence. Medical professionals must know how to distinguish between reliable and unreliable (or good and bad) evidence. Although evidence can aid decision making, the evidence itself does not make decisions.

4   Align our evaluation of the evidence with our own expertise and the details of the particular patient. We must understand how the evidence will apply to particular people. As noted above, this means taking into account people's rights and preferences and any contra-indications for specific treatments.

5   Evaluate steps 1 to 4 in a process of continual feedback, refinement, and flexibility. It is important to evaluate not only the outcomes (i.e. whether the chosen treatment was successful), but also the processes of integrating the evidence with clinical judgement. Through such self-evaluation, the process of evidence-based practice should become more effective.

Ideally, steps 1 to 5 form a feedback loop whereby our evaluation of the processes and outcomes of medical decision making informs the development of more appropriate question formulation, better evidence-gathering, better evaluation, and better integration of evidence with clinical expertise (see Figure 12.1).

These five steps represent an ideal pattern, which may not be followed by all clinicians all of the time (Straus et al., 2018). Clinicians may shift between different modes of evidence-based practice depending on the nature of their work and the presenting condition. Often the third step may be skipped, with clinicians preferring to use others' evaluations. However, all modes of evidence-based practice will involve formulating the right questions and integrating evidence with clinical expertise, patient characteristics, and circumstances.

12.1.2 A Hierarchy of Evidence

In terms of finding the best evidence to answer appropriate treatment questions, some have identified a **hierarchy of evidence** for evidence-based practice (Straus et al., 2018). The components of this hierarchy are systems, synopses, syntheses, and studies. These will be described in an order of decreasing utility for evidence-based practice.

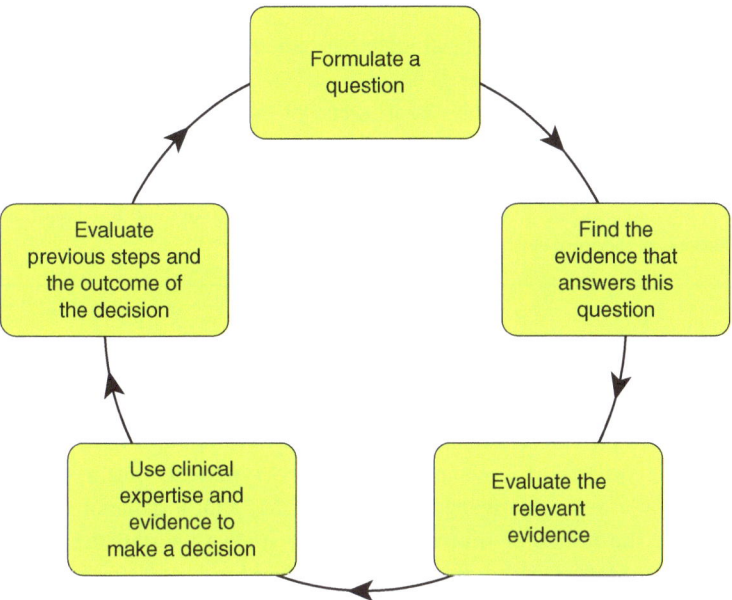

Figure 12.1 The cycle of activities in evidence-based practice (based on Straus et al., 2018)

Source: Straus, S.E., Richardson, W.S., Glasziou, P., & Haynes, R.B. (2018) *Evidence-Based Medicine: How to Practice and Teach EBM* (5th edition). Copyright Elsevier

Systems

These are computerised decision-support systems which contain up-to-date information about different treatments and allow for the input of details of particular people to aid identification of the most appropriate treatment.

Synopses

These consist of brief, up-to-date summaries of current best practice. Health professionals may benefit from investing in evidence-based practice journals and online resources (see Clinical Notes 12.1).

—Clinical Notes 12.1—

Finding Up-To-Date Research Evidence

- Use synopses of research such as the Database of Abstracts of Reviews of Effects (DARE), the journal *Evidence Based Medicine*, or the American College of Physicians' *ACP Journal Club*.
- Look for recent systematic reviews and/or meta-analyses of the evidence.

(Continued)

- Use the Cochrane evidence synthesis database to find up-to-date reviews of different treatments (www.cochrane.org).
- Be sure you know how to find the relevant primary research evidence using databases like PubMed (www.pubmed.gov) and develop the skills required to read research reports critically.
- You can also access Healthtalk online (www.healthtalk.org) for case studies of people's experiences of different illnesses and treatments.

Syntheses

Systematic reviews provide summaries of published research, and there are several ways in which reviews can synthesise this evidence. **Narrative synthesis** outlines the main findings from the evidence in a text narrative, without conducting additional analysis. **Meta-analysis** is used to combine the results of similar quantitative studies for statistical data analysis (see Highlight Box 12.1). **Meta-synthesis** or meta-ethnography is used to analyse the results of qualitative studies and extract over-arching themes (Melendez-Torres et al., 2015). In all cases there is usually also an evaluation of the quality of studies, so that studies with weaker research designs have less influence on the findings and conclusions than studies with more robust methodologies.

—Highlight Box 12.1—

What is Meta-Analysis?

- Meta-analysis is a statistical procedure used to combine the results and samples of several similar studies into one larger analysis. It is particularly useful for evaluating intervention studies because small sample sizes can affect the likelihood of finding statistically significant results.
- The first step in meta-analysis is to identify relevant studies – usually via a systematic search of electronic databases. Once relevant studies have been identified, it is important to determine which studies are of a suitable quality for inclusion. Then the data can be extracted and analysed to find the overall effect size – i.e. not only whether a treatment has a statistically significant effect on clinical outcomes, but also the magnitude of that effect.
- Meta-analysis can only be as good as the studies that are entered into it. Furthermore, meta-analysis may be affected by the 'file drawer effect', where studies that do not find significant effects may never be published and thus are likened to the analogy of remaining in a filing cabinet. The real effect size may therefore never be known. This has led to the increasingly common practice of clinical trials needing to be registered before data are collected so that the extent of the 'file drawer effect' can be estimated (International Committee of Medical Journal Editors, 2024).

Studies

These include individual research studies and clinical trials as reported in peer-reviewed journals. A disadvantage of relying on single studies is that no single research study will be perfect in terms of its design and execution. Even with good studies, the characteristics of the sample may not be the same as those of the people to whom you want to apply the findings. Thus, you will need to read and evaluate several papers in order to find the appropriate evidence to answer your questions. This is a difficult task with more than a million English-language records being added to the PubMed database each year for biomedical sciences alone. Finding the best and most relevant evidence therefore requires the development of good search skills and devoting a considerable amount of time to this endeavour. The hierarchy of evidence (Straus et al., 2018) suggests that individual research papers found via searches of databases such as PubMed have a low priority for health professionals. However, research syntheses, synopses, and systems are all based, one way or another, on original research.

Research studies may employ one of several study designs. In a **randomised controlled trial** (**RCT**), the efficacy of a treatment or intervention is assessed by comparing clinical outcomes in a group receiving the target treatment (the intervention group) with a control group which may receive routine care or a placebo treatment. People are randomly allocated to treatment or control groups and statistical checks can be conducted to ensure that the groups do not differ in important characteristics at the start of the study (baseline characteristics). Methodological rigour is enhanced by ensuring that the people receiving treatment and the researchers measuring clinical outcomes are 'blind' (do not know) as to whether a person received the treatment or a placebo.

Other common study designs include **case-control studies**, which compare people with a particular condition (cases) to a group of healthy people (controls), and **cross-sectional surveys**, where standardised questionnaires are used with a group of patients or a sample of the general population.

Qualitative methods are used to examine people's experiences, and typically involve individual interviews or group interviews (focus groups). Qualitative analysis is typically based on the systematic interpretation of oral accounts, rather than statistics. Important information can also be gleaned from case series or **case reports**, but because these are based on small numbers of people in specific contexts it may be inappropriate to apply their results to other clinical settings.

12.1.3 How to Read a Paper

It is important to know how to read and critically evaluate individual research papers. Medical research papers usually follow a set structure. The introduction should provide an accurate summary of current knowledge of the topic covered in the paper, give a rationale for the current study, and state clear research aims or hypotheses. The methods section should describe the study methods in sufficient detail that other researchers could replicate the study if they wanted to. The results section should present the results of any statistical or qualitative analyses conducted to address the stated research questions or hypotheses. The discussion should give an accurate description of how the results of the study relate to existing knowledge and the implications for clinical practice and research.

Highlight Box 12.2 outlines several questions to ask when critically reading research papers. These questions cover all four sections of the research papers just described. The list was adapted from Greenhalgh's (2019) book, *How to Read a Paper: The Basics of Evidence-Based Medicine and Healthcare*, which also provides useful tips for reading the different types of papers that appear in healthcare journals.

—Highlight Box 12.2—

How to Read a Research Paper

The following questions may be helpful for guiding critical reading of papers reporting original research. Not all of them will apply to all study designs. You may not be able to answer all of these questions at this stage of your education, but you should aim to be able to.

- Where was the paper published?
  - o Journal esteem is a good first indicator of the quality of a study.

- Was the study original?
  - o Does the introduction give thorough coverage of existing knowledge of the topic?
  - o What does the study offer in terms of new information?

- Who were the participants?
  - o How were people selected for the study?
  - o Who was included/excluded?
  - o Was it a 'real life' study or an experimental study?

- Was the study design appropriate?
  - o What was done and how was it assessed?

- What was done to reduce bias?
  - o Was it necessary to have a control group (or groups)?
  - o Were participants randomised to groups?

- Was the treatment/intervention complete?
  - o Did all participants complete all requirements?
  - o Was there differential attrition (i.e. did people who dropped out differ from those who completed the study)?

- Was the assessment/analysis blind?
  - o Did the researchers know who was getting which treatment?

- Were the preliminary statistical issues addressed?
  - o Was the sample size big enough?
  - o Was the duration of follow-up long enough to detect effects on key outcomes?

- Were appropriate analyses conducted?

  o Were the appropriate statistical or qualitative analyses conducted?
  o Where necessary, was there adjustment for differences in the number of participants who dropped out?

- Were the conclusions supported by the analysis?

  o Did the authors 'cherry pick' results that supported their argument?
  o Were alternative explanations of the results considered?
  o Was the influence of unmeasured confounding factors considered?

- Were all conflicts of interest declared?

  o Were all sources of funding and all researchers' competing interests stated clearly?

Summary 12.1

- Evidence-based practice means integrating the best research evidence with clinical judgement and knowledge of each patient.
- Different sources of information may be more or less useful for evidence-based practice. The availability of research syntheses may facilitate evidence-based practice.
- For evidence-based practice, health professionals need to be able to assess the quality of individual research papers.

12.2 Adherence to Treatment

One important focus of evidence-based practice is an understanding of **adherence** to treatment. Better adherence to treatment results in better clinical outcomes (DiMatteo et al., 2002). It is therefore worrying that around a quarter of patients across a range of medical conditions do not take their medication as prescribed (Thier et al., 2008). Non-adherence results not only in poorer outcomes for people, but also huge avoidable healthcare costs.

Most adherence research has focused on adherence to medication, but the notion of non-adherence can also apply to other forms of medical treatment or therapy (e.g. exercise or physiotherapy) or behaviour modification (e.g. diet). The terms 'adherence' and 'compliance' are often used interchangeably. However, it has been argued that 'adherence' is preferable because it implies the active involvement of the person in treatment processes, whereas 'compliance' implies that people simply follow health professionals' orders.

The relationship between adherence and non-adherence should be thought of not in binary terms but rather in terms of a continuum of more or less adherence. This approach counters the idea that there is a 'non-compliant patient' type and acknowledges that adherence may not be perfect even in those who are strongly motivated to adhere to their treatment programme. It also means we need to think of adherence in broad terms and consider the various ways in which people may deviate from a prescribed treatment:

- Taking too little of the prescribed treatment (e.g. too little of recommended exercise).
- Taking too much of the prescribed treatment (e.g. exceeding prescribed drug dosages).
- Not taking the treatment at the prescribed intervals (e.g. exercising too frequently or not as frequently as required).
- Not taking the treatment for the prescribed duration (e.g. stopping antibiotic medication when one feels better).
- Taking other medication without the knowledge of the prescribing health professional.

─Activity 12.1─

Adherence to Medication

Think back to the last time you were prescribed medication.

- Did you take all the doses?
- Did you take all of the doses at the prescribed times?
- If not, why not?

12.2.1 Reasons for Non-adherence: Unintentional or Intentional?

It is useful to distinguish between intentional and unintentional reasons for non-adherence. There may be various reasons for **unintentional non-adherence**. People may not understand the instructions for treatment or may forget the instructions. Non-adherence may occur because people find it difficult to follow their regimen or simply forget to take doses. To reduce non-adherence, we need to consider:

- People's understanding and recall of information (see Chapter 10).
- People's motivation (see Chapter 2).
- The provision of resources to facilitate adherence.

Poor communication between health practitioners and patients often contributes to unintentional non-adherence (see Chapter 13).

Intentional non-adherence occurs when people decide not to follow a treatment regimen. A useful model of behaviour in the domain of adherence is the **self-regulation model** of illness representations (see Chapter 4), which has also been referred to as the common-sense model of self-regulation (Leventhal et al., 2016). This model highlights the need to pay attention to a person's understanding of their illness, including its cause, consequences, and treatment. According to this model, there are three important aspects of self-regulatory processes. The first is beliefs about the illness (illness representations). The second is emotional responses to illness and its treatment. The third component is the person's appraisal of their behaviour and of the progress of treatment. The model therefore emphasises the person's ability to reflect on their actions and the consequences of their actions. It also highlights the constant interaction between the three components – beliefs, emotions, and appraisal. The model helps to explain various reasons for non-adherence, including defensive coping or denial of the threat posed by the illness, missing medication doses to avoid unpleasant side effects, or stopping treatment early when symptoms subside.

12.2.2 Reasons for Non-Adherence: Multifaceted Models

Although the intentional/unintentional distinction discussed above is helpful, multifaceted models of adherence are probably more useful in prompting clinicians to identify and address a range of barriers to adherence. Reviews of research have identified several important characteristics of individuals, medical conditions, and treatment regimens (Beatty & Binnion, 2016; Dimova et al., 2019; Salvador et al., 2023). These are illustrated in Figure 12.2 and Case Study 12.1.

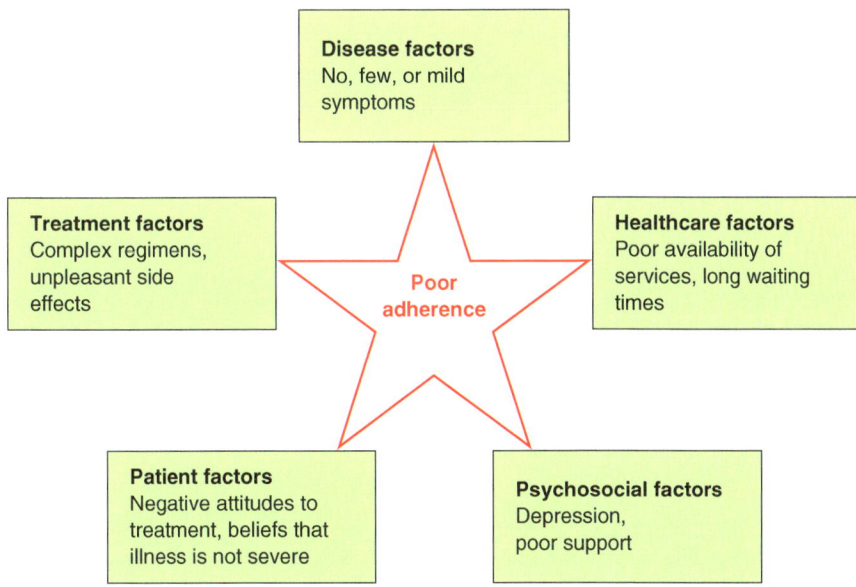

Figure 12.2 Multidimensional model of barriers to adherence

Disease Factors

Adherence tends to be better when people experience the symptoms of illness. This has clear implications for medical conditions with fluctuating symptoms (e.g. asthma) or no symptoms (e.g. hypertension). For less serious conditions, better adherence is found among people with poorer health. For serious conditions, worse adherence is found among people with poorer health. This difference may arise because people with more serious conditions have more physical, practical, and psychological barriers to adherence.

Case Study 12.1

Barriers to Adherence to HIV Treatment

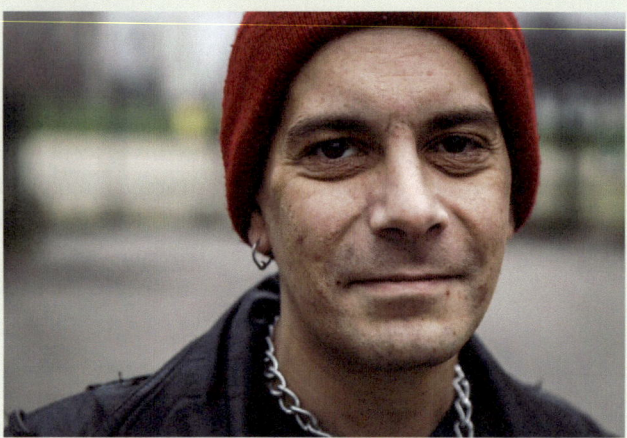

Figure 12.3   Ben's adherence to antiretroviral therapy

Source: © tinx/Adobe Stock

Ben was diagnosed with HIV 15 years ago. He has developed AIDS and his health has generally been good. He has been using combination antiretroviral therapy (ART) since his diagnosis. He has changed medication several times to make it easier to manage the timing and number of the doses of drugs. He is currently taking two antiretroviral medications – one of which is a combination of two drugs – in three doses. Ben finds this combination much easier to adhere to than earlier prescriptions:

> It's so much easier having the combination pill. Before I started this, I had to take three different drugs – one twice a day, one three times a day, and the other one once a day. I also had to try to have some on an empty stomach.

Like many people using ART, Ben has experienced unpleasant side effects, such as nausea and headaches. When changing to his current medication, he initially developed a rash, insomnia, and lipodystrophy – a redistribution of body fat caused by a disturbance in the fat metabolism.

> Obviously, I haven't been really sick yet, and I want to stay that way. Taking these drugs is probably the best way for me to stay healthy, but the side effects do sometimes make me wonder … I'm also worried about what all these drugs are doing to my liver.

Although Ben tries to maintain his adherence to his medication, and this has been helped by a simpler drug regimen, he does still sometimes miss doses:

Sometimes you go out and you meet someone, and one thing leads to another, and you end up going back to their house, and you don't take your medication. But that's usually only one or two doses.

Ben's case illustrates how adherence can be affected by a range of factors, including a rational consideration of the potential benefits, concerns about the immediate and long-term side effects, and the difficulties of matching treatment regimens and lifestyles.

Treatment Factors

Adherence reduces as the complexity or burden of dosing regimens increases. It is generally easier for people to adhere to single daily doses than multiple daily doses and their associated timing schedules. It is also easier to adhere to regimens that do not involve multiple medications, specific times, or dietary requirements. Adherence rates are lower when people experience unpleasant medication side effects.

Patient Factors

Adherence is not strongly influenced by demographic factors such as age, sex, or socioeconomic status. However, as noted in the discussion of intentional non-adherence, people's beliefs exert an important influence on adherence. As predicted by conceptual frameworks such as the Health Belief Model (see Chapter 5), better adherence is found when:

- People believe their condition is serious.
- People perceive more benefits from adherence.
- People perceive or experience fewer barriers to adherence.
- People are more motivated to adhere.

Barriers to treatment include people not agreeing with their diagnosis or treatment plan. They may also include concerns about side effects or the long-term effects of medication (Horne et al., 2013).

Psychosocial Factors

Psychosocial factors are also important. Adherence tends to be poorer in people who are depressed (Lassen et al., 2024; Poletti et al., 2022). Adherence tends to be greater in people who have better support (Babygeetha & Devineni, 2024), although this may vary depending on the condition and treatment (Sousa et al., 2019). In addition to direct practical or emotional encouragement for treatment adherence, social support may have more general effects. For example, adherence is greater among people in households that are more cohesive and have less conflict (Killian et al., 2018).

Healthcare Factors

Practical issues such as accessibility of services and waiting times may affect adherence. One aspect of healthcare systems that has received much attention is **practitioner–patient communication** and the **practitioner–patient relationship**. A fuller consideration of the importance of practitioner–patient communication is given later in this chapter and Chapter 13, but adherence

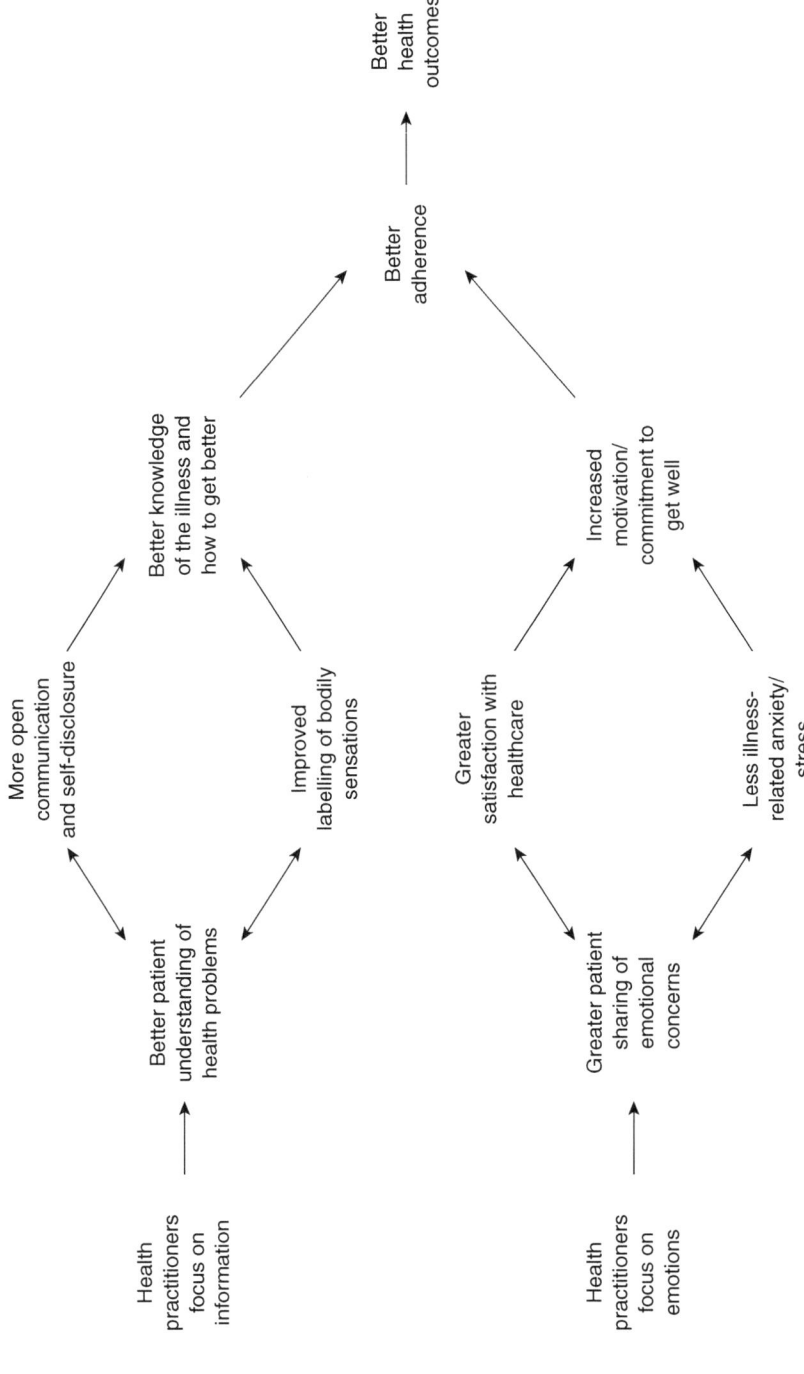

Figure 12.4 How better practitioner–patient communication leads to better adherence (adapted from Squier, 1990)

tends to be better if people have longer consultations and a trusting relationship with a health practitioner who expresses a genuine interest in their health. Similarly, better practitioner–patient relationships lead to better adherence. Figure 12.4 displays the ways in which better practitioner–patient communication can lead to better adherence and better outcomes for patients.

Adherence is also influenced by the provision of information by health professionals and the efficient use of this information. The exchange of information should not just focus on facts about illness and its treatment, but also on the emotional concerns of the patient (see Chapter 13). Good communication skills are required to elicit people's concerns and beliefs, to respond to them sensitively, and to include these when developing a treatment plan that will most likely be adhered to (see Chapter 13).

Adherence is better when people are more satisfied with the amount of information given and when they are better able to understand and recall this information (see Clinical Notes 10.2). People need information to:

- Help them to be adherent.
- Counter fears or misconceptions about their treatment.
- Counter feelings that they have not been adequately listened to and/or that their symptoms have not received adequate attention.

However, more information is not always a good thing. Too much information can hamper efficient decision making. Information about low treatment efficacy or side effects may lead to lower adherence rates.

—Clinical Notes 12.2—

Agreeing Treatment Plans

- Discuss the person's beliefs, concerns, and intentions relating to treatment. Where possible, customise the regimen in accordance with their wishes.
- Simplify the treatment regimen as much as possible.
- Provide simple, clear instructions for taking medication.
- Elicit the person's feelings about their ability to follow the regimen and discuss strategies for enhancing adherence.
- Consider the use of medication-taking systems, including electronic reminders.
- Emphasise the value of the prescribed regimen and the importance of adherence for producing the best treatment outcomes.
- Obtain any necessary help from family members, friends, etc.

(Osterberg & Blaschke, 2005)

The value of recorded information – in print, digital, or video format – is widely acknowledged, particularly for complex treatment regimens. Although written information, such as instructions or leaflets, may help to increase adherence, such information needs to be discussed with people to ensure that they understand the content. Combinations of verbal and written information may be more effective than either verbal or written information in isolation. Combined approaches can repeat and reinforce information, as well as emphasise that the practitioner is interested in the person's understanding of the information and the importance of adherence. The benefits of written information can be further enhanced if that information can be customised or tailored to each patient (as opposed to generic letters, leaflets, or video resources).

12.2.3 Strategies for Improving Adherence

Various methods can be used to help people to follow through on their intentions to adhere to treatment. These include specific action plans or implementation intentions, clearly written or printed information, and the use of electronic reminders, smartphone apps, or monitors of medication use (Anderson et al., 2020; King et al., 2023). A systematic review of interventions for improving adherence found that effects were inconsistent and successful interventions only produced modest improvements in adherence (Nieuwlaat et al., 2014). Many of these interventions are complex and multifaceted, meaning it is difficult to determine the relative importance of various components. Nevertheless, the evidence suggests that to increase adherence it may be necessary to provide information, reminders, counselling, support, and reinforcement, to explore the patient's beliefs about their condition and its treatment, to discuss the severity of the person's illness, and to emphasise the importance of adherence before treatment begins.

Adherence tends to be better when the practitioner and patient are able to talk about it in a non-judgemental way (Young et al., 2016). It is preferable that such discussions happen when treatment is being decided on, rather than after the non-adherence has occurred. It is also important to monitor adherence and to give appropriate feedback to people (see Clinical Notes 12.3).

─Clinical Notes 12.3─

Increasing Adherence

- Monitor adherence. Watch for the markers of non-adherence, such as missed appointments, missed prescription refills, and lack of a response to treatment.
- Express approval of adherence and encourage continued adherence. When appropriate, include objective measures of improvement due to treatment.
- Ask the person about non-adherence and barriers to adherence in an understanding, non-judgemental way.
- If adherence appears unlikely, consider prescribing more 'forgiving' treatments or medications (i.e. medications whose efficacy is less affected by missed doses). Options may include medications with long half-lives, depot (extended-release) medications, or transdermal medication.

(Osterberg & Blaschke, 2005)

Summary 12.2

- Many people find it difficult to adhere to treatment regimens.
- Poorer adherence is related to poorer health outcomes.
- A range of factors affect the likelihood of adherence to treatment regimens, including the characteristics of the disease, treatment, and patient and healthcare factors.
- Adherence should be discussed at the time treatment is prescribed. People should also be given feedback on their adherence.

12.3 Practitioner–Patient Communication

In addition to helping improve adherence, practitioners who communicate well with their patients are more likely to detect emotional distress in people and respond to it appropriately, make accurate, comprehensive diagnoses, and have patients who are more satisfied with their care (Shields et al., 2023). People often receive less information than they desire from health professionals, and practitioners tend to overestimate the time they spend giving information and answering questions.

Information given to patients should be tailored to their needs and capacities. Practitioners must pay attention to the complexity of their language and the speed of delivery. They should check that a person understands the information they have been given. They should also attend to how a person's emotions may affect their capacity to take in information and recall it after a consultation. A fuller description of clinical consultation skills is given in Chapter 13.

To understand why practitioner–patient communication is such a powerful phenomenon you need to consider the purposes of medical communication, the communication behaviours practitioners use, and the influence of communication skills on patient outcomes. Each of these aspects of communication is described below.

12.3.1 Purposes of Clinical Communication

Communication is fundamental to good clinical practice and forming a positive practitioner–patient relationship. This topic is covered in more detail in Chapter 13. Here we briefly look at a few aspects of clincial communication, including the practitioner–patient relationship, medical decision making, and communicating risk.

Practitioner–Patient Relationship

One purpose of medical communication is to develop a good practitioner–patient relationship. In psychotherapy, it is understood that a good therapeutic relationship is essential for successful interventions. Although Rogers' (1951) 'client-centred' approach was developed for psychotherapy, several of its principles also apply to practitioner–patient relationships. As practitioners, we should aim to be non-judgemental, respectful, and empathic by eliciting and responding sensitively to people's concerns. Practitioners need to be aware of the appropriate use of silence and nonverbal behaviours (see Chapter 13). We also need to be attentive to what a patient is saying through active listening, paraphrasing, or reflecting back to the person what they have said. In addition, we need to be aware of what a patient is *un*able to say. Practitioners who employ these and other communication techniques are more likely to detect underlying and undeclared emotional concerns (e.g. Mitchell et al., 2020). Practitioners who attend to patients' emotional wellbeing are better able to reduce anxiety or other heightened emotions that can impair a person's attention to medical information and the later recall of such information (see Chapter 10). Research shows that patients are more satisfied with practitioners who take a person-centred, partnership approach to treatment, which facilitates patient autonomy and involvement through activities such as active listening and explanation on the part of the practitioner (see Chapter 13) (Tak et al., 2015).

—Activity 12.2—

Health Professional Communication

Think back to the last time you consulted a health professional.

- How many of the positive behaviours mentioned above were displayed by the health professional?
- Was the health professional empathic? If so, how did they display their empathy?
- Which undesirable behaviours did they display?

Reflecting on your own experiences as a patient can be used to improve your own communication skills as a health professional.

Exchanging Information

The person-centred approach emphasises that people should feel able to express all of their reasons for consulting a health professional, whether these relate to physical symptoms or emotions. The ideal consultation will be collaborative, and will integrate person-centred and practitioner-centred approaches (see Figure 13.2).

Just because a patient is given information, there is no guarantee that there will be a transfer of knowledge or skills, or changes in behaviour. Any information given to a person must be understood and used in positive and productive ways. People actively process information according to their pre-existing beliefs and understanding. As noted in Chapter 10, memory is an active process with a limited working capacity. Therefore, information provided to a person may not be remembered:

- If it is not understood in the first place.
- If too much information is given.
- If the information is not stored in memory (i.e. through repetition or rehearsal).

Much of the information given to patients does get forgotten or cannot be recalled accurately (Kessels, 2003). One way to increase the likelihood that information is understood in the first place is to ask patients to put into their own words what they have been told and to then correct any inaccuracies. However, this kind of checking of patients' comprehension is rare (Katz et al., 2012).

As noted elsewhere (see Chapters 10 and 13), it is also important to consider how strong emotions, such as someone's fear and anxiety about their health, can affect memory processes by limiting their attentional focus during consultations, and thereby reducing the amount of information that they can recall (Kessels, 2003). Recall of information can be improved by developing and using recordings of important information and/or written materials prepared in a patient-friendly style (Watson & McKinstry, 2009). For example, one review of research found that pictures that are relevant to written or verbal information can markedly increase the attention people pay to health information, and their recall of it later (Schubbe et al., 2020). Another review found that written, audio-visual, interactive digital, and multicomponent materials can enhance understanding and recall of information relevant to informed consent procedures for treatment (Glaser et al., 2020).

Medical Decision Making

In recent decades the paternalistic approach to practitioner–patient relationships – where the practitioner directed the care and made decisions – has been largely replaced by a person-centred and **shared decision-making** approach. This term should not be taken to imply a 50/50 share in decision making, because patients may not feel capable of making decisions and may be worried about being responsible if they choose a treatment that does not work. However, patients should be given as much information as they want about different treatment options before a final decision is made.

In a seminal model, Charles et al. (1997) identified four characteristics of shared decision making:

- *Shared decision making involves at least two participants*: the minimum requirement is that a health professional and patient are involved. Other parties may include relatives (e.g. parents), advocates, interpreters, or legal guardians. In complex cases, more than one health professional may be involved in decisions about treatment.
- *Both parties must share information*: the minimum requirement is that health professionals give information about a treatment in order to gain informed consent. However, people may bring important information about their circumstances and may have also gathered their own information about treatment options (some of which will be valid, some of which will not). It is important to bear in mind that people may want information for reassurance rather than to become involved in decision making.
- *Both parties must make an effort to be involved*: although both the health professional and patient should be involved in decision making, different patients may prefer different levels of involvement.
- *A decision must be made and both parties must agree to it*: it is important to consider both the process and outcome of shared decision making. Possible outcomes of shared decision making include no decision, disagreement between the health professional and patient, or agreement about a treatment plan.

Different patients will approach medical encounters in different ways, so health professionals need to be adaptable when it comes to decision making. Shared decision-making is complex, and in some situations, patients may not want to share the responsibility for decision making, and will instead prefer an 'informed' model, in which they are provided with as much information as they want, but can leave the decisions to the health professional (Gregório et al., 2021). Because patients and communities vary in their desire for involvement in decision making, health professionals must have the necessary skills, patient knowledge, and time to determine when and how patients wish to be involved (MacFarlane, 2020; Witkop et al., 2021). However, the research evidence suggests that the behaviour of many health professionals precludes shared decision making (Stevenson et al., 2000). To some extent this reflects health professionals' beliefs and behaviour, but structural factors, such as the short duration of consultations, may also hamper them.

Research Box 12.1

Interventions to Improve Adherence to HIV Treatment

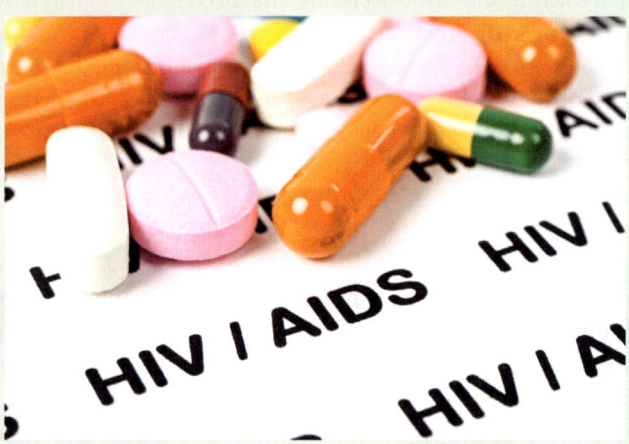

Figure 12.5　Antiretroviral therapy

Source: © gamjai/Adobe Stock

Background

High adherence to antiretroviral therapy is critical to the successful treatment of HIV. This review was conducted to inform the World Health Organization's guidance on interventions to increase adherence to HIV treatment.

Method and Findings

A systematic review and meta-analysis of randomised controlled trials (RCTs) up to 2015 identified 85 RCTs with 16,271 participants. It was found that short text messages improved adherence to antiretroviral medication (odds ratio (OR) 1.48), but that interventions with multiple components were more effective than single interventions at increasing adherence. Increased viral suppression was found following cognitive behavioural therapy (OR 1.46) and supportive interventions (OR 1.28) overall, but not when analysis was restricted to low- and middle-income countries.

Significance

This review and meta-analysis shows that interventions can increase adherence to antiretroviral treatment and, in some instances, improve viral suppression. However, the effect sizes are modest.

Kanters, S., Park, J.J.H., Chan, K. et al. (2017) Interventions to improve adherence to antiretroviral therapy: A systematic review and network meta-analysis. *Lancet HIV, 4*(1): e31–e40.

12.3.2 Communication Behaviours in Medical Settings

Analyses of clinical consultations indicate that asking questions is one of the most common practitioner behaviours after giving information and instructions (Bensing et al., 2003). However, such questions are most likely to be closed 'yes/no' questions during the history-taking phase and are more likely to be **instrumental behaviour** (exchanges of facts) rather than **affective behaviour** (sharing emotions) (Mjaaland & Finset, 2009). Time pressures are often cited as a reason for a lack of attention to affective behaviours, as well as a barrier to shared decision making. However, longer consultations do not necessarily mean that greater attention is being paid to people's emotions and concerns. One comparative study of US and Dutch physicians identified four different communication patterns which varied in their relative attention to affective and instrumental behaviours (Bensing et al., 2003). There was also variation between countries, suggesting that medical training and professional cultures influence practitioners' attention to affective issues.

Reviews of the research reveal some important sex differences in practitioner–patient communication. Female practitioners are more likely to engage in patient-centred behaviours, whether this relates to shared decision making or affective behaviour. In turn, patients speak more in consultations with female physicians (Jefferson et al., 2013), which may mean that fewer consultations are possible. However, not only do patients share more emotional/affective information in longer patient-centred consultations, but they also share more biomedical/instrumental information.

For both male and female practitioners, communication skills can be enhanced by communication skills interventions and training (Baniaghil et al., 2022; Gelis et al., 2020). Such training should include active, practice-orientated strategies such as role-play, feedback, and small group discussions. There is also evidence that interventions aimed at patients can improve practitioner–patient communication (D'Agostino et al., 2017). Although research has tended to focus on verbal behaviour, nonverbal behaviour is also very important, particularly for communicating emotions. The full range of communication behaviours employed in medical consultations and their effects is covered in more detail in Chapter 13.

12.3.3 The Influence of Communication Skills on Patient Outcomes

Research reviews confirm that better clinical communication results in a range of better patient outcomes, including better emotional wellbeing, the resolution of symptoms, improved functioning, better physiological measures, and better pain control (Boerebach et al., 2014; De Vries et al., 2014). The verbal behaviours that appear to be related to better patient outcomes include person-centred questioning and empathic responses to patients, along with summarising and clarifying information given to, and received from, patients. The main nonverbal behaviours include adopting an open and direct posture, leaning towards the patient, and nodding where appropriate (Chapter 13).

Better clinical communication appears to lead to better patient outcomes via several routes (Street et al., 2009). Better communication leads to better proximal outcomes, including mutual understanding, patient satisfaction, trust, decision making, agreement about treatment, and patient motivation (De Vries et al., 2014; Henry et al., 2012). Better intermediate outcomes include better adherence and self-care by patients, both of which lead to improved health outcomes (DiMatteo et al., 2002). These processes are reflected in Figure 12.4, which was introduced in the section on adherence. It has been suggested that better practitioner–patient relationships may act as a form of social and physiological support (Adler, 2002). As a result, it has been argued that for the best outcomes, clinicians and patients should focus on the proximal and intermediate outcomes of respect, trust, and a commitment to adherence (Street et al., 2009).

12.3.4 Communication About Risk

One significant aspect of medical communication is the discussion of risk. However, there are many aspects to people's understanding of risk. People do not passively receive risk information; rather, they actively process it according to their pre-existing knowledge, beliefs, and preferences (Bayne et al., 2020). Although many models of health behaviour are based on rational decision making (see Chapter 5), it is necessary to consider the emotional content and context of medical information. We must also consider whether people can understand risk information in the forms in which it is communicated.

Understanding Risk Information

One difficulty in communicating risk information is that there are numerous ways to calculate and present risks. Information is often presented in the form of a **relative risk** (e.g. 'Smokers are ten times more likely than non-smokers to develop lung cancer'). Such information is derived from population-based research which compares the relative likelihood of an outcome (e.g. lung cancer) in people exposed or not exposed to a risk factor such as smoking. Although such data are extremely useful at a population level, it is difficult to convert them into numbers that apply to individuals.

Individuals are more likely to be persuaded by an **absolute risk** (e.g. 'If you continue to smoke, there is a 20% chance you will develop lung cancer in the next ten years'). However, absolute risks may be difficult to calculate because you will need to incorporate a range of individual risk factors.

Regardless of whether risk information is presented in relative or absolute terms, risk figures are always estimates that have margins of error, which are often given as **confidence intervals**.

However, providing patients with risk estimates as well as confidence intervals may in fact hinder, rather than aid, comprehension. Simpler numerical information may be preferable because it is easier for people to understand.

Many people have difficulty understanding health statistics and probabilities. The fact that many health professionals also have difficulty understanding probabilities makes it even harder to convey such information accurately to patients (Wegwarth & Gigerenzer, 2018). This difficulty with medical statistics is reflective of a broader phenomenon. It can be argued that lotteries and the gambling industry rely on the fact that people do not understand probability and statistics! However, patients need to understand risk information in order to participate in decision making and to maximise adherence to treatment. To help people understand numerical risk information it is recommended that health professionals use 'real' numbers rather than percentages and probabilities (Hashim, 2024) (see Table 12.1). Decision aids, such as pictorial representations, may also help people to understand different event likelihoods (Zipkin et al., 2014).

Table 12.1 Recommendations for communicating risk information (adapted from Gigerenzer et al., 2008)

	What to aim for	What to avoid
Use frequency statements instead of single-event probabilities	Four out of 10 patients taking this medication will experience insomnia	There is a 40% likelihood of insomnia from taking this medication
Use absolute risks instead of relative risks	Mammograms reduce the risk of dying from breast cancer from five in 1,000 to four in 1,000	Mammograms reduce the risk of dying from breast cancer by 20%
Use mortality rates instead of survival rates	There are three prostate cancer deaths per 1,000 men in the USA, compared to two per 1,000 men in the UK	The five-year survival rate for men with prostate cancer is 98% in the USA and 71% in the UK

Emotional Responses to Risk Information

Even when people understand statistical risks, they do not necessarily apply these probabilities to themselves. Affective responses to risk information are an important influence on subsequent behaviour. People can often find exceptions to statistical risk information and apply these to their own preferred patterns of behaviour. For example, a heavy smoker who does not want to follow a recommendation to quit may say: 'My grandmother smoked all of her life, and she lived to 94'. Implicit biases in how risk information is processed can mean that people feel more or less likely than other people to experience negative health outcomes (Bayne et al., 2020). Unrealistic optimism about health and risk reduces the likelihood that people will engage in a healthy behaviour change, particularly when they believe they have some control over health outcomes (Shepperd et al., 2015).

To counter implicit biases such as unrealistic optimism and to promote health behaviours, we must convince people that the risks are real and serious (Floyd et al., 2006). Some health promotion campaigns use shockingly graphic images in order to emphasise the seriousness of health risks and prompt behaviour changes (e.g. images of fatty deposits being squeezed from the arteries of deceased smokers, or graphic images of a motor vehicle accident). In one-to-one medical consultations, techniques based on shock or fear may be employed (e.g. 'If you don't stop smoking, you'll die before you're 60'). However, a paradox of risk communication is that although a certain amount of anxiety may be necessary to motivate a change in behaviour, too much anxiety can lead to inappropriate responses, such as the denial of risks. If information or images are too shocking or frightening, they may cause defensive avoidance of the issue – that is, people will stop thinking about their behaviour and its associated risks because they do not want to think about the feared outcome. Health campaigns using shock or fear are more likely to be successful when they are accompanied by clear information about what people can do to avoid undesirable outcomes (Ruiter et al., 2014). However, positive health promotion campaigns and those that encourage coactive behaviours are more likely to be effective (Yousef et al., 2023).

Summary 12.3

- Good clinical communication serves many purposes and is an important aspect of patient-centred care.
- If people receive the information they need and are able to use it as part of decision making about treatment, they are more likely to be satisfied with consultations, adhere to treatment, and experience positive outcomes.
- Better clinical communication will result in improved practitioner–patient relationships and exchanges of important information, better medical decision making, and more positive outcomes.
- Communication about risk is an important aspect of medical communication. However, many patients (and health professionals) have difficulty understanding the meaning of risk data. In addition, people's emotional responses to risk information may help or hinder healthy behaviour.

Conclusion

This chapter has provided an overview of evidence-based practice, highlighting the importance of ensuring that clinical decisions are grounded in reliable and sound evidence. By examining the key sources of information used in evidence-based practice, it is clear that integrating research findings, clinical expertise, and patient preferences is essential for optimal healthcare. Additionally, the chapter explored the factors influencing adherence to treatment, emphasising that patient adherence to treatment is shaped by a complex interplay of individual, social, and contextual factors. Lastly, the discussion on practitioner-patient communication underscored the critical role of effective interaction in fostering trust, understanding, and adherence.

Understanding and applying evidence-based practice is therefore vital for improving patient outcomes and building more effective healthcare systems. With this foundation, the next chapter will delve further into the communication skills necessary for clinicians to enhance patient engagement and outcomes, bridging the gap between knowledge and practice.

Further Reading

Goldacre, B. (2008) *Bad Science*. London: Fourth Estate. Written by a journalist, this book is an accessible critique of the use and misuse of evidence in mainstream media reporting of health and science issues.

Greenhalgh, T. (2019) *How to Read a Paper: The Basics of Evidence-Based Medicine and Healthcare* (6th edition). Oxford: Blackwell. A useful guide on how to approach and make sense of research papers. Includes how to approach different kinds of papers, literature searches, and statistics.

Straus, S.E., Richardson, W.S., Glasziou, P. & Haynes, R.B. (2018) *Evidence-Based Medicine: How to Practice and Teach EBM* (5th edition). London: Elsevier. Although written mainly for experienced practitioners, it includes some useful information that is suitable for students.

Revision Questions

1   Give a definition of evidence-based practice.
2   Why is it important for health professionals to use evidence-based practice?
3   What is meant by the hierarchy of evidence in evidence-based practice? What distinguishes sources of evidence higher in the hierarchy from those further down?
4   Describe the differences between intentional and unintentional non-adherence.
5   Outline the range of factors which influence adherence to a prescribed treatment.
6   Describe the different purposes of practitioner–patient communication.
7   Describe some of the characteristics of shared decision making.
8   Better clinical communication leads to better patient outcomes. Outline the mechanisms that explain this link.

13

CLINICAL COMMUNICATION

---**Learning Objectives**---

This chapter is designed to enable you to:

- Describe the different ways in which we communicate.
- Recognise the importance of each person's agenda in clinical consultations.
- Outline communication skills for the different stages of clinical consultations.
- Describe some effective ways to deal with strong emotions in clinical consultations, such as anger, anxiety, and distress.
- Consider important factors when giving bad news.

Most clinicians undertake between 140,000 and 160,000 clinical consultations during their career (Frankel & Sherman, 2015). As we have seen in Chapter 12 on evidence-based practice, how we communicate in clinical consultations is an important part of good clinical practice. Good communication is associated with increased confidence, more accurate diagnoses, better clinical management, adherence to treatment, patient satisfaction, and improved outcomes for patients (Georgopoulou et al., 2018; Venktaramana et al., 2022). Good communication is also associated with fewer complaints and less litigation (Domino et al., 2014).

Communication in clinical settings requires particular skills, and training is usually available to health professionals during and after qualifying. Communication skills training can involve mock clinical interviews, role-play, video-recording, and feedback. Some people find this kind of simulated training awkward and unnatural, but evidence shows that it is an effective and cost-efficient way to learn these skills (Gelis et al., 2020). For example, studies evaluating healthcare students' performance in clinical examinations (OSCEs) before and after communication skills training show that students who have communication skills training do better in their OSCEs (e.g. Baniaghil et al., 2022). In a randomised controlled trial, students who had training were rated as more competent, having a better relationship with the patient, and being better at clinical assessment, negotiation, and decision making. They also showed better organisation and time management during the consultation (Yedidia et al., 2003).

In this chapter we start by examining how we communicate through verbal and nonverbal behaviour. Then we look at clinical consultations, including different models of clinical consultations as well as the specific skills and techniques to use. The final sections consider the communication skills required in difficult encounters, such as how to cope with angry or upset people, or when giving bad news. In this chapter we use the terms 'clinical consultation' and 'communication' rather than 'interview'. This is because 'interview' implies the clinician is active and the patient is passive in the consultation process, whereas 'clinical consultation' more accurately reflects the two-way communication between the clinician and patient.

13.1 How We Communicate

Communication is the process through which people provide and exchange information through a common system of signs, symbols, or behaviour. Communication is frequently thought of in terms of verbal and nonverbal behaviour in one-to-one, in-person consultations. However, the increase in e-health and tele-health means that care is increasingly provided through technology such as online video calls, text or in-app messaging, email, or telephone consultations. The use of technology raises further challenges in terms of communication in clinical practice.

13.1.1 Verbal Communication

Verbal communication includes both *what* we say and *how* we say it. Speech is often surprisingly disjointed, but we are still able to understand the message being conveyed. The example below is a person talking about the doctor explaining what happened to them:

> Um, and he just came back and sort of said, 'Do you know what's happened to you?' (Laughs) And I said (High voice), 'Ooh no, I don't think I do.' (Laughs) I was very emotional. [Pause] And then he explained it all to me, and that actually made me feel a thousand times better, just him taking five minutes just to explain that to me.

In day-to-day interaction, many factors are used to interpret the meaning of what is said, including nonverbal behaviour and the social context. Consequently, even if *what* we say is very clear, people may still misinterpret it because of their expectations, beliefs, social context, and our speech characteristics (e.g. our tone of voice) and nonverbal behaviour.

At a simple level, communication can be conceptualised as a messaging process where a message is encoded, transmitted, and received. It is possible for communication to break down at each of these stages. The message might be ambiguous, that is, difficulty can result from the way we write or say the message (*encoding*), the message may not transmit properly through faulty technology, delivery, or noise (*message transmission*), or the other person may misinterpret the message (difficulty *decoding*).

In medical practice, the words we use and the way we say things are both important. The way in which questions are asked can influence how people respond (see Figure 13.1). **Closed questions**, which tend to start with words like *did, is, have, can*, require people to respond in fixed ways (typically, by saying *yes* or *no*). Such questions are useful for obtaining specific information or clarifying points, such as *'Have you taken any medication for this?'* or *'Is the pain sharp or dull?'* The disadvantage of closed questions is that you only get very limited amounts of information in response. **Open questions** encourage respondents to talk freely and tend to start with *what, how, when, why*, etc. Such questions are useful because they encourage the person to express what is important in their own words, for example *'What have you come to see me about today?'* or *'What does the pain feel like?'* The disadvantage is that they are less well suited for reaching definite goals or clarifying points.

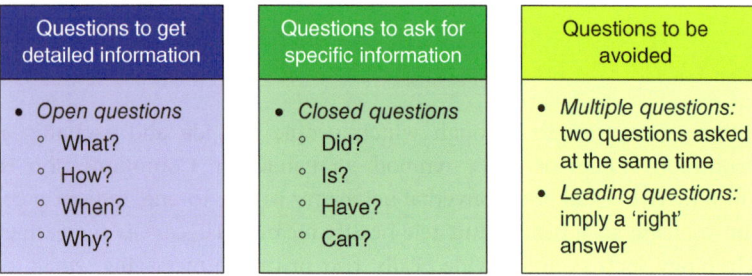

Figure 13.1   Different types of questions

Open and closed questions are both useful in clinical consultations. A common approach is the '**open-to-closed cone**' or '**funnel approach**', in which open questions are used at the start of a consultation and closed questions are used later. Open questions are used first to obtain a broad picture of the problem from the person's perspective. This provides an opportunity for the health professional to listen and consider what other information may be important. The use of open questions at the beginning of a consultation is extremely helpful to explore problems: their power as an information-gathering tool cannot be over-emphasised. A common mistake in clinical consultations is to move to closed questions too quickly. As the consultation progresses, however, using more specific open questions, probes, and closed questions can clarify information and find out details that the person may not mention otherwise.

There are some types of questions that need to be avoided. The main ones are multiple and leading questions. **Multiple questions** are those in which two or more questions are asked together – for example, *'Have you seen a doctor about this and what treatment did they prescribe?'* Such questions often result in people answering only one part of the question. **Leading questions** are those that imply an expected answer – for example, *'You don't have any pain, then?'* or *'There's no history of heart problems?'* Questions of this type impose our own assumptions on the person and make it difficult for them to disagree. Research on forensic interviews has shown that even slight variations in the words we use can influence people's judgements. For example, assessing how fast a car was going when it collided with a wall will be influenced by the choice of verb used in the question (e.g. 'smash' or 'hit'): people will estimate that the car was going faster if you ask 'how fast was the car going when it *smashed* into the wall?' (Wright & Loftus, 2008). Leading questions or questions using words that imply the extent of something can therefore influence a person's responses and should be avoided.

Characteristics of speech also influence the interpretation of meaning. Features such as tone, pitch, pauses, sighs, and speed influence how speech is interpreted. These features may completely change the meaning of a sentence. For example, using a sarcastic tone of voice indicates that a person means the opposite of what they are actually saying. Speech characteristics may also be used as a guide to a person's mood. Fast, high-pitched speech usually indicates arousal, such as excitement or anxiety, whereas slow speech can be characteristic of depression. These characteristics of speech can be used in clinical practice to gauge and influence a person's mood. For example, if you are talking to a person who is angry or anxious, deliberately slowing your speech and using a lower pitch may help to calm them.

In healthcare practice, the characteristics of our speech can also influence the relationship we have with the person and the confidence they have in us. A study of 1,411 patients or carers in Japan found that speech characteristics (way of speaking, volume, tone, pitch, etc.) were more important than a doctor's reputation, title, dress, age, or gender in how much confidence people had in the doctor (Kurihara et al., 2014). Similarly, a study in the USA in which surgeons' speech in consultations was rated for warmth, hostility, dominance, concern, and anxiety found that surgeons who were rated as high on dominance and low on concern or anxiety were almost three times more likely to have been sued by patients (Ambady et al., 2002).

13.1.2 Nonverbal Communication

Nonverbal communication plays a crucial part in communication. It includes facial expression, eye movements, spatial behaviour, posture, gestures, touch, and bodily contact. **Facial expression** is important in indicating mood or emotions, as shown in Chapter 2 (see Figure 2.4). **Eye movements** and eye contact are important in social interactions (Birmingham & Kingstone, 2009). They help to establish a rapport with another person. People look more at people they like, and frequent or sustained eye contact is usually a sign of attentiveness, liking, or being attracted to someone (Montoya et al., 2018). Conversely, reduced eye contact may signal stress, avoidance, emotional problems such as depression, or autism (Cañigueral & Hamilton, 2019). It is necessary to get the balance of eye contact right. On the one hand, we want to appear attentive, so we need to have plenty of eye contact, especially at the beginning of a consultation. On the other hand, prolonged eye contact can be interpreted as too intimate or aggressive (Wieser et al., 2009). After all, long and direct eye contact can be observed in courting couples, and boxers may try to intimidate their opponents by 'staring them down' before a fight.

Spatial behaviour is a form of nonverbal behaviour that may be either supportive or intimidating (see Chapter 9 for information on social roles). In a seminal theory, anthropologist Edward Hall (1966) suggested that personal space can be divided into four zones:

1   Intimate zone (0–45 cm): only lovers, close relatives, and very close friends are normally allowed into this zone.
2   Personal zone ranges (45–120 cm): friends and family members are allowed into this zone.
3   Social zone (120–360 cm): conversations with acquaintances and work colleagues usually take place in this zone.
4   Public zone (360–760 cm): this zone is often used when someone is giving a talk to an audience.

These distances apply to North American and Northern European cultures. However, there are large cultural differences in the demarcation of zones. For example, many cultures favour smaller distances in ordinary conversations. This variation in norms can create problems when people from different cultures meet, because the person who is used to more space may feel uncomfortable, or think that the other person is assuming a closer relationship than they have. There can also be differences between certain patient groups, or under particular circumstances. For example, feeling threatened is associated with a need for greater personal space in most people (Stamps, 2012). There is evidence that people with schizophrenia often need a larger personal space zone around them, which may be due to symptoms of paranoia (Schoretsanitis et al., 2016). In contrast, people with autism spectrum disorders often have a reduced personal space zone (Asada et al., 2016). Zones can also shift rapidly within cultures in response to events, as observed during the COVID-19 pandemic, where social distancing was important to reduce the spread of disease.

Cultures have implicit rules about the use of space which affect everything from which seat we take in a classroom to where we put our towels on a beach. If someone's personal space is invaded, they will usually withdraw. If this is not possible, people may use other nonverbal behaviour to diffuse the situation. For example, Goffman's concept of 'civil inattention' proposes that if we are in crowded situations, we are able to tolerate it better if eye contact is reduced because avoiding eye contact is a culturally accepted way to self-distance ourselves from others (Goffman, 1972). It probably explains why commuters on crowded trains rarely look at each other.

Activity 13.1

Spatial Behaviour

- Next time you are on a train or in a cinema, pay attention to where people sit. As long as the space is not completely full, people will usually try to keep a certain distance from people they do not know.

Spatial behaviour has a number of implications for clinical practice. First, we must be careful how we position ourselves in relation to the patient. We must not be so close that we invade their personal space, or so far away that we signal that this is a formal 'public zone' encounter. The traditional consultation room set-up, where the health professional sits behind a desk, is not conducive to good rapport. If a desk is necessary, it is far better to position yourself at the corner so that there is no barrier between you and the patient. Second, physical examinations and procedures need to be performed with a lot of care because we are in a person's intimate zone. Uncaring remarks or a lack of acknowledgement of the person during this time can have a particularly negative impact because they have allowed us into their intimate space (Cream, 2019). Finally, personal space varies between individuals, so we should not assume we know what is appropriate. Instead, we should watch for nonverbal cues that a person may not be comfortable with our proximity.

Posture is an indicator of attentiveness, interest, a social relationship, and someone's attitude towards us. A **closed posture** is one where people have their arms or legs crossed or are hunched over. These types of posture indicate a lack of engagement or defensiveness. An **open posture** is best for clinical consultations and includes:

- Not crossing legs or arms.
- Facing your body towards the person.
- Leaning forwards (showing attentiveness).
- Being relaxed (which sends the message 'I am relaxed; I have time for you').

People rate clinicians who use open postures as having more empathy and better rapport. For example, research shows that something as simple as sitting by a person's bedside rather than standing is associated with better ratings of doctors' communication, the interaction, and understanding of the person's condition, despite there being no difference in the amount of time spent with the person (Merel et al., 2016). In social situations, posture also indicates personal alliances. When people like each other, they often mimic each other, including mirroring each other's posture (Chartrand & Larkin, 2013). Research shows that mirroring strengthens rapport with patients in clinical consultations (Sharpley et al., 2001), although it needs to be used judiciously. It is obviously not helpful to mirror the posture of a highly anxious person who has crossed their arms and legs or is fidgeting.

Finally, **touch** can be a very powerful human response, particularly when someone is distressed. Touch must always be used appropriately, with due regard to the sensitivities of the person and professional codes of conduct. People vary greatly on what they consider to be acceptable touch, and there are strong cultural differences (Green, 2017). **Clinical examinations** involve touch – sometimes of very intimate areas. This will be accepted by most people because of the socially accepted roles of patients and health professionals. Making sure the person consents to the examination is essential. Touch in clinical consultations raises potential ethical, legal, and professional issues, so many factors need to be considered (Griffith, 2015). Four basic factors are important for using touch positively:

1. The therapeutic encounter must have clear boundaries.
2. The touch must be appropriate to the circumstances.
3. The person should feel they have control over physical contact.
4. The touch must be for the person's benefit, not the therapist's benefit.

Guidelines for physical examinations are given in Clinical Notes 13.1.

Clinical Notes 13.1

Physical Examinations

When carrying out clinical examinations, it is basic good practice to:

- Explain what you are going to do before you do it.
- Ask the person's permission.
- Ask if they have any concerns.
- Respect their modesty.
- Never comment on their anatomy or state while carrying out the examination.
- Watch the person's body language for any signs of discomfort.

Summary 13.1

- We communicate through verbal and nonverbal behaviours.
- Verbal communication includes both *what* we say and *how* we say it.
- Communication can break down at the stages of (1) encoding, (2) message transmission, or (3) decoding.
- The way we say things (e.g. tone of voice) can override the meaning of what we say, such as when using sarcasm. Speech characteristics are often good indicators of emotional state.
- Nonverbal behaviours include facial expression, eye movements, spatial behaviour, posture, and touch.
- Good clinical consultation skills include a relaxed, open posture, good eye contact, and the appropriate use of space and touch.

13.2 Clinical Consultations

Models of clinical consultations have been developed to help health professionals to understand the processes involved and to improve their clinical communication and consultation skills. These models can be broadly divided into those that focus mainly on the different perspectives of clinicians and patients, and encourage a more person-centred approach to consultations and relationship-building; and those that break down the clinical consultation into different stages and consider which communication skills and techniques may be useful for each stage. Here we look at examples of each of these approaches, although there is obviously some overlap, and these approaches are complementary rather than competing. They are both useful in improving clinical consultations and communication skills.

13.2.1 Person-Centred Approaches to Clinical Consultations

An example of a person-centred approach to clinical consultations is shown in Figure 13.2. This approach was first developed by McWhinney (1989) and highlights the importance of considering different agendas during the clinical consultation. The first is the **clinician's agenda**: the clinician needs to explore and identify any underlying disease. For this reason, they need to ask about symptoms, carry out investigations, and consider differential diagnoses. The second is the **person's agenda**: this arises from the person's concern with their illness (e.g. their experience of sickness). As we have already seen in Chapter 4, people come to consultations with ideas and beliefs about what is wrong and they may have concerns about the illness and the impact it will have on them. Examples of models focusing on a person-centred approach are the E4 model of clinical communication (Keller & Caroll, 1994), the REDE model of healthcare communication (Windover et al., 2014), and the Four Habits model (Frankel & Stein, 2001).

One strength of the person-centred approach is the equal emphasis placed on the patient's agenda. Substantial evidence confirms the necessity of considering each person's agenda and using person-centred communication. For example, person-centred care has been shown to lead to more improved outcomes for patients, better use of resources, decreased costs, and increased

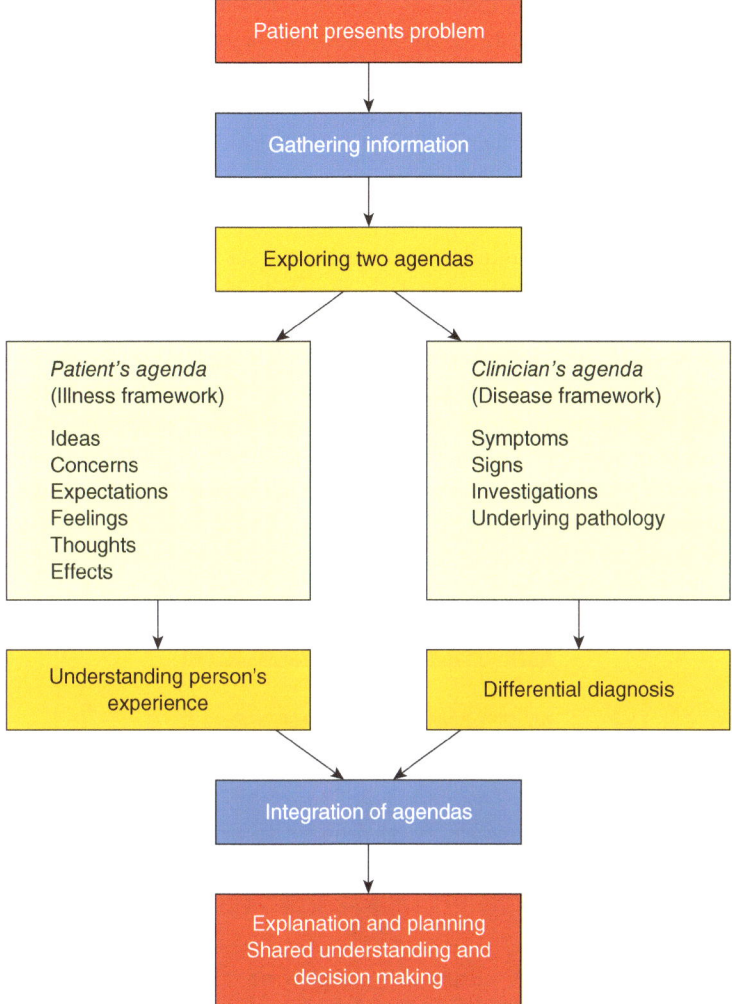

Figure 13.2   Person-centred approach to clinical consultations (McWhinney, 1989)

satisfaction with care (Gluyas, 2015; Shields et al., 2023). People are also more likely to discuss difficult issues, such as a prognosis in cancer, and be able to discuss their values, needs, and preferences (Mitchell et al., 2020).

Another strength of the person-centred approach is the focus on collaboration between the clinician and patient. The approach specifies that after considering the different agendas, there should be an integration of these agendas and shared planning and decision making about the treatment. Evidence confirms that collaborative approaches to treatment are more effective. For example, a review of studies found that consultations with a collaborative relationship, where the person's perspective was considered, led to better adherence in paediatric and adult samples, as well as in primary and secondary care (Arbuthnott & Sharpe, 2009). Similarly, a review of studies of patient experience across a wide range of services found that a good experience is associated with better health outcomes, adherence to treatment, preventative care, resource use, and possibly fewer adverse events (Doyle et al., 2013). Unfortunately, it is still sometimes the case that the patient's perspective is not always considered. A review of surgeons' communication found that although surgeons were good at providing information about surgical conditions and treatment, they rarely explored the person's concerns or feelings (Levinson et al., 2013).

13.2.2 Skills for Different Stages of Clinical Consultations

Other approaches to clinical communication focus on the skills needed at different stages of the consultation. Examples of models using this approach are the Calgary-Cambridge model (Silverman et al., 2013), the Three-function model (Cole & Bird, 2014), and the SEGUE Framework for teaching and assessing communication skills (Makoul, 2001). The Calgary-Cambridge model is shown in Figure 13.3. It breaks down the consultation into different parts and suggests which skills are most relevant to each stage of the consultation. It provides a clear structure that is useful because it helps us to concentrate on learning skills that are most relevant to each stage. Health professionals can therefore build up their skills as they become more competent at each stage.

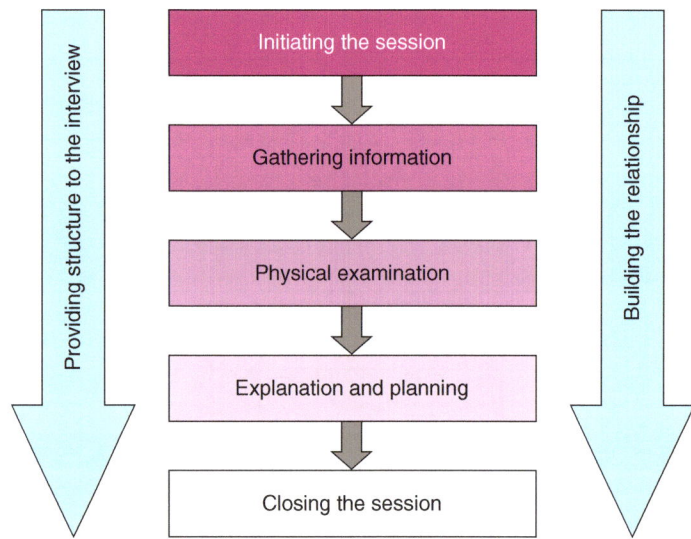

Figure 13.3 Calgary-Cambridge model of clinical consultations

Initiating the session involves starting to establish a rapport with the person and identifying the reason for the consultation. The skills that the Calgary-Cambridge model lists as key at this stage are shown in Highlight Box 13.1. It is always important, especially in hospital settings, to get your introduction right and not to assume the person knows either who you are or what the consultation will involve. Getting the introduction right is not as easy as you might think. A study in the USA observed medical students' consultations in emergency medicine to see whether students acknowledged the patient, introduced themselves, identified they were a student, and explained the care plan, that other providers would be involved in their care, and the duration of care. This study showed that students were good at introducing themselves in consultations (91%), but did not always remember to identify themselves as a student (58%), or acknowledge the patient (61%). Only one consultation out of 246 managed to cover all these elements (Turner et al., 2016). In the UK, a doctor who had a terminal illness initiated the *#hellomynameis* campaign to remind health professionals to introduce themselves, which she saw as the first step in person-centred compassionate care (Case Study 13.1).

Highlight Box 13.1

Initiating the Clinical Consultation

Establish an initial rapport:

- Greet the person and ask for or check their name.
- Introduce yourself and tell the person what your role is in their care.
- Show interest and respect for the person.
- Maintain good eye contact and body posture.

Identify the reasons for the consultation:

- Use open questions to find out about the problems the person would like to discuss.
- Listen carefully to what the person says and do not interrupt.
- Check whether there is anything else the person wants to discuss (e.g. 'so you've come about these headaches, is there anything else you'd like to discuss today?')

(Adapted from Silverman et al., 2013)

Case Study 13.1

The Importance of Introducing Yourself

Dr Kate Granger was a consultant in elderly medicine who was diagnosed with terminal cancer. During the course of her treatment, she found that many of the health professionals involved in her care did not introduce themselves. She said it made her feel that she was not a person but 'just a diseased body in a hospital bed'. Kate started the *#Hellomynameis* campaign to remind health professionals to introduce themselves to every patient they care for. She said:

(Continued)

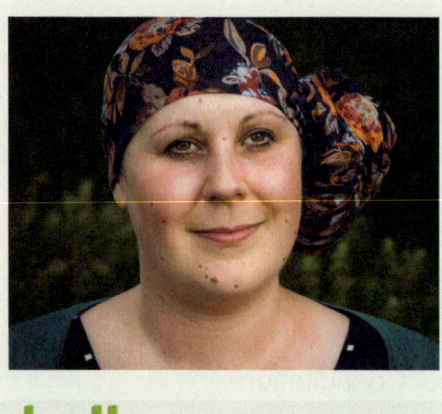

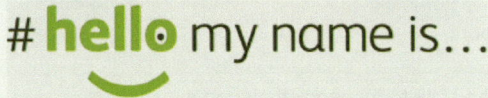

Figure 13.4 Dr Kate Granger and the *#Hellomynameis* campaign

Source: Paul Clarke

The *#Hellomynameis* campaign … is about inspiring and reminding healthcare staff about the importance of introductions. They're much more than a common courtesy in my mind: they're about starting a human connection, about breaking barriers, building trust and rapport, and really building that therapeutic relationship that's all-important in the healthcare relationship.

The campaign was hugely successful in the UK and in other countries, with staff and students joining the campaign to make introducing yourself the norm. Hospitals used *#Hellomynameis* badges, lanyards, and poster boards to promote this practice. When Kate died, her husband Chris continued her work with the *#Hellomynameis* campaign. Kate said that if she left a legacy of inspiring health professionals to provide more person-centred care, then 'it means I can die proud'.

See www.hellomynameis.org.uk

Using open questions at the beginning of the consultation is a good way to obtain maximum information from the person – providing we then listen to what they say. Research shows that on average doctors interrupt a person 18 seconds after they start talking (Coyle et al., 2022). Some of these interruptions may be supportive rather than intrusive but, contrary to popular belief, the more a doctor interrupts, the longer a clinical consultation will take (Menz & Al-Roubaie, 2008). Interruptions disrupt a person's concentration and lead them to expect they will only have a few seconds to say what they want to say. Attentive listening to what people say is therefore as important as asking the right kind of questions.

Active or attentive listening is a skilled process that involves listening, facilitating responses, and picking up on cues from the person. A number of skills can be used to help the person tell their 'story' or expand on their situation. These include:

- **Encouragement**: nonverbal and verbal encouragement, such as '*uh-huh*', '*go on*', or '*I see*', signal that the person should go on with their story. Such interjections involve only minimal interruption and give the person the necessary confidence to keep going. Facilitative comments should be **neutral** and not use words like '*right*' or '*good*', which can be misinterpreted as meaning that what the person is saying is correct or positive.

- **Silence**: verbal facilitation is ineffective unless it is followed by an attentive silence. However, many of us find silences uncomfortable and tend to leap in quickly if a response is not forthcoming. A useful skill, therefore, is to leave a slightly longer pause after the person has finished speaking before you start speaking, which may encourage them to continue.

- **Reflection** (**echoing**): reflecting back or echoing the last few words the person has said may encourage them to expand or continue talking. Students sometimes worry that echoing will sound unnatural, but it is remarkably well accepted by people. Repetition encourages the person to continue with their last phrase so is more directive than encouragement or silence.

- **Paraphrasing**: paraphrasing involves restating in your own words the content or feelings of the person's message. It is not quite the same as summarising or checking because it is intended to sharpen rather than just confirm your understanding. Paraphrasing helps to check whether your *interpretation* of what the person said is correct.

Gathering information is the second stage of the clinical consultation and involves exploring the problem further, understanding the person's perspective, and providing structure to the consultation. The communication skills that the Calgary-Cambridge guide identifies as important for this stage are shown in Highlight Box 13.2.

—Highlight Box 13.2—

Gathering Information

Explore the problem further:

- Facilitate and clarify the person's story of the problem.
- Use open and closed questions.
- Use active listening.
- Summarise the person's points from time to time to check your understanding.
- Use clear, concise questions or comments and avoid jargon.

Understand the person's perspective:

- Explore and acknowledge the person's ideas and concerns about the problem.
- Determine how it affects the person's life.
- Explore the person's goals and expectations.
- Encourage the person to express feelings and thoughts.
- Pick up on the person's verbal and nonverbal cues, and check and acknowledge as appropriate.

(Continued)

Provide a structure to the consultation:

- Summarise the person's points at the end of a line of enquiry to check understanding before progressing.
- Signpost moving from one section to another (e.g. 'We'll come back to that in a minute, but first I would like to ask you a few questions about your family history').
- Sequence the consultation logically.
- Use appropriate timing to keep the consultation on task.

(Adapted from Silverman et al., 2013)

Physical examination is the third stage of the model and should follow clinical guidelines, with clear explanations of what the examination involves, as well as checking the patient consents to the examination.

Explanation and planning is the fourth stage and involves the aspects covered in Chapter 12. These include providing the correct amount and type of information, aiding accurate recall and understanding, achieving a shared understanding that incorporates the person's perspective, and shared decision making. The communication skills that the Calgary-Cambridge guide lists as important for this stage are shown in Highlight Box 13.3.

—Highlight Box 13.3—

Explanation and Planning

Provide the correct amount and type of information:

- Establish what the person knows already.
- Give information in manageable chunks.
- Check for understanding.
- Ask what other information might be helpful.
- Make sure information is given at appropriate times.

Aid accurate recall and understanding:

- Organise information into logical, discrete sections.
- Use explicit categorisation or chunks (e.g. *There are three things that are important …*').
- Repeat and summarise information.
- Use concise statements that are easily understood and avoid jargon.
- Check their understanding at the end and clarify where necessary.

Achieve a shared understanding:

- Link explanations to the person's agenda.
- Encourage the person to contribute.
- Pick up on verbal and nonverbal cues.
- Elicit the person's beliefs, reactions, and feelings about the information given.

Shared planning and decision making:

- Share your own thoughts, ideas, and dilemmas as appropriate.
- Involve the person by offering suggestions rather than orders and giving the person a choice.
- Negotiate a mutually acceptable plan.
- Check with the person if the plan is acceptable and whether they have any concerns.

(Adapted from Silverman et al., 2013)

The final stage of the consultation consists of **closing the consultation**. This stage can have a dis-proportionate effect on what people take away from the consultation (see primacy and recency effect in Chapter 10, section 10.4.1). Providing a summary of what has been discussed and agreed is an opportunity to check that understanding has been shared and that the person is happy with the agreed treatment. In addition, **safety netting** – where we tell the person what to do if the treatment plan does not work or if other symptoms arise – may prevent future difficulties. Simple things, such as asking whether there is anything else the person wants to discuss and saying goodbye properly, can make a big difference to the person's experience of the consultation. The communication skills that the Calgary-Cambridge guide identifies as important for this stage are shown in Highlight Box 13.4.

—Highlight Box 13.4—

Closing the Clinical Consultation

- Briefly summarise the session and agreed treatment plan.
- Lay out and agree with the person the next steps, both for you and them.
- Provide a safety net: explain any possible unexpected outcomes and what to do if the plan doesn't work – as well as how and when to seek help.
- Make a final check that the person agrees and is comfortable with the plan.
- Ask if there are any questions or other items to discuss.

(Adapted from Silverman et al., 2013)

In many consultations, people raise a new problem in the final stage of the clinical consultation (Rodondi et al., 2009). This will often be the problem the person is most worried about. One way to avoid the problem being raised only at the end of the consultation is to gather information as skilfully as possible earlier on. Research confirms that health professionals who ask about people's beliefs, who are responsive to people, give plentiful information, and discuss treatments with people are less likely to find such new problems being raised during the closing stage of consultations (Rodondi et al., 2009).

The Calgary-Cambridge and other models using this approach provide useful frameworks of strategies that health professionals can use during different stages of a consultation. These models form the basis for training programmes in many countries, as well as rating scales that can be used for self-evaluation, peer evaluation, and examination of communication skills (Boucher et al., 2020). Researchers have also expanded the number of strategies that can be included. For example, Lefroy et al. (2014) identified over 200 strategies that students can use to improve their consultation skills, either alongside or separate from the Calgary-Cambridge or other models. Although originally developed for medical students, models of communication in clinical consultations have since been widely used in training for health and care professionals in many disciplines, including nursing, dentistry, dietetics, midwifery, pharmacy, and social work (Baniaghil et al., 2022; Kerr et al., 2021; Knight et al., 2024; Moore 2022; Reith-Hall & Montgomery, 2023).

However, criticisms of the approach include that medical consultations often do not follow the stages outlined (Noble et al., 2022) and that the approach does not explicitly include relationship factors that are highly important, such as the quality of the therapeutic relationship, trust, and empathy. Empathy is commonly mentioned in healthcare training and is a core learning objective of the American Association of Medical Colleges. However, the concept of empathy is complex and widely debated (Jeffrey, 2016). Empathy can be simply defined as the ability to understand and identify with another person's feelings. There are different ways in which we can be empathic, including cognitive (i.e. you can imagine what it might feel like to be in their situation), emotional (i.e. you feel what they feel), or compassionate (i.e. you understand their feelings and feel concern). There is ample evidence that empathy is associated with better therapeutic relationships and outcomes for health professionals and patients (X. Zhang et al., 2024) (see Research Box 13.1). However, a minority of studies find that empathy can be associated with burnout (Wilkinson et al., 2017), so the type of empathy we develop may be important. It has been suggested that compassionate empathy is most functional because it enables health professionals to be empathic without being too emotionally detached (as in cognitive empathy) or emotionally overwhelmed (as in emotional empathy) (Perez-Bret et al., 2016).

Research suggests that health professionals and students can be trained to be more empathic through communication skills training (Menezes et al., 2021). Research Box 13.2 gives an example of empathy training for nursing students. Models of clinical communication, such as those outlined in this chapter, are useful aides for developing communication skills and conducting consultations that are in line with good practice and consider a person's agenda. However, non-specific factors, such as empathy, are also important and need to be maintained with appropriate training.

─Research Box 13.1─

Empathic Person-Centred Approach and Recovery from Surgery

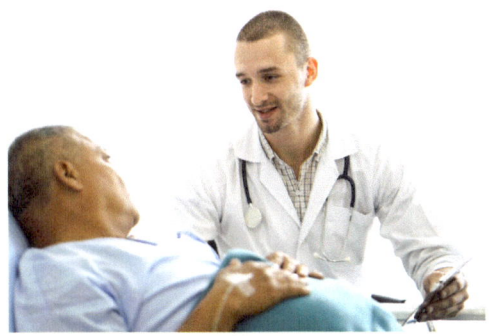

Figure 13.5   An empathic, person-centred approach

Source: © Pormezz/Adobe Stock

Background

Empathy is a key component of the therapeutic relationship. This research evaluated how pre-operative anxiety and post-operative recovery were affected by an empathic, person-centred approach to pre-operative consultations.

Method and Findings

In this randomised controlled trial, 104 patients having general surgery at a hospital in Portugal were randomly allocated to receive a personalised, person-centred pre-operative consultation (intervention) or standard information (control). People who experienced the person-centred consultation were found to have lower levels of anxiety before the operation. Following surgery, they reported less pain, better post-operative recovery (including wound healing), and greater daily activity. They also reported greater satisfaction with their care compared to those who had received standard information.

Significance

This study is consistent with other literature showing the positive impact that empathic, person-centred approaches have on a wide range of clinical processes and patient outcomes.

Pereira, L., Figueiredo-Braga, M. & Carvalho, I.P. (2016) Preoperative anxiety in ambulatory surgery: The impact of an empathic patient-centered approach on psychological and clinical outcomes. *Patient Education & Counselling, 99*(5): 733–738.

—Research Box 13.2—

Empathy Training in Healthcare

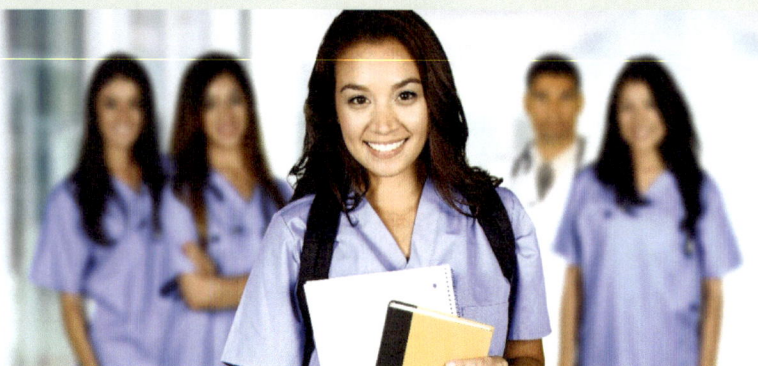

Figure 13.6 Teaching empathy to healthcare students

Source: © Rob/Adobe Stock

Background

Empathy is associated with better patient health, so it is a necessary skill for health profession-als to develop. This study evaluated the effectiveness of empathy training for nursing students.

Method and Findings

This randomised controlled trial (RCT) included 116 nursing students. They were randomly allocated to receive empathy training immediately (intervention group) or at the end of the project (control group). At the end of the project all students completed a simulated clinical consultation at which four measures of empathy were taken, including self-reports of empathy and observations made by others. Results showed that the students who had received empa-thy training reported greater self-esteem and were rated as significantly more empathic by both patients and independent observers. However, students' own ratings of their empathy did not differ between groups.

Significance

This study shows that training in empathy is effective and can result in more empathic clinical communication and greater self-esteem in students. However, the results also indicate that our beliefs about our own empathy may not always agree with the opinions of others.

Bas-Sarmiento, P., Fernández-Gutiérrez, M., Díaz-Rodríguez, M. & iCARE Team (2019) Teaching empathy to nursing students: A randomised controlled trial. *Nurse Education Today, 80*: 40–51.

Summary 13.2

- Person-centred approaches to clinical consultations highlight the importance of considering each patient's agenda.
- Models that outline the different stages of clinical consultations provide a useful guide to the communication skills that are important at each stage of the clinical consultation.
- Good clinical skills include thorough introductions that encompass an explanation of who you are, what the consultation is about, and gaining consent.
- Gathering information is best achieved using a funnel of open-to-closed questions.
- Physical examinations should involve an explanation, respect, and sensitivity to a person's verbal and nonverbal cues.
- Explanation and planning involve providing the right amount and type of information in a way that achieves a shared understanding and a treatment plan.
- Closing a consultation should include a summary, checking for understanding and agreement, and providing a safety net.
- Relational factors, such as empathy and the clinician's attitude, are also critical and need to be developed and/or maintained during training.

13.3 Difficult Consultations

In healthcare, we work with people from cradle to grave. Consequently, care often involves working with others' extreme emotions in response to events such as birth, traumatic events, illnesses, life-threatening events, and death. Some of the most difficult consultations for health professionals are those that involve high levels of negative emotions, such as anger, distress, grief, anxiety, or fear. Consultations may also be difficult because people have difficulty communicating (e.g. people with language or hearing difficulties). These raise challenges for health professionals, because it is hard to discuss and make decisions about treatment with a person who is highly emotional or has difficulty communicating.

In this section we focus on the communication skills health professionals need to help people who are angry, anxious, or distressed, or those who have communication difficulties. Then, in the final section of the chapter, we look at how to give bad news.

13.3.1 Communicating with Angry People

Although anger and aggression are linked, they are not the same. Anger is an emotion, whereas aggression is a behavioural response involving some form of attack towards an object or person. The link between anger and aggression means that when we are confronted with an angry person, it is normal to feel under attack, particularly if the anger is directed at us. However, the true cause of the anger may be something completely different, such as illness, disability, or frustration.

When confronted with an angry person, some responses may escalate the situation and make it worse. Trying to ignore the anger and to keep going with the consultation as normal, getting angry back, or telling the person to calm down are likely to make the anger worse.

Ignoring someone's anger rarely diffuses it, and consequently the consultation is likely to go badly. Although getting angry in return is an understandable human response, it merely escalates the situation. In addition, trying to pacify the person (e.g. by telling them to calm down) may potentially inflame the situation.

As we saw in Chapter 2, anger has a range of effects on us. It is associated with strong physiological arousal and a narrowed focus on what provoked the anger. Until the anger has dissipated, it will be hard for the person to think about or deal with anything else. Common underlying reasons for anger include:

- Feeling hurt or let down: if people are emotionally hurt, they may try to protect themselves by being angry about it. In this case, the anger will usually be directed at a particular person or group.
- Perceived injustice or broken rules: perceived injustice can lead to anger and can arise in situations where a particular treatment is given to some people but not others. Cognitive theory suggests that we all have our own 'rules' about how both we and other people should behave (see Chapter 14). If people break our rules, we may get angry. For example, I might have a rule that 'I must always be there for people when they need me'. If a health professional is then not there for me when I need them (e.g. cancels an appointment or keeps me waiting for a long time), I might get angry.
- Goal frustration: if we are prevented from doing things or reaching goals that are important to us, it is common to feel frustration and angry (see Chapter 9). Injury and illness often prevent people from attaining their goals, so anger and frustration may be common.

Activity 13.2

Understanding Anger

Think back to the last time you were really angry with someone.

- Why did you feel angry?
- Were you hurt, frustrated, or had they broken one of your rules?
- What could they have done that would have stopped you feeling angry?

Like all strong emotions, anger needs to be expressed and diffused before a clinical consultation can continue. The following points can be helpful when trying to achieve this outcome:

- **Check your own emotional response**: if you feel angry, anxious, or upset, it will be harder for you to calm the person. Remind yourself that anger is an emotion and not necessarily an attack, and that the source of their anger can be the illness or hurt and so is not necessarily about you.

- **Acknowledge the anger**: recognise that the person is angry and that it is important to deal with this anger. For example, you may say, *'I can see you're angry and I think it's important we talk about this first'*.

- **Find out the source of the anger**: let the person talk. Giving them space to verbalise and vent what they are angry about is the first step towards diffusing that anger. People cannot remain angry forever, especially when they are with a sympathetic person.

- **Empathise**: the most effective way to tackle anger is to sympathise or understand. You do not have to agree with the person to be able to understand why they might be angry. Simple statements such as *'I can understand why you're angry'* or *'I would be angry too in your situation'* may prove very effective.

- **Disarm**: many people who are angry say all they want is for the person they are angry at to understand and apologise. Some health professionals worry that an apology means they are admitting fault or liability, but it is possible to express regret without agreeing that the person is right by saying something like *'I'm sorry if that/I upset you'*. If appropriate, a clear apology is powerful at disarming a situation.

13.3.2 Communicating with Anxious People

Anxiety and fear are normal responses to perceived threats, and illness or injury often comprise a threat to a person. Thus, anxiety and fear are common in healthcare settings. People differ temperamentally in their anxiety levels and responses. Those with the personality trait of neuroticism will be more prone to anxiety and have higher levels of anxiety (see Chapter 2).

Anxiety makes people hypervigilant for signs of threat. Consequently, they are likely to react strongly to unexpected events, symptoms, or negative news. Anxiety also makes people less flexible in their coping strategies, so specific strategies become more rigidly applied. For example, anxious people may need to know exactly what will happen next so that the additional threat of unexpected events is reduced. Reassurance on its own rarely works with anxious people – in fact, it can backfire because they may feel that you do not understand. In dealing with an anxious person the following may help:

- **Use your body language and speech**: as we saw at the beginning of this chapter, characteristics of speech and nonverbal communication can help someone to calm down. Adopt a relaxed and open body posture (non-threatening), lower the tone of your voice slightly, and slow down your speech.

- **Acknowledge the anxiety**: as with anger, recognise the person's anxiety (e.g. *'You seem worried'*).

- **Find out the main source of the anxiety**: anxiety can become generalised, so asking someone why they are anxious may elicit only a general or defensive response. Use a more focused question, such as *'Are you worried about anything in particular?'*, *'What is it you are particularly worried/anxious about?'*, or *'What was it that brought on your anxiety?'*

- **Empathise**: as with anger, empathy and understanding can be very helpful responses to strong emotion. In cases of terminal illness, where the threat of death is inevitable, empathy is crucial. In these cases, we cannot 'fix' anxiety or any other strong emotion – we can only empathise and provide support.

- **Minimise the threat**: anxiety is based on a perceived threat. Therefore, one way to lower anxiety is to reduce or remove that threat. This is best done by providing information as opposed to reassurance. For example, a pregnant woman may be anxious about her baby dying. In this instance, finding out why she believes this will happen and giving her information about the actual risk of it happening (or not) will be more effective than telling her not to worry. If there is a high risk, then involve her in planning her care so that the risk of adverse consequences is minimised.
- **Increase feelings of safety**: a related technique is to increase feelings of safety through information and control. For example, you may tell the person about self-monitoring or other things they can do to prevent complications developing, or about medical tests that can be done to check whether the perceived threat is real or likely.

Fear and panic are extreme forms of anxiety and require a different approach. They invoke very strong physical and behavioural responses, such as fight, flight, freezing, or turning to the group (see Chapter 3). Soothing responses in these circumstances are similar to those we might use with a frightened animal. Our body language and voice can be used to calm the person. Offer support and empathy and, if something triggered their fear or panic, remove it from the situation or stop the procedure. Strong fear or panic rarely last long, so should subside after a few minutes. Be prepared to stay with the person and remain calm while their fear or panic reduces. Distraction can be useful, when it is sensitively timed, because it can help the person to refocus their attention away from the threat.

13.3.3 People with Communication Difficulties

People can have difficulty communicating for a wide range of reasons. Common difficulties are people who have hearing, speech, or language difficulties. This means consultations may have to involve interpreters or a family member to facilitate communication. These consultations raise specific challenges but do not need to be difficult if you are patient and take time to communicate in the best way possible for that person. Remember that difficulties in communicating do not mean the person is not intellectually capable. Guidance for communicating with various groups, such as people with hearing loss or speech and language difficulties, has a few core things in common:

- **Find out about the person's communication difficulties** so you know how to best adapt your communication style to help them. For example, if someone is hearing impaired, you may ask if they need to lip read.
- **Check whether the person would prefer to be seen alone or with a companion** for part or all of the consultation.
- **Get the person's attention before you start talking to them**. For example, address them by name, wave, or tap them on the arm.
- **Address the person directly**: it is important to address the person directly and treat them with respect in the same way you would with someone without

communication difficulties. Talk directly to them, not to the interpreter or a family member. For people with hearing impairments, face-to-face contact is important for lip reading so look at them directly when you talk and do not cover your mouth with your hand or clothing.

- **Speak clearly but naturally**: do not shout, excessively slow down, or exaggerate your words or movements. Although it can help to slow your speech to make words clearer, it can appear patronising if you overdo it. Shouting may appear aggressive and is uncomfortable for people wearing hearing aids. Natural facial expressions and gestures are easier for people to understand and interpret, so do not over-exaggerate them.
- **Listen to the response**: give the person enough time to respond and do not try to finish their sentences or words for them, or cut them off. Be patient, and if you do not understand something it's fine to ask them to repeat it. If the person has a speech problem, such as a stammer, do not tell them to slow down or start again as this can increase their stress.
- **Pay attention to nonverbal communication**: you can pick up a lot from the person's facial expressions, gestures, and other responses that they may not be able to verbalise.
- **Check that the person understands**: use plain language and don't over-elaborate or repeat things. If the person doesn't understand, try saying it in a different way.

In addition, there are specific aspects that need to be considered. For example, if someone has a hearing impairment, it helps if there is no background noise and the room is well lit so they can clearly see your face.

13.3.4 Dealing with Distress

Distress is a general term and is used here to describe situations in which people are upset or crying. Distress can result from anger, anxiety, or fear, so dealing with distress draws on similar principles to dealing with those emotions. Two particular points should be borne in mind:

- Although it is natural to want to stop someone crying, it is not helpful to tell the person to stop. Even if you say it sympathetically, the underlying message is that you think they should not be upset or crying.
- Although empathy and understanding are important, too much empathy can *increase* someone's distress. If they are really distressed, they will be consumed by their feelings, so in these circumstances too much empathy can keep them focused on these feelings and they may feel overwhelmed. In such cases, it is more useful to try to get them to focus on specific events or facts which will lower their distress. This is not to say you need to be completely unempathetic, only that you need to help them to focus. For example, you might say '*I can see it's really upsetting – can you tell me exactly what happened?*' or '*Is there someone I can call who can come and be with you?*' This will encourage them to focus on specific details or actions rather than their emotions.

Clinical Notes 13.2

Dealing with Strong Emotions

- If strong emotions are ignored, the consultation will be difficult and ineffective.
- Anger is associated with aggression/attack but people can express anger safely if helped to do so.
- Useful techniques include acknowledging the emotion, identifying the reason for the emotion, empathising/understanding, and disarming.
- Anxiety is the result of a perceived threat and is associated with hypervigilance and inflexible coping.
- Anxiety can be helped by reducing the perceived threat and increasing feelings of safety.
- Consultations with people with hearing, speech, or language difficulties require that you adapt your communication style accordingly.
- High levels of distress will reduce if the person is sensitively asked to focus on specific events or facts.

Activity 13.3

Dealing with Distress

Think about a time when you were really upset about something important.

- When someone was sympathetic, did it make you more or less upset?

13.4 Giving Bad News

One of the hardest tasks in healthcare is to give bad news to people. This can range from telling them they have a chronic or terminal illness to giving news about death or disability. However, any news that brings with it some restriction or potential loss can be sad or bad news. A useful definition of bad news is that it is 'any information that produces a negative alteration to the person's expectations about their present and future' (Fallowfield & Jenkins, 2004: 312). This definition recognises the subjective nature of bad news and the importance of each individual's perception of what the news means for them. Thus, a sprained ankle can be bad news for someone who has a job that requires them to be on their feet all day; an infectious illness can be bad news if it is diagnosed the day before someone has planned to go away on the holiday of a lifetime.

Reviews of research in this area identify three key factors when giving bad news. First, people appreciate it if the health professional is kind, confident, sensitive, and caring. People also prefer health professionals to show concern and distress rather than being aloof and detached. Second, people appreciate it if the news is given clearly, using simple terms, and if they have time to talk about it with the health professional and ask questions. Third, people appreciate a quiet and private setting (Joekes, 2019).

A number of things can affect a health professional's ability to give bad news sensitively. These include burnout, fatigue, stress, and if the health professional has a fear of death (R. Brown et al., 2009; Dzierżanowski & Kozlowski, 2019). Training for health professionals in giving bad news is increasingly available, with some evidence that it improves their competence at giving bad news (Alelwani & Ahmed, 2014). Many guidelines for how to give bad news are available and the principles in these guidelines overlap. The SPIKES approach (Baile et al., 2000) advocates the following six steps and appears to be an effective learning aid for health professionals (Mahendiran et al., 2023):

1. **Setting up**: prepare thoroughly for the consultation. Make sure you have all the relevant information. Locate the consultation somewhere private, where you will not be interrupted. Allow yourself the time to give the news and then deal with the person's response and questions.

2. **Person's perception**: start by checking how much the person already knows and understands so you can tailor the bad news appropriately. Use an open question here, such as 'What have you been told so far?'

3. **Information needed**: ask the person how much they want to know about the diagnosis, prognosis, and treatment. This helps to tailor the type and amount of information you give in this session to what the person wants and is able to cope with.

4. **Knowledge given**: impart knowledge of the bad news. It can help to pre-warn the person by saying something like 'It's not the good news we hoped for', and then pausing. This allows the person a short time to prepare for the bad news. Give the bad news clearly and in simple language. Ambiguous statements should be avoided (e.g. saying a test was 'positive' means the opposite in pathology to lay language). Give the information in small, manageable chunks.

5. **Emotional response**: a range of emotional responses may arise when giving bad news, including shock, disbelief, fear, anxiety, distress, grief, and anger. As discussed in the previous section, the best way to deal with strong emotions is to recognise them and sympathise. With very bad news there is little you can do but offer sympathy and support. Evidence suggests that people appreciate this.

6. **Summarising and strategy**: towards the end of the consultation, the clinician should summarise the main points or outcomes of the consultation and consider or agree a future strategy, such as curative or palliative treatment. This helps to focus the person on the next steps, gives some certainty, provides a known support structure, and provides hope where possible.

Case Study 13.2

Giving Bad News

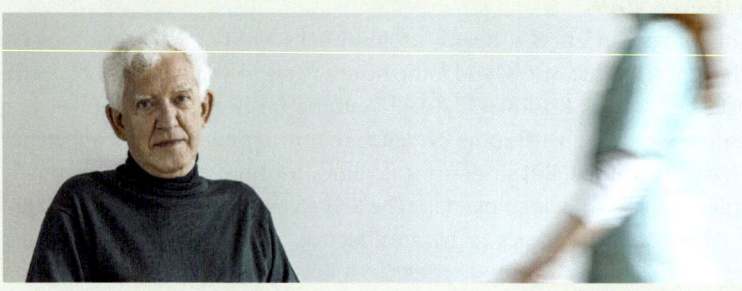

Figure 13.7   Jack's difficult diagnosis

Source: © Photographee.eu/Adobe Stock

Jack is a 70-year-old man who has been diagnosed with secondary progressive multiple sclerosis.

When I was first diagnosed in the hospital, a consultant, who I'm glad to say has now retired, said to me, 'Oh, we've got your diagnosis. I'm sorry, you've got an incurable disease and we can't treat it'.

The way my current consultant did it was much better. He sat on the side of the bed, he had a pad of plain paper and a pencil, and he drew the spinal column, right, and he showed the scarring as much, as near as he could, as my particular scarring.

He explained how messages travelled and he said, 'The trouble is when they hit a scar they're delayed, they go to the next scar and they're delayed a bit further, and further and further and further.' Unfortunately, I've got quite severe scarring, and so the messages are delayed quite a bit.

I think that difficult information should be given in the way that my present consultant has given me other news. He sits you down, and he smiles at you, and first of all you realise that he's on your side, he's with you, and he understands you as a person, and when he tells you or gives you news – like when he gave me the final diagnosis – it was done in a way that, in fact he held my hand, you know, and he built up to it, he didn't just blurt it out.

He gave the information gently, but factually … in a very sympathetic, that's the word I think, in a sympathetic way and that you realise, as the patient, that the person giving you that information understands that you're going to have to come to terms with that, which for me has been very difficult.

It doesn't really matter how brave you are or how not brave you are, if you're going to have bad news of any sort, any sort of bad news, I'm sure there must be a way of, of easing it so that you can make it as gentle as you can to the person that's going to have to receive it.

(Adapted from www.healthtalk.org © Dipex)

—Clinical Notes 13.3—

Giving Bad News

- Give bad news in a private setting.
- Give the news clearly and make sure there is enough time to talk about it.
- Be kind and caring.
- **SPIKES** is a useful mnemonic to remember the **S**etting, **P**erson's perception (what do they know), **I**nformation needed (what do they want to know), **K**nowledge giving, **E**motional response, **S**ummarising and strategy.

Conclusion

This chapter has explored the different ways we communicate and how they can be used in clinical practice to be more effective. Person-centred approaches remind us that each person's agenda is as important as the health professional's agenda, and that the relationship should be collaborative. Models of clinical consultations, such as the Calgary-Cambridge model, provide useful frameworks to think about the different stages of a clinical consultation and which skills are relevant to each. These approaches have been used in the training and assessment of clinical communication in a range of disciplines. This chapter has covered a variety of techniques and skills that can be useful in both routine and difficult clinical consultations. However, as with any skills, they need to be practised in order to learn them. They may feel awkward and demanding initially, but with practice they will feel more natural. Usually, when learning skills, we move from (1) unconscious incompetence to (2) conscious incompetence to (3) conscious competence to (4) autonomous competence (see also Chapter 10). Clinical skills are a good example of this, so the more you practise the more quickly you will reach unconscious competence.

—Further Reading—

Llewellyn, C.D. et al. (eds) (2019) *The Cambridge Handbook of Psychology, Health and Medicine* (3rd edition). Cambridge: Cambridge University Press. Includes short chapters on communicating risk, health professional–patient communication, breaking bad news, medical interviewing, and communicating health information.

Platt, F.W. & Gordon, G.A. (2004) *Field Guide to the Difficult Patient Interview* (2nd edition). Philadelphia, PA: Lippincott Williams & Wilkins. A pocket guide to communication skills for difficult clinical consultations, it is an easy-to-read, accessible book with useful tips.

Silverman, J., Kurtz, S. & Draper, J. (2013) *Skills for Communicating with Patients* (3rd edition). Oxford: Radcliff Medical Press. Describes the Calgary-Cambridge approach to communication skills in detail and is written in an accessible style.

Revision Questions

1   Describe three types of nonverbal behaviour and discuss how they are relevant to clinical practice.
2   How do the characteristics of speech influence communication?
3   Describe the person-centred approach to clinical consultations.
4   Discuss the evidence that health professionals' communication affects patient outcomes.
5   Outline the Calgary-Cambridge model of clinical consultations and illustrate it with the communication skills that are relevant to the different stages of the consultation.
6   Describe the key communication skills for effective information gathering in clinical consultations.
7   Outline the six main points for good clinical practice when conducting a physical examination.
8   What communication skills are useful for diffusing anger in clinical settings?
9   Discuss the key communication skills for closing a clinical consultation.
10 Outline the six steps of the SPIKES model for giving bad news.

14

PSYCHOLOGICAL INTERVENTION

Learning Objectives

This chapter is designed to enable you to:

- Outline the different psychological specialisms and their applications to medical settings.
- Understand the theoretical basis of psychological therapies.
- Describe cognitive behavioural therapy, third wave therapies, psychodynamic therapy, and counselling.
- Understand the use of psychotherapeutic techniques in healthcare practice.

Mental illness is surprisingly common. It is estimated that one in eight people worldwide have a mental health disorder, mostly depressive or anxiety disorders (World Health Organization, 2022). Less severe problems, such as mild or moderate symptoms of depression or anxiety, will be experienced by many more people at some point in their lives. Psychological interventions have the potential to make a huge difference to individuals and society, and are likely to play an increasing role in healthcare practice. However, the range of psychological professionals and interventions can be confusing. Many professions are involved in psychotherapy, such as psychiatrists, psychologists, counsellors, mental health nurses, and psychotherapists, and it is not always clear who does what. As with medicine, psychology includes many specialisms. Table 14.1 summarises some of the main psychological specialties. In practice, an individual's work may span two or three specialisms: for example, a clinical psychologist may also work in a forensic setting.

In most countries, psychology is regulated by organisations such as the European Federation of Psychologists' Associations or the American Psychological Association. These organisations regulate the content of psychology degrees and training in the same way that medicine is regulated by organisations such as the General Medical Council (UK) or the Liaison Committee on Medical Education (USA). Psychologists need to be registered with the relevant organisation and apply for professional status in order to practise.

This chapter focuses on the use of psychotherapy in healthcare settings. First, it explains some of the main types of psychotherapy used to treat mental health problems. Then it looks

Table 14.1 Psychology specialisms

Specialism	What do they do?	Where do they work?
Clinical psychologist	Assess and treat mental health problems such as depression, schizophrenia, and personality disorders	Health and social care settings such as hospitals and community mental health teams
Counselling psychologist	Assess and treat moderate mental health problems such as depression and anxiety	Wide variety of places, such as hospitals, prison services, education, and industry
Health psychologist	Health promotion, health services research, treat health problems such as obesity, smoking, and pain management	Health and social care settings such as hospitals, health centres, and other health-related organisations
Forensic psychologist	Work in legal processes, criminal behaviour, and investigations, including rehabilitation work with offenders	Prison services, secure hospitals and rehabilitation, police and probation services
Educational psychologist	Assess and provide remedial work for children with behavioural or learning difficulties	Schools, education departments, and local authorities
Occupational psychologist	Work with individuals and organisations to increase the effectiveness of employees and organisations	Industry, commerce, and other large organisations
Neuropsychologist	Assess and rehabilitate people with brain injury or disorders	Healthcare settings such as hospitals and neurological and community rehabilitation services
Sport and exercise psychologist	Work with athletes, sports people, and teams to enhance performance	Health services, professional sports teams, and national governing bodies

more specifically at interventions for physical health problems, such as motivational interviewing to help people to change their behaviour, and the provision of support groups for people with cancer.

14.1 Different Approaches to Psychotherapy

Here we use the term 'psychotherapy' very broadly to mean any form of therapy that involves talking and exploring psychological issues. The aims of **psychotherapy** are to resolve mental health problems and help people to thrive. Psychotherapy usually involves one-to-one sessions in which people talk through their problems. However, there are different types of psychotherapy, each with its own theoretical foundations. As a consequence, the content of psychotherapy can differ hugely, and in addition to talking therapies may involve writing, drawing, imagery work, role-play, and homework.

The main theories on which psychotherapies are based include psychodynamic (Freudian) theory, humanistic and existential theory, behaviourism, and cognitive theory. Figure 14.1 shows how these theories have resulted in different approaches to psychotherapy, each with their own philosophical assumptions and techniques. For example, **humanism** assumes (1) that humans are essentially good, (2) that we strive for personal growth and development, and (3) that we have free will and can therefore make choices. The humanistic approach to therapy, which was very

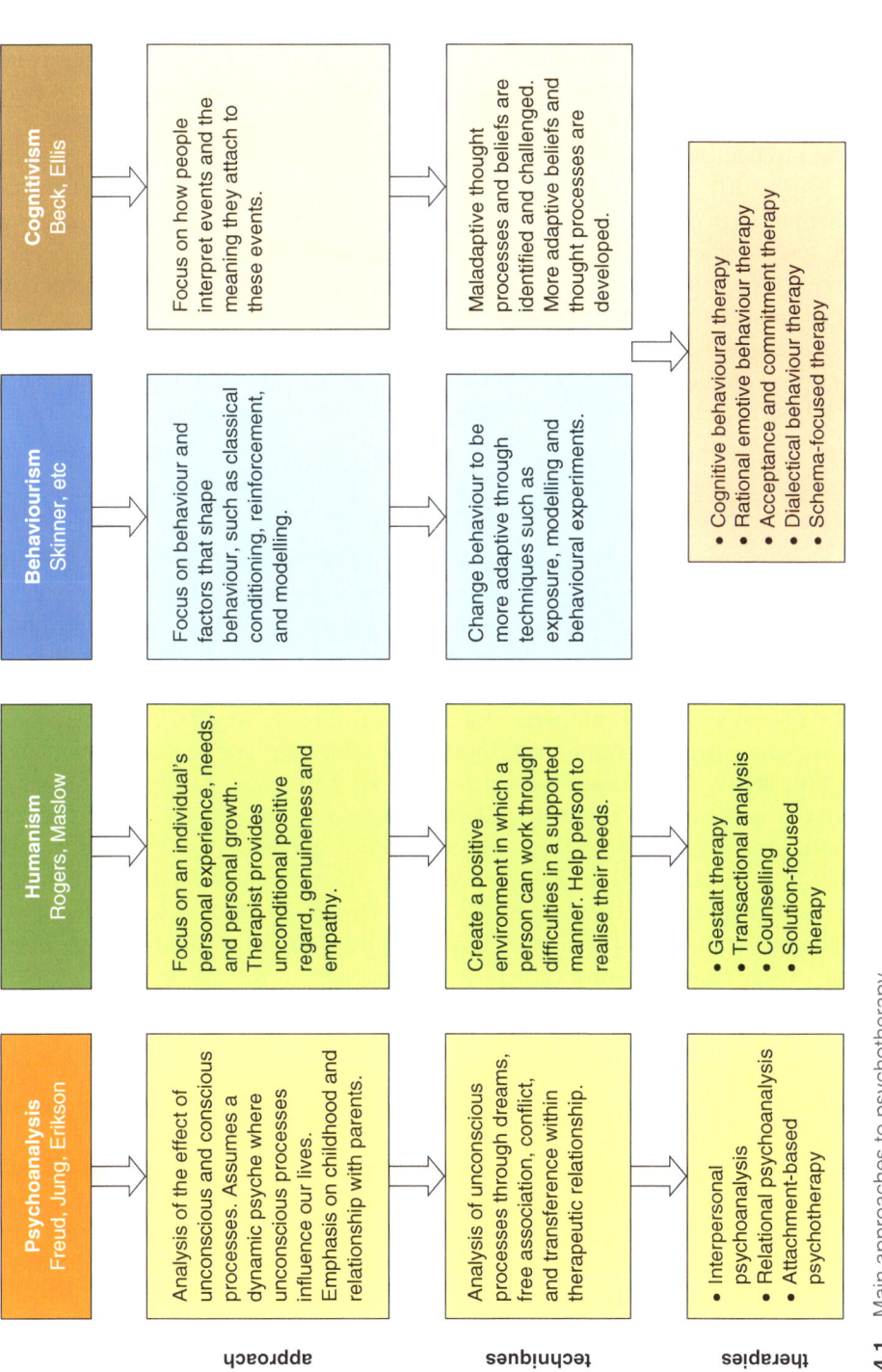

Figure 14.1 Main approaches to psychotherapy

	Psychoanalysis Freud, Jung, Erikson	Humanism Rogers, Maslow	Behaviourism Skinner, etc	Cognitivism Beck, Ellis
Broad approach	Analysis of the effect of unconscious and conscious processes. Assumes a dynamic psyche where unconscious processes influence our lives. Emphasis on childhood and relationship with parents.	Focus on an individual's personal experience, needs, and personal growth. Therapist provides unconditional positive regard, genuineness and empathy.	Focus on behaviour and factors that shape behaviour, such as classical conditioning, reinforcement, and modelling.	Focus on how people interpret events and the meaning they attach to these events.
Therapeutic techniques	Analysis of unconscious processes through dreams, free association, conflict, and transference within therapeutic relationship.	Create a positive environment in which a person can work through difficulties in a supported manner. Help person to realise their needs.	Change behaviour to be more adaptive through techniques such as exposure, modelling and behavioural experiments.	Maladaptive thought processes and beliefs are identified and challenged. More adaptive beliefs and thought processes are developed.
Specific therapies	• Interpersonal psychoanalysis • Relational psychoanalysis • Attachment-based psychotherapy	• Gestalt therapy • Transactional analysis • Counselling • Solution-focused therapy	• Cognitive behavioural therapy • Rational emotive behaviour therapy • Acceptance and commitment therapy • Dialectical behaviour therapy • Schema-focused therapy	

popular in the 1960s and 1970s, is founded on the principle that the therapist provides an **unconditional positive regard**: in other words, whatever a person has done will be understandable given that person's experience. The focus in humanistic therapy is on the person's unique experience, needs, and personal growth. The humanistic approach continues to be used in therapy today and is also evident in patient-centred approaches to medicine.

Modern psychotherapy draws on a range of theoretical approaches, including cognitive behavioural therapy (CBT), third wave CBT therapies, psychodynamic therapies, and counselling. Psychotherapies often overlap with each other and so are not always easy to classify. For example, cognitive analytic therapy (CAT) combines CBT and psychoanalytic principles in therapy. Interpersonal therapy focuses on relationship processes and draws on psychodynamic principles and CBT techniques. Eye-movement desensitisation and reprocessing is a specific therapy used to treat post-traumatic stress disorder (PTSD): it is referred to as integrative but incorporates a lot of CBT principles. The next section looks in more detail at the most historically influential and widely used psychotherapies in healthcare settings: CBT, psychodynamic therapy, and counselling.

14.1.1 Cognitive Behavioural Therapy (CBT)

Cognitive behavioural therapy (CBT) is founded on behaviourism and cognitivism. CBT is not a single therapy but rather a group of therapies that have shared core principles. Consequently, some argue that the term 'cognitive and behaviour therapies' is a more accurate label (Eagle & Worrell, 2019). These therapies have developed in three waves (Hayes, 2004). The first wave derived from **behaviourism**, which focuses on people's behaviour and how it is learned and shaped by events. Behaviourism describes the processes through which people's behaviour is shaped, including classical conditioning, operant conditioning, and modelling (outlined in Chapter 10). Behavioural therapy uses these processes to change maladaptive behavioural responses and substitute them with new adaptive behaviours. For example, phobias are often conditioned responses to an object that is associated with fear because of a negative or traumatic experience in the past. Behaviour therapy involves trying to counter-condition this response through techniques such as exposure to the feared object, systematic desensitisation to the object, relaxation training, modelling of adaptive behaviour, and reinforcement of adaptive behaviour. A well-known example of positive reinforcement is the use of reward charts and stickers with children to encourage good behaviours. Wearable technology that monitors health behaviours, such as exercise, can encourage behaviour modification using principles of behavioural monitoring and reinforcing healthy behaviour (Davison & Garcia, 2019).

Behaviourism emphasises scientific, or empirical, testing. Behavioural therapy therefore includes carrying out **behavioural 'experiments'**, in which people test their views of what will happen under certain circumstances. Consider, for example, the case of a person who has social phobia and avoids social situations because they make them highly anxious and they assume that everyone notices and thinks they are odd. This can lead to a vicious cycle where social situations are avoided. The more these situations are avoided, the more anxious the person will become about attending them. The person's assumptions are not challenged or disproved because there is no opportunity for them to have a good experience of a social situation. The combination of negative assumptions and avoiding social events (avoidance behaviour) creates a negative cycle that perpetuates the phobia. In these circumstances, a behavioural experiment might be for the person to attend a social situation, monitor their anxiety (which should reduce over time), monitor how they act, and also to notice how other people respond to them – whether that is positively or negatively. Another possibility might be to ask other people how they feel in social situations and whether they ever get anxious. This technique can normalise a certain degree of social anxiety. Behavioural experiments can reduce anxiety in many ways: the increased exposure to social situations can reduce anxiety through habituation, challenge negative beliefs, and break the negative cycle. We once heard of a therapist who went out and acted in bizarre ways in an attempt to show a patient how *little* other people would notice!

Behavioural experiments can affect a person's thoughts as well as their behaviour. From a cognitive viewpoint, behavioural experiments encourage people to become aware of underlying assumptions, specify and test them, and then revise their thoughts and behaviour accordingly. There is ongoing debate about whether behavioural experiments work mainly through behavioural or cognitive means (McMillan & Lee, 2010; Ougrin, 2011) but, regardless of how they work, behavioural experiments can be powerful tools of change and are particularly effective for anxiety disorders. They are also useful when treating people with reduced cognitive abilities, such as young children or people with learning difficulties. Case Study 14.1 provides an example of how cognitive and behavioural methods were used to treat a woman with PTSD after a difficult birth.

Case Study 14.1

Cognitive Behavioural Therapy for Postpartum PTSD

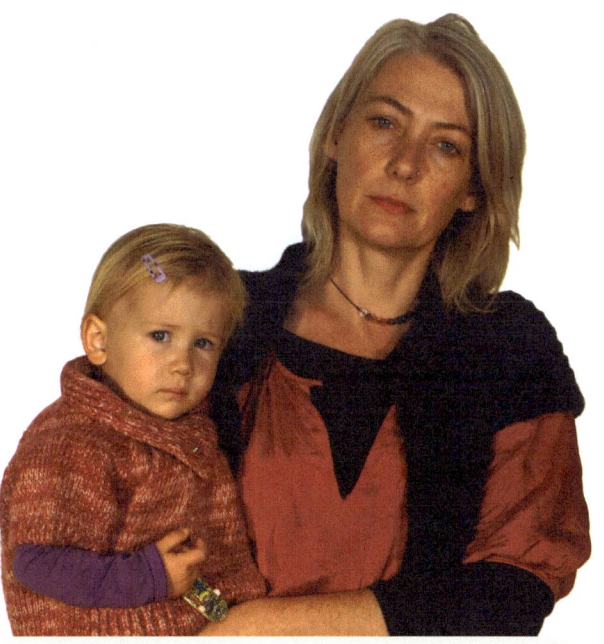

Figure 14.2 Sarah's postpartum PTSD

(Continued)

Sarah's labour was induced and there was confusion over when it would happen. Sarah panicked because she was unprepared and her husband was not there. The midwife was not sympathetic to Sarah's anxiety. After a painful internal examination, during which Sarah cried and asked the midwife to stop, the midwife said 'If you think that's painful, what are you going to be like giving birth?' From this point on Sarah's labour was characterised by pain, extreme distress, and fear of the midwife. Sarah's daughter was delivered by emergency caesarean section after a long labour, during which Sarah thought she might die. Sarah started to feel the surgery half way through and was given morphine. She reported dissociating (feeling detached from herself and like the labour was unreal) and cannot remember anything for 12 hours after the delivery.

Sarah said that the first few months after the birth were 'a blur' and it took her a year to bond with her daughter. Sarah suffered from postpartum PTSD and depression, and was prescribed antidepressants. Sarah first attended CBT 14 months after giving birth. She was highly distressed, appeared to be reliving the birth experience, and was crying and shaking. She had the full range of PTSD symptoms, including flashbacks, nightmares, and strong physical and emotional reactions to reminders of birth, feeling emotionally numb yet crying all the time. Her flashbacks were of seeing herself lying in the delivery room feeling helpless and terrified as the midwife came into the room.

Cognitive and behavioural techniques were used to help Sarah to process what happened during the birth:

1   *Mild exposure in the form of reliving exercises*. Sarah was asked to imagine the birth as if it were currently happening and to talk through the events in detail.
2   *Stronger exposure*, through visiting the labour ward with the therapist to help Sarah overcome her fear and avoidance.
3   *Cognitive exercises* to change Sarah's appraisals of difficult events in the birth, such as using a role-play to act out confronting the midwife and reducing Sarah's fear.
4   *Visualisation exercises* to rewrite her flashbacks. For example, she imagined the anaesthetist, with whom she felt comfortable and safe, with her in the delivery room.
5   *Formulation and positive reformulation* were used to help Sarah to understand and challenge maladaptive beliefs and to consolidate positive changes in beliefs.

After ten sessions of CBT, Sarah's PTSD symptoms had gone and her maladaptive beliefs about herself and others had changed.

(Adapted from Ayers et al., 2007)

The second wave of CBT derived from cognitivism, which sees thoughts as central to how we feel and behave. Cognitivism was the dominant paradigm in psychology for many years, and the importance of cognition is apparent in many of the theories and research outlined in this book. The first main cognitive theory of mental illness was proposed by Aaron Beck (1967), who argued that appraisal and the personal meaning of events are central in the development and maintenance of psychological problems. According to Beck, early experiences lead to sets of **core beliefs** or **schema** about ourselves, the world, and others. These beliefs are not necessarily rational because most of them are formed in childhood without the benefit of adult logic. Core beliefs can lead to **maladaptive assumptions**, which are sometimes referred to as 'rules for living'.

Beck was particularly interested in depression. He argued that people become depressed when they have a depressogenic triad of negative beliefs about themselves (e.g. they are deficient in some way), others and the world (e.g. others don't like them or treat them badly), and the future (e.g. negative expectations or hopelessness about the future). Evidence supports the existence of this depressogenic style of thinking, which has been observed in adults and children during depression (Marchetti & Pössel, 2023). It led to the cognitive content-specificity model, which proposes that, although anxious and depressed people have maladaptive cognitions, the content of these differ for each disorder. Following on from Beck's work, it has been suggested that depressive cognitions are largely focused on negative beliefs about the self, the future, and loss, whereas anxious cognitions are largely focused on perceived danger or threat. There is some evidence to support this. For example, a study of anxiety and depression from childhood to early adulthood in over 1,600 pairs of twins found that anxiety sensitivity (fear of bodily sensations) was associated with anxiety but not depression (H.M. Brown et al., 2014). However, the same study found that social concerns (fear of publicly observable symptoms) were associated with both anxiety and depression, and so were not disorder-specific. The authors therefore concluded that there are both specific and shared thought patterns in anxiety and depression (H.M. Brown et al., 2014). This is consistent with transdiagnostic approaches to psychopathology, which led to therapy techniques being developed to target problems observed across different psychological disorders, such as negative thinking (Hirsch et al., 2020) or rumination (Watkins, 2016).

CBT is used to treat a wide range of psychological problems, not only depression. Cognitive theories have been developed for different psychological disorders, including depression (Golonka et al., 2023), panic (Kyriakoulis & Kyrios, 2023), anxiety (V.M. Brown et al., 2023; Wells, 2010), PTSD (Brewin & Holmes, 2003), and personality disorders (Bora, 2021). These theories and the evidence for content-specificity have informed the development of cognitive therapy protocols for different psychological disorders. The defining features of CBT are given in Highlight Box 14.1. CBT has been applied to an increasing range of mental and physical disorders and has developed over the years to incorporate newer techniques based on mindfulness, meditation, and acceptance. These are collectively referred to as the third-wave therapies and are outlined in the next section.

However, the underlying theory can be applied to most of us, even when we are functioning well. Consider, for example, a person whose core beliefs include that they are unlovable and that other people will judge them, which could stem from having overly judgemental or unloving parents. This person might compensate for these core beliefs by having rules for living such as:

'If I do everything perfectly, then people will love me.'

'If I do what people want, they will not criticise me.'

'I must not show negative emotions or people will judge me.'

These rules help the person to function well and feel good about themselves as long as they adhere to these high standards. However, keeping up these standards will put them under considerable strain and make them vulnerable if something happens to make them think they've failed, such as not doing well in an exam or being made redundant from work. Under these circumstances, it is possible that they will develop depression because they have violated their rules and so activated their underlying belief that they are unlovable.

One difficulty with cognitive therapy is that people are not consciously aware of their own core beliefs and rules for living. However, these beliefs are usually reflected in the moment-to-moment **automatic thoughts** people have, especially in difficult situations. Thus, CBT involves monitoring automatic thoughts to help uncover a person's rules and core beliefs. Their core beliefs are put together in a formulation, which can be written or in diagrammatic form. The formulation is then used as a guide for the therapist and person to understand the problem and work out ways to test and challenge existing beliefs and build new, more adaptive beliefs. Testing beliefs can be done using cognitive and behavioural methods. Cognitive methods include guided discovery or Socratic questioning, where the therapist helps the person to examine and question their existing beliefs by considering evidence of whether or not they are correct.

—Activity 14.1—

Automatic Thoughts and Distress

Think about the last time you felt upset or angry and write down the following:

- What was the situation or trigger?
- What thoughts went through your mind (automatic thoughts)?
- How did these thoughts influence how you felt?
- Can you identify any of your rules (assumptions) that might have been broken?

—Highlight Box 14.1—

Core Features of CBT

1. It is a collaborative relationship between the therapist and the client.
2. The client is educated about the CBT approach so that they can become their own 'therapist'.
3. The focus is on the present problem, i.e. 'here and now'.
4. Structured sessions with content (an agenda) are agreed between the therapist and the client at the beginning of each session.
5. It is goal-directed, with aims for therapy being stated at the beginning. Work in therapy is directed towards achieving these aims.
6. It is short-term therapy, typically between six and 24 sessions.
7. It includes examination of maladaptive beliefs.
8. Maladaptive beliefs are cognitively challenged through Socratic questioning.
9. Behavioural experiments are used to test maladaptive beliefs (empirical approach).
10. General and specific formulations are used to guide understanding and change.

There is little doubt that CBT is a popular and effective treatment for a variety of conditions. It is now the recommended treatment for many psychological disorders, including depression, PTSD, generalised anxiety disorder, panic, and obsessive-compulsive disorder (e.g. National Institute for Health and Care Excellence, 2022). The widespread use of CBT is based on evidence that it is an effective treatment for these disorders. Reviews of CBT show that it is better than waiting-list or placebo controls and as effective as pharmacological treatment in reducing depression, generalised anxiety, panic, social phobia, PTSD and insomnia (Butler et al., 2006; van Dis et al., 2020; Y. Zhang et al., 2022). In addition, CBT has lower dropout rates than pharmacological treatment (Mitte, 2005).

CBT is also increasingly used as an adjunct to treatments of chronic illnesses. Reviews of randomised controlled trials have generally found positive effects of CBT treatment for illnesses as diverse as chronic pain (Williams et al., 2020), fibromyalgia (Cojocaru et al., 2024), sleep problems (Trauer et al., 2015), and asthma (Kew et al., 2016). However, the assessment of the effects of CBT is often limited to psychological outcomes, such as quality of life and measures of distress, rather than to physical functioning.

The popularity of CBT means that it is now in danger of being applied in a blanket fashion to areas where there is inconsistent evidence of its efficacy. For example, there are instances where CBT appears helpful but does not result in clinically significant change, such as trying to reduce harmful sexual behaviours in young people (Sneddon et al., 2020), domestically abusive men (Dennis et al., 2012), or treating the psychological consequences of child sexual abuse (Caro et al., 2023). There is also evidence that other therapies can be just as effective as CBT (Zhu et al., 2023). A more considered view may be to recognise that CBT works very well for *some* disorders, where it can lead to an improvement in *some* outcomes, but that it is by no means a panacea.

14.1.2 Third Wave CBT Therapies

More recent developments in CBT have been referred to, collectively, as third wave cognitive and behavioural therapies (Hayes, 2004). These therapies focus less on challenging the *content* of thoughts and more on the *relationship* that an individual has with their thoughts and emotions. Techniques such as acceptance, mindfulness, and cognitive diffusion help a person to accept their thoughts and emotional responses and not see them as all-defining or permanent. Being able to accept thoughts and emotional responses prevents psychological symptoms from becoming worse through negative appraisals of those thoughts and emotions. There is also a focus on life values and spirituality in many third wave therapies.

Various third wave therapies have been developed. A review identified 17 therapies classified in the literature as 'third wave' (Dimidjian et al., 2016). The most widely cited were mindfulness, Acceptance and Commitment Therapy (ACT), and Dialectical Behaviour Therapy (DBT), which are described below. Other third wave therapies include functional analytic psychotherapy, behavioural activation, compassion-focused therapy, metacognitive therapy, and integrative behavioural couples therapy.

Mindfulness is based on meditative practices which have been used for centuries. In its contemporary form, mindfulness has been defined as bringing non-judgemental awareness to an object of attention, being receptive, and being in the present moment (Kristeller, 2019). Mindfulness interventions involve regular meditation to practise raising awareness of factors such as breathing, bodily sensations, or thoughts and emotions. Specific techniques, such as guided meditation, walking meditation, body scan meditation, or mindful eating, can be incorporated into a range of different psychotherapeutic approaches. These techniques involve focusing on a particular task (e.g. walking or eating meditation) or different parts of the body (e.g. body scan meditation) in order to be focused in the present moment, to notice and pay attention to what we are doing or feeling.

There are also stand-alone mindfulness therapies which have been widely used and evaluated. The most common are Mindfulness-Based Stress Reduction (MBSR) (Kabat-Zinn, 1990) and Mindfulness-Based Cognitive Therapy (MBCT) (Segal et al., 2002). Both of these therapies consist of around eight weekly sessions of mindfulness meditation with daily mindfulness practice in between to teach people mindfulness skills with the goal of reducing stress or depression. The therapist or instructor provides psychoeducation about mindfulness and emotions, guides mindfulness practice in person or via audio-recordings, and provides specific content relevant to the intervention (e.g. risk factors for stress or depression).

Many mindfulness interventions have been developed for specific health problems or illnesses, with mixed evidence for efficacy. Interventions have been developed for changing health behaviours such as smoking (Maglione et al., 2017) or obesity (Ruffault et al., 2017), for symptoms such as chronic pain (Soundararajan et al., 2022), for psychological disorders such as attention deficit/hyperactivity disorder (Mitchell et al., 2015) or psychosis (Aust & Bradshaw, 2017), for physical illnesses such as breast cancer (X. Wang et al., 2024), cardiac disorders (Wankhar et al., 2024), respiratory disorders (Harrison et al., 2016), and diabetes (Fisher et al., 2023), and for specific groups of people, such as carers (e.g. Rayan & Ahmad, 2017) and health professionals (Kriakous et al., 2021).

Mindfulness interventions have been widely evaluated and there is evidence that they are effective compared to waiting-list controls or treatment as usual. A review of 47 randomised controlled trials found that mindfulness meditation programmes, such as MBSR and MBCT, result in small to moderate improvements in anxiety, depression, and pain (Goyal et al., 2014), but there was poor or insufficient evidence of effects on positive mood or stress-related behaviours, such as substance use, eating habits, sleep, or weight. Mindfulness interventions are not more effective than other active treatments, such as behavioural therapies or exercise (Goyal et al., 2014). Similar results are found for mindfulness apps (Gál et al., 2021). There is also interesting evidence about physiological responses to mindfulness interventions (see Research Box 14.1).

Research Box 14.1

Effect of Mindfulness Interventions on Biomarkers in People Who Have Cancer

Background

This systematic review looked at the effect of mindfulness-based interventions on biomarkers in people with cancer and cancer survivors.

Method and Findings

A systematic review of the evidence published up to 2022 found 25 research studies with a total of 1,603 participants. These studies examined 35 different biomarkers that fell within eight categories:

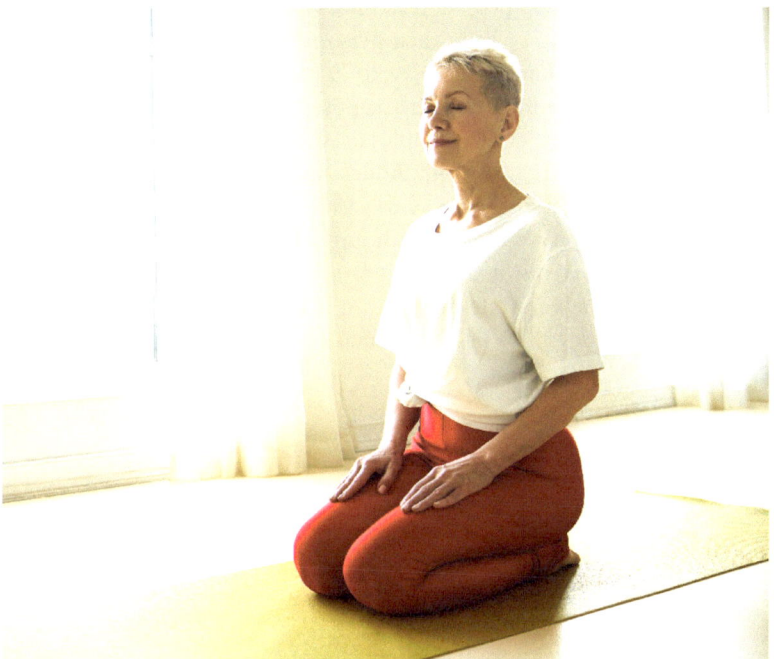

Figure 14.3 Practising mindfulness

Source: © shurkin_son/Adobe Stock

cortisol, blood pressure, heart rate, and respiratory rate; C-reactive protein; telomere length and telomerase activity; genetic signature; cytokines and hormones; leucocyte activation; leucocyte count; and cell subpopulation analysis. The results showed that mindfulness-based interventions had positive effects on biomarkers in seven of the eight categories. The most promising results were obtained for cortisol, blood pressure, telomerase activity and pro-inflammatory gene expression.

Significance

The authors say the review 'confirms the potential for mindfulness-based interventions for improving physiological health in cancer patients and survivors'. They suggest that the changes in biomarkers observed after mindfulness interventions may be due to the reduction of stress. However, they raise a number of limitations, including large variability between studies included in the review – for example, in type of cancer, type and duration of mindfulness intervention, type of control conditions, and type of biomarker. It limits the confidence with which conclusions can be drawn and highlights the need for additional evidence to confirm the impact of mindfulness interventions on biomarkers.

Matiz, A., Scaggiante, B., Conversano, C., Gemignani, A., Pascoletti, G., Fabbro, F. & Crescentini, C. (2024) The effect of mindfulness-based interventions on biomarkers in cancer patients and survivors: A systematic review. *Stress & Health*, 23 January: e3375. doi: 10.1002/smi.3375. Epub ahead of print.

Acceptance and Commitment Therapy (**ACT**) (Hayes et al., 2013) incorporates mindfulness and other techniques to help people to accept events, thoughts, and feelings that are outside their control and instead to identify their personal values and commit to acting on these. ACT rests on the assumption that trying to avoid or get rid of symptoms perpetuates negative emotions and suffering – hence the focus on accepting these symptoms and making a commitment to living a valued life. The core principles of ACT are shown in Highlight Box 14.2. The evidence for ACT is similar to that for mindfulness in that it appears to be an effective treatment but no more effective than standard CBT. A meta-analysis of 60 randomised controlled trials of ACT for stress and physical and psychological disorders found a small effect of ACT compared to waiting-list controls or treatment as usual (Ost, 2014). Similar results are found with internet-based ACT interventions (Han & Kim, 2022). However, ACT was not significantly better than other forms of cognitive or behavioural therapy.

Highlight Box 14.2

Core Features of ACT

ACT uses six core principles to help people to develop psychological flexibility:

1   **Cognitive diffusion**: helping people to realise that their thoughts, emotions, and memories are not necessarily true or define them.
2   **Acceptance**: helping people to allow their thoughts and feelings to come and go rather than struggling with them.
3   **Present moment**: helping people to be aware of the here and now, and to experience it with openness, interest, and receptiveness.
4   **Observing the self**: helping people to develop a transcendent sense of self and a continuity of consciousness that is unchanging.
5   **Values**: helping people to discover what is most important to them.
6   **Committed action**: helping people to set goals according to their core values and acting on them.

Dialectical Behaviour Therapy (**DBT**) (Linehan, 2014) was originally developed as a treatment for suicidal people and then tailored for people with borderline personality disorder. Since then, it has been used as a treatment for a range of psychological and behavioural problems. DBT uses standard CBT techniques for emotion regulation along with mindfulness and acceptance. DBT has four components: (1) individual therapy to address problem behaviours, set goals for quality of life, and to work towards them; (2) group sessions to teach the core skills of mindfulness, emotion regulation, tolerance of distress, and interpersonal skills; (3) a therapist consultation team to support therapists providing DBT; and (4) telephone coaching to help people to apply skills in their daily life. As with other third wave therapies, reviews of the evidence suggest that DBT is an effective treatment for borderline personality disorder and suicidality (Hernandez-Bustamante et al., 2024) as well as eating disorders and treatment-resistant depression (Hatoum & Burton 2024). However, DBT is not necessarily more effective than other psychotherapies.

Third wave therapies such as mindfulness, ACT, and DBT share a number of similarities. Common characteristics are the focus on mindfulness, acceptance, and cognitive diffusion. There is substantial evidence that these third wave therapies are effective. A review of meta-analyses conducted for common third wave therapies (including those described here) concluded that they have 'at least moderate to large effects' for treatment of anxiety, depression, eating disorders, borderline personality disorder, and suicidal behaviours compared to waiting-list controls or treatment as usual (Dimidjian et al., 2016). For example, a review of psychological therapies for depression found that third wave therapies and standard CBT approaches were equally effective and acceptable treatments (Schefft et al., 2023). Third wave therapies therefore provide a useful extension of cognitive and behavioural therapies to include new techniques and approaches that are as effective as standard CBT.

14.1.3 Psychodynamic Therapy

Psychodynamic therapy is based on Freud's theory of the psyche and psychopathology. The central idea is that we have a dynamic unconscious – hence the term psycho*dynamic* therapy. This dynamic unconscious involves a continuous conflict between drives and impulses on the one hand (the 'id'), and internalised social constraints and normative standards (the 'super-ego') on the other hand, as reflected in our 'ego', which is the component of personality through which we engage with reality. Conflict, suppression, and a building up of psychological defences then influence our behaviour, thoughts, and feelings, which can lead to psychopathology.

Psychodynamic theory has been extensively developed and refined and there are now many different types of psychodynamic therapy. These include interpersonal psychoanalysis, relational psychoanalysis, and attachment-based psychotherapy. Carlyle (2007) outlines three common principles in psychodynamic therapies. The first is the importance of early childhood experience. Modern psychodynamic theory incorporates work on **early attachments**, which indicates that the relationship a child has with their primary caregiver between the ages of six months and three years of age is fundamental in forming a person's early experience and their expectations of social relationships (see Chapter 8). Attachment is not the only important early experience. Research suggests that playing helps children to learn about the rules for appropriate behaviour and social roles. It also helps them to test their own abilities and regulate their emotions. For example, a child play-fighting with a parent will learn about acceptable and unacceptable levels of aggression.

Psychodynamic theory puts forward two processes by which early experiences affect development. These are introjection, where the child internalises aspects of their parents or other significant people into themselves. The other process is projection, where people project aspects of their own internal world onto others. The most well-known example of projection is when you view another person negatively because they do something or represent something you dislike about yourself. For example, a father may react angrily when his son does not achieve top grades at school because the father is frustrated by his own lack of achievement and success. The father is therefore projecting a part of himself that he dislikes onto his son and reacting strongly because of this.

Psychopathology in adults is therefore thought to result from early experiences being negative in some way, such as having neglectful or over-intrusive parents or a childhood that involved trauma, loss, or separation. These negative experiences then result in difficulties coping with life or relationships. As a result, the second common principle in psychodynamic therapies is the importance of relationships, particularly the **therapeutic relationship**. The therapeutic relationship is thought of as a regular, contained space for people to work through and understand their difficulties. This means that psychodynamic therapy is regular and intensive – often happening more than once a week for more than a year – to provide the person with a frequent and predictable time in their life to deal with their difficulties.

Through the therapeutic relationship, it is thought that the therapist starts to symbolise a parent for the patient. The therapeutic relationship therefore becomes a 'stage' on which interpersonal difficulties are played out. This is known as **transference**, where the way the patient views and relates to the therapist is thought to represent their underlying issues or interpersonal difficulties with parents or other significant people. A psychodynamic therapist therefore remains as neutral as possible and is not supposed to bring their own characteristics or feelings into therapy. This aspect of psychodynamic therapy is summed up by the (often untrue) stereotype of the therapist who says nothing while the person lies on the couch and talks.

The third common principle in psychodynamic therapies is the importance of **personal defences**, which are the ways in which people avoid difficult or painful thoughts. There are many different types of defences, including denial, repression, humour, rationalisation, escapism, and regression. Like coping strategies, defences are not necessarily maladaptive. For example, a person who needs complicated surgery may well deny or repress thoughts of possible complications or a painful recovery, which will minimise the threat of surgery and reduce their anxiety beforehand. The defining features of psychodynamic therapy are given in Highlight Box 14.3. Case Study 14.2 illustrates psychodynamic therapy for sexual dysfunction.

—Highlight Box 14.3—

Core Features of Psychodynamic Therapy

1   It assumes that we have a dynamic unconscious.
2   It is focused on the past, particularly early childhood experience and conflict, and on the suppression or psychological defences that have resulted.
3   The therapist remains neutral so transference can occur and the underlying issues can be explored.
4   The focus is on interpersonal relationships and how these are influenced by childhood experience, subsequent defences, projection, etc.
5   Maladaptive personal defences are explored.
6   It is an intensive therapy, typically comprising one or more sessions a week for at least a year.

Case Study 14.2

Psychodynamic Therapy for Sexual Dysfunction

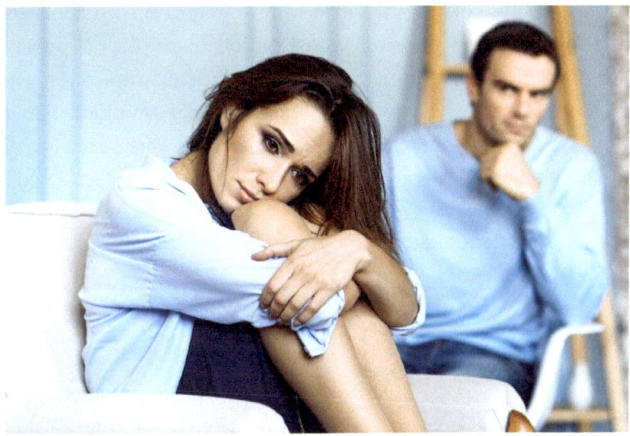

Figure 14.4   Laura and Dan's symptoms of sexual dysfunction

Source: © zinkevych/Adobe Stock

Laura is 38 and suffers from pain during intercourse (dyspareunia) and an inability to have sexual intercourse. Dan suffers from indigestion (dyspepsia) and backache. His mother died when he was five. Laura and Dan had a son who died of a hereditary brain disorder at 15 months. When he died, Laura was pregnant and this baby also died of the same disorder when 10 months old. The following year Laura had an ectopic pregnancy and chose to be sterilised. At the funeral of their first child, Laura said she felt 'numb'. Laura and Dan went on to foster and adopt two children. Their sexual dysfunction started after the death of their first child.

Psychodynamic Therapy

Laura and Dan's symptoms were interpreted as physical manifestations of the distress caused by the loss of their children and fertility. Their problems were therefore thought to be due to unresolved loss and bereavement. Dan and Laura were seen individually and as a couple by the same therapist for a year.

The therapist described Laura as 'wooden and lifeless' when discussing her experiences. This was interpreted as a defence mechanism, where Laura was no longer in touch with her feelings but projected them onto others so that they felt distress. Fostering, adoption, and work with disabled children were her way of escaping from the pain of bereavement.

The therapist explored Dan's relationship with his mother, who died when he was five years old. The therapist suggested that his marriage was an attempt to replace the relationship he had

(Continued)

with his mother. Dan therefore felt rivalry with his own children while they were alive because they took away Laura's attention. When the babies died, he felt responsible and guilty, so reacted negatively to Laura's distress because it reminded him of his guilt. Laura's dyspareunia and inability to have intercourse may therefore have been her angry attempt at retribution because he did not allow her to grieve.

Following this insight, the couple were able to have intercourse again. After Laura had an orgasm, she broke down and said it was as if she was 'crying from the deepest depths of herself'. She reported recovering mental images of her babies when they were dead, whereas previously she could only picture them alive. By the end of therapy, Dan's symptoms had disappeared and Laura's dyspareunia was intermittent but tolerable. The couple were sexually active and reported that their marriage had improved greatly.

(Adapted from Lewis & Casement, 1986)

The emphasis on unconscious processes means that psychodynamic theory is difficult to test scientifically. However, advances in neuroscience and research using imaging, such as functional magnetic resonance imaging (fMRI), have demonstrated that unconscious neural activity in the brain often pre-empts our voluntary action (Bonn, 2013). Because of various criticisms and the lack of consistent evidence, psychodynamic therapy is not as commonly recommended in guidelines for the treatment of mental health disorders as CBT. Proponents of the psychodynamic approach argue that this dismissal of psychodynamic therapy by clinical guidelines is premature and unjustified (Smith, 2007). Reviews of research into the effectiveness of psychoanalysis for disorders such as personality disorders and depression conclude that it is effective. For example, a review of randomised controlled trials of short-term psychodynamic psychotherapy concluded that there is evidence for 'modest to large gains' for common disorders such as anxiety, depression, and interpersonal problems (Abbass et al., 2014). Reviews and meta-analyses of the effect of manualised or internet psychodynamic therapy conclude that psychodynamic therapy is as effective as CBT and other types of psychotherapy for reducing depression and other psychological outcomes (Lindegaard & Berg, 2020; Smith & Hewitt, 2024).

14.1.4 Counselling

Counselling is an integrative approach that draws on various psychotherapeutic techniques, which makes counselling difficult to summarise. However, broad principles and core skills can be identified. The first is that it is **client-focused**. The needs of the client are put first and the aim of counselling is to increase or protect the person's psychological wellbeing.

A second principle is that counselling is **non-directive** and the emphasis is on the person exploring, clarifying, and solving their problems. The role of the counsellor is to facilitate this process. A third core principle is that counselling aims to provide a safe and accepting environment in which the person can explore and reflect on their difficulties. This is partly based on the principle of providing people with empathy, **unconditional positive regard**, and congruence to facilitate self-acceptance and feelings of self-worth. For example, parents and society place expectations on us about performance, achievement, and what is seen as successful or worthwhile. It means that many people may only feel worthwhile if they reach expectations and perform well in these areas. A counsellor might explore this with a person while at the same time accepting them regardless of their achievements or failures. This approach provides the person with an insight into their behaviour and feelings at the same time as allowing them to experience a relationship where they are liked and accepted for who they are.

Various core skills used in counselling have been outlined by different counselling organisations and training programmes. Skills include a focus on the therapeutic relationship through a working alliance, empathy, rapport building, and using nonverbal communication, as well as facilitative skills such as active listening, reflection, questioning, summarising, and providing feedback (e.g. British Association for Counselling and Psychotherapy, 2020).

Counselling tends to be used for treating people with mild to moderate anxiety and depression, or people who are experiencing difficult life circumstances or crises. Counselling is also increasingly used in healthcare settings to help people to adjust to and cope with difficult events, such as a diagnosis of HIV, coronary heart disease, a late miscarriage or stillbirth, or to help people make difficult decisions, such as during fertility treatment or genetic testing (Bor & Eriksen, 2019). The defining features of counselling are given in Highlight Box 14.4.

Currently, evidence for the efficacy of counselling is limited. This is partly because it is difficult to define a 'standard' approach to counselling, so research has focused on evaluating more clearly outlined therapies, such as CBT. Research into counselling is often methodologically limited because counselling is poorly defined or not compared to other forms of therapy. However, where evidence is available, it suggests that counselling is evaluated positively by participants and can improve some outcomes in the short term. For example, a review of counselling for psychological and psychosocial problems in primary care settings concluded that it was more effective than usual care in the short term (Bower et al., 2011). Similarly, a review of face-to-face and web-based counselling for university students concluded that it led to improved mental health and academic achievements for students (Cerolini et al., 2023).

Highlight Box 14.4

Core Features of Counselling

1   The therapist provides unconditional positive regard and accepts the person for who they are.
2   The therapist is non-judgemental and provides a safe space in which the person can work through their problems.
3   The needs of the client are primary.
4   The person explores their problems and solutions and the therapist facilitates this.
5   Sessions are directed towards the overall aim of improving a person's psychological wellbeing.
6   An integrative or eclectic approach is taken towards therapeutic techniques. These are drawn from various psychotherapeutic approaches, such as CBT and psychodynamic therapy.
7   It is a short-term therapy, typically consisting of between six and 16 sessions.

14.2 Which Therapy is Best?

The issue of whether one type of therapy is better than another is contentious. There is evidence that various different psychotherapies are effective treatments for depression and anxiety disorders. Richardson (2006) argued that 'where one therapy appears to have an advantage over others in terms of empirical research, this is usually because the others have failed to accumulate the relevant evidence'. It may be that different therapies are equally effective for some disorders. Indeed, there is evidence that this may be the case. For example, a review of 257 meta-analyses of the effect of psychotherapy on a range of outcomes showed that the majority (80%) reported a significant effect on outcomes. The authors concluded that the most convincing evidence was for CBT, meditation, cognitive remediation, counselling, and mixed psychotherapy (Dragioti et al., 2017). Similarly, a review of randomised controlled trials comparing CBT with mindfulness-based therapy for depression found both were equally effective (Sverre et al., 2023).

This evidence suggests that non-specific factors, such as the therapeutic relationship or placebo effect, may play an important role in the effectiveness of psychotherapy. As in all areas of healthcare, the importance of a good relationship between the person and therapist is well established, and evidence shows that it leads to better outcomes, regardless of the type of psychotherapy (Department of Health, 2001). Whether therapy partly works through a placebo effect is less widely considered, despite the fact that psychotherapy involves no active physiological substances and relies on a person's experience of therapy, and beliefs about therapy to treat illness. Thus, some have called for greater exploration of possible placebo effects in psychotherapy (Enck & Zipfel, 2019).

So what can we conclude from this? There is little doubt that psychotherapy is effective in the treatment of mental health. Which type of psychotherapy is best is likely to vary for different psychological problems and individuals. Although the current guidelines favour CBT and third wave therapies, this position may change as the evidence accumulates for counselling and psychodynamic approaches. It would be nice to think that in the future psychotherapy will move away from a 'winner takes all' mentality, where one type of therapy has to prove itself as better than the others, and will integrate those approaches and techniques that are shown to be effective under different circumstances. This approach is already evident in counselling, which draws on techniques from many different approaches to therapy.

Summary 14.1

- There are many different types of psychotherapy.
- Therapies have developed from theories of psychoanalysis, humanism, behaviourism, and cognitivism.
- Common approaches to therapy are CBT, third wave cognitive therapies, psychodynamic therapy, and counselling.
- CBT is a structured, short-term therapy that focuses on the present problem and changes maladaptive beliefs and behaviour.

- Third wave cognitive therapies focus on the relationship people have with their thoughts and changing this relationship through techniques such as mindfulness, meditation, acceptance, and cognitive diffusion.
- Psychodynamic therapy is an intensive, long-term therapy that focuses on a person's early childhood experience, interpersonal relationships, and unconscious conflicts.
- Counselling is a short-term therapy that can consist of one approach to therapy, such as psychoanalysis, but is often more integrative or eclectic.
- There is some indication that different types of therapy may be equally effective for some disorders. This may be due to the importance of non-specific factors such as the therapeutic relationship or a placebo effect.

14.3 Psychological Interventions in Medical Settings

Psychological interventions in medical settings extend beyond psychotherapy. They do not purely aim to resolve mental health problems but include any intervention to promote physical or mental health in medical settings. This includes health promotion, pain management, self-management in chronic illnesses, crisis intervention, stress management, and support groups. Descriptions of some of these interventions are given in Table 14.2. Examples and case studies of these interventions can be found throughout the chapters in this book.

There is general support for the effectiveness of psychological interventions for promoting health and wellbeing, although this varies according to the type of intervention and target group. Interventions can be broadly grouped into:

- Those that aim to change health behaviours.
- Those that aim to help people cope with difficult or stressful circumstances.
- Those that target particular symptoms or illnesses, such as pain management.

14.3.1 Interventions for Changing Behaviour

Interventions to change health behaviours include health education, health promotion, and motivational interviewing. **Health promotion** is a broad area, ranging from national advertising campaigns to interventions with people who have a particular illness. Its effectiveness varies according to the method chosen and the people targeted. Providing blanket information to everyone is less effective than targeting information. Evidence has clearly shown that educational interventions are more effective if they are relevant to the people they target, are individualised, can provide feedback on people's learning, facilitate change by explaining how people can take action, can help people to develop the required skills to change, and can reinforce the desired behaviour (Kok, 2007). This evidence has informed health promotion campaigns and there are many examples of health promotion advertising that targets specific groups, such as that in Figure 14.5, which was aimed at increasing activity in people with long-term health conditions.

Table 14.2 Psychological interventions in medical settings

Psychological intervention	Aims	What it consists of	Use	See example
Assessment	Assess an individual's psychosocial needs	Interview and questionnaires to assess people's needs and mental state	For severe or chronic illnesses that require multidisciplinary management	
Pain management	Help people to manage their pain to increase activity levels and wellbeing	Education about pain and CBT techniques such as monitoring activity and pain, setting goals, empowering people	For chronic pain of any kind, e.g. back pain, pelvic pain, arthritis, etc.	Chapter 4
Motivational interviewing	Help people to change risky health behaviours	Exploring and understanding a person's current beliefs and behaviour, facilitating change through developing the discrepancy between a person's values and current behaviour, and building confidence that change is possible	For smoking, alcohol use, other drug addictions, eating disorders, and depression	Chapter 2
Self-management	Help people to manage their illness or recovery, including adherence to medication, rehabilitation, and facilitating psychological wellbeing	Examining beliefs about illness, illness behaviour, and emotions, and facilitating change to promote good self-management of illness	For chronic illnesses, e.g. multiple sclerosis, diabetes, heart disease, asthma, irritable bowel syndrome, arthritis, etc.	Chapter 4
Health promotion	Promote health and positive health behaviours and reduce risky health behaviours	Education and promotion of health through information and interventions to reduce risky behaviours	With the normal population, e.g. people attending primary care, antenatal clinics, sexual health clinics, and smoking cessation	Chapter 5
Crisis intervention	Support people in times of crisis and help them to adjust and cope	Supporting people to work through what has happened and encourage positive adjustment	After a diagnosis of a serious illness, such as cancer, heart disease, multiple sclerosis, etc., and in palliative care	Chapters 6, 15 & 16
Stress management	Help people to manage stress effectively	Education about stress: understanding and breaking down stress, appraisal processes and responses, and exploring more adaptive ways to cope	When stress may exacerbate conditions such as heart disease, premenstrual tension, and for professionals in high-stress jobs (including health professionals)	Chapter 3
Support groups	Encourage contact with, and support from, other people in similar circumstances	Small groups of people with similar problems, which are usually facilitated by a health professional	With groups such as people with cancer, heart disease, or following stillbirth	Chapter 15
Bereavement counselling	Help people to cope with and come to terms with their loss	Individual or couple counselling to help people to mourn their loss and find ways to cope	For the loss or bereavement of a significant other, e.g. a stillbirth, relatives of people who are dying	Chapter 6
Neuropsychological rehabilitation	Assess, treat, and rehabilitate people with a brain injury to reduce disability and increase quality of life	Examination of cognitive, behavioural, emotional, and social function, and rehabilitation through various techniques, e.g. goal setting, skill training, and increasing awareness	Following brain injury or neurodegenerative diseases such as dementia	Chapter 7

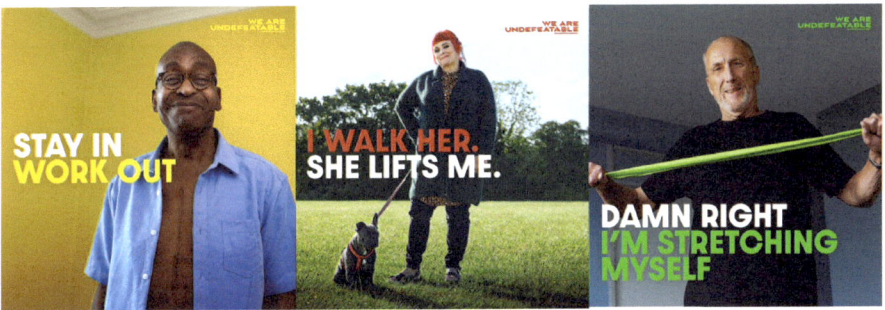

Figure 14.5   Targeted health promotion: increasing activity in people with long-term health conditions

Source: Used with permission of the 'We Are Undefeatable' campaign and Age UK

Motivational interviewing is used to change risky behaviour and promote healthy behaviour. Motivational interviewing was developed as a treatment for substance misuse, where people often have positive and negative attitudes towards the problem behaviour. It is a form of directive counselling that helps people to explore their reasons for a behaviour and their ambivalence towards a problem behaviour in order to resolve it. Motivational interviewing is more focused and goal-directed than normal counselling, although the emphasis here is not on *persuading* someone to change but on *helping* them to develop their own motivation to change. This is done through (1) empathising with the situation the person is in, (2) avoiding argumentation or persuasion, (3) examining the discrepancy between what the person wants to do and what they are actually doing, (4) examining resistance, and (5) bolstering the person's self-efficacy (Miller & Rollnick, 2023). An example of motivational interviewing is given in Chapter 2 (see Case Study 2.2).

Evidence suggests that motivational interviewing can be highly effective. Reviews of clinical trials of motivational interviewing across a wide range of behaviours show that it is effective in the short term (Crosby et al., 2023; X. Huang et al., 2023; Kao et al., 2023). In the long term, the effect of motivational interviewing appears to be more limited and change may be more likely when motivational interviewing is used in addition to a standard treatment (Hettema et al., 2005). It is therefore a worthwhile approach for health professionals to use to help people change behaviours, such as substance abuse and non-adherence to treatments.

14.3.2 Interventions for Stressful or Difficult Circumstances

Interventions to help people to cope with stressful or difficult circumstances include stress management, critical incident debriefing, crisis intervention, bereavement counselling, and support groups. **Stress management** has been used with occupational groups, patient groups, and health professionals. It is based on an understanding of the processes of stress and coping (see Chapter 3) and helps people to identify the factors that are contributing to their stress and to find more adaptive ways to cope. In healthcare settings, stress management has most often been provided for people with cancer or heart disease. In this context, stress management reduces anxiety, depression, perceived pain, and increases quality of life for people (Tang et al., 2020). However, it may have no effect on the course of illness or morbidity (Kenny, 2007).

Activity 14.2

Coping with Stress

Think of a time you found really stressful or difficult.

- How did you cope with it?
- What did you find most helpful?

Critical incident debriefing was initially developed to help emergency service workers cope with the traumatic events they attended, such as disasters, homicides, or road traffic accidents. Debriefing was carried out in groups and the approach was rapidly applied to a range of traumatic situations. However, evidence has shown that debriefing is *not* effective, and in some cases can make people worse. As a result, many clinical guidelines recommend against using it. Despite this, debriefing is still used in some settings in varying forms. For example, most hospitals in the UK offer some form of midwife-led debriefing to women after difficult or traumatic birth experiences (Thomson & Garrett, 2019). However, the content of midwife-led debriefing is different from critical incident debriefing so these services are usually referred to by other names, such as 'Birth afterthoughts' or 'Birth stories'.

Debriefing shares some similarities with **crisis intervention** and bereavement intervention in that they all try to reduce the impact of a situation rather than prevent it happening in the first place. Crisis intervention is used in situations where there has been threat of harm or violence, mental health crises, or suicide attempts. It draws on a range of psychological theories and techniques to support people through a critical period (Huber et al., 2024). Evidence for crisis interventions in medical settings is mixed, partly because of the wide range of approaches that are used. There are promising approaches, particularly those focusing on risk-reduction in suicidality (Otis et al., 2023) or crisis intervention following traumatic events (Lotzin et al., 2023).

Bereavement interventions are used following the death of a significant other, such as a spouse, parent, or child. Bereavement interventions vary according to which theoretical view is taken of bereavement. The psychodynamic view focuses on unresolved conflicts or issues with the deceased. Stage theories of bereavement emphasise the different stages a person needs to go through, such as numbness, yearning, despair, and recovery. Stress theories of bereavement emphasise the stress of bereavement and the loss of resources to cope. Support theories emphasise the loss of social support and the disruption of support networks (see Chapter 6).

A review of bereavement interventions considered the different theoretical viewpoints and whether they can account for the evidence that (1) men are more affected by the death of a spouse than women; and (2) how the person dies affects the nature of grief – for example, an unexpected death is likely to result in more severe grief than an expected death. The review concluded that these facts were best accounted for by stress or support theories of bereavement (Kato & Mann, 1999). However, this and more recent reviews of the evidence suggest that bereavement interventions as a whole are limited in their impact (Harrop et al., 2020). Although they may improve short-term outcomes compared to no treatment, these differences are not observed in the longer term, which may be because grief tends to reduce naturally over time in those who have no treatment. There is also evidence that bereavement interventions are only really effective for high-risk individuals – for example, in cases where the death was unexpected or where there was a high level of dependency in the relationship, or if the person has a history of psychological problems (Currier et al., 2008; Jordan & Neimeyer, 2003).

Clinical Notes 14.1

Psychotherapy Techniques and Clinical Practice

- Recognise that individuals come to you with their own emotional baggage, core beliefs, past experience, and relationship history.
- Do not underestimate the effects of a good therapeutic relationship and placebo.
- Give people unconditional positive regard to improve the therapeutic relationship and the patient's psychological wellbeing.
- Be on the patient's side, understand their experience, and work with them to encourage change.
- Help people to accept and distance themselves from negative thoughts (e.g. to accept their thoughts and think of them as a wave that will just wash over them and recede).

14.3.3 Interventions for Specific Illnesses or Symptoms

Interventions targeted at specific illnesses or symptoms are wide-ranging and include self-management interventions, support groups for people with particular problems or illnesses, pain management, and neuropsychological rehabilitation.

Self-management interventions draw on the theories outlined in Chapters 4 and 5 to help people to manage their illness or rehabilitation effectively, with the aim of improving their psychological and physical wellbeing. Self-management interventions have been designed for many illnesses, such as arthritis, asthma, diabetes, hypertension, chronic obstructive pulmonary disease (COPD), headache, and back pain (Mulligan & Newman, 2019). Generic self-management programmes for chronic disease have also been developed (Lorig et al., 2007). Most self-management programmes involve five key components to increase people's skills at managing their illness. These are: problem solving, decision making, how to find and use resources, forming partnerships with health professionals, and taking action (Lorig & Holman, 2003).

Evidence shows that self-management interventions are effective in the short term and can improve health behaviours and the management of an illness, such as adherence to medication. Self-management interventions can also lead to improved physical and emotional wellbeing. For example, a review of 969 randomised controlled trials of self-management interventions for different conditions found strong evidence that self-management interventions for diabetes improved blood glucose control, self-management interventions for rheumatoid arthritis led to improved disability and psychological wellbeing, and self-management interventions for asthma reduced hospital admissions and emergency healthcare services (Taylor et al., 2014). However, these effects are not always maintained over the long term (Mulligan & Newman, 2019).

Support group interventions are based on substantial evidence that social support is associated with better health and wellbeing and that, conversely, social isolation is a risk for many illnesses. Support interventions usually consist of a group of up to 12 people with similar problems or circumstances who meet eight to ten times. Groups can be facilitated by a health professional or be patient-led. Support groups aim to increase the support available to people, increase education and the sharing of knowledge about relevant circumstances, and increase the sharing and modelling of positive coping strategies.

Historically, the popularity of support groups in medical settings was boosted by a study that found that women with breast cancer who attended a support group lived on average 18 months longer than those who did not attend a support group (Spiegel et al., 1989). Since then, the evidence has been less consistent, and although support groups usually improve psychological wellbeing and quality of life, they do not have a consistent impact on morbidity or mortality (Gottlieb, 2007; Z. Li et al., 2024). It is possible that this is because they work better for some people than for others. For example, if a person has a poor social network and does not express their emotions or cope particularly well, then a support group can be very helpful by increasing their social network, helping them to talk about their feelings, and exposing them to other group members who might model better ways of coping. Conversely, a person who already has many close friends and family members to support them may not benefit from a support group.

There are many other interventions for specific illnesses. Evidence shows that **pain management** programmes based on CBT can lead to short-term reductions in pain, disability, negative mood, and catastrophising compared to usual treatment (Williams et al., 2020; see also Chapter 4). **Neuropsychological rehabilitation** uses a range of psychological theories and techniques to treat and rehabilitate people with neuropsychological problems, such as brain injury (see Chapter 7). Families are usually highly involved in this process. Technologies such as computer programs, virtual reality training, electronic reminders, and memory aids are also available to help people to adapt and function in the community. Research into the effectiveness of neuropsychological rehabilitation has focused on specific techniques. For example, there is evidence that memory rehabilitation and specific attention skills training can be effective, but that general attention training is not (Rohling et al., 2009).

Summary 14.2

- Psychological interventions in healthcare settings include health promotion, interventions for stressful or difficult circumstances, and interventions for specific illnesses or groups of people.
- These interventions are wide-ranging and draw on a range of psychological theories and techniques.
- Evidence shows that health promotion, motivational interviewing, self-management, pain management, and neuropsychological rehabilitation are effective.
- However, the beneficial effect of many psychological interventions in healthcare settings can be short-term and limited to psychosocial outcomes.
- Critical incident stress debriefing is the only intervention where there is evidence that it should not be used.
- Bereavement interventions are of limited use but may be effective with high-risk individuals.

14.4 Technology and Psychological Intervention

The limited availability and cost of psychological services in many contexts means there is an increasing use of technology to support or deliver psychological interventions. The advantages are that treatment is accessible, convenient, and can be provided over a wide geographical area. Online interventions are often more easily available, accessible, and affordable. Some online interventions may also provide anonymity, which can reduce barriers to accessing treatment, such as the stigma associated with some illnesses.

Tailored psychological interventions are increasingly accessible through the worldwide web, smartphones, and tablets. Online resources are available to treat illnesses, such as computerised therapy for anxiety and depression. Technology can be used to facilitate support groups through online forums, email discussion groups, and social media. People generally rate online groups positively, but there is a lack of high-quality evidence for the effectiveness of online groups (Cheng et al., 2023; Y. Huang et al., 2022). Technology-assisted programmes are also available to assist people in lifestyle change or therapy, such as exercise trackers, mood trackers, and meditation apps.

Technology-mediated psychotherapy programmes are usually self-directed, that is, people work through a series of modules in their own time. Some are supported by an AI assistant or trained person who oversees a person's progress via telephone, email, or messaging. Programs and apps are available for a range of common psychological problems, such as insomnia, stress, depression, anxiety, phobias, etc. Many are based on CBT or third wave cognitive therapy techniques, which are easily adapted for this medium. There is now substantial evidence that online and computerised programs can be effective treatments for less severe psychological problems. Reviews and meta-analyses show that web-based treatments for stress, depression, and anxiety disorders are more effective than no treatment or placebo controls, and in some cases are as effective as face-to-face psychotherapy treatment (Olthuis et al., 2016).

The advantages and potential efficacy of programmes delivered through technology mean that this is an area of rapid growth and development. However, not all programmes have evidence that they are effective (Ashford et al., 2016). Web-based interventions have also been developed to help people to manage long-term physical health conditions, such as diabetes (Hofmann et al., 2016), and to encourage healthier behaviours. However, programmes that are available via the internet vary in quality and content. It is clear from reviews that some web-based programmes are more effective than others, and that not all of them are founded on validated theories of psychological disorder or behaviour change (Murray, 2012). Similarly, there are vast numbers of health apps available, but many lack a theoretical basis or evidence of efficacy. Apps that do have a theoretical basis, such as self-monitoring for behaviour change, have been positively evaluated, but the evidence is limited (Payne et al., 2015; Yau et al., 2022). It is therefore important that people are directed to programmes that have evidence they are effective.

Other technological developments include the use of games and virtual reality to monitor or improve health. Games such as *Wii Fit* promote physical activity and have been used in neuropsychological rehabilitation (e.g. with people who have had a stroke) as part of rehabilitation to regain mobility. Although improvements are similar to those observed after conventional rehabilitation, people were less likely to drop out from programmes using exercise-based games (Perrochon et al., 2019). Games have also been developed for specific health issues. These can be to help patients, such as *Bobby got a Burn*, which prepares children for standard medical procedures, or *iSpectrum*, which aims to improve social interaction skills in people with autism or Asperger's syndrome.

Games have also been developed to help healthcare students learn procedures in surgery, radiology, dentistry, nursing, cardiology, dietitians, and first aid (Xu et al., 2023).

Virtual reality programs enable scenarios to be simulated, and therefore have potential applications in psychological interventions such as neuropsychological rehabilitation and psychotherapy for anxiety disorders. Virtual reality has been used in rehabilitation for conditions such as dementia (Stavropoulou et al., 2024), multiple sclerosis (J. Zhang et al., 2024), cerebral palsy (Hao et al., 2024), and in end-of-life care (Xia et al., 2024), with evidence that it is a promising method in terms of increasing mobility and motor skills, as well as decreasing distress and psychological symptoms. Virtual reality has also been used as part of exposure treatment for anxiety disorders. As mentioned earlier, an effective behavioural treatment for fears and phobias is to expose people to the feared object until their anxiety reduces. Obviously, being exposed to fearful situations can be very challenging for people, so virtual reality is a useful medium through which to 'expose' someone to their feared object or situation but where the person knows it is not real. Virtual exposure has been used as part of treatment for a range of problems, including fear of flying, dental phobia, spider phobia, social anxiety, and PTSD (Kim & Kim, 2020). Several reviews show that virtual reality exposure is an acceptable and effective treatment for phobias and anxiety disorders (Shahid et al., 2024). For example, a review of virtual reality exposure for phobias found it resulted in improved outcomes and that improvements are maintained over time (Krzystanek et al., 2021).

Conclusion

In this chapter we have looked at different types of psychotherapy and the theories underlying them. First, we looked at cognitive behavioural therapy and third wave therapies such as mindfulness, ACT and DBT. Then we looked at different approaches of psychodynamic therapy and counselling. There is now extensive evidence that psychotherapy is more effective than no treatment for common affective disorders such as anxiety and depression. Non-specific factors, such as the relationship between the therapist and client, are likely to be important in the efficacy of psychotherapy. In the future, psychotherapies may therefore move away from focusing on one particular approach to using techniques that are shown to be effective for different symptoms under different circumstances.

Psychological interventions in medical settings draw on psychotherapy and health behaviour change techniques to promote physical and mental health. These interventions aim to (1) reduce negative health behaviours, such as health promotion and motivational interviewing; (2) help people to cope with stressful circumstances, such as stress management, debriefing, crisis intervention, and bereavement interventions; or (3) target specific illnesses or symptoms, such as pain, self-management of chronic illnesses, or neurological rehabilitation. The evidence for the effectiveness of such interventions is mixed – probably due to the wide range of interventions and target populations. For example, there is good evidence that motivational interviewing and self-management programmes are effective, but little evidence that bereavement interventions are effective unless targeted at high-risk individuals.

Technology is increasingly used to provide computerised or app-based psychotherapy. These are usually based on CBT and third wave cognitive therapy techniques, which lend themselves to self-directed psychotherapy. There is substantial evidence that computerised psychotherapy is effective for less severe affective symptoms, such as mild or moderate depression and anxiety. Games and virtual reality are also used to improve psychological and physical health in specific groups, such as people with phobias or neurological disorders.

Further Reading

Llewellyn, C.D. et al. (eds) (2019) *The Cambridge Handbook of Psychology, Health and Medicine* (3rd edition). Cambridge: Cambridge University Press. Includes short chapters on behaviour therapy, cognitive behavioural therapy, behavioural couples therapy, biofeedback, counselling, group therapy, technology-assisted interventions, hypnosis, mindfulness, motivational interviewing, pain management, peer support interventions, psychodynamic therapy, self-help interventions, stress and crisis management, and worksite interventions.

Bramber, M.R. (2006) *CBT for Occupational Stress in Health Professionals*. Hove: Routledge. Outlines the use of CBT to help cope with problems such as performance anxiety, health anxiety, perfectionism, and burnout.

Rollnick, S., Miller, W.R. & Butler, C.C. (2008) *Motivational Interviewing in Health Care: Helping Patients Change Behavior*. New York: Guilford Press. Outlines the basic principles and core skills required for motivational interviewing.

White, C.A. (2001) *Cognitive Behaviour Therapy for Chronic Medical Problems*. Chichester: Wiley. Provides an introduction to using CBT with a wide range of medical problems, including surgical, cardiac, dermatological, cancer, pain, and diabetes.

Revision Questions

1 Describe third wave cognitive therapies, illustrating your answer with an example of one such therapy.
2 Describe the core features of cognitive behavioural therapy (CBT).
3 Outline the cognitive theory of depression and discuss the role of the depressogenic triad of negative beliefs.
4 Briefly compare and contrast behavioural and cognitive techniques for treating psychological problems.
5 What is a formulation and what is its role in psychotherapy?
6 Briefly outline the three core principles of psychodynamic therapy.
7 Describe the five core features of counselling.
8 Outline three psychological interventions used in medical settings and discuss whether they are effective.
9 What is unconditional positive regard and from which theory or theories does it originate?
10 Outline three psychological specialisms and discuss their potential application to healthcare.

SECTION IV
BODY SYSTEMS

15

IMMUNITY AND PROTECTION

──Learning Objectives──

This chapter is designed to enable you to:

- Understand the effect of stress and emotion on the immune system.
- Describe the role of psychological factors in immune disorders.
- Describe aspects of psycho-dermatology.
- Outline the psychosocial risk factors for cancer.
- Explain how psychological factors can affect the progression of cancer.

Do you get sick around exam time? Your greater susceptibility to infections at such times may be related to inadequate sleep, a lack of exercise, and a poor diet. It can also be affected by prolonged stress. Links between emotions and health have long formed a part of medical thinking. Pre-modern medical thought was based on the beliefs that optimal health depended on a balance of the four humours (blood, yellow bile, black bile, phlegm) and that imbalances influenced disease and behaviour. For example, the depressive melancholic personality is named after the Latin words for black bile.

Our understanding of disease is now very different, but modern medicine continues to find evidence of links between psychological and physical wellbeing. In a classic early study, Ishigami (1919) found decreased phagocyte function among people with tuberculosis when they were emotionally agitated. Since then, understanding of the links between psychological states and immune function has increased. Over the same period, there has been increasing evidence of pathogenic involvement in diseases previously not thought to involve the immune system (e.g. *Helicobacter pylori* infection is often implicated in peptic ulcers and myocardial infarctions) (see Chapters 16 and 17).

Psychoneuroimmunology (PNI) examines how psychological states affect our immune function. Although most PNI research has focused on negative psychological states such as stress and depression, recent research has examined the beneficial effects of positive moods. In this chapter, we first look at the effect of psychological factors on the immune system and immune disorders. The next section looks at our main protective organ – the skin. Finally, the large body of knowledge on psychosocial factors and cancer is examined as an illustration of how immune impairment can lead to disease.

15.1 Infection, Inflammation, and Immunity

The presence of protein molecules called antigens on the surface of each cell allows the immune system to distinguish body cells from potentially harmful foreign cells. There are two broad types of barriers to infection – non-specific and specific. The non-specific barriers include mucous membranes, which destroy many foreign micro-organisms, and phagocytes, which consume and destroy foreign micro-organisms and debris. The specific immune barriers involve the action of specialised white blood cells called lymphocytes. There are two components to this type of immune response. The **cell-mediated immune response** involves T lymphocytes. The **antibody-mediated immune response** (also called the humoural response) involves B lymphocytes. In each case, a response to an immune challenge is usually reflected in an increase in proliferation of T lymphocytes and B lymphocytes.

15.1.1 Stress and Immune Function

Stress has measurable effects on our immune function, susceptibility to infections, severity of infections, response to vaccinations, and wound healing (Haykin & Rolls, 2021; Sørensen et al., 2023). Whether these effects are beneficial or detrimental is determined by the duration of stress. The immune response to stress is affected by activation of the sympathetic nervous system and hypothalamic-pituitary-adrenal axis (HPA axis) (see Chapter 3). The sympathetic nervous system increases some immune system activity, particularly large granular lymphocyte activity such as natural killer cells. However, the HPA axis suppresses some immune activity through the production of cortisol, which has an anti-inflammatory effect and reduces both the number of white blood cells and the release of cytokines.

Acute (i.e. short-term) threats, challenges, or stress produce protective inflammatory immune responses – particularly non-specific barriers – which revert to normal levels fairly quickly after the stressor ends (Rohleder, 2019). Thus, stressful events such as physical activity may temporarily enhance our immune function: they invoke the fight-or-flight response and the body prepares adaptively to deal with potential infection and/or injury arising from that challenge. Problems arise because, although this is an adaptive response to physical challenges, it is not an appropriate response to the very different sorts of threats that we experience today. The stress we experience today tends not to arise from acute physical challenges, but from longer-term psychosocial experiences: we have a stone-age response to modern stress. Chronic stress tends to impair immune function. Chronic stress can arise from various causes: study, work, unemployment, financial concerns, difficult relationships, and caring for others. More severe and longer-lasting stress is associated with a continuation of the acute inflammatory immune response, which contributes to the metabolic syndrome and more global immunosuppression. Immune down-regulation due to chronic stress can lead to impaired wound healing, poorer responses to infectious diseases, autoimmune diseases including skin disorders, and the progression of cancer (K. L. Chan et al., 2023; Eckerling et al., 2021; França & Jafferany, 2017; Rohleder, 2019).

A different pattern can be seen in people who have been exposed to traumatic events, such as natural disasters, war, or terrorism, particularly people who also develop symptoms of post-traumatic stress disorder (PTSD). In these instances, exposure to a severely traumatic event is associated with increased immune measures, such as antibodies, lymphocytes, interleukins, and natural killer cell activity, which may persist many years after the traumatic event. This is an intriguing contrast to the effect of chronic stress and other negative affect (e.g. depression). It may be explained by the observation that PTSD leads to a dysregulation of the HPA axis and reduced cortisol responses (Yang & Jiang, 2020). Paradoxically, people with PTSD have elevated rates of physical illnesses (Peruzzolo et al., 2022).

Substantial evidence of the effect of stress on the immune system has led to interest in whether interventions that alleviate stress can counter the disruption of immune function caused by chronic stress. There is some evidence that emotional disclosure (e.g. writing about negative emotions and experiences), hypnosis, and conditioning can reduce stress and may produce positive changes in immune function (Deleemans et al., 2023; Guo, 2023; Tekampe et al., 2017). Furthermore, there is evidence that physical activity can reduce the harmful effects of stress, and reduce the effects of stress on cortisol (Gerstberger et al., 2023; Pauly et al., 2019). There is also substantial evidence to show that psychological interventions such as stress management, mindfulness, meditation, and relaxation are effective, and can reduce the harmful immune effects of chronic stress (Antoni & Dhabhar, 2019; B. Chen et al., 2023; Koncz et al., 2021; Pascoe et al., 2017; Tang et al., 2020; van Loon et al., 2022). An example of the impact of a stress management intervention is provided in Research Box 15.1.

Research Box 15.1

Online Stress Management for People with Cancer

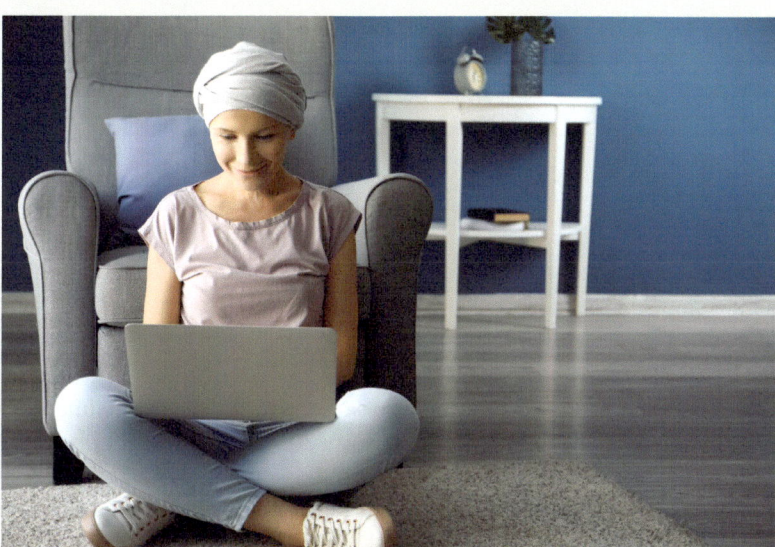

Figure 15.1   Using an online stress management programme

Source: © Pixel-Shot/Adobe Stock

(Continued)

Background

A diagnosis of cancer can be a cause of major psychological distress, but most newly-diagnosed people lack psychological support during this critical period. Psychotherapeutic interventions can be effective in this domain, but they may not be available or affordable for all patients. Web-based stress management programmes may be a way to make stress management interventions more accessible.

Method and Findings

In this randomised controlled trial, 129 people who had started first-line treatment for newly-diagnosed cancer within the past three months were randomly assigned to the therapist-guided web-based intervention or to a waiting-list control group (meaning that they were offered the treatment at the end of the study). The intervention ran for eight weeks, and a psychologist provided personal guidance for each person every week.

The analyses took into account initial distress levels, and the key measures of the intervention impact were quality of life, distress, and anxiety or depression. At the end of the intervention, quality of life was significantly higher, and distress was significantly lower in the intervention group.

Significance

The study indicates that online stress management programmes that include individual guidance or supervision from psychologists are feasible and are effective for reducing the psychological distress that often accompanies a cancer diagnosis. Such programmes may be more cost-effective than individual face-to-face therapy.

Urech, C. et al. (2018) Web-based stress management for newly diagnosed patients with cancer (STREAM): A randomized, wait-list controlled intervention study. *Journal of Clinical Oncology*, *36*: 780–788.

15.1.2 Emotions and Immune Function

There is evidence that positive and negative emotions have different effects on immune function and health outcomes.

Negative Emotions

Negative emotions, such as depression, are associated with impaired immune function: clear evidence of this relationship has been available for over 30 years (Herbert & Cohen, 1993; Kiecolt-Glaser & Glaser, 2002). The effect of negative emotions on the immune system may be the common pathway between negative emotions, a range of illnesses (including cardiovascular disease, rheumatoid arthritis, Type 1 diabetes, and some cancers) and premature mortality (Barry et al., 2020; Polityńska et al., 2022). There is substantial evidence that negative emotions are associated with dysregulation of the immune system, an increased susceptibility to infections, and slower wound healing. To emphasise the importance of the links between negative emotions and physiology noted in the previous section, there is also evidence that chronic inflammation may be a key causal factor in the development of depression (Cruz-Pereira et al., 2020).

Depression is associated with several changes in the immune function (see Highlight Box 15.1) as well as changes in clinical outcomes. For example, depressive symptoms have been linked with the more rapid progression of disease and poorer responses to treatment among people with immune disorders (Bortolato et al., 2017; Leserman, 2008; Matcham et al., 2018) and heart disease (Chapter 16). There may be direct physiological effects of depression on immune function, and there may also be indirect effects: depression may be linked to impaired immune function because of less healthy behaviours among depressed people, including poorer adherence to treatment (Gonzalez et al., 2011; Yussof et al., 2022).

─Activity 15.1─

Symptoms and Emotions

- The last time you were ill, what was the relationship between your physical symptoms and your emotions?
- Do you think one caused the other, that they influenced each other, or that they were separate?

─Highlight Box 15.1─

Changes in Immune Function Associated with Depression

- Lower total numbers of lymphocytes.
- Reduced proliferation of lymphocytes in response to mitogens that usually promote lymphocyte production.
- Reductions in the numbers and functioning of natural killer cells.
- Increased CD4/CD8 ratios.
- Increases in pro-inflammatory cytokines.
- Increases in interleukin-6 (an important mediator of fever and inflammation).

Given the association between depression and immune function, it is not surprising that psychotherapy and other treatments for depression are not only effective for alleviating depression, but they may also affect the course of immune disorders (Mundle et al., 2021; Passchier et al., 2018; Wan et al., 2022).

Positive Emotions

The good news on the link between psychological states and immune function is that positive moods and personalities appear to be associated with enhanced immune function and slower disease progression (Panagi et al., 2019; Pressman et al., 2019). For example, early research in this domain revealed that optimism, emotional expressiveness, and extraversion are associated with greater numbers of helper T lymphocytes and greater natural killer cell cytotoxicity (Segerstrom et al., 1998). Such results suggest that mood may be an important moderator of the impact of stress and negative affect on immune function. More recent research has shown that experience of more positive moods is associated with better viral control in HIV/AIDS (Wilson et al., 2017), and that people who report more positive moods on the day that they receive a vaccination have stronger enduring immune responses to vaccination (Ayling et al., 2018).

Whereas some studies have examined optimism as a dispositional characteristic of individuals that is fairly stable, other studies have examined the effect of positive psychological experiences, such as watching humorous videos, and have found significant improvements in immune function. A meta-analysis of good-quality studies indicated that brief interventions to boost positive mood (e.g. comedy video- or audio-recordings, massage, listening to music, group drumming, relaxation exercises, and recall of positive memories) can lead to enhancements in some immune parameters (Ayling et al., 2020). More research is required to determine the causal mechanisms through which positive moods affect immunity.

The promising data that are available have informed the inclusion of positive mood interventions such as laughter medicine and laughter yoga, which may have positive effects that arise from addressing mood and also modifying breathing. Intervention studies indicate that laughter yoga reduces cortisol response to stress, and that these physiological benefits may be observed even if people do not report feeling less stressed (Meier et al., 2021; Ozturk & Tezel, 2021). There is also some evidence that laughter medicine can be successfully administered remotely using digital technology, thereby increasing access (Ozturk & Tekkas-Kerman, 2022).

15.1.3 Immunisations

Immunisations are an important part of tackling disease and promoting health. Immunisations prime the immune system to respond to a disease by giving a small, usually disabled, form of the virus or bacterium. The ability of vaccines to protect against the disease depends on the strength of the immune response to the vaccine. Given the relationship between negative psychological states and immune functioning, it is perhaps not surprising that people who are stressed, upset, or anxious have weaker, delayed, or less enduring responses to vaccines (Ballesio et al., 2023).

In recent decades there has been some controversy over vaccines for young children, which has led to reduced uptake. For example, the uptake of measles/mumps/rubella (MMR) immunisation has fallen to below the levels required for 'herd immunity' (May, 1982; McClure et al., 2017). Whether parents decide to immunise their children is determined by beliefs about the perceived risks associated with the disease and with vaccination, and such beliefs can be shaped by misinformation (Cooper et al., 2021; Díaz Crescitelli et al., 2020). Parents are less likely to immunise children if they think there are dangers associated with the vaccine, have doubts the vaccine will be effective, believe they can protect their children from exposure, or think their children are unlikely to catch the disease.

Many health professionals are concerned that social media platforms have provided spaces in which anti-vaccination beliefs are encouraged, and which act as 'echo chambers' in which such attitudes are reinforced (Kalichman & Eaton, 2023). As noted in Chapter 9 (section 9.3), the phenomenon of polarisation means that agreement about a topic within a group tends to intensify over time so that each individual's attitude becomes stronger. Analyses of social media posts indicate that the existence of online 'echo chambers' that reject alternative views lead to more polarised pro- and anti-vaccination stances and help to explain why campaigns that provide accurate information may have limited impact (Mønsted & Lehmann, 2022).

Many of the influences on childhood vaccination just described were also found to affect uptake of COVID-19 vaccination among adults (Lun et al., 2022; Roy et al., 2022). Reviews of the research indicated that willingness to be vaccinated was lower among people who had less knowledge or less positive beliefs about the vaccine's efficacy, safety, and side effects. However, providing information about the vaccine was not sufficient to increase uptake, because broader beliefs about all vaccines were also important. There was also a strong influence related to less trust in medicine, less trust in politicians, greater endorsement of conspiracy beliefs, and greater reliance on social influences, including social media.

Vaccinations and other medical procedures involving needles can cause substantial anxiety and distress in children, adolescents, and many adults (Alsbrooks & Hoerauf, 2022; Orenius et al., 2018). Needle-related distress and anxiety have adverse short- and long-term psychological effects, including anticipatory nausea, disrupted sleep and eating patterns, and avoidance behaviour, including avoidance of treatment. Furthermore, needle-related fear and pain are important barriers to the uptake of vaccinations (Taddio et al., 2022). Effective management of needle distress in children is therefore critical. Pharmacological management involves analgesics during or after the injection, which can be topical (applied to the skin) or oral. However, it must also be noted that parents and health professionals can have a strong influence on children's distress during needle procedures (DiLorenzo-Klas et al., 2023; Mahoney et al., 2010). A review of intervention studies revealed that although there is a need for further high-quality research, there is evidence that psychological strategies including distraction, hypnosis, and breathing exercises can help to reduce children's pain, distress, and fear of needles (Birnie et al., 2018). An example of a psychological intervention for distress related to vaccinations is included in Research Box 15.2. Learning (and unlearning) fear of needles is also covered in Chapter 10.

Research Box 15.2

Managing COVID-19 Vaccination-Related Pain and Fear

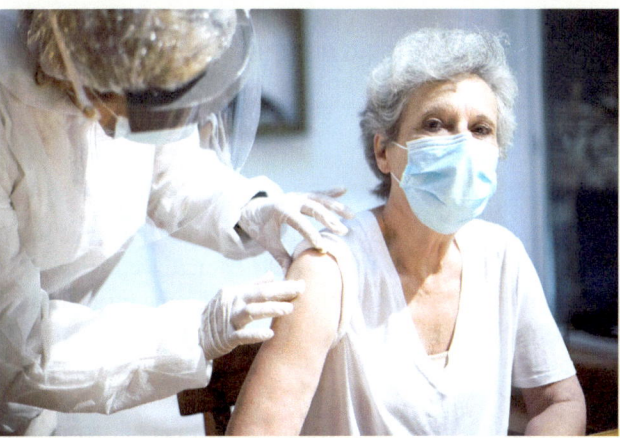

Figure 15.2   Stress reduction during a COVID-19 vaccination

Source: © Kampus Production/Pexels

(Continued)

Background

Vaccinations and other procedures involving needles can cause distress, fear, and pain. The aims of this study were to examine whether a stress-reduction process would lead to more positive experiences of COVID-19 vaccinations and to see whether the process was acceptable to staff.

Method and Findings

Participants were 2,488 people aged 12+ years receiving COVID-19 vaccines: 1,118 before the intervention and 1,370 post-implementation. The name of the intervention was CARD, which reflected the four key components: Comfort – check whether people want to stand, sit, or lie down; Ask – check whether people have any questions about the vaccine or the process; Relax – make the situation as relaxing as possible (e.g. keep needles out of sight); Distract – draw attention away from the injection using music, conversation, etc. Vaccine recipients reported their level of pain, fear, and dizziness during vaccination. Clinic staff reported their opinions on the CARD interventions. CARD improved client symptoms across genders and ages with an average reduction in needle pain, fear, and dizziness of 75%, 40%, and 44%, respectively. Clinic staff reported positive attitudes about CARD and uptake of selected CARD interventions.

Significance

The CARD system reduced stress-related responses of pain, fear, and dizziness in a general population undergoing COVID-19 vaccinations in a mass vaccination clinic. It was also feasible and acceptable to staff to implement the programme. CARD and similar approaches may be one way to reduce vaccine hesitancy and increase vaccine uptake.

Tetui, M., Grindrod, K., Waite, N., VanderDoes, J. & Taddio, A. (2022) Integrating the CARD (Comfort Ask Relax Distract) system in a mass vaccination clinic to improve the experience of individuals during COVID-19 vaccination: A pre-post implementation study. *Human Vaccines & Immunotherapeutics, 18*(5): 2089500. doi:10.1080/21645515.2022.2089500

15.1.4 Preventative and Protective Behaviours

In addition to immunisations, there are numerous behaviours that affect immunity and the risk of infection. Some of these are activities that we take because we live in societies, meaning that our individual behaviour may affect those with whom we come into contact. Most of us experienced 'lockdown' or 'shelter in place' rules and guidance for self-isolation, social distancing, and other protective behaviours during the COVID-19 pandemic. Some people considered these measures to be restrictive, limiting, and frustrating, but they appear to have been effective for reducing transmission rates and subsequent deaths (Nussbaumer-Streit et al., 2020). There was established evidence pre-COVID that encouraging hygiene behaviours, such as handwashing, and facilitating them by providing hand sanitiser can lead to behaviour change that leads to lower transmission rates (Gaube et al., 2020; Jefferson et al., 2011). Research based on psychological models, such as the COM-B (see Chapter 5), indicated that people were more likely to engage in protective behaviours if they felt confident about carrying them out, had opportunities to do so that were facilitated by the social context (e.g. providing hand sanitiser and being reminded to use it), and were motivated to protect themselves and others (L.G. Brown et al., 2022).

Section 15.1.1 began by explaining how stress and emotions can affect immunity, and how psychological interventions can boost immunity and reduce the harmful effects of difficult psychological experiences. In addition, many elements of people's lifestyles can enhance their immune function. For example, immune function appears to be worse in people who sleep fewer hours per night and who have more disturbed sleep (Besedovsky et al., 2019; Garbarino et al., 2021), but it may be enhanced by regular physical activity (Kurowski et al., 2022; Simpson et al., 2021). In relation to diet and dietary supplements, there is little evidence that mega-doses of vitamin C reduce the risk of developing a cold (Hemilä & Chalker, 2013). Preventative mega-doses of vitamin C may reduce the duration of colds that do develop, but they are not effective after the onset of a cold.

15.2 Psychological Aspects of Immune Disorders

So far we have focused on how psychological states can affect immune function. Of course, the reverse is also true: changes in immune function can lead to changes in psychological wellbeing. Many of us find that when we have a cold or other illness our mood can also be affected. This may be due to the direct effects of the illness and/or the indirect effects if the illness prevents us from doing things that are important or meaningful to us. In the case of more serious and/or chronic infections, the psychological consequences can be more severe. Anxiety and depression are more common among people with chronic illnesses than in the broader population (Renaud-Charest et al., 2021; Siegmann et al., 2018; Vargas-Roman et al., 2020). As noted in section 15.1, there is also evidence that chronic inflammation may be a key causal factor in the development of depression (Cruz-Pereira et al., 2020). In general, fatigue is more common among people with chronic autoimmune disorders, and self-reported quality of life also tends to be lower (Kharawala et al., 2022; Möller et al., 2021; Tanaka et al., 2024). Such experiences of depression, stress, and anxiety resulting from disease may in turn impair immune function.

Autoimmune diseases occur when the body's immune system mistakenly identifies self-cells as foreign cells and mounts an immune response against initially healthy tissues. Some examples of autoimmune diseases and their psychological impact are given below. Others include coeliac disease and lupus erythematosus. The mechanisms involved in many immune diseases are not fully understood. Thus, people may have no hope of a cure, and must adjust physically and psychologically to the long-term management of symptoms (see Chapter 6).

Rheumatoid arthritis is a chronic systemic inflammatory autoimmune disorder which can affect many tissues and organs, but principally attacks the synovial lining of joints. There is no known cure for rheumatoid arthritis, but different treatments may be used to alleviate symptoms, including pain, and/or to try to prevent future joint destruction. People with rheumatoid arthritis are more likely than healthy controls to report anxiety and depression (Tanaka et al., 2024). Longitudinal research indicates that greater anxiety and depression are associated with increased perceptions of pain, and that higher levels of pain and/or disability in turn predict higher levels of distress. These findings suggest a reciprocal relationship between psychological wellbeing and experiences of pain or disability (Machin et al., 2020).

There is a paradox in the role of stress in inflammatory diseases like rheumatoid arthritis. Physical responses to stress involving the HPA axis and autonomic nervous system can play a vital role in inflammation. As we have seen, the release of cortisol via the HPA axis should reduce inflammation. Thus, in theory, stress should improve the symptoms of rheumatoid arthritis. However, stress actually results in worse immunological markers, physical symptoms, and disability (de Brouwer et al., 2010). This seems to be due to a physical hypo-responsiveness to stress: people with rheumatoid arthritis have consistently reduced autonomic nervous system responses to stressful events. HPA responses to stress also appear blunted and out of proportion to corresponding immune activity. There is a need for further longitudinal prospective research (i.e. research that follows people over time) with larger samples to determine the effects of different kinds of stressors on the autonomic nervous system, HPA axis, and immune function (de Brouwer et al., 2010).

Type 1 diabetes mellitus (also called insulin-dependent diabetes mellitus) is an autoimmune disease in which the insulin-producing cells of the pancreas are destroyed by an inappropriate immune response. As a result, the body is unable to regulate blood sugar levels. There is no known cure for Type 1 diabetes, and people must use insulin replacement therapy to avoid potentially fatal diabetic ketoacidosis. The prevalence of depression is higher in people with Type 1 diabetes than in the general population (van Duinkerken et al., 2020). Among people with diabetes, hyperglycaemia resulting from poor glycaemic control has been linked to depression (Lustman et al., 2000), but the mechanisms and casual links are not fully understood (Habib et al., 2022).

Syntheses of research shows that there are bi-directional associations between depression and a range of diabetes-related complications, including retinopathy, neuropathy, renal disease, coronary artery disease, and sexual dysfunction (Nouwen et al., 2019). Depressive symptoms are associated with lower levels of treatment adherence, and treatment adherence has an important influence on disease progression, so it is important to address the psychological wellbeing of people with diabetes (Gonzalez, 2008; Kongkaew et al., 2014). A review of randomised controlled trials revealed that pharmacological treatment and various forms of psychotherapy can be effective for alleviating depression in adults with diabetes, and that this can have a significant positive effect on glycaemic control (van der Feltz-Cornelis et al., 2021).

Case Study 15.1

Living with HIV

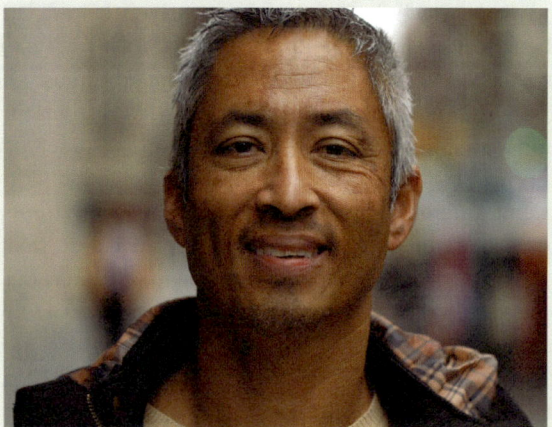

Jose was diagnosed with HIV seven years ago. HIV has had a marked influence on Jose's plans for the future. He had initially worried about an early death, but he is now more concerned about the prospect of living with a chronic condition and managing the emotional aspects of the antiretroviral therapy.

Before I found out I was HIV positive, I was determined to live forever – and that was how I lived my life. I had great expectations of making a fortune with the company I was running.

Figure 15.3   Jose on living with HIV

Source: © blvdone/Adobe Stock

At first, I thought the diagnosis meant I was dying. I hadn't really thought about it before, and I didn't know much about what treatment was available. But then I learnt about how good some treatment is now. So now I do feel that I have a future, but it is not the kind of future I had planned, and I have had to adjust to that … and it hasn't been easy because it has affected my sense of who I am, and my relationships.

I've struggled at times with depression, and it wasn't always easy to get the help I needed. It was never *really* bad – I could still get out of bed and get work done – so I was referred to online counselling, but it didn't really suit me. I just found it a bit impersonal. I discussed this with my doctor and they suggested face-to-face counselling, which has been really helpful. What I really needed was to have someone listen to my story, just listen to know that they were interested in my life, and then start to think about practical issues. So it was good to get that, and it has really helped me get a better perspective.

Unlike the autoimmune diseases discussed above, **HIV/AIDS** is an acquired immune deficiency. There is clear evidence that the course and development of HIV/AIDS is affected by psychosocial factors such as stress, depression, and social support (Schuster et al., 2012). Depression is more common among people with HIV/AIDS than among the general population, probably because of the impacts of the virus on people's health and social lives (Hoare et al., 2021). HIV can have profound and long-lasting impacts on health, work, finances, and sexual relationships (Groß et al., 2016). These affect how people experience their current health and wellbeing, and how they plan for the future (see Case Study 15.1). The net effect is that people with HIV/AIDS tend to have a lower quality of life. However, it is important to note that physical activity interventions and psychosocial interventions may help to reduce stigma, alleviate depression, manage stress, improve quality of life, and may result in better outcomes for people with HIV/AIDS (Dianatinasab et al., 2020; T. Jiang et al., 2021; Scott-Sheldon et al., 2019; L. Zhang et al., 2023).

Summary 15.1

- Acute stress leads to enhanced immune responses, but chronic stress impairs immune functioning.
- Negative emotions, such as depression, are associated with reduced immune functioning.
- Conversely, positive emotions appear to have a positive effect on immune function.
- Immune disorders are associated with reduced quality of life, increased anxiety, and increased depression.
- There is a reciprocal relationship between negative mood, pain, and disability.
- Some psychological interventions, such as disclosure and conditioning interventions, may result in improved immune function in disorders such as HIV/AIDS.

15.3 Skin

The skin is a key protective organ that is made up of many layers of epithelial tissues. It protects the body against pathogens, insulates the body, prevents dehydration, and protects the internal organs, muscles, etc. against damage from external sources. The impact of psychological factors on skin has mainly been examined in relation to wound healing and skin disorders.

15.3.1 Wound Healing

Wound healing research typically creates small puncture wounds or suction blisters on volunteers, and then monitors immune activity and healing over time. It has consistently shown that stressed people heal 20–40% slower than people who are not stressed, apparently because of an interaction between glucocorticoids (e.g. cortisol) and proinflammatory cytokines (Walburn et al., 2009). Evidence of these links has been clear for some time. For example, Marucha, Kiecolt-Glaser, and Favagehi (1998) made small punch biopsy wounds in students' oral hard palates: once during the summer vacation and once just before exams. In the exam period, students took 40% longer for their wounds to heal and had 68% less interleukin 1ß messenger RNA than during the vacation, because they were more stressed at exam time.

Wound healing is slower when we experience difficult circumstances, such as caring for chronically ill people or having relationship difficulties. However, wound healing is not only affected by stress. Wounds also heal more slowly in people who are depressed, anxious, or have poor anger control, and also those who have less healthy lifestyles (Avishai et al., 2017; Gouin et al., 2008; Wynn & Holloway, 2019). Positive factors that speed up wound healing – including surgical site wound healing – include emotional disclosure, close personal relationships, and exercise (Emery et al., 2005; N. Wang et al., 2024).

The prospective experimental design of wound healing studies makes it possible to establish a causal link between stress and healing. This is relevant to many areas of medicine, but particularly surgery. There is substantial evidence that negative emotions, such as fear and anxiety, are associated with worse outcomes after surgery, including more post-operative distress, more pain, greater use of analgesia, a longer hospital stay, and a slower return to normal functioning. Similarly, research shows that preparing people for surgery by providing more information, coping skills, or relaxation techniques can result in lower post-operative pain, shorter hospital stays, and better psychological outcomes (Powell et al., 2016). This is an area of medicine where psychological preparation has the potential to make a real difference to clinical outcomes, but there is a need for more robust evidence about what works, and how.

Clinical Notes 15.1

Immunity, Vaccinations, and Surgery

- Negative emotions are associated with poorer immune function. This is especially important for people who have serious health conditions.
- It is therefore important to address negative emotions via appropriate psychosocial interventions.
- You can have a strong influence on people's distress during invasive procedures, so use distraction, humour, and give them strategies to help them cope.

- Wound healing is slower when people are stressed.
- Surgical outcomes are better if people feel prepared for surgery and are relaxed. Anxiety and distress lead to worse outcomes.
- Give people undergoing surgery as much information as they want, help them to develop coping sills, and encourage them to use relaxation techniques.

15.3.2 Skin Disorders

The field of psychodermatology acknowledges that many dermatological disorders have a psychosomatic or behavioural aspect, and that the skin and the mind are linked through psychoneuroimmunoendocrine mechanisms and behaviours that can strongly affect the onset or progression of skin disorders (Shenefelt, 2011). Psychological factors can affect the course of dermatological disorders in several ways. First, stress is associated with increased symptoms in disorders such as psoriasis, atopic dermatitis, alopecia areata, and urticaria (França & Jafferany, 2017). This is likely to be due to physiological mechanisms such as those detailed above and changes in behaviour that are also associated with stress, such as scratching and increased tobacco or alcohol use. Scratching can exacerbate symptoms and cause further skin damage and is usually a conditioned response (see Chapter 10).

Second, people with various skin disorders have higher than average levels of anxiety, depression, suicidal ideation, and dysfunctional coping strategies, such as avoidance (Chang et al., 2022; Dalgard et al., 2015). The likelihood of depression or anxiety is especially high for people with psoriasis, atopic dermatitis, hand eczema, and leg ulcers. However, there is little prospective research into the causal relationship between negative emotions and symptoms of skin disorders. It is therefore difficult to know whether negative emotions make physical symptoms worse or whether worse physical symptoms cause people to become more anxious or depressed. Regardless of the direction of causation, we need to recognise how common and difficult psychological comorbidity is in dermatology. The objective severity of skin disorders is not associated with the level of subjective distress a person feels. Instead, distress and quality of life are more closely related to physical appearance, disfigurement, fear of negative evaluation, and social stigma, because they are visible conditions (Baker & Billick, 2022; Harcourt, 2017).

—Activity 15.2—

Treating a Conditioned Response

- If scratching is partly a conditioned response, how might you go about reducing scratching behaviour in someone with eczema? (it may help to refer to Section 10.3)

Educational interventions are an effective component of the clinical management of skin disorders, but psychological interventions appear to be more effective (Hua et al., 2023; Qureshi et al., 2019). Interventions draw on a variety of techniques, such as education, relaxation training, biofeedback, cognitive restructuring, and social skills training to manage stigma (see Chapters 6 and 14). An important part of these interventions appears to be improving self-control of scratching through habit-reversal training. This involves helping people to:

- Recognise scratching cues or triggers.
- Interrupt and prevent the automatic scratching response.
- Use a competing response, such as relaxation, to reduce the itching sensation.

The ability to use relaxation techniques, such as progressive muscle relaxation and calming imagery, helps people to manage stress, improves self-control, and may provide a good substitute for scratching. Evidence for the effectiveness of psychological therapies has driven interest in the development and use of simple screening tools for skin-related distress, and the provision of accessible treatment using digital technologies (Blom et al., 2023; Dahy et al., 2020).

Summary 15.2

- Stress and negative emotions are associated with slower wound healing.
- Distress and anxiety are associated with poorer psychological and physical recovery from surgery.
- Stress is also associated with increased symptoms of skin disorders.
- A substantial minority of dermatological outpatients report psychiatric symptoms, which are less influenced by the severity of the skin disorder than by physical appearance, disfigurement, the fear of a negative evaluation, and social stigma.
- Psychological interventions add significantly to the effectiveness of the clinical management of skin disorders, resulting in fewer psychiatric and physical symptoms.

15.4 Cancer

There are over 100 different types of cancer. It has been estimated that around a quarter of all people in the world will develop cancer at some point in their lives, with a higher incidence (38%) in high-income countries (Zheng et al., 2023). The development of cancerous tumours is a complex process that involves a cascade of events that is a bit like cellular anarchy. At least three different types of gene damage or mutation are necessary for cancer to develop. Cancer cells have to avoid the normal process of programmed cell death (apoptosis) that usually protects against the proliferation of abnormal cells. Normal cells have a fixed capacity of division and growth, but cancer cells manage to divide indefinitely. As the tumour grows, it requires nourishment and the removal of waste products, so it has to encourage blood vessel growth around it. The tumour also has to be able to invade other areas of the body. This requires the inactivation of a whole series of factors that will usually restrict cells to a specific site. In the later stages of the disease, cancer cells may break off (metastasise) and migrate to other areas of the body.

Psycho-oncology examines (1) psychosocial risk factors that influence the development of cancer, (2) psychological responses to cancer, and (3) interventions for people with cancer. These are discussed in turn.

15.4.1 Psychosocial Risk Factors for Cancer

Cancers are often caused by the interplay between internal factors, such as genetic vulnerability and hormones, and external factors, such as toxins, viruses, and lifestyle. Psychosocial factors that influence cancer onset include demographic factors, lifestyle and health behaviour, social support, and coping and adjustment (see section 15.2).

Demographic factors that influence cancer include ethnicity, country of residence, and socioeconomic status (SES). Ethnic differences include the observation that malignant melanoma (skin cancer) is more common in white people, and that Japanese people are up to ten times more likely to get stomach cancer than white Americans or Europeans. Figure 15.4 shows the most common cancers for men and women in different countries. There is also demographic variation within countries. In many countries, lung cancer is more common among people of lower SES (reflecting higher rates of smoking in this group) and breast cancer is more common among people of higher SES (Arık et al., 2021; Bryere et al., 2018; Fantin et al., 2020). However, the links between SES and other types of cancers often varies between countries, and may reflect an interaction of both genetic and behavioural factors.

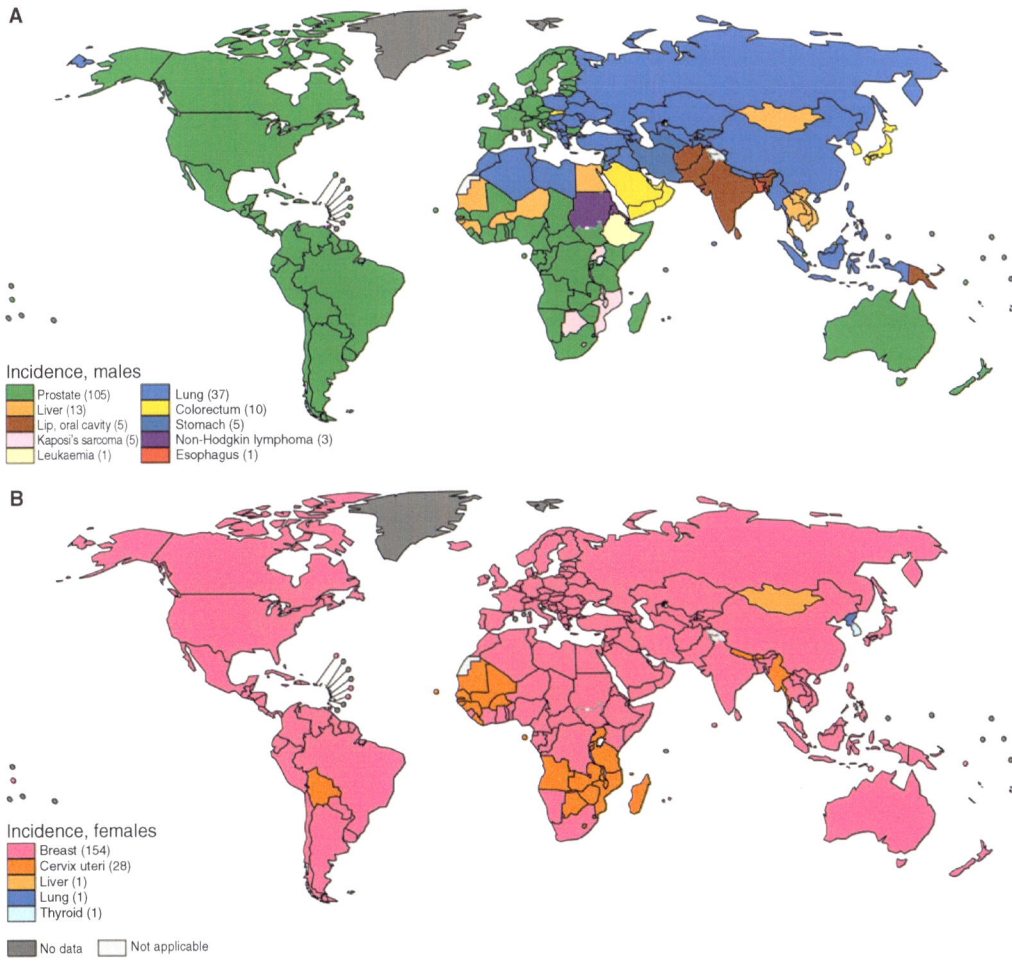

Figure 15.4   Most common cancers across the world

Source: GLOBOCAN 2018 © World Health Organization

The observed differences in cancer rates for people of different ethnicity, SES, and country of residence are often due to differences in lifestyle. For example, higher rates of stomach cancer are observed among Asian people who live in Asia than among Asian Americans and white Americans (Mok et al., 2024). This suggests that behavioural patterns in the country of residence, including the intake of salt and pickled foods, can affect a person's health risks. Similarly, higher rates of melanoma in people from higher SES groups may reflect the fact that they are more able to afford vacations in sunny locations, but do not always properly protect their skin.

Lifestyle factors include *health behaviours* such as smoking, diet, exercise, and alcohol use. They also include *exposure to toxins or infections* such as asbestos (lung cancer), *H. Pylori* (stomach cancer), and human papilloma virus (cervical cancer). Tobacco use, diet, and infections alone are thought to be responsible for half of all cancers in developed countries. Changing people's behaviour so that they live healthier lifestyles could prevent up to 50% of cancer deaths, particularly smoking-related and gastrointestinal cancers (World Health Organization, 2020a). Risk factors vary for different cancers and many cancers have multiple risk factors. For example, risk factors for breast cancer include genetic vulnerability, greater age, the early onset of periods, being childless or not having children until over 30, using hormone replacement therapy, and greater alcohol consumption.

Stress contributes to the progression of some cancers through its effect on the immune system (Eckerling et al., 2021). Increased tumour growth and metastases are observed in non-human animals that have been implanted with tumour cells and then put in stressful situations. Research in humans indicates that chronic stress may increase the likelihood of cancer incidence, but there is stronger evidence that chronic stress can result in faster cancer progression.

Social support is important for psychological health and adapting to chronic illness (see Chapter 6). Thus, it is not surprising that support can influence the onset and progression of cancer. Reviews of published research reveal that people with less social support and more social isolation tend to be diagnosed with cancer at a later stage of progression, experience more rapid cancer progression, and have higher rates of cancer mortality (Coughlin, 2020). One meta-analysis revealed that the risk of premature cancer mortality was 25% lower in people with higher levels of perceived social support and 20% lower in people with larger social networks (Pinquart & Duberstein, 2010). Cancer mortality rates were also 12% lower among married people, with never-married people at greater risk of premature death than those who were widowed, divorced, or separated. Further research is required to fully determine the causal links between social support and cancer mortality for different cancers at different stages, but it has been proposed that various social factors, such as relationships and friendships, social ties and social integration, social norms, and social resources are important (Kroenke, 2018). More supportive social networks may affect cancer mortality through direct physiological pathways involving inflammation (Uchino et al., 2018). There are also indirect pathways that include encouragement to lead healthier lifestyles, to make more appropriate use of health services, and to adhere to treatment and advice (Meng et al., 2021).

15.4.2 Psychological Responses to Cancer

Cancer can pose severe threats to health that may require extensive adjustment on the part of individuals and their loved ones (see Chapter 6). A diagnosis of cancer should therefore be given carefully and sensitively (see Chapter 13, section 13.4). Many people with cancer report significant levels of anxiety, depression, or PTSD, and for many people these reactions appear for the first time as a consequence of their cancer diagnosis (Abbey et al., 2015; Osmani et al., 2023;

Walker et al., 2021). The likelihood of developing psychological disorders is related to medical factors, such as cancer type, severity, and prognosis, and is also partly due to individual factors, such as a younger age, a history of psychological problems, life stress, and poor support (Abbey et al., 2015; L.C. Brown et al., 2020). The vulnerability-stress model is a useful framework for thinking about how individual vulnerability interacts with medical factors to determine a person's distress (see Figure 3.5).

Although anxiety and depression are both common responses to a cancer diagnosis, the relationship between cancer and depression has been more widely studied. Depression is associated with cancer onset and mortality, but it is difficult to tease out whether depression causes cancer or is a response to cancer. In fact, there appear to be reciprocal links between the severity of depressive symptoms and the *progression* of cancer. Prospective studies suggest that people with a history of depression may have an increased risk of getting some cancers, but not others (Batty et al., 2017; Cowdery et al., 2022). Depression probably plays a more important role in the *progression* of cancer. Prospective research indicates that people who develop anxiety or mood-related disorders after a cancer diagnosis have a higher risk of earlier death from cancer (Hamer et al., 2009; Zhu et al., 2017).

Case Study 15.2

Managing the Stress of Cancer

Hannah was diagnosed with breast cancer six months ago. She had a double mastectomy two months ago, but there were indications the cancer might have spread, so Hannah has started chemotherapy. She is frightened of cancer, tearful, and does not feel she is coping. She thinks she is going to die, has stopped going out, and does not want to talk about it. Hannah is convinced that no one will want to be in a relationship with her now because of the mastectomy. Chemotherapy makes her feel

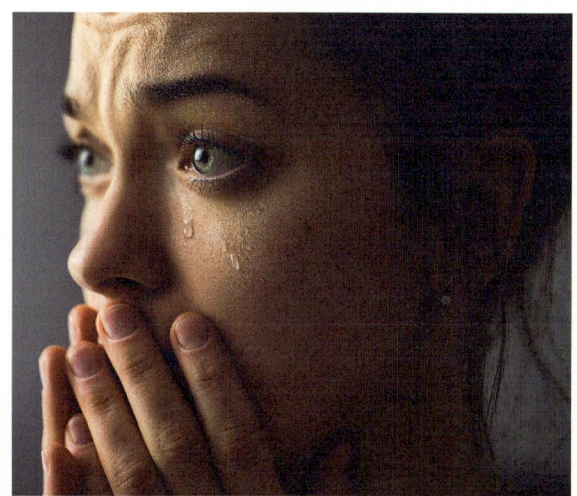

Figure 15.5 Stress management for Hannah's cancer diagnosis and treatment

Source: © Goffkein/Adobe Stock

worse and she can't bear the thought of losing her hair. She has missed her two most recent chemotherapy appointments.

(Continued)

Stress Management

Stress management involves education about stress and coping, exploring the person's ways of coping, and facilitating more adaptive coping. Stress management has many forms. In this example, we use the transactional model (see Chapter 3) to examine the role of perceived demands, appraisal, resources, and coping.

Demands: Explore the Demands of Cancer So They Are Explicit

- What are the triggers to this situation (e.g. breast cancer, chemotherapy)?
- What demands does it place on Hannah (e.g. cancer threatens her life, identity, attractiveness)?
- Which of these demands are based on facts or fears?

Appraisal: Examine Her Appraisals and How They Affect Her Feelings and Coping

- When she is feeling overwhelmed and unable to cope, what is she thinking?
- How can she think differently to help her to feel and cope better?
- For example, 'Many women go through breast cancer and chemotherapy and are fine'.
- For example, 'Breasts are not the only quality that make women attractive'.

Resources to Cope: Explore the Resources She Has to Cope

- What support does she have available to her?
- How has she coped with previous stressful situations?
- How can she use these strategies to cope now?
- What new ways of coping might help her now?

Coping

Drawing on the previous stages, explore practical steps and strategies that would help Hannah to cope with her diagnosis and treatment.

The relationship between depression and cancer is bi-directional and involves physiological and behavioural mechanisms. First, neuroendocrine and immune changes that accompany depression may contribute to the progression of cancer. Second, depression may interact with lifestyle to contribute to the onset and progression of cancer (see section 15.1.2). Indeed, reviews of research evidence indicate that when links between depression and cancer are found, they are at least partially explained by associations between depression and smoking, alcohol consumption, and being overweight (van Tuijl et al., 2023). Third, having cancer may contribute to or exacerbate depressed mood.

The coping strategies people use are influenced by their appraisal of cancer. As noted in Chapter 3, our appraisal of events determines the extent to which we find them stressful and how we attempt to cope with them. This is also the case in response to cancer (see Case Study 15.2 and Chapter 6). People who appraise the cancer as a threat or challenge to be addressed are more likely to use problem-focused coping strategies, such as information gathering, problem solving, accepting responsibility, and seeking support. People who appraise the cancer as involving harm or loss are more likely to use avoidant strategies, such as denial, distancing, wishful-thinking, and substance use (Richardson et al., 2017).

Coping strategies can be either adaptive or maladaptive, depending on the individual and the context. For example, a review of the use of denial by people with cancer found that it was more likely to be used by elderly people or those in the terminal phase of cancer (Vos & de Haes, 2007). The effect of denial on physical and psychological function was inconsistent. However, this may be because there are reciprocal relationships between quality of life and coping strategies among people with cancer (Danhauer et al., 2009). A review of the impact of coping strategies in advanced cancer found that avoidance of thoughts, feelings, and emotions can alleviate distress in the short term, but it may impair longer-term social functioning and quality of life (Davis et al., 2023).

Although the way people cope influences their emotional response to cancer and quality of life, the role of coping in cancer progression is less obvious (Richardson et al., 2017). Evidence reviews have shown that there is little consistent evidence that coping styles play an important part in cancer survival or cancer recurrence (Morris et al., 2018; Petticrew et al., 2002). However, this does not mean we should dismiss coping as completely unimportant. Coping is important in promoting psychological wellbeing and self-help behaviour. For example, one qualitative study of people with incurable cancer who had outlived their diagnosis by two to 12 years found that they had common coping styles of:

- Authenticity: a clear understanding of what was important in their lives.
- Autonomy: a perceived freedom to shape their lives around what they valued.
- Acceptance: more peaceful, joyful experiences and greater emotional closeness to others.

These people were also more involved in their own self-help soon after diagnosis than those who did not survive (Cunningham & Watson, 2004).

Responses to cancer are not always negative. There is increasing evidence that many people experience positive personal changes in response to cancer. Reviews of published research indicate that psychological and social factors are important influences on whether people experience post-traumatic growth following cancer diagnosis or treatment (Knauer et al., 2022; Marziliano et al., 2020; Z. Wang et al., 2023). Personality characteristics such as resilience, hardiness, optimism, and gratitude may be important, but so too are behaviours such as positive reframing and self-reflection, and interpersonal factors linked to the availability and use of social support.

A meta-analysis of research with people with cancer and HIV showed that personal growth is associated with lower levels of distress, better mental health, and better self-ratings of physical health (Sawyer et al., 2010). Furthermore, the positive aspects of personal growth increased over time: people who believed their cancer had led to positive changes in their life continued to do well in terms of their mental health and perceived physical health.

15.4.3 Interventions for Cancer

As noted earlier in this chapter, more rapid progression of cancer arises from immune dysregulation due to chronic stress, depression, and other negative emotional states. It is therefore important to ensure that effective treatment is provided to those people who experience psychological distress.

Research generally confirms that psychological interventions can increase psychological and physiological adaptation in people with cancer, and there is also some evidence that effective interventions also lead to better outcomes in relation to tumour growth, cancer recurrence, or survival (Antoni et al., 2023; Thornton et al., 2020). Various psychosocial interventions for cancer can be used, including counselling, cognitive behavioural therapy, mindfulness interventions, and support groups (see Chapter 14).

Cognitive behavioural therapy (CBT) for cancer usually focuses on reducing stress and negative emotions, helping people to manage pain, fatigue, appetite control, and the side effects of treatment. CBT can be delivered as individual or group programmes, and usually involves education, an examination of stress and coping styles, and the use of cognitive and behavioural techniques to improve coping with the difficult and stressful aspects of cancer and its treatment. Research shows that CBT interventions delivered in-person or online can lead to improved quality of life, reduced distress, and reduced fatigue (Abrahams et al., 2017; Antoni et al., 2023). However, a meta-analysis found no clear effect of CBT-based mobile health interventions on breast cancer survivors' mental health, which suggests that the in-person aspects of standard CBT may explain at least part of its effects (Horn, Jírů-Hillmann et al., 2023).

Mindfulness interventions encourage people to experience life fully by paying attention to moment-to-moment experiences (see Chapter 14). People are encouraged to be aware of the world, other people, their own thoughts and emotions, and to accept these emotions and thoughts without judgement. Because mindfulness focuses on the present, it is a good way to prevent people from ruminating about the past or future. Mindfulness-based interventions (MBIs) include education and training about mindfulness and meditation. Evaluations of MBIs in people with cancer have shown promising results, suggesting that they may contribute to reductions in psychological distress, sleep disturbance, and fatigue, and may help to promote personal growth. MBIs can also have positive effects on activity in the immune system, HPA axis, and ANS, but there is not yet clear evidence of whether these always translate into clinically relevant health benefits (Chayadi et al., 2022; Cillessen et al., 2019).

Support interventions include individual support, telephone support, support groups, and internet support. The support can be provided by health professionals or by peers, and can be provided in-person or online. Early research into support interventions suggested that they could prolong survival (Spiegel et al., 1989). However, subsequent reviews of research indicate that although support interventions are positively evaluated, lead to high levels of satisfaction, and can have positive effects on self-efficacy, distress, and psychological wellbeing, there is less evidence for significant physical benefits (Hong et al., 2012; Ihrig et al., 2020). Mixed findings are probably due to a wide variation in support interventions and individuals. Support groups do not appeal to everyone: many people with cancer will refuse to attend or will drop out. People with less severe cancer may be more distressed by attending support groups with people who are at the end-stages of the disease. Support interventions are therefore only likely to be beneficial for a subgroup of people, such as those with high levels of distress, poor personal resources, and little existing support. People who *do* choose to attend support groups usually report improved psychological wellbeing and quality of life (Hong et al., 2012).

Expressive writing involves writing down one's feelings with the aim of reducing feelings of emotional trauma, and it has been found to help to reduce anxiety and depression and increase self-efficacy among people with cancer (C. Zhang et al., 2023). There is also evidence that music therapy offered by trained music therapists may have beneficial effects on fatigue and quality of life in adults with cancer, but that music medicine (i.e. listening to pre-recorded music offered by medical staff interventions) is not as effective (Bradt et al., 2021). Other more active interventions have been used with positive results. For example, graded physical exercise programmes help to improve quality of life, physical functioning, and emotional wellbeing, and can also reduce fatigue (Ehlers et al., 2020; Mustian et al., 2017).

In addition to considering the content and the theoretical basis of interventions, the mode of delivery is also important. Telephone interventions provide a convenient way of supporting the self-management of cancer-related symptoms for adults with cancer (Ream et al., 2020). Reviews have also highlighted that technology-based interventions can be an effective approach to improving quality of life in people with cancer and their carers, and that interventions that treated patient–carer pairs as a unit were even more effective (Low et al., 2024).

Clinical Notes 15.2

Coping with Cancer

- Psychosocial factors influence the onset and progression of many cancers.
- Encourage people to change risk factors, such as lifestyle, stress, emotions, and psychological problems.
- It is important to treat psychological disorders in people with cancer.
- Encourage the partners and relatives of people with cancer to engage actively in discussions about cancer to find constructive ways of coping with it.
- Generally, it is not helpful if the partners of people with cancer hide their concerns.
- Support groups are helpful for some people with cancer, but be aware that many people do not find them to be beneficial.

Summary 15.3

- Psychosocial risk factors for cancer include demographic factors, lifestyle, stress, and support.
- Tobacco use, diet, and infections are responsible for up to half of all cancers.
- Poor social support and depression are associated with the onset and progression of some cancers, but it is unclear whether depression causes cancer or is a response to cancer.
- Many people with cancer report clinically significant levels of anxiety, depression, or PTSD.
- Psychosocial interventions for cancer include cognitive behavioural therapy, mindfulness-based interventions, and support groups.
- These interventions usually improve quality of life and psychological wellbeing, but there is little consistent evidence that they affect physical outcomes.

Further Reading

Llewellyn, C.D. et al. (eds) (2019) *Cambridge Handbook of Psychology, Health and Medicine* (3rd edition). Cambridge: Cambridge University Press. Includes short chapters on psychoneuroimmunology, immunisation, and many specific skin disorders and cancers.

Breitbart, W.S., Butow, P.N., Jacobsen, P.B., Lam, W., Lazenby, M. & Loscalzo, M.J. (eds) (2021) *Psycho-Oncology* (4th edition). New York and Oxford: Oxford University Press. A comprehensive book covering all aspects of psycho-oncology, including lifestyle factors and risk, screening, responses to treatment, psychiatric comorbidity, psychosocial intervention, cancer in special groups such as children, and those with other special needs.

Jafferany, M. (2022). *Handbook of Psychodermatology: Introduction to Psychocutaneous Disorders.* Cham, Switzerland: Springer Nature. Contains an array of chapters that provide a practical guide to the management of people with psychocutaneous conditions. It considers issues from the perspectives of dermatologists and psychiatrists.

Revision Questions

1   How do the immune effects of acute stress differ from those of chronic stress?
2   Describe the links between negative emotions and immune function.
3   Describe the links between positive emotions and experiences and immune function.
4   How does stress affect responsiveness to vaccinations?
5   Compare the prevalence of depression in people with immune disorders to the prevalence in the general population. How can we explain the observed differences?
6   What do the results of wound healing studies tell us about the impact of negative psychological states on immune function?
7   Why are psychological interventions useful for treating skin disorders?
8   Outline the important psychosocial risk factors for cancer onset.
9   How do psychosocial factors such as coping and social support affect cancer progression?
10   'Every person with cancer should join a support group'. Give arguments for and against this statement.

16

CARDIOVASCULAR AND RESPIRATORY HEALTH

─Learning Objectives─

This chapter is designed to enable you to:

- Describe the role of psychosocial factors in the development of cardiovascular disease.
- Outline the various pathways through which psychosocial factors affect cardiovascular disease.
- Describe the role of psychosocial factors in respiratory infections and asthma.
- Discuss the efficacy of psychological interventions for cardiovascular and respiratory disorders.

The first part of this chapter examines how psychosocial factors can affect the development and progression of cardiovascular disease (CVD). Cardiovascular health is affected by a range of psychosocial risk factors, including lifestyle, stress, emotions, and social circumstances. These factors can influence the development of CVD, as well as the prognosis in people who already have CVD. Coronary heart disease (CHD) – also called ischaemic heart disease or coronary artery disease – is the leading cause of death worldwide (World Health Organization, 2020a). It is a life-threatening condition in which the heart's blood supply becomes restricted due to atherosclerosis. The second most common cause of death is stroke, which occurs when the blood supply to the brain is restricted because blood vessels become blocked or rupture. Both conditions require extensive lifestyle changes. Unsurprisingly, acute CVD events, such as myocardial infarction (MI, or 'heart attack') or stroke, may result in high levels of fear, distress, anxiety, and depression, which in turn may affect both health and prognosis. Cardiac rehabilitation supports people to reduce their risk of future illness.

The second part of this chapter examines psychological factors in respiratory health. Breathing and emotions are strongly interlinked. Furthermore, psychosocial factors can influence the onset and progression of respiratory disorders. After CVD, respiratory disorders are the second most common cause of death worldwide (World Health Organization, 2020a). Given the range and variety of respiratory disorders, it is not possible to cover them all. Here we focus on common examples of respiratory infections and asthma to illustrate the role of psychological factors in acute and chronic respiratory disorders.

16.1 Cardiovascular Health

Psychosocial factors affect heart disease through four pathways:

- Sociodemographic factors are associated with risk and the accessibility of services.
- Lifestyle factors, such as smoking, diet, and exercise, affect the risk of developing CVD.
- Psychosocial factors can trigger acute cardiac events in people with existing cardiovascular pathology.
- Beliefs influence the use of healthcare services by people with cardiovascular disease.

This section examines the key psychosocial risk factors that influence CVD: lifestyle, stress, depression, hostility or anger, and social connectedness or isolation.

16.1.1 Psychosocial Risk Factors for Cardiovascular Disease

Chronic risk factors exert their influence over prolonged periods and include things like smoking, hypertension, and high cholesterol. Acute risk factors are transient physical changes that occur following exposure to physical or psychological triggers, such as exercise or stress, and which cause clinical events such as ischaemia, infarction, or sudden death. Chronic and acute risk factors combine to increase the overall risk of a cardiac event. In other words, people with high chronic risk (e.g. a smoker with a family history of CHD) have the greatest risk of a problem occurring when acute risk factors arise (e.g. intense exercise or stress). Table 16.1 shows the main chronic and acute risk factors for CHD.

Table 16.1 Chronic and acute risk factors for coronary heart disease (Emdin et al., 2016; Smith, 2022; Tsao et al., 2023)

	Chronic risk	Acute risk
Physical	Genetic susceptibility	Cardiovascular reactivity
	Cholesterol	
	Hypertension	
	Diabetes	
Demographic	Age (older)	
	Sex (male)	
	Socioeconomic status	
Lifestyle	Smoking	Intense exercise
	Obesity	
	Sedentary lifestyle	
Psychosocial	Stress	Intense stress
	Hostility/anger	Intense anger
	Depression	
	Anxiety	Anxiety
	Social isolation	

Many physical and psychosocial risk factors overlap, so separating out the impact of physical, lifestyle, and psychological risk factors can be a challenge. For example, a study that followed 2,272 men over ten years found that those with the lowest incomes were more than twice as likely to die of CHD than men with higher incomes (Lynch et al., 1996). However, the effect of socioeconomic status on CHD was due to 23 different physical (e.g. cholesterol, blood pressure, body mass index), lifestyle (e.g. smoking, alcohol use, and physical activity), and psychosocial factors (e.g. depression and social support). More recent studies have shown that depression, less education, living in a more deprived area, and having a low income all individually increase the risk of major cardiac events, but that individuals with depression and also less education, greater deprivation, or lower income were at particularly elevated risk (Prigge et al., 2022). Furthermore, although cardiovascular disease is declining in many countries, health inequalities in CVD appear to be widening (Leyland & Dundas, 2020). It is therefore important to consider all areas of risk in the prevention and treatment of CVD.

Lifestyle and Health Behaviours

Lifestyle has a powerful impact on cardiovascular health. A study of more than 20,000 men and women over ten years identified four behaviours that made a dramatic difference to mortality, particularly deaths from cardiovascular causes. People who did not smoke, were physically active, had moderate alcohol intake, and ate five or more servings of fruit or vegetables a day were three times less likely to die prematurely from CVD or have a first stroke than people who did none of these behaviours (Khaw et al., 2008; Myint et al., 2009). The differences remained even after taking into account age, sex, body mass index, and socioeconomic status. In fact, the impact of doing these four health behaviours was equivalent to being 14 years younger.

Changes in lifestyle factors explain a large proportion of the reduction in CVD over recent decades (Ahmadi & Lanphear, 2022; Marasigan et al., 2020). Figure 16.1 shows that population-level prevention-focused interventions were at least as important as treatment-focused clinical interventions (Ahmadi & Lanphear, 2022).

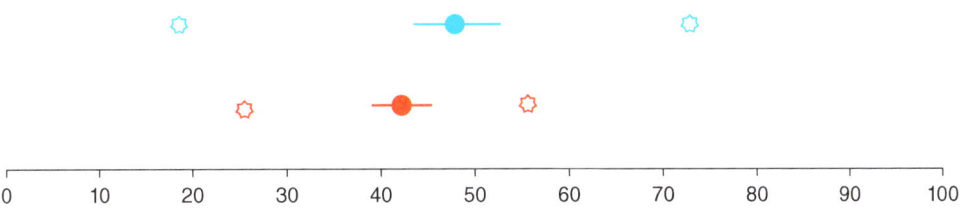

Blue: proportion of decline in CHD attributable to population (prevention) interventions
Red: proportion of decline in CHD attributable to clinical (treatment) interventions

The circles indicate the proportion of decline attributable to each approach, the lines indicate the 95% confidence intervals, and the asterisks indicate the highest and lowest estimates across the studies

Data from 500 million people in 20 high-income countries 1980–2012

Figure 16.1 The relative importance of prevention and treatment for declines in CVD (Ahmadi & Lanphear, 2022: 14, reproduced under a CC BY 4.0 license)

However, there is still room for improvement in areas such as obesity. Figure 16.2 shows the contribution of medical treatments and lifestyle to CHD mortality in the UK at the end of the last century: decreases in smoking, hypertension, and high cholesterol made a larger contribution to reducing CHD than did advances in medical treatment. Reductions in smoking alone had a greater impact than all the advances in medical treatments during this time (Ünal et al., 2005). Smoking is therefore the single most important lifestyle risk factor to address. Smokers are twice as likely to die from CHD and two to four times more likely to have an MI. Quitting smoking is more important than trying to cut down, because even light smoking increases the risk of CVD (Hackshaw et al., 2018). Compared to people with CVD who continue to smoke, those who stop smoking reduce their risk of premature death, CVD death, major adverse cardiac events (e.g. MI), and stroke by over 30% (Wu et al., 2022).

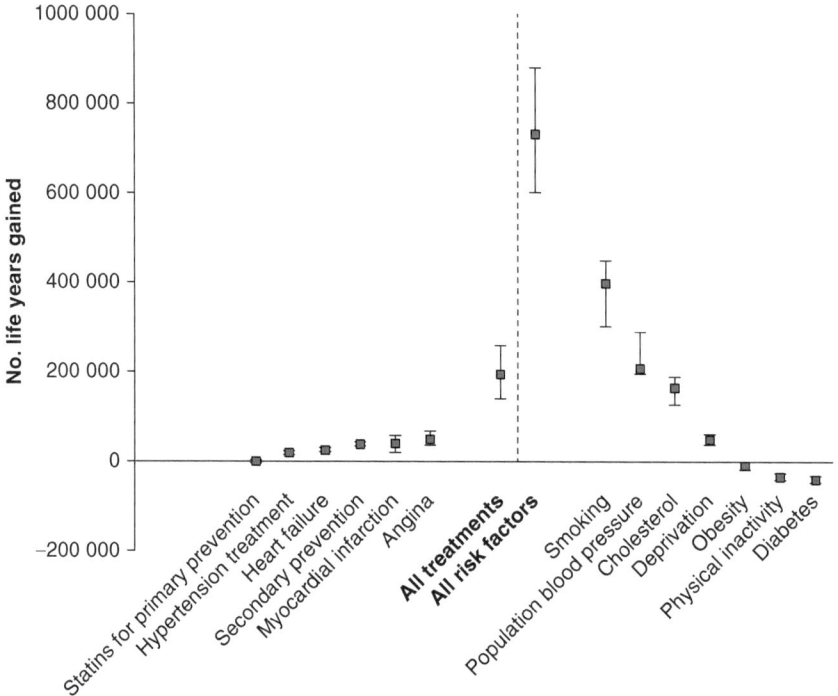

Figure 16.2 Effect of treatment and risk factors in the decline in CHD (England and Wales, 1981–2000)

Source: Ünal, B., Critchley, J.A., Fidan, D. & Capewell, S. (2005) Life-years gained from modern cardiological treatments and population risk factor changes in England and Wales, 1981–2000. *American Journal of Public Health, 95*(1): 103–108. Reused with permission of American Journal of Public Health

Diet and exercise are important because CVD risk is increased by high cholesterol levels, obesity, and high blood pressure (Bechthold et al., 2019). Although there have been beneficial changes in smoking, the trend for increasing obesity and physical inactivity is adversely affecting rates of CHD (Figure 16.2). The World Health Organization (2020c) advises people to aim for healthier diets by:

- Reducing the level of salt/sodium added to food.
- Increasing the availability, affordability, and consumption of fruit and vegetables.
- Reducing saturated fatty acids in food and replacing them with unsaturated fatty acids.
- Replacing trans-fats with unsaturated fats.
- Reducing the consumption of free and added sugars in food and drinks.
- Limiting excess calorie intake by avoiding energy-dense foods and reducing portion size.

It is commonly thought that moderate alcohol consumption reduces the risk of cardiovascular disease. However, recent analyses of the available data do not provide clear evidence of the protective effects of moderate alcohol consumption (Larsson et al., 2016; Rehm et al., 2017). Furthermore, many people incorrectly believe that their alcohol intake is 'moderate' when it is in fact greater. Regular moderate physical activity reduces the risk of CVD, and is effective as part of efforts to reduce weight, body fat, blood pressure, and cholesterol, and to improve psychological wellbeing (D.J. Chu et al., 2020).

Being aware of a person's risk factors and helping them to stop smoking, to exercise more, and to eat healthily are important parts of cardiac disease prevention and rehabilitation. However, people who have experienced CVD often underestimate the importance of modifiable lifestyle-related risk factors such as hypertension, stress, and being overweight (Timmermans et al., 2018). Furthermore, one study found that less than 20% of cardiology notes covered all the major risk factors (Gravely-Witte et al., 2008). Although smoking and cholesterol were reported in 80% of the notes, other risks, such as obesity and family history, were reported in less than 50% of notes. Careful screening of risk behaviour is an important first step toward reducing CVD and improving the prognosis in people with CVD. Various evidence-based techniques for health behaviour change can contribute to effective intervention and rehabilitation (see Chapter 5).

The physical and lifestyle risk factors referred to above account for about half of new cases of heart disease, but they leave much of the risk unaccounted for. Researchers have therefore focused on other potential risk factors, such as stress and differences in cardiovascular responses to stress, emotions, and social isolation.

Activity 16.1

Stress and Lifestyle

- When you are stressed, how does it affect your lifestyle (e.g. health behaviours such as smoking, drinking, diet, sleep, and exercise)?
- How do you think we can separate the effect of stress from the effects of lifestyle?

Stress

There is substantial evidence from epidemiological and experimental studies that stress affects CVD onset and can also trigger cardiac events (Booth et al., 2015; Osborne et al., 2020; Sara et al., 2018; Spencer et al., 2024). Epidemiological studies show that stressors such as natural disasters, war, terrorism, and even sporting events can be associated with increased cardiac morbidity and mortality. For example, a national survey in the USA showed that diagnosed CHD increased by 53% after the 9/11 terrorist attacks, even after taking into account existing risk factors (Holman et al., 2008). Watching sporting events is also linked to increased risk of acute cardiac events (L.-L. Lin et al., 2019). It has been argued that cultivating resilience and adaptive responses to stressful situations should be an important part of primary and secondary prevention of CVD (Chinnaiyan, 2019). An example of one kind of intervention is given in Research Box 16.1. Experimental studies have shown that stressful tasks, such as giving a public speech, increase both heart rate and blood pressure and can trigger ischaemia (restricted blood flow to the heart) in people with CHD (Mehta et al., 2022; Osborne et al., 2020). Ischaemia is easily provoked, reversible, and clinically important, so it is a good way to study the effects of stress on the heart. Studies of naturally-occurring ischaemia show that it is more likely to occur during intense physical activity, stressful mental activity, or when people feel angry.

—Research Box 16.1—

Group Psychosocial Stress-Reduction Intervention Improves Survival in Women with CHD

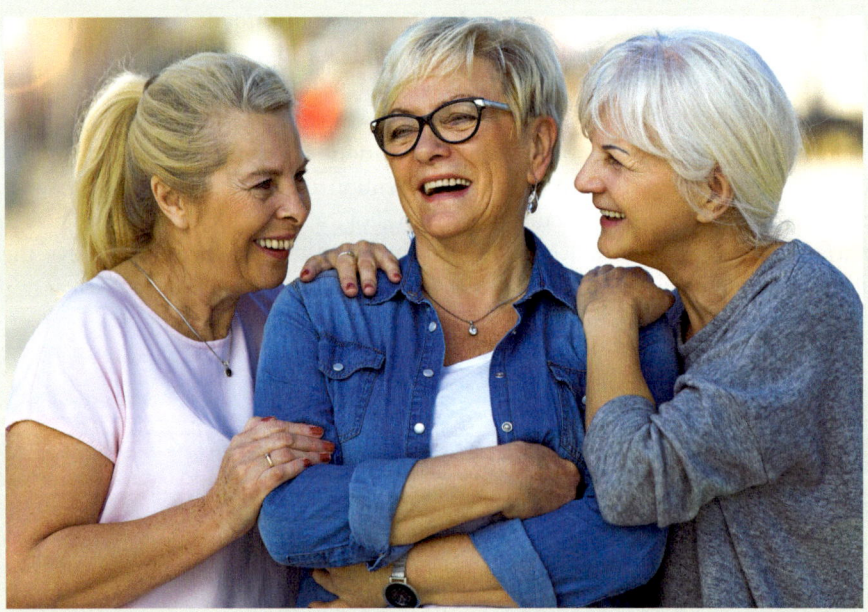

Figure 16.3   Intervention to reduce stress in women with coronary artery disease

Source: © pikselstock/Adobe Stock

Background

Psychosocial stress can accelerate atherosclerosis progression and worsen the prognosis in women with coronary artery disease. There is a need to identify interventions that can reduce stress and to determine whether this improves survival.

Method and Findings

Study participants were 237 women aged 75 or under who had experienced an extreme coronary event. They were randomly allocated to receive usual care or a novel psychosocial intervention. The intervention was delivered as one-hour sessions in groups of four to eight women. The 20 sessions were spread over one year and covered a range of psychosocial components: knowledge of heart health, skills for coping with serious illness, managing marital stress, counteracting anxiety and depression, relaxation techniques, improving social relations, and social support. Women were followed-up for an average of seven years. The likelihood of death among the intervention group was one-third of that among the control group (7% versus 20%). The intervention effect was significant even after taking account of clinical prognostic factors such as medication prescription and use.

Significance

The intervention may have been effective because of its extended duration, the session content, and/or the group participation, which may have provided motivation and social support. Further research could usefully explore the relative influence of these different aspects of the intervention.

Orth-Gomér, K., Schneiderman, N., Wang, H.X., Walldin, C., Blom, M. & Jernberg, T. (2009) Stress reduction prolongs life in women with coronary disease: The Stockholm Women's Intervention Trial for Coronary Heart Disease (SWITCHD). *Circulation: Cardiovascular Quality & Outcomes*, 2(1): 25–32.

Hostility and Anger

The study of hostility and anger originated from research into the association between CHD and the Type A behaviour pattern. Type A personalities are characterised by competitiveness, impatience, and hostility or aggression. Early research in the 1950s found that Type A men were more at risk of CHD. However, later research revealed that hostility and anger were the most important components of Type A in the development and prognosis of CHD. Meta-analyses show that anger and hostility are associated with an increased risk of CHD in healthy people, particularly men, and with a poor prognosis in people with CHD, even after taking into account the severity of the disease (Chida & Steptoe, 2009; Smaardijk et al., 2020).

Anger and hostility are therefore chronic risk factors for CHD. Anger is also a potent trigger of acute cardiac events. In two large studies of MI in the USA and Sweden, anger was found to be a particularly strong trigger. People were between two and four times more likely to have an MI after an angry episode compared to when they were not angry (Steptoe & Brydon, 2009). Interview studies of people after MI show that between 2% and 17% of them reported being angry in the two hours before their MI symptoms. Anger and hostility also predict worse outcomes in people with existing heart disease. A meta-analysis revealed that among people with known ischaemic heart disease, subsequent major adverse cardiac events were more likely for men with higher levels of anger and hostility (Smaardijk et al., 2020). A smaller study followed people with heart failure over three years and found that subsequent hospitalisation rates were greater for those with higher levels of hostility, and also those with higher levels of specific aspects of anger, for example, the expression of angry feelings towards others and a trait measure of how often people get angry (Keith et al., 2017).

At the population level, there is some evidence that anger can trigger stroke, with the association appearing to be stronger among people of lower socioeconomic status (H. Chen et al., 2019; J. Liu et al., 2023; Smyth et al., 2022).

Depression and Other Negative Psychosocial States

Cardiovascular disease is more likely to develop among people who have been diagnosed with and/or are being treated for various psychological conditions (Trajkova et al., 2019; Zivkovic et al., 2019). There is substantial evidence that depression is associated with CVD onset and prognosis, and that CVD is in turn associated with the onset of depression (Cai et al., 2023; Pan et al., 2011; Smaardijk et al., 2020). It has been argued that depression should be considered to be a major modifiable risk factor for CVD in the same way that smoking, hypertension, and hyperlipidaemia are.

The link between depression and CVD may be due to both physical and behavioural pathways (see Table 16.2). People with depression after CVD onset show physiological changes in HPA axis function, platelet activation, inflammatory responses, and impaired vascular function that increase the risk of further adverse CVD outcomes (Warriach et al., 2022). There is also evidence that acute experiences of negative moods, such as sadness, upset, and worry, can trigger MI (Olsson et al., 2023).

Table 16.2 Mechanisms through which depression affects the prognosis of CVD

Biological	Hypothalamic-pituitary-adrenal (HPA) axis dysfunction
	Reduced heart rate variability
	Increased inflammatory response
	Impaired vascular function
	Increased platelet activation
Behavioural	Poor adherence to medication and treatment regimes
	Lack of participation in cardiac rehabilitation
Lifestyle	Smoking
	Diet
	Sedentary lifestyle
Psychosocial	Social isolation
	Chronic stress
	Comorbid anxiety disorders

Socioeconomic Status and Social Support

Cardiovascular disease morbidity and mortality are more likely among people of lower socioeconomic status (SES) (Potter et al., 2019; S. Wang et al., 2020). This is partly explained by people of lower SES tending to have less healthy patterns of behaviour and more CVD risk factors

(Wang, Li & Zheng, 2024). However, even when these behavioural differences are accounted for, an association between CVD and low SES remains (Y.B. Zhang et al., 2021).

The effect of low social support, negative interpersonal relationships, and isolation on increased CVD risk is well established (Cené et al., 2022; Teshale et al., 2023). For example, some physiological studies indicate that responses to acute stress are greater when people are prompted to think about negative or ambivalent relationships (Carlisle et al., 2012), whereas others indicate that the size of social networks may be less influential than the quality of these networks and feelings of loneliness (Gallagher et al., 2024).

Social isolation and loneliness are direct predictors of coronary heart disease and stroke mortality (Cené et al., 2022). Syntheses of research have revealed better cardiovascular outcomes for married women and men, the benefits of marriage appearing to be greater for men (Dhindsa et al., 2020; Y. Wang et al., 2020). The influence of relationships and social support on CVD is partly due to single people being more likely to have unhealthy lifestyles and greater distress. For example, a study of over 13,000 Scottish adults showed that 59% of the risk of dying of cardiovascular causes was explained by health behaviours, metabolic dysregulation, and distress (Molloy et al., 2009). It is important to note that many of the studies referred to above explicitly or implicitly focused on people in heterosexual relationships. Although studies of people in lesbian, bisexual, or gay relationships show broadly similar patterns to those found for heterosexual relationships, there are some more nuanced results – notably, formal marital status appears to be less important than relationship status (Solazzo et al., 2020).

Social isolation is highly pathogenic: it is associated with morbidity and mortality in healthy people and people with CHD. In relation to morbidity, one study followed more than 5,000 people for over five years and found that loneliness was associated with a significantly increased risk of CVD (Valtorta et al., 2018). In relation to mortality, a study of 430 people with CHD found that those who had fewer than four close friends or family were more than twice as likely to die from CHD or other causes, even after controlling for disease severity, age, hostility, smoking, and psychological distress (Brummett et al., 2001). A more recent study of over 30,000 people with stable coronary artery disease found that living alone significantly increased the risk of CVD death, MI, and stroke among men, but not among women (Gandhi et al., 2019).

In sum, psychosocial factors such as stress, depression, anger, and social isolation are influential risk factors for CVD morbidity and mortality. Depression and social isolation, in particular, are equivalent to other major risk factors, such as smoking. The physical processes through which stress, emotions, and social isolation can affect CVD onset and progression are believed to include stress-induced autonomic nervous system dysfunction, haemodynamic responses, neuroendocrine activation, inflammatory responses, and prothrombotic responses (notably platelet activation). These factors contribute to coronary plaque disruption, ischaemia, cardiac dysrhythmias, and thrombus formation (Steptoe & Brydon, 2009). The role of cardiovascular reactivity and other haemodynamic responses is therefore examined in the next section.

16.1.2 Cardiovascular Reactivity

To understand the links between psychosocial factors and CVD, we need to understand cardiovascular responses to emotions and how these are moderated by other risk factors. There is a wealth of evidence that people vary in the magnitude of their cardiovascular responses to stress (Whittaker et al., 2021). In such research, the term 'reactivity' is used to describe the magnitude of changes in blood pressure, heart rate, ischaemia, or endothelial function while people complete stressful tasks.

Cardiovascular reactivity appears to be an enduring individual trait: people's responses are fairly consistent over time and with different stressors. A key question is whether hyper-reactivity causes future heart disease or whether it serves as a marker of future risk (without necessarily being causal). Reviews of research indicate that hyper-reactive responses to stress are related to a greater risk of developing hypertension, atherosclerosis, and abnormal left ventricular mass, which may be precursors to CVD (Howard, 2023; Whittaker et al., 2021).

Cardiovascular reactivity therefore differs between people and is associated with long-term risk factors for CVD and a higher clinical risk in people with CHD. However, reactivity is influenced by a number of other factors, including physical fitness, family history, and support. People of lower SES do not necessarily have greater reactivity to stress, but they have been found to have poorer recovery from stress (Boylan et al., 2018). A review of research evidence indicated that aerobic exercise to enhance fitness can attenuate cardiovascular reactivity to stress, and may reduce the incidence of stroke and myocardial infarction (Mücke et al., 2018).

Another area of interest is vascular endothelial reactivity. Endothelial function contributes to vessel tone, dilation, platelet aggregation, and inflammation, and affects CVD outcomes (Widmer et al., 2020). Stressful situations typically result in a reduction in endothelial-dependent vasodilation, whereas positive emotions, such as laughing, result in increases. In one study, people who watched a comedy film had a 22% increase in vasodilation whereas those who watched a harrowing war film had a 35% decrease (Miller et al., 2006). Thus, it has been proposed that vascular reactivity may be a critical link that explains the impact of positive and negative emotions on cardiovascular health.

16.1.3 Impact of Cardiovascular Disease

Cardiovascular disease can have a severe impact on a person's wellbeing and lifestyle: MI and stroke are sudden, unexpected, and potentially life-threatening events which require significant adjustment (see Research Box 16.2). Around 30% of people who have experienced a major cardiac event meet the diagnostic criteria for major depressive disorder, and many experience anxiety. Rates may be higher among those who undergo cardiac surgery (Feng et al., 2019). Depression and anxiety appear to be more common in people with CHD who are younger, female, experience greater pain or disability, perceive more serious consequences of CVD, have less coherent understanding of CVD, have a history of psychological problems, or have less social support (Bennett, 2007; Pai et al., 2019). In addition, 12% develop clinically relevant symptoms of PTSD. Post-traumatic stress disorder is bad enough in itself, but it also doubles the risk of subsequent acute cardiac events (Vilchinsky et al., 2017). As with most illnesses, there is little association between the objective severity of CHD and psychological distress: what matters more is how people experience, make sense of, and respond to CVD. For example, one study found that the following factors were strong predictors of the development of PTSD:

- A history of psychological problems.
- A belief that the MI had negative consequences (e.g. problems in relationships or dealing with medication and self-care).
- Dysfunctional coping techniques (e.g. trying to numb emotions or distract themselves from upsetting thoughts).

These factors were more strongly associated with PTSD than the perceived severity of the MI (Ayers et al., 2009).

Research Box 16.2

The Psychological Impact of Acute MI

Background

For people who survive MI, secondary prevention primarily focuses on optimising clinical outcomes. However, there is a clear need to understand the psychological impacts of MI, and how these affect engagement with secondary prevention activities.

Method and Findings

Qualitative methods can provide useful insights into people's experiences

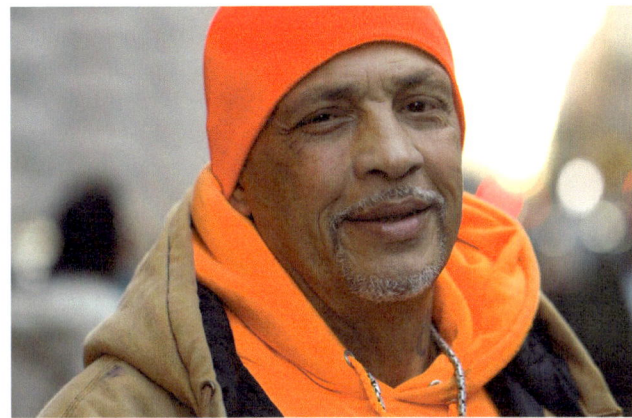

Figure 16.4   Psychological wellbeing post-MI

Source: © blvdone/Adobe Stock

and understanding of health and illness, but individual studies often have small samples. Meta-synthesis of the findings of multiple qualitative studies can highlight important similarities and differences across samples. In this study, the authors analysed the accounts of over 200 people from 17 studies in four countries. The analysis revealed that when MI was an acute event, it had intrusive and disruptive effects on long-term psychological and physical wellbeing. It required people to make sense not only of what had happened to them, but also how they could gain control and establish a lifestyle that also gave them meaning and purpose.

Significance

This meta-synthesis highlights that whereas clinicians may focus on clinical aspects of recovery post-MI, for patients, there is an ongoing need to develop healthier lifestyles while at the same time enhancing their psychological wellbeing and sense of control. The findings indicate that rehabilitation activities should focus not only on physical factors, but also on existential and motivational issues.

Dreyer, R.P., Pavlo, A.J., Hersey, D., Horne, A., Dunn, R., Norris, C.M. & Davidson, L. (2021) 'Is my heart healing?' A meta-synthesis of patients' experiences after acute myocardial infarction. *Journal of Cardiovascular Nursing, 36*(5): 517–530. doi:10.1097/JCN.0000000000000732.

Psychological distress is also more common among stroke survivors than the general population. Depression affects about 30% of stroke survivors (Knapp et al., 2020; L. Liu et al., 2023). Depression increases the risk of earlier death among stroke survivors, but timely diagnosis and management of post-stroke depression can facilitate motor recovery and improve independence (Cai et al., 2019). Reviews indicate that anxiety is present in around 20% of stroke survivors (Knapp et al., 2020).

Reviews of studies of people with CVD have shown that those who experience depression, anxiety, or PTSD have a higher risk of subsequent cardiac events and premature mortality (Baumeister et al., 2015; Flygare et al., 2023). Comorbid psychological conditions in people with CHD result in greater healthcare use and higher overall and outpatient healthcare costs. Much of this is due to worry and health concerns rather than cardiac problems. Symptoms of anxiety, such as a racing heart or palpitations, may be a particular issue because they mimic the symptoms of cardiac problems, and therefore perpetuate distress.

Psychological problems therefore affect people's wellbeing, quality of life, and use of health services. They may also affect whether people change unhealthy behaviours. People with CVD who also develop depression-, anxiety- or stress-related disorders are less likely to adhere to medication or make healthy lifestyle changes (Poletti et al., 2022). This means that they have a worse prognosis (Gathright et al., 2017; Wen et al., 2021). Many studies show a clear dose–response relationship between the severity of depression and cardiac morbidity. This relationship is evident even after physical risk factors are considered.

Given these links, it is important to identify and treat depression in people with CVD. In particular, the American Heart Association recommends that all people with CHD are screened for depression. Those with mild symptoms should be followed up during subsequent routine visits. Those with moderate or severe symptoms should be referred for comprehensive evaluation and treatment by a mental health professional. However, many clinicians do not routinely ask people about depression, and even when depression is identified, it is not always treated (Feinstein et al., 2006; Hare et al., 2020). Although there is currently no consensus on the optimal screening tool for depression in people with CVD, there is a clear need to increase the use of any of the existing screening tools (Ren et al., 2015). Table 16.3 shows a brief screening questionnaire that can be used with people with CHD to identify depression and other forms of psychological distress.

Table 16.3 Screening tool for psychosocial distress (STOP-D)

Over the last two weeks, how much have you been bothered by:

Feeling sad, down, or uninterested in life?	Not at all	0	1	2	3	4*	5	6	7	8	Extremely
Feeling anxious or nervous?	Not at all	0	1	2	3	4*	5	6	7	8	Extremely
Feeling stressed?	Not at all	0	1	2	3	4	5*	6	7	8	Extremely
Feeling angry?	Not at all	0	1	2	3	4	5*	6	7	8	Extremely
Not having the social support you feel you need?	Not at all	0	1	2	3	4	5*	6	7	8	Extremely

*Recommended cut-off indicating those people who need referral to psychological services for further assessment and treatment for psychological distress. Reproduced courtesy of Quincy Young from Young et al. (2007)

It should also be noted that the effect of heart disease on psychological wellbeing is not always negative. Positive changes can also occur after illnesses such as MI. Studies have revealed that in the months after MI some people report post-traumatic growth as reflected in coping responses, perceptions of social support, improved close relationships, psychological wellbeing, and a greater appreciation of life (Hegarty et al., 2021).

16.1.4 Treatment and Rehabilitation

The prognosis following MI or stroke is much better if treatment is obtained quickly. However, many people take several hours to go to hospital for treatment. It is interesting to note that the amount of physical pain a person feels does not affect how quickly they obtain treatment, but that psychosocial factors do influence speed of help-seeking (Arrebola-Moreno et al., 2020; Perkins-Porras et al., 2009; Walsh et al., 2004). People who believe that a heart attack has serious consequences, who attribute their symptoms to a cardiac event, and who have active or problem-focused coping styles are quicker to attend hospital (Arrebola-Moreno et al., 2020; Walsh et al., 2004). Women tend to be slower to attend hospital, perhaps because they believe that CVD is a male condition, and this belief affects their interpretation of symptoms. Single people are also slower to attend hospital, perhaps because they do not have a partner to encourage or help them to get treatment.

People's beliefs about CVD can also affect relevant longer-term behaviours. Those who believe that their lifestyle affects the development of CVD, that lifestyle change can improve prognosis, and that they are capable of making behaviour changes are more likely to change their behaviour (Mercer et al., 2018; Zanatta et al., 2024). For example, in one study, older people who considered their recent MI or stroke to be an inevitable consequence of 'old age' were less likely to make healthy lifestyle changes during a three-year follow-up period, but they were more likely to consult health professionals or to be hospitalised (Stewart et al., 2016).

As noted above, psychological distress following MI or stroke can impair quality of life and lead to premature death. Although effective pharmacotherapy and psychotherapy are available, a review of the research indicated that fewer than one-quarter of MI and stroke patients with depression receive treatment (Ladwig et al., 2018).

Clinical Notes 16.1

Treating Cardiovascular Disease

- Careful screening of risk behaviour is an important step toward reducing CVD and improving the prognosis in people with CHD.
- When taking a cardiovascular history, it is important to ask about:
  - Lifestyle factors of smoking, physical activity, alcohol intake, and diet.
  - Current stress, depression, anxiety, anger, relationship quality, and social isolation.

  These factors can be as important as physical risk factors in the progression of illness.
- Depression occurs in 30% of people with CHD and increases the risk of death. Anxiety and PTSD are also prevalent.

(Continued)

- Depression is more likely in younger, female, socially isolated people or those with a history of psychological problems.
- Guidelines recommend screening for depression and referring moderately or severely depressed people for appropriate treatment.
- Cardiac rehabilitation reduces mortality, but attendance is poor. Make sure you refer all patients and strongly encourage them to attend.
- You may want to consider using a home-based psychological rehabilitation programme that can be facilitated by a specialist nurse, such as the Heart Manual.

CVD Rehabilitation

Rehabilitation programmes vary widely between countries and regions. Programmes may give different attention to diet, exercise, or other factors. They may also vary in the extent to which they focus on education or other psychological variables known to improve adherence to therapeutic advice. It is therefore important to identify which programmes and which component parts are most effective. Meta-analyses indicate that lifestyle modification programmes can lead to significant improvements in diet and physical activity, as well as benefits across intermediate health outcomes, including blood pressure and blood cholesterol (Dibben et al., 2021; Patnode et al., 2022; Shi et al., 2023).

Higher intensity interventions result in greater improvements, and programmes are more effective if they incorporate self-regulation techniques such as goal setting, self-monitoring, planning, and feedback techniques. Changes in lifestyle during rehabilitation are associated with reductions in all-cause mortality, cardiac mortality, cardiac readmissions, and non-fatal reinfarctions. A key issue is that attendance at rehabilitation programmes and adherence to recommended lifestyle changes are poor. Lower attendance is seen in people with ischaemic heart disease, older people, women, and people from ethnic minority groups. Beliefs about the illness can also influence attendance and other measures of recovery. A systematic literature review that examined the relationship between illness perceptions and attendance at cardiac rehabilitation found that people are more likely to attend rehabilitation if they feel that they understand their condition more, and if they view their condition as more controllable, more symptomatic, and having more severe consequences (see Chapter 4, section 4.4) (French et al., 2006).

One key marker of successful rehabilitation is return to work. Important psychosocial facilitators of returning to work include having greater self-efficacy and motivation to return to work, and perceiving more employer support, whereas barriers to returning to work include high physical job demands and/or job strain, psychological or physical comorbidities, and perceiving CVD to be an obstacle to a return to work (Gragnano et al., 2018; Salzwedel et al., 2020). Attending to these facilitators and barriers can help people to obtain the financial, psychological, and social benefits that many people find in work.

Despite the importance of beliefs and emotions in whether people attend rehabilitation, adhere to treatment, and recover, there is mixed evidence about the use of psychological intervention in rehabilitation programmes. Various rehabilitation programmes with psychological components have been developed, such as the MULTIFIT programme in the USA (Taylor et al., 1997) and the Heart Manual in the UK (Lewin et al., 1992). Such programmes were originally designed to be administered in the home by a trained facilitator, but they may now also include online and/or smartphone components as well as monitoring behaviour via wearable or portable technology. They use cognitive behavioural therapy or self-efficacy approaches for positive coping, changing maladaptive beliefs, stress management (see Chapter 3), self-management (see Chapter 4), and relaxation training (see Chapter 14). An example of this kind of programme is given in Case Study 16.1. To maximise both initial and ongoing engagement with such programmes, it is important to tailor components to the needs of individuals (Antypas & Wangberg, 2014; Bostrom et al., 2020; Pfaeffli Dale et al., 2015). Such programmes can be as effective as hospital-based rehabilitation on numerous psychological, behavioural, biological, service, and cost outcomes (Clark et al., 2011; Munro et al., 2013). Systematic reviews conclude that psychological interventions can produce benefits in physical activity and psychosocial wellbeing, with less clear evidence of the effect on clinical outcome such as re-hospitalisation or premature death (McGregor et al., 2020; Munro et al., 2013; Whalley et al., 2011; Zou et al., 2021).

Case Study 16.1

Cardiac Rehabilitation

Omar was 42 when he had an MI and surgery to insert a stent into the blocked artery. He is married with a daughter and manages a regional finance office. After Omar was discharged from hospital, he participated in a home-based rehabilitation programme using the Heart Manual. This is a six-week course based on CBT principles that involved working through manuals and audio-recordings to increase understanding and promote lifestyle changes, supported by a nurse.

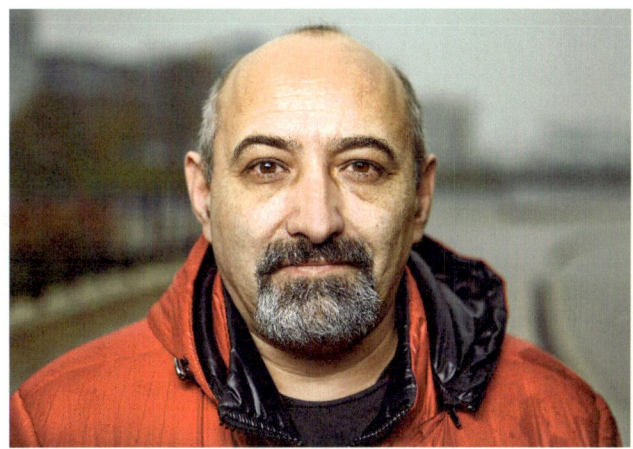

Figure 16.5 Omar's rehabilitation programme after an MI and surgery

Source: © grigvovan/Adobe Stock

First, Omar was assessed to find out what his needs were with regard to medication adherence and lifestyle changes. Unhealthy behaviours and maladaptive beliefs were explored, and Omar was encouraged to challenge these throughout his rehabilitation.

- Part 1 of the Heart Manual provides information and education about heart attacks and heart health. Part 1 also includes information on common psychological reactions to heart attacks and how to manage distress or seek help, if necessary.

(Continued)

- Part 2 of the Heart Manual is a six-week rehabilitation programme, which includes an exercise programme, health education, risk factor reduction, stress management, and sections on low moods, sleep problems, anxiety, and depression. During these six weeks, Omar used a diary to monitor his lifestyle and set his own weekly goals. He also used recorded relaxation exercises.
- Part 3 of the Heart Manual gives facts and advice to help recovery. Topics include medicines, tests, revascularisation procedures, chest pains, anxiety, stress, and depression.

Omar's wife was involved throughout the rehabilitation programme and was encouraged to help Omar to achieve his goals and change. She was given a carer's booklet about the impact of a heart attack on relationships and intimacy, and how best to support Omar.

Omar met the nurse every week for the first few weeks and then continued to complete the Heart Manual programme on his own. He was followed-up two months later so that any depression or unhealthy behaviour could be picked up on.

Summary 16.1

- Psychosocial factors affect heart disease through three pathways: (1) the impact of health-related behaviours, (2) direct or chronic physiological changes that contribute to heart disease, and (3) accessing medical care and treatment.
- The main psychosocial risk factors for heart disease are lifestyle (smoking, exercise, diet), stress, depression, hostility/anger, and social isolation.
- People differ in their cardiovascular reactivity to stress. Reactivity may be a critical link between stress/emotion and cardiovascular health.
- Heart disease is associated with psychological disorders: many people develop depression or anxiety, or experience PTSD.
- Psychological problems are associated with a reduced quality of life, a reduced uptake of rehabilitation programmes, poor adherence to treatment, and the increased use of health services.
- Cardiac rehabilitation programmes significantly reduce cardiac mortality, but are not attended by the majority of people who are referred to them.
- Psychological interventions for heart disease can reduce non-fatal reinfarctions, depression, and anxiety, but do not influence mortality.

16.2 Respiratory Health

The remainder of this chapter addresses the importance of psychological factors in different respiratory disorders and interventions. It is not possible to cover *all* respiratory disorders. Here we focus on two common examples – acute respiratory infections and chronic asthma – which differ widely in terms of their management and prognosis. These disorders illustrate the different applications of psychological knowledge to respiratory disorders.

16.2.1 Breathing and Emotions

Breathing is closely linked to our psychological state: it is the only vital bodily function that can be controlled voluntarily or by reflexes. Controlled slow breathing is the basis for many relaxation exercises and meditation techniques, and it can reduce physiological arousal, tension, and distress. Fast breathing and hyperventilation are common when we are stressed, anxious, or panicked. Our emotions, thoughts, and behaviour therefore both *influence* breathing and are *influenced by* breathing. For example, if people are asked to breathe quickly – to hyperventilate voluntarily – they will report a significant increase in anxiety. This shows that how we breathe affects our emotions and vice versa.

Activity 16.2

Simulating Hyperventilation

- Take short, shallow breaths – at least 30 per minute – for five minutes.
- What symptoms did you notice? How did you feel physically and emotionally?

Hyperventilation may play a role in panic disorder. Symptoms of hyperventilation (e.g. shortness of breath) are common during panic. Exaggerated respiratory responses are associated with spontaneous panic attacks and people with panic disorder often have low arterial carbon dioxide (CO_2) caused by chronic hyperventilation. Experimental studies in which people are given CO_2 show that those with a panic disorder or a family history of panic disorder respond with greater anxiety (Zvolensky & Eifert, 2001). This effect remains even when they are compared with people with a generalised anxiety disorder or other mood disorders. Thus, it may be that people with panic disorder are more sensitive to changes in CO_2 levels. Physical vulnerability to panic is compounded by psychological factors, particularly thoughts and the interpretation of physical symptoms. Panic disorder is strongly associated with anxiety sensitivity, which is a relatively stable personal characteristic that means that people become frightened, worried, or embarrassed by physical symptoms of anxiety.

The reciprocal relationship between breathing and emotion means that controlled breathing can be useful when treating stress-related disorders, anxiety, and panic. It can also be useful in promoting emotional wellbeing in chronic lung diseases (F.-L. Lin et al., 2019; Santino et al., 2020).

16.2.2 Upper Respiratory Tract Infections

Upper respiratory tract infections (URI), such as colds and influenza, account for 50% of all acute illnesses and are a major cause of morbidity and mortality worldwide. Colds are the most common URI and are caused by over 200 viruses (Cohen et al., 2019). The economic impact of the common cold is enormous, as it includes not only the direct costs of treatment, but also the indirect costs associated with people taking time off work.

Exposure to a virus does not necessarily mean people will develop the clinical symptoms and illness that go with it. In fact, only one in three people exposed to a cold virus will develop a cold (Galanti et al., 2019). The most obvious variables to consider are the degree of exposure to a virus and the strength of someone's immune system and overall health. For example, the fact that colds are most prevalent in children may be due to a relative lack of resistance and increased exposure to viruses through contact with other children at school or nursery.

Contrary to folklore, catching a cold is not affected by cold weather. Evidence shows that putting people in cold conditions has little or no effect on the development or severity of a cold, unless these are extreme conditions (Eccles & Wilkinson, 2015). Nor is susceptibility related to factors such as exercise, diet, or enlarged tonsils or adenoids. The use of mega-doses of vitamin C does not prevent people catching colds, but it can have a small effect on speeding up recovery (Hemilä & Chalker, 2013; see also Chapter 15). There is evidence that vitamin D may reduce the risk of colds, but only among people who are already deficient (Jolliffe et al., 2021). Whereas aerobic exercise is known to enhance immune function (see Chapter 15), there is inconclusive evidence the exercise protects against developing colds (Grande et al., 2015).

Psychosocial factors associated with susceptibility to URIs include stress, poor social relationships, disrupted or short sleep, negative emotions, and lower socioeconomic status (Cohen, Alper et al., 2008; Cohen, Chiang et al., 2020; Prather et al., 2015; Robinson et al., 2021). The evidence is most convincing for stress. The impact of stress on immune function is well established (see Chapter 3), but it seems to be particularly related to a susceptibility to upper respiratory tract infections.

Social relationships also affect our susceptibility to URIs. Interpersonal stresses such as conflict with family, friends, or colleagues increase the susceptibility to colds. However, people with good social networks (both in terms of size of network, integration, and sociability) are protected to some extent from developing colds, and there is evidence that positive interpersonal relationships can reduce the harmful impact of lower SES referred to above (Cohen, Chiang et al., 2020). It is notable that more sociable people appear to be less at risk of developing colds. Although greater exposure to other people may increase the risk of contracting a virus, sociability and the immune-enhancing aspects of social support appear to be more important in determining whether a person develops a cold.

16.2.3 COVID-19: A Biopsychosocial Phenomenon

The upper respiratory tract is the key entry portal for the severe acute respiratory syndrome coronavirus 2 (SARS-CoV-2). The evidence of the impact of psychosocial factors being key in URIs became apparent following the onset of the COVID-19 pandemic. Many of the variables found to affect susceptibility to the common cold were also found to influence susceptibility to COVID-19, such as poor sleep (Shafiee et al., 2023) and chronic stress (Bienvenu et al., 2020; Lamontagne et al., 2021).

However, COVID-19 was a truly biopsychosocial phenomenon, and the absence of effective medical interventions to prevent infection highlighted the importance of individual and social behaviour, such as social distancing and the use of masks and other protective barriers (D.K. Chu et al., 2020). Reviews of research into the impact of psychosocial interventions provide some support for their impact on lowering transmission rates, but the evidence is affected by inconsistent adherence and the simultaneous impact of other legal and social measures (Jefferson et al., 2023). A meta-analysis revealed that enactment of hand hygiene, face-mask wearing, and physical distancing during the COVID-19 pandemic was significantly related to the key components of models of health behaviour (see Chapter 5): people were more likely to engage in these behaviours if they had better knowledge, more positive attitudes, and perceived stronger social norms (Liang et al., 2022). The COVID-19 pandemic also highlighted the important interactions between general beliefs and emotions (e.g. general health anxiety, conscientiousness, trust in science) and COVID-19-specific beliefs and emotions (e.g. social norms, responses to conspiracy theories, empathy for people with COVID-19) (Peters, 2022; van Mulukom et al., 2022).

Other research based on the COM-B model indicated that protective behaviours were significantly influenced by perceived and actual capability, opportunity, and motivation (L.G. Brown et al., 2022). This highlights the need to look beyond individual factors to also consider how to establish positive feedback loops that facilitate and enable healthy behaviour (e.g. installing dispensers of hand sanitiser), and thereby establish healthy norms.

16.2.4 Asthma

Asthma is one of the most common chronic diseases in the world and it is the most common chronic disease among children in developed countries. Over 260 million people worldwide – over 3% of the global population – have asthma (Shin et al., 2023). The highest prevalence is found in the UK, Ireland, New Zealand, and Australia, but most asthma deaths occur in low- and middle-income countries. Asthma attacks incur large economic costs in terms of lost productivity, medical treatment, and social security costs. In the past, asthma was thought of as a psychosomatic disease – that is, due to, or influenced by, psychological factors. We now know that numerous factors can contribute to the condition, including genetic predisposition, diet, and lifestyle factors, as summarised in Table 16.4. It can be seen that, in comparison to the CHD risk factors in Table 16.1, there are fewer lifestyle and psychosocial causes of asthma. However, psychosocial factors are very important triggers for asthma attacks in people who already have the condition.

Genetic vulnerability and parental smoking are strong risk factors for the initial onset of asthma. Although there is no specific gene that causes asthma, a combination of genes passed from parents to children approximately doubles the likelihood of children having asthma. Environmental factors are also important: around 15% of new cases of childhood asthma are attributable to traffic-related air pollution (Anenberg et al., 2022). Lifestyle factors are also important, particularly maternal smoking. Analyses of 10,860 participants in five European birth cohort studies show that children whose mothers smoked during pregnancy are more likely to develop transient or persistent asthma, especially if their mothers are heavier smokers (Thacher et al., 2018). Reducing parental smoking is therefore one of the most important modifiable risk factors for the development of asthma. Psychological knowledge can be used to develop health promotion interventions that encourage parents to give up smoking (see Chapter 5).

Stressful life events may be involved in triggering asthma symptoms or exacerbating symptoms in people who already have asthma (Liu et al., 2013; Plourde et al., 2017). Research has also shown that children who are exposed to, or experience, conflict report more symptoms and have an increased risk of complications (Bierstetel et al., 2021; Tobin et al., 2015). The core pathological process of inflammation of the airways has led to the proposal that stress-induced changes in immune responses may contribute to this exacerbation and triggering of asthma (see Chapter 3).

Table 16.4 Risk factors for developing asthma or triggering asthma episodes

	Development of asthma	Factors that trigger asthma attacks or exacerbate symptoms
Physical	Genetic vulnerability (family history)	Allergens, e.g. pollen, dust mites
	Air pollution	Food allergies, e.g. nuts, shellfish
		Chest infections
		Chemical fumes or pollution
		Cold weather
Demographic	Age (younger)	
	Sex (male)	
	Socioeconomic status	
	Ethnic minority	
	Maternal age (younger)	
Lifestyle	Maternal smoking in pregnancy	Smoke
	Maternal anxiety	
	Smoking in the home	Intense exercise
	Violence in the home	
Psychosocial	Childhood adversity or stress	Stress
		Anxiety
		Exposure to conflict

For example, in one study, children with and without asthma were asked to make a speech and do mental arithmetic in front of an audience (Buske-Kirschbaum et al., 2003). The children did not differ in their heart rate responses to this stress, but those with asthma showed a significantly reduced cortisol response. Cortisol is anti-inflammatory, so dysregulation of the cortisol response may be important in chronic asthma. There are similar findings for other chronic inflammatory diseases, such as rheumatoid arthritis (see Chapter 15).

Section 16.2.2 explained that chronic stress makes people much more vulnerable to respiratory infections. The role of respiratory tract infections in triggering asthma is well established: it is another important pathway between stress and asthma attacks (Trueba & Ritz, 2013). Section 16.2.1 highlighted the links between breathing and emotions, particularly anxiety. Research syntheses suggest that breathing training for asthma leads to improved outcomes in quality of life, hyperventilation symptoms, and lung function in adults, but the lack of similar clear evidence among children may be because breathing training is often presented as part of broader intervention programmes that are effective (Macêdo et al., 2016; Santino et al., 2020).

There is evidence that anxiety and anxiety-related disorders can exacerbate asthma symptoms. For example, a study of self-reported asthma attacks after the 9/11 terrorist attacks showed that among people with asthma, those who also had PTSD were three times more likely to have symptoms and visit their doctor, and six times more likely to visit hospital emergency departments. This increased risk was irrespective of pre-9/11 asthma symptoms, demographic characteristics, or the amount of physical exposure to the attacks (Fagan et al., 2003). It therefore appears that anxiety disorders are important in the triggering and perception of asthma symptoms. Meta-analysis indicates that people with asthma are more likely than the rest of the population to have anxiety disorders (Ye et al., 2021), and evidence reviews indicate that CBT for anxiety may be an effective way to target the mechanisms thought to maintain this comorbidity (McGovern et al., 2023; Pateraki & Morris, 2018).

Psychological factors are very important when it comes to managing asthma. People with asthma are expected to monitor their symptoms and use inhaler medication when they need it. However, many people with asthma are unable to reliably detect changes in their lung function (Still & Dolen, 2016). Some evidence suggests that providing people with feedback on their lung function can lead to more accurate estimates of lung function, which may result in better adherence to controller medications (Feldman et al., 2012).

The perception of symptoms and medical outcomes is associated with various psychological factors, including anxiety, pessimism, and perceived stigma (Feldman, Arcoleo et al., 2023; Feldman, Becker et al., 2021). Compared to objective measures of asthma symptoms, these factors are better predictors of outcomes, such as the number of times a person is hospitalised for asthma, how long they stay, and their medication prescription. Thus, there is a strong role for psychological factors in the management of asthma symptoms and their consequences. This is illustrated in Case Study 16.2, which shows how someone's illness representations can affect how they manage their symptoms (see Chapter 4, section 4.4).

Case Study 16.2

Illness Representations and Asthma Symptoms

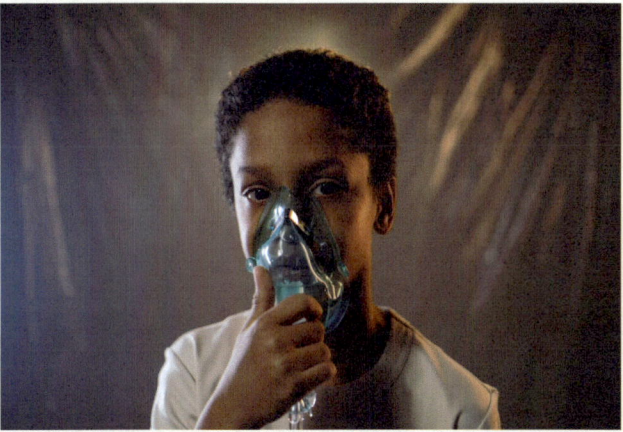

Figure 16.6   Different representations of asthma

Source: © cottonbro studio/Pexels

(Continued)

Consider the following differences in how a young boy thinks about his asthma.

Table 16.5   Illness representations related to asthma symptoms

Illness identity	Asthma is a mild condition.	Asthma is a severe condition
Cause	Caused by infections and a pet allergy	I inherited it from my dad
Timeline	It's something that many people grow out of	It'll never go away
Control	I can control the symptoms and exposure to triggers	I can't control it
Consequences management	It is unlikely to kill me	If it gets bad it could kill me
	Relaxed attitude but avoids triggers where possible; will increase medication when he has an infection. Low anxiety, so will only visit the doctor when his own attempts to manage his symptoms do not work	Tense and anxious about asthma symptoms. Has not thought about what might trigger his asthma, so is constantly worried and hypervigilant. Takes regular preventive medication and visits his doctor at the first sign of breathlessness

Global guidelines for asthma suggest that self-management should be incorporated into a continuous cycle of assessment, treatment, and review (Global Initiative for Asthma, 2018). Psychological interventions to help people manage asthma include: education, objective monitoring of lung function, self-monitoring of lung function and triggers, developing an action plan to help the patient to know what to do during an asthma episode, and exploring and modifying illness beliefs. There is evidence that patient-centred self-management interventions are highly effective and result in reduced hospitalisation, fewer visits to health professionals, and fewer days off school or work (Normansell et al., 2017). There is also sufficient evidence to show that asthma self-management apps and other digital interventions can produce similar benefits (A. Chan et al., 2022), as in Research Box 16.3, which shows how digital psychological interventions can promote adherence and management of asthma.

Research Box 16.3

A Mobile Phone Intervention to Increase Asthma Control

Background

To best manage asthma, people must take at least 80% of their preventative doses of inhaled corticosteroid medication. People with asthma often fail to meet this requirement. It is therefore important to identify ways to promote healthier beliefs among people with asthma: digital interventions can be an accessible, low-cost method of enhancing self-management.

Method and Findings

This study compared a fully-functional asthma management app to a version of the app with limited functionality. The participants were 411 adults whose scores on the Asthma

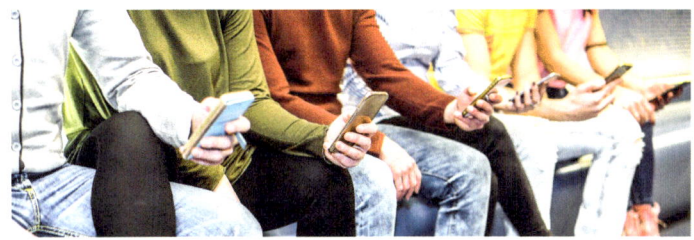

Figure 16.7   Using mobile phones to manage asthma

Source: © DisobeyArt/Adobe Stock

Control Test (ACT) indicated uncontrolled asthma. They were randomly allocated to the intervention or the control group. The intervention app presented participants with personalised weather, pollen, and air pollution data, and used passively-gathered smartphone data to provide personalised recommendations about healthy behaviours. At the eight-week follow-up, the participants in the intervention group had significantly higher mean ACT scores than the control group, and were significantly more likely to have a clinically meaningful improvement in their ACT score. There were no significant differences in the worsening of asthma or health-related quality of life.

Significance

Digital apps appear to be a cheap and effective way of improving asthma control. It may be an efficient way to deliver interventions to people who find it difficult to engage with face-to-face interventions. However, the authors also noted that high drop-out rates indicate a need to identify barriers to both initial engagement and continued engagement.

Kandola, A., Edwards, K., Straatmen, J., Dührkoop, B., Hein, B. & Hayes, J. (2024) Digital self-management platform for adult asthma: Randomized attention-placebo controlled trial. *Journal of Medical Internet Research, 26*: e50855. doi:10.2196/50855.

Clinical Notes 16.2

Treating Respiratory Disorders

- Smoking and passive smoking are among the most important, modifiable risk factors.
- Most people cannot reliably detect changes in their lung function. It is important to confirm people's self-reports with physical measures, such as a spirometer.
- Anxiety is strongly implicated in respiratory symptoms. Symptoms can be triggered or exacerbated by stress and anxiety.
- Symptoms are strongly affected by anxiety and beliefs about illness – these factors are more predictive of health outcomes than objective physical health.

(Continued)

- Self-management programmes are very effective at helping people to manage their illness better.
- Self-management programmes involve education, self-monitoring of lung function and triggers, using action plans to cope during episodes, and exploring and changing people's beliefs about illness.
- Guidelines state that self-management programmes should be incorporated into regular medical care.

Summary 16.2

- The reciprocal relationship between breathing and emotion means that controlled breathing can be useful when treating stress-related disorders and panic.
- Susceptibility to URIs is affected by stress, social relationships, sleep, emotions, and socioeconomic status. The effect of stress and social relationships on susceptibility to URIs is probably mediated by changes in immune function.
- Traditionally, asthma has been viewed as a psychosomatic illness, but the evidence shows that the initial onset is mainly determined by biological factors (genetic vulnerability, age, sex) and parental factors (e.g. being exposed to smoking or violence in the home).
- Anxiety is strongly implicated in respiratory symptoms. In those who have asthma, symptoms can be triggered or exacerbated by stress and anxiety.
- Although psychological factors are not strongly implicated in the onset of asthma, they are very important when it comes to managing it. Self-management interventions are highly effective, and can result in fewer hospitalisations, visits to the doctor, or days off.

Conclusion

This chapter has examined the role of psychosocial risk factors in cardiovascular and respiratory disease. There are similarities and differences in the role of psychosocial factors in disorders of these two body systems. Psychosocial factors are extensively associated with cardiovascular disease: lifestyle, stress, and negative emotions are critical in the development of disease and the subsequent prognosis. Depression and anger/hostility are particularly implicated in heart disease. Respiratory disorders are also affected by lifestyle, stress, and emotions, but research shows that anxiety is especially important. In the respiratory disorders addressed here, psychosocial factors are less involved in the development of pathology but are implicated in triggering or exacerbating symptoms. Of course, we have only looked at URIs and asthma, and it is true to say that lifestyle factors – particularly smoking – are critical in the development of other respiratory diseases, such as chronic obstructive pulmonary disease (COPD) and lung cancer. Furthermore, whereas it is too soon to quantify the long-term damage to lungs caused by electronic cigarettes or vapes, the short-term harms are clear (Jonas, 2022).

Psychological intervention in cardiac or respiratory rehabilitation has various positive effects. In cardiac rehabilitation, psychological intervention improves psychological wellbeing and can reduce overall mortality, but it does not always affect specific cardiac outcomes. In chronic respiratory disorders, there is strong evidence that interventions that address psychological components, including self-management, can improve symptom management and healthcare use.

Further Reading

Llewellyn, C.D. et al. (eds) (2019) *Cambridge Handbook of Psychology, Health and Medicine* (3rd edition). Cambridge: Cambridge University Press. Includes short chapters on cardiovascular disease, coronary heart disease, and hypertension, as well as specific respiratory disorders (asthma, lung cancer, COPD, colds).

Levenson, J.L. (ed.) (2019) *The American Psychiatric Publishing Textbook of Psychosomatic Medicine: Psychiatric Care of the Medically Ill* (3rd edition). Arlington, VA: American Psychiatric Association Publishing. Covers many of the topics discussed in this and other chapters, including heart disease, lung disease, oncology, and psychological interventions.

Revision Questions

1 Describe three pathways by which psychosocial factors influence the onset and progression of cardiovascular disease.
2 Outline the major psychosocial risk factors for cardiovascular disease and the magnitude of their effect.
3 How do individual differences in cardiac reactivity to stress affect the risk of cardiovascular disease?
4 Describe the common psychological responses to cardiovascular disease. Outline the impact of psychosocial interventions on physical and psychological wellbeing in cardiovascular disease.
5 Outline the factors associated with delays to seeking treatment for CHD and non-adherence to treatment regimens.
6 How is the relationship between breathing and emotions reciprocal? What is the clinical relevance of this observation?
7 Describe how psychosocial factors influence susceptibility to upper respiratory tract infections.
8 Compare the relative importance of psychological and biological factors for asthma onset and episodes.
9 Outline why self-management interventions are effective in treating asthma.
10 Compare and contrast the role of psychosocial factors in cardiovascular and respiratory disease.

17

GASTROINTESTINAL HEALTH

┌─Learning Objectives─┐

This chapter is designed to enable you to:

- Outline the physiological basis for the relationship between psychological factors and gastrointestinal (GI) health.
- Describe the role of stress in GI function and illness.
- Consider the impact of diet and alcohol use on GI health and illness.
- Outline the role of psychosocial factors in specific GI disorders.

There are clear links between psychology and the gastrointestinal (GI) system. This close relationship is illustrated in common language. Common expressions of psychological states include (to follow the sequence of the GI tract) *choking* on information, not *digesting* difficult news, having butterflies in the *stomach*, someone making us *sick*, having a *gut* feeling, or being scared *shitless*. Direct bi-directional physiological links exist between the brain, autonomic nervous system, and enteric nervous system. This is called the brain–gut axis. The four main links between psychological states and the GI system are:

1   Brain–gut axis.
2   Effect of stress on GI function.
3   Effect of lifestyle on GI function and wellbeing (e.g. diet, alcohol use, smoking).
4   Psychological impact of GI disorders.

The relative importance of these links varies. Functional GI disorders, such as irritable bowel syndrome (IBS) and dyspepsia, are strongly affected by psychosocial factors such as stress and symptom perception. Organic disorders, such as cirrhosis or cancer, have stronger associations with lifestyle factors, such as diet and alcohol use. GI medicine is therefore an area that certainly requires a biopsychosocial approach to prevention and treatment.

We start this chapter by examining how psychological factors interact with GI functioning through the brain–gut axis and the role of stress. We then examine the role of lifestyle factors on GI health, concentrating on diet and alcohol use. Finally, disorders of the GI system are examined to illustrate the complex interplay between psychology and the gut, and the profound impact of GI disorders.

17.1 Psychological Factors and the GI System

Physiological responses to stress involve the central nervous system (CNS), autonomic nervous systems (ANS), and immune and neuroendocrine responses (see Chapter 3). All of these are implicated to varying degrees in GI function or disorders (Alexander & Turnbaugh, 2020; Maier & al'Absi, 2017).

17.1.1 The Brain–Gut Axis

The **brain–gut axis** comprises the CNS, ANS, and enteric nervous system (see Figure 17.1). The sympathetic and parasympathetic branches of the ANS innervate GI organs such as the stomach, liver, spleen, pancreas, and bowel. Under stress, the sympathetic nervous system and subsequent release of adrenaline (epinephrine) increases blood supply to the muscles, but reduces GI blood flow and peristalsis, and inhibits the contraction of the rectum. Sympathetic activation is also associated with reduced food intake and weight loss. Under normal conditions, the parasympathetic nervous system restores blood flow and peristalsis to the usual functioning when the stressor is removed.

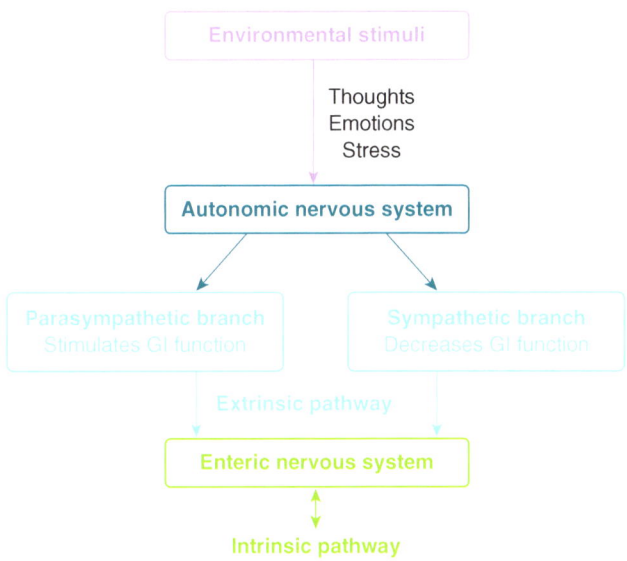

Figure 17.1 The brain–gut axis

The **enteric nervous system** is embedded in the lining of the GI system and has been referred to as the '*brain of the gut*' or '*second brain*' because it is large and complex (approximately 100 million neurons) and uses the same neurotransmitters as the CNS (Abdullah et al., 2020). Although it is connected to the CNS, it is able to operate independently without conscious control. It controls all the functions of the GI tract. Sensory information is sent from the enteric system to the CNS via the 'vagal nerve' or 'vagus nerve' (the tenth cranial nerve). The longest nerve in the ANS, the vagus nerve contains both sensory and motor fibres, and is thought to comprise 80% afferent fibres (Goyal & Hirano, 1996).

The existence and influence of the brain–gut axis means that psychological and gastric phenomena influence each other (Keightley et al., 2015; Maier & al'Absi, 2017; Makris et al., 2021). For example, placebos and suggestion may increase or decrease GI activity (Meissner, 2009), and the symptoms of nausea and vomiting can be classically conditioned, such as when people having chemotherapy develop anticipatory nausea (see Chapter 10). People with functional GI disorders are more likely to have psychological disorders or to have had past traumatic experiences. Furthermore, a high prevalence of functional GI disorders is found in people with mental health problems, especially depression and anxiety disorders (Makris et al., 2021).

This reciprocal relationship between emotions and GI function is found not only in people with GI disorders. For all of us, emotions such as anxiety and disgust are linked with GI symptoms. Disgust tends to be accompanied by physiological movements that mimic retching or vomiting. Products of the GI system (e.g. vomit, faeces) are universal triggers of disgust across cultures (Rozin et al., 2018). Anxiety is associated with changes in GI function. In one study, healthy volunteers were asked to recall experiences that had made them feel anxious, or experiences that were neutral. These were recorded and then played back to them while they underwent various tests of gastric function. When listening to the recording of their anxious experience, volunteers had reduced gastric function and more reports of bloating and fullness (Geeraerts et al., 2005).

In functional GI disorders the brain–gut axis may become dysregulated. This is analogous to ANS and HPA-axis dysregulation in stress disorders (see Chapter 3), or dysregulation of immune responses in autoimmune disorders (see Chapter 15). Dysregulation of the brain–gut axis leads to altered sensation, symptoms, motility, and other aspects of GI function. Other alterations include an increased sensitivity to GI symptoms and altered pain pathways. Permanent changes may occur to the distribution of neurons in the enteric nervous system in chronic disease, such as Crohn's disease or ulcerative colitis (Villanacci et al., 2008). It has been noted that whereas many treatments for these conditions target inflammatory pathology, better understanding of enteric nervous system processes may allow the development of alternative treatment options (Stavely et al., 2020).

17.1.2 Stress and the GI System

As the brain–gut axis is intricately connected with stress responses, it is not surprising that stress affects GI function in healthy people and exacerbates existing GI disorders, particularly functional disorders such as irritable bowel syndrome (IBS) (Schaper & Stengel, 2022), and stomach ulcers (Fink, 2017). Most people report changes in bowel function in response to stress, and experimental studies indicate that stress can produce changes in bowel function (Pritchard et al., 2015). Stress leads to numerous changes in the gut, including increased motility, altered ion secretion, increased intestinal permeability, low-grade inflammation, epithelial abnormalities, and enteric neuron dysfunction. In people with GI disorders, stress can contribute to gastric erosions and ulcers, and increase the severity of colitis (Fink, 2017). Stress may interact with pathogens such as *Helicobacter pylori* or non-steroidal anti-inflammatory drugs (NSAIDs) to increase the likelihood of GI disorders (Fink, 2017).

The relationship between stress and GI function is complex because stress is also associated with psychological factors, such as an increased sensitivity to GI sensations and symptoms, decreased pain tolerance, and changes in behaviour that can affect GI function (Ferdousi & Finn, 2018; Jennings et al., 2014). Emotional distress, increased sensitivity, and an increased perception of symptoms may play a role in this. For example, in addition to reporting more anxiety, depression, and reduced quality of life, people with constipation are also more likely to monitor symptoms, are more sensitive to rectal distension and urge sensations, and are less tolerant of bowel volume (Chan et al., 2005). In a more recent study, people reporting high functional GI symptoms had heightened perceptions of various bodily sensations alongside a reduced trust in bodily signals (Gajdos et al., 2021). As for other conditions, it appears that for GI disorders, there are important associations between symptom perception, pain, psychological wellbeing, and coping strategies that may be mutually reinforcing (Dent et al., 2022; Knowles et al., 2017).

Although the relationship between stress and GI symptoms is well established, the exact causal mechanisms through which it occurs are complex, and are likely to involve many factors, including physiological changes, emotional wellbeing, sensitivity, and symptom perception (see Figure 17.2). Stress may interact with other factors, such as exposure to pathogens, unhealthy lifestyles, and individual differences in coping style. This means that treating GI disorders can be particularly challenging: health professionals must assess which physical and psychosocial factors are contributing to the disorder and then treat them appropriately. In recent years, interventions focused on psychotherapeutic practices and processes have been found to alleviate pain and improve quality of life in many people with GI disorders (Lackner & Jaccard, 2021). Research Box 17.1 indicates that the availability and accessibility of online and smartphone interventions mean that more people may be able to experience the benefits of such interventions.

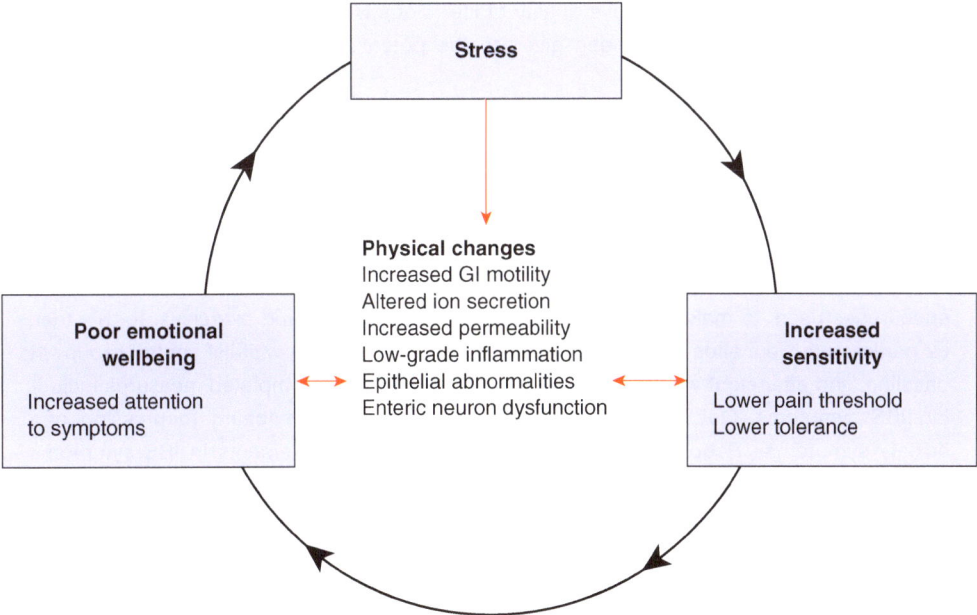

Figure 17.2   Stress and GI function

Research Box 17.1

Mobile Digital Cognitive Behavioural Therapy for Irritable Bowel Syndrome

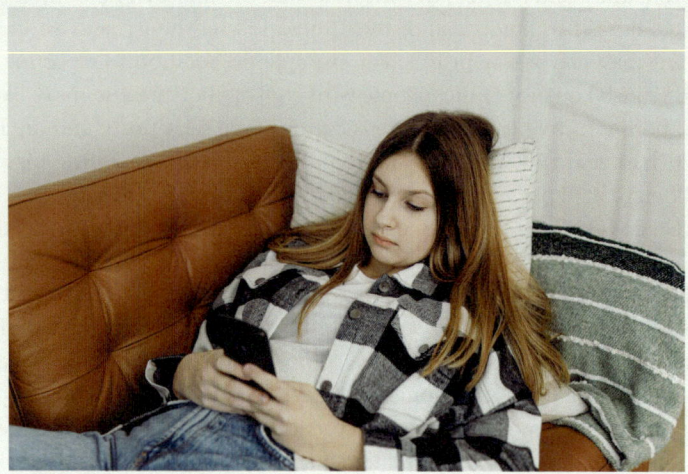

Figure 17.3　Mobile phone therapy for IBS

Source: © kaboompics.com/Pexels

Background

Cognitive behavioural therapy (CBT) has been shown to reduce the symptoms of irritable bowel syndrome (IBS) and improve quality of life (QoL). Because access to qualified therapists is limited, attention has been given to the potential for smartphone-based digital CBT for IBS.

Method and Findings

The mobile phone app Zemedy delivers an eight-week programme that addresses knowledge, relaxation skills, stress management, exercise, and behavioural experiments to encourage new ways of living with IBS. An integrated chatbot presents the app content and encourages users to make specific plans, including homework and exercises. In this trial, 62 participants were allocated to use the app or were placed in a wait-list control group. At baseline, and after eight weeks and three months, participants completed measures including IBS symptoms, QoL, general health, and psychological wellbeing (depression and anxiety symptoms). People in the intervention recorded improvements in IBS symptoms and QoL that were generally maintained at three months post-treatment. The improvement in QoL was partially explained by reductions in visceral sensitivity and catastrophic thinking about IBS. There was less strong evidence of improvements in psychological wellbeing.

Significance

The authors noted some limitations to the study, such as the relatively small sample and the lack of a placebo control group. However, the results of this trial are promising. Because the app requires no in-person input from health professionals, and is not restricted by schedules or geography, it can increase the accessibility of CBT, which is an effective evidence-based treatment in IBS.

Hunt, M., Miguez, S., Dukas, B., Onwude, O. & White, S. (2021) Efficacy of Zemedy, a mobile digital therapeutic for the self-management of irritable bowel syndrome: A cross-over randomized controlled trial. *JMIR mHealth and uHealth, 9*(5): e26152. doi:10.2196/26152.

17.1.3 A Biopsychosocial Approach to GI Disorders: The Case of Peptic Ulcers

One clear example of the need to take a biopsychosocial approach to GI health is the history of our understanding of peptic ulcers. Historically, suggested causal factors included vascular occlusion, gastric acid, friction/abrasion, psychosomatic factors, and stress, but in the early 1980s Robin Warren and Barry Marshall conducted Nobel Prize-winning research which identified the role of the bacterium **Helicobacter Pylori** in stomach ulcers (Marshall & Warren, 1984). Marshall used himself as a guinea-pig and infected himself with *H. pylori*, after which he developed gastritis. This discovery changed our understanding of what causes peptic ulcers. Since then, research has shown that *H. pylori* can be associated with a range of GI problems, including dyspepsia (heartburn, bloating, and nausea), gastritis, ulcers, and stomach cancer. Treatment of *H. pylori* with antibiotics has resulted in a steady decline in the incidence of peptic ulcers.

However, not all people with *H. pylori* develop disease, and up to 20% of people with ulcers do not have *H. pylori*. It is now thought, therefore, that *H. pylori* alone does not cause ulcers, but interacts with other factors, including genetic vulnerability, diet, excess stomach acid, and use of non-steroid anti-inflammatory drugs (NSAIDs) and aspirin (Katelaris et al., 2023; Lanas & Chan, 2017). Importantly, it has been estimated that psychosocial factors such as stress and lifestyle contribute to 30–65% of ulcers, regardless of whether they are caused by *H. pylori* or NSAIDs (Levenstein et al., 2015). Thus, research into *H. pylori* and peptic ulcers illustrates how we have moved from a purely biological explanation to a biopsychosocial explanation of peptic ulcer disease.

Summary 17.1

- The brain–gut axis comprises the CNS, ANS, and enteric nervous system, which means psychological and GI states influence each other quickly and easily.
- The enteric nervous system is connected with the CNS but is able to operate independently.

(Continued)

- In functional GI disorders, the brain–gut axis may become dysregulated.
- The relationship between stress and GI function and symptoms is well established, but this complex relationship involves many physiological and psychological factors.
- Stress leads to changes in GI motility and physiology. It is also associated with lower pain tolerance, increased sensitivity to GI sensations, greater perception of symptoms, and changes in lifestyle that may further affect GI function.
- A biopsychosocial approach is vital in GI medicine, as illustrated by the interaction between *H. pylori* and psychosocial factors in peptic ulcers.

17.2 Lifestyle and GI Health

Lifestyle factors such as diet, smoking, alcohol use, and exercise affect GI health. Smoking is associated with an increased risk of Crohn's disease, peptic ulcers, and cancers of the upper GI tract, but a reduced risk of ulcerative colitis. What we eat influences our risk of developing many disorders, including cancer, diabetes, and the intermediate outcome of obesity: it is estimated that approximately 30% of cancers in developed countries are caused by unhealthy diets. Furthermore, the increase in cancers of the GI system in low- and middle-income (developing) countries reflects the increased consumption of animal products and more sedentary lifestyles (Sung et al., 2021). The liver has a key role in filtering toxins, and alcohol consumption is therefore a risk factor for liver disorders. Ethanol is a carcinogen, and alcohol use is a risk factor for numerous cancers of the GI tract (cancer of the oropharynx, larynx, oesophagus, liver, colon, and rectum) as well as breast cancer (Connor, 2017). In this section we therefore examine diet and alcohol use in more detail.

17.2.1 Healthy and Disordered Eating

Diet is important to GI health. However, the links are complex because our diet consists of different nutrients that can affect our health directly or in combination with each other.

Diet and GI Health

Various aspects of diet are important to health (see Highlight Box 17.1). Although there are some areas where evidence is incomplete or inconsistent, the following aspects of diet are known to be important for GI health:

- *High fibre* reduces bowel cancer risk by up to 40%. This may be due to the effect of fibre on bowel function (i.e. stools spend less time in the bowel), so there is less time for food-related chemicals and antigens to damage the bowel lining. It may also be due to the creation of short-chain fatty acids when fibre is broken down, which may make it harder for tumours to develop.

- *Fruit and vegetables* reduce the risk of cancers, particularly of the upper GI tract. This may be because they are a good source of fibre (as above) or because they provide vitamins A, B, and C, which may protect against cancer.
- *Oily fish*, such as salmon and mackerel, decrease the risk of GI cancers.
- *Salt* is associated with an increased risk of stomach cancer, which is more prevalent in countries that have a very salty diet, such as Japan.
- *Red meat* increases the risk of stomach and bowel cancer, particularly if the meat is processed (e.g. bacon, salami). The increased risk is thought to be due to chemicals contained in red meat, such as haem, that damage the bowel when broken down. Carcinogens are also created when meat is cooked at high temperatures.

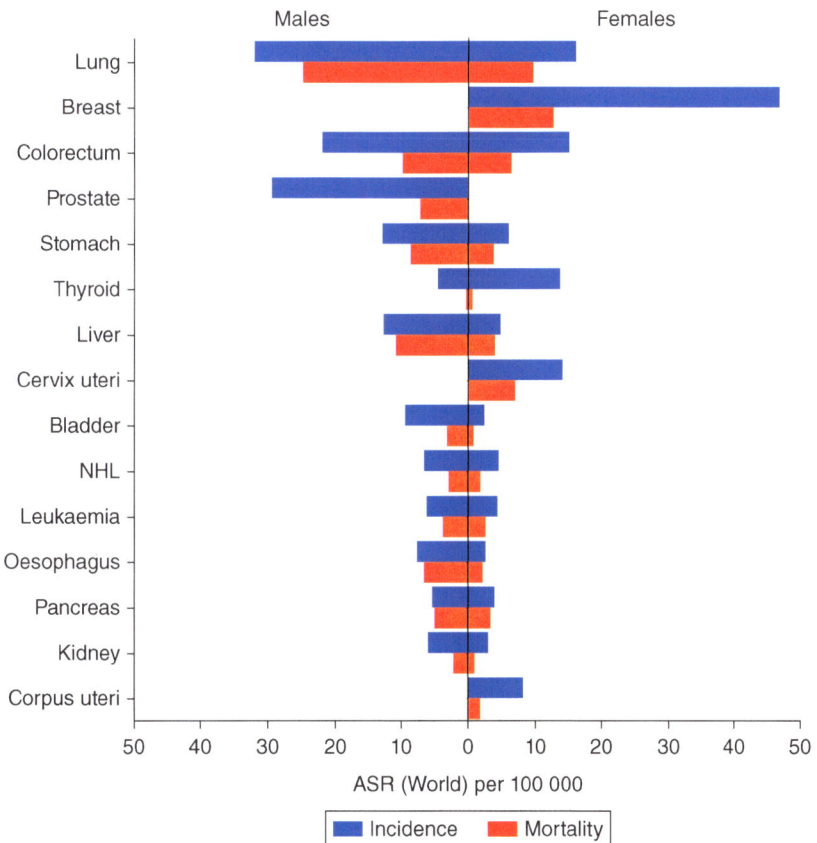

Figure 17.4 Age-standardised cancer rate (world) per 100,000, incidence and mortality, males (left of zero line) and females (right of zero line), in 2022

Source: Cancer TODAY | International Agency for Research on Cancer - https://gco.iarc.who.int
© World Health Organization

Highlight Box 17.1

Guidelines for a Healthy Diet

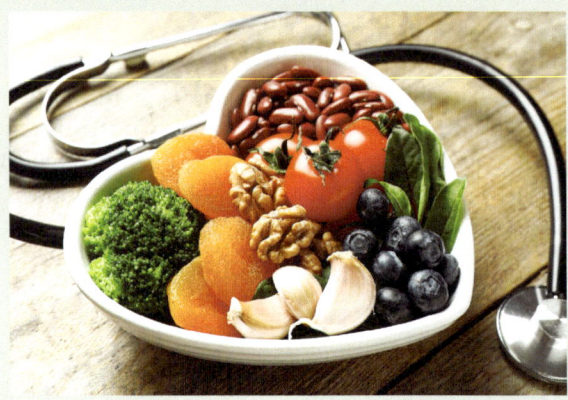

Figure 17.5 Heart-healthy foods

Image credit: © New Africa/Adobe Stock

- Diet should be high in fibre: it should include fruit, vegetables, pulses, rice, and wholegrain foods.
- Eat 5+ portions of fruit and vegetables per day.
- Eat 2+ portions of oily fish a week.
- Decrease the intake of red or processed meat.
- If you drink alcohol, do so in moderation.
- Limit salt intake.
- Avoid refined sugar.
- Avoid saturated fats.

Activity 17.1

How Healthy is Your Diet?

- How does your diet compare to the recommendations given in Highlight Box 17.1?
- What kinds of factors influence the types of food you eat and when?

Why Do We Eat What We Eat?

Given the evidence outlined above, it is a public health concern that many people do not have a healthy diet (GBD 2017 Diet Collaborators, 2019; Qiao et al., 2022). In addition, although there is some variation in diets between countries, globalisation has resulted in an increasing homogenisation of diets. Whatever the norm for a particular country, women usually eat more fruit, vegetables, fibre, and less saturated fat than men. This appears to be because women have more concerns about weight, and healthier food-related attitudes and beliefs.

With obesity increasing (World Health Organization, 2023b), it is important to understand how poor dietary habits develop. Research suggests that we are not born with a tendency to overeat or have a poor diet. Studies of infants and young children suggest that if they are offered a variety of healthy food and allowed to eat what they want, they will naturally choose a balanced diet (Tanofsky-Kraff et al., 2007). Poor dietary habits therefore appear to be learnt. This learning occurs through the processes of exposure, reinforcement, modelling, and imitation during childhood (see Chapter 10). For example, reviews indicate that although peers and siblings can have positive influences on healthy eating, their overall effect tends to be negative (Ragelienė & Grønhøj, 2020).

Dietary habits are also influenced by attitudes, beliefs, and weight concerns in adolescence and adulthood. Children will eat the food they are exposed to, and will prefer those foods they are exposed to regularly. Therefore, the more that unhealthy food is available and accessible in the environment (e.g. fast food), the more likely it is that children will eat and prefer this type of food. Eating habits are also shaped through imitating friends and family. Modelling good eating behaviour can be used to promote healthy eating. For example, studies in several countries have assessed the impact of peer role models or 'food dudes' – older children who were filmed enthusiastically eating healthy food – and found that exposure to such modelling can successfully change children's preferences for foods and increase their fruit and vegetable intake (Laureati et al., 2014; Marcano-Olivier et al., 2021).

The meaning of food in interactions between children and parents can shape children's eating behaviour. Food used as a reward or a treat will be liked more and preferred over food that is seen as a non-reward. This means that strategies such as telling children they can only have a dessert if they eat their vegetables may result in children learning to prefer pudding and dislike vegetables. Parental control over what children eat may have different effects depending on how the control is exercised. Hidden or covert control, such as making sure unhealthy food is not available in the child's environment, is associated with less snacking on sweets or energy-dense foods, and can lead to lower BMI (Say et al., 2023). Overt control, such as telling the child what they can and cannot eat, is associated with an increased intake of healthy foods like fruit. However, parental restrictions may lead to a child eating more 'bad' foods when not in the home environment or under parental control.

For children and adults, food consumption is influenced by the availability of healthy and less healthy food options, which has led to growing interest in the impact of 'nudge' strategies to encourage healthier behaviour by changing the 'choice environment' (Ensaff, 2021; Turner et al., 2021). When applied to dietary behaviour, this may mean making healthy food options more visible, easier to choose, or the default options on menus, and making less healthy food options less easy to obtain. There is evidence that such approaches are effective in relation to children's choice of meals at school, and adults' fruit and vegetable intake (Lindstrom et al., 2023; Marcano-Olivier et al., 2020; Yi et al., 2022). However, as is the case in many other domains, nudging is only one strategy, and sustained and widespread behaviour change requires multifaceted approaches (Wright & Bragge, 2018).

In adolescence and young adulthood, diet is increasingly affected by body dissatisfaction and weight concerns. One longitudinal study in the USA followed adolescents and young adults over a 15-year period and found that dieting was common, and increased over time for young women and young men. At the start of the study, 56% of women and 29% of men had been on a diet to lose weight in the last year, but 15 years later it had increased to over 65% of women and 44% of men (Haynos et al., 2018). Although extreme dieting behaviours such as fasting and self-induced vomiting were less common, they were as common in young adulthood as adolescence. A separate US study used a 30-year follow-up from age 20 to age 50 and found that at all ages women had a greater drive for thinness, and were more likely to report eating disorders. Notably, whereas drive for thinness and eating disorders became less common as women aged, no such age-related changes were found among men (T.A. Brown et al., 2020).

A meta-analysis of over 1 million people worldwide revealed that at least one-third were trying to lose weight (Santos et al., 2017). The likelihood of trying to lose weight was greater among those who were overweight or obese. However, large-scale studies of university students in high-, low- and middle-income countries indicate that many people with healthy weights want or intend to lose weight, and that many people with unhealthy weights do not want or intend to change their weight (Gorbeña et al., 2021; Peltzer & Pengpid, 2015).

Dietary restraint or restrained eating does not always lead to attainment or maintenance of a healthy weight (Clark, 2015). It is therefore important to note that restrained eating outside validated weight-loss programmes is often associated with a range of negative psychological states, including body dissatisfaction, food cravings, preoccupations with food, guilt about food/eating, over-estimating body size, low self-esteem, anxiety, and depression, and may contribute to eating disorders such as anorexia and bulimia (Gorrell et al., 2019; Schaumberg et al., 2016; Stewart et al., 2022). Conversely, disinhibited or uncontrolled eating – where people find it hard to control their eating in response to environmental cues, including festive periods – may play a role in overeating and obesity (Bryant et al., 2019; Zorbas et al., 2020).

The following sections take a biopsychosocial approach to different eating disorders, but it is important to note the effect that emotions can have on the eating behaviour of people of normal weight who do not have eating disorders. For example, meta-analyses indicate that stress, depression, and sadness tend to elicit eating behaviours that are unhealthy because of the amount that people eat and/or the types of foods that people choose to eat as part of efforts to make themselves feel better – that is, 'comfort foods' that are high in fat and/or sugar (Devonport et al., 2019; Hill et al., 2022).

Disordered Eating: Anorexia, Bulimia, and Binge Eating

Paradoxically, as food has become more widely available, there has been an increase in disordered eating: anorexia nervosa, bulimia nervosa, and binge eating disorder. Estimates of lifetime prevalence are 1–2%, but many more people may have symptoms of eating disorders without meeting the full criteria for diagnosis. Eating disorders are associated with an increased risk of other psychiatric problems, such as phobias, anxiety disorders, substance misuse, and personality disorders (Dolan et al., 2022; Dufresne et al., 2020; Fornaro et al., 2021; Keski-Rahkonen, 2021; Schaumberg et al., 2021; van Eeden et al., 2021). Eating disorders can lead to a variety of physical problems, especially GI tract disorders such as gastric reflux, peptic ulcers, and constipation. Severe cases can lead to other problems, such as cardiac arrhythmias or cardiac arrest. Furthermore, eating disorders may increase the risk of premature death by a factor of five or more (van Eeden et al., 2021).

Anorexia nervosa is a refusal to maintain a healthy body weight. Anorexia has a lifetime prevalence of approximately 4% of women and 0.3% of men, and cases are increasing. It is most likely to occur in women during their teenage years or early adulthood, and it is rare for new cases to occur after age 25 (see Case Study 17.1). White women from wealthy families are most at risk. Anorexia is also more prevalent in certain occupational groups, such as models and dancers, where there is pressure to be thin. Anorexia has the highest mortality rate of any psychiatric disorder, with suicide a common cause of death.

Many potential causes of anorexia have been proposed, including genetic vulnerability, biological abnormalities in noradrenaline or serotonin systems, mood disturbances, a need for control, low self-esteem, perfectionism, the internalisation of thin body ideals, dysfunctional family dynamics, and childhood sexual abuse. Although these factors have been found to be *associated* with anorexia, there is little prospective research that allows us to determine whether such factors are the causes or consequences of anorexia. Twin studies indicate that genetic and environmental factors are both important (Paolacci et al., 2020).

Bulimia nervosa is characterised by binge eating followed by compensatory behaviours. These usually take the form of purging (e.g. self-induced vomiting or the use of laxatives) or non-purging (e.g. excessive exercising or fasting). Bulimia nervosa affects around 3% of women and 1% of men (van Eeden et al., 2021). People with bulimia are often of an average weight, which means that the condition can often go undetected.

Most evidence supports a social-cognitive explanation of bulimia, where the promotion of thin body-ideals in the media leads to increased body dissatisfaction, negative feelings, and low self-esteem. These negative feelings can trigger dieting and bulimic behaviours. Bingeing and purging are thought to be used by bulimics to deal with or distract from their negative feelings and thoughts. This then becomes self-reinforcing because it temporarily removes negative feelings. Evidence supports this explanation. Research confirms that binge eating is usually preceded by negative emotions, such as anxiety, depression, or loneliness, and may also be influenced by the ability to control impulses (Zanella & Lee, 2022).

Binge eating disorder (BED) or **uncontrolled eating** is increasing. The prevalence of BED is around 2–4% of women and 1–2% of men (Keski-Rahkonen, 2021; Kjeldberg & Clausen, 2023). BED differs from other eating disorders in a number of ways. In contrast to anorexia, new cases of BED have a broader age of onset (Favaro et al., 2019). BED also tends to last longer than anorexia and bulimia (Schaumberg et al., 2019). Furthermore, sex differences are less marked than for other eating disorders.

People with BED are not necessarily obese, although BED is more common in obese people than in the general population. Its aetiology is unclear, but it is thought to be due to factors similar to those associated with bulimia: initial increases in weight can lead to body dissatisfaction, dietary restraint, negative emotions, and emotional eating, which increases the risk of BED. Experimental studies indicate that compared to other people, the eating behaviour of people with BED, and their sense of control over eating, may be more likely to vary in response to negative affect, suggesting that food intake may be varied as part of efforts to regulate negative emotions (Bottera et al., 2018; Russell et al., 2017).

Whereas anorexia, bulimia, and BED are of concern because of unhealthy behaviours and psychological states linked to food quantity, other conditions are of concern because of a potential unhealthy focus on food quality. **Orthorexia** is not identified as an eating disorder in psychiatric classifications such as the ICD-11 (World Health Organization, 2019a) or DSM-5 (American Psychiatric Association, 2013) but it is characterised by an excessive focus on 'healthy' or 'clean' eating that is paradoxically unhealthy for nutritional reasons and/or psychological reasons. There is some evidence that orthorexia is related to restraint and to weight loss efforts that may reflect unhealthy attitudes to eating. However, the lack of clear links between orthorexia and body dissatisfaction or dysregulated eating suggests that it is distinct from other eating disorders (Atchison & Zickgraf, 2022; Zagaria et al., 2022).

Case Study 17.1

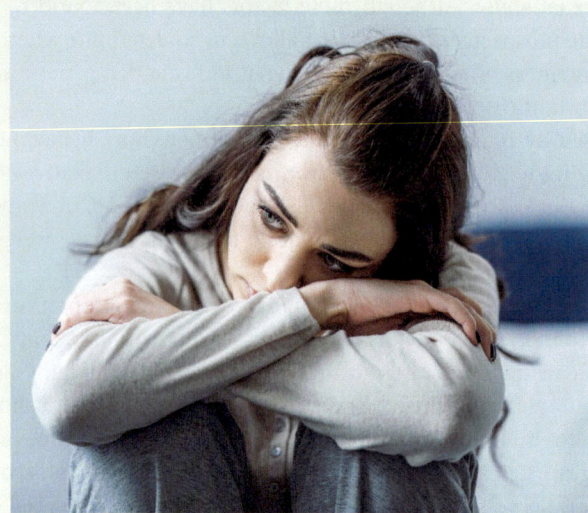

Figure 17.6   Andrea's anorexia nervosa

Source: © Lightfield Studios/Adobe Stock

Anorexia Nervosa

Andrea developed anorexia nervosa at the age of 15 and suffered from it for four years before finally returning to a healthy weight. Although she was always slim, Andrea said she felt 'deeply uncomfortable about my body and under-confident about who I was'. Comparing herself to girls at school and models in maga-zines, she felt overweight and became determined to get thin. She started to restrict her food intake and exercise exces-sively. Eventually her weight fell to less than 4.5 stone (29 kg). Her BMI was 10.8.

The anorexia led to heart palpitations. Tests showed extreme malnutrition, so Andrea was admitted to hospital. After inpatient treatment, her weight increased to six stone (38 kg), and she was allowed to go home. She said being ill and in hospital 'was a turning point as it made me realise the damage I was doing to myself. I had to help myself'. Andrea had several months of psychotherapy to help her develop a better relationship with food, a healthier and more realistic view of her body, and a more critical view of media representations of women.

Activity 17.2

Triggers for Overeating

- When are you most likely to overeat and consume a large number of highly calorific foods?
- What factors do you think are significant in triggering overeating?

Preventing and Treating Eating Disorders

To be effective, the prevention of eating disorders should be based on our understanding of what causes these disorders. Simple educational approaches are not effective; it is also important to encourage attitude change and to develop skills. Prevention programmes are most likely to be effective if they are interactive, involve more than one session, promote body acceptance, address personal, familial, and social factors, and are facilitated by a health professional (Stice et al., 2021).

Treatment of eating disorders varies according to the disorder. Of course, programmes are most likely to have a beneficial effect if people complete them. However, systematic reviews reveal that dropout from treatment is mostly in the range of 20–40% (Kan et al., 2020). This is an important statistic in itself, but it also hampers the ability to draw strong conclusions about the efficacy of interventions for eating disorders (see Research Box 17.2).

Research Box 17.2

Digital Interventions to Reduce Binge Eating

Background

Digital interventions can increase access to treatment for eating disorders. Such interventions are typically 'multi-target': they address multiple processes and influences on eating behaviour. However, it has been suggested that if multi-target interventions focus on topics that are not relevant for all users, it may reduce motivation to continue using them. Consequently, there is a need to determine whether more focused digital interventions can boost adherence without reducing treatment impact.

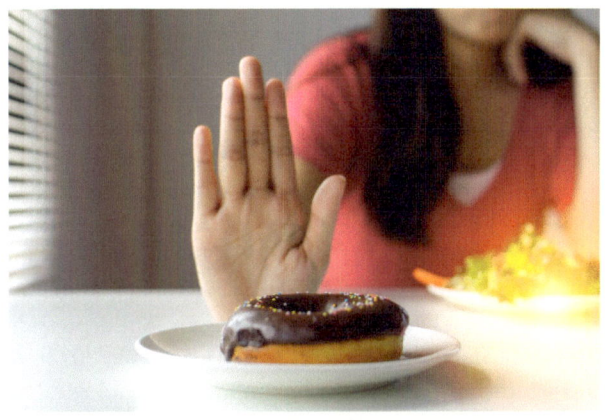

Figure 17.7 Interventions to reduce eating disorders

Source: © Vittaya_25/Adobe Stock

Method and Findings

The aim of this study was to compare a focused digital intervention with a multi-target intervention. The focused intervention addressed dietary restraint, whereas the multi-target intervention also addressed body image disturbances and mood intolerance. Six hundred participants with recurrent binge eating were randomly allocated to one of the two interventions or to a wait-list control group, and were followed up after four weeks and eight weeks. The results revealed that both interventions were successful, and that impact of the targeted intervention was broadly comparable to the multi-target intervention. However, people who received the targeted

(Continued)

intervention were less likely to comply with all elements of the programme and were more likely to discontinue its use.

Significance

Like studies in other domains of health behaviour change, this study demonstrated that further work is needed to determine how to increase uptake of interventions and adherence to them.

Linardon, J., Shatte, A., McClure, Z. & Fuller-Tyszkiewicz, M. (2023) A broad v. focused digital intervention for recurrent binge eating: A randomized controlled non-inferiority trial. *Psychological Medicine, 53*(10): 4580–4591. doi:10.1017/S0033291722001477.

Physical therapy in the form of aerobic and resistance training may increase weight in people with anorexia nervosa (Vancampfort et al., 2014). Aerobic exercise, massage, body awareness therapy, and yoga may also improve psychological and physical quality of life in people with anorexia (Minano-Garrido et al., 2022). There is modest evidence to support the use of family therapy (especially for younger people) and individual psychological therapies (Datta et al., 2023; Jansingh et al., 2020; Solmi et al., 2021). There is some evidence that psychopharmacological medications may be effective for anorexia, but their efficacy for bulimia or binge eating disorders is less clear (Muratore & Attia, 2022). There is a lack of studies of the effects of combining pharmacotherapy and psychotherapy for eating disorders (Reas & Grilo, 2021).

Reviews of the research evidence indicate that cognitive behavioural therapy (CBT) and self-help strongly based on CBT can be effective for bulimia and BED (Atwood & Friedman, 2020). Such programmes counter dysfunctional thoughts about weight and body shape to reduce binge–purge cycles and enhance self-esteem. Antidepressants can also reduce the symptoms of binge eating and purging (Crow, 2019; Duan et al., 2022). Aerobic exercise, massage, basic body awareness therapy, and yoga may improve psychological and physical quality of life in people with bulimia (Vancampfort et al., 2014).

Whichever approach is taken, it is important to initiate treatment early. A systematic review of published research indicated that earlier initiation of treatment of eating disorders is related to better outcomes (Austin et al., 2021; Kaidesoja et al., 2023).

Summary 17.2

- What we eat affects our risk of many disorders, including cancer, diabetes, and the intermediate outcomes of obesity.
- A healthy diet includes high fibre, fruit, vegetables, and oily fish, and reduced salt, red meat, sugars, and saturated fat.
- Poor dietary habits are learned during childhood through modelling, exposure, reinforcement, and family interactions.
- In adolescence and adulthood, dieting and body dissatisfaction is common, even in those who are not overweight.

- Restrained eating is associated with body dissatisfaction, food cravings, preoccupations with food, guilt, overestimating body size, low self-esteem, anxiety, and depression.
- Eating disorders occur in approximately 3% of the population and include anorexia nervosa, bulimia nervosa, and binge eating disorder.
- Bulimia and binge eating disorder are influenced by a social pressure to attain the thin-ideal, increased body dissatisfaction, negative emotions, and low self-esteem. Less is known about the causes of anorexia.
- CBT is currently the most effective treatment for bulimia and binge eating disorder.

17.2.2 Obesity

Obesity has been labelled an epidemic by health organisations. It is associated with an increased risk of chronic diseases, including Type 2 diabetes, cardiovascular disease, and cancer. It is defined using the body mass index (BMI), which is a person's weight in kilograms divided by the square of their height in metres (see Table 17.1). The prevalence of being overweight and obese has increased in recent decades (World Health Organization, 2023b). Over the last 50 years, the prevalence of obesity in children and adults has more than doubled. Today around one in seven adults – over half a billion adults – are obese. Figure 17.8 shows that being overweight or obese is most common in the Americas, Europe, and the Eastern Mediterranean region, but is also increasing in Africa and Asia.

Table 17.1   Levels of obesity

Classification	BMI (kg/m^2)	Treatment
Overweight	BMI 25–29.9	Self-directed diet and exercise; behavioural weight-loss programmes
Obese (I)	BMI 30–34.9	Behavioural weight-loss programmes
Obese (II)	BMI 35–39.9	Pharmacotherapy; very low-calorie diet
Obese (III)	BMI ≥ 40	Bariatric surgery

A basic explanation of weight gain is that it occurs because the intake of energy is greater than the energy expended. This balance is influenced by a complex system of physiological, psychological, and social factors (Masood & Moorthy, 2023). Such factors include:

- *Genetic vulnerability*: a number of genes have been identified that are associated with obesity. It is thought that these genes predispose people to weight gain and interact with other physiological feedback systems, such as the hormone leptin, which is released by adipose tissue and has a role in appetite regulation. Genes are important, but they are not the most important influence on obesity, and gene–environment interactions must also be considered (Pérusse et al., 2022; T. Wang, Xu et al., 2018).

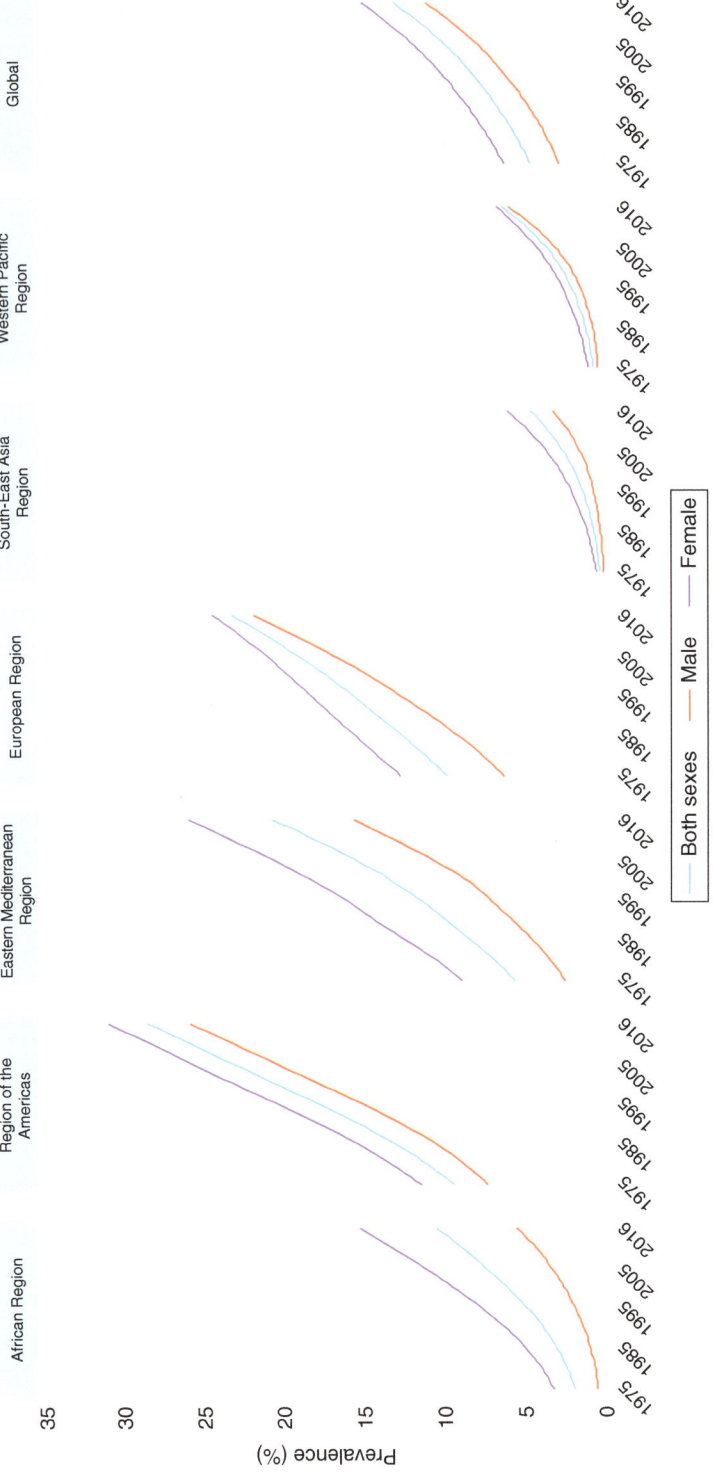

Figure 17.8 Global rates of obesity in adults, 1975–2016

Source: World Health Organization (2023b) *World Health Statistics 2023: Monitoring Health for the SDGs, Sustainable Development Goals.* Geneva: WHO

Physiological appetite control: processes of homeostasis should regulate food intake according to need – as seen in the eating behaviour of infants and young children. However, it is clear that many people eat more than they need. This is probably due to food cues in the environment overriding physiological cues.

Early development and parental obesity: parental obesity is strongly associated with children's obesity. This is likely to be due to a combination of genetic and environmental factors. Birth weight and development in early infancy are important in later chronic diseases such as diabetes and heart disease. Rapid weight gain in early childhood is associated with adult obesity.

Eating behaviour: eating behaviour is determined by motivation (see Chapter 2) and the availability of food. Animal research shows that internal drives (i.e. satiety) are overridden when a variety of palatable food is available. In our society, the wide availability of various palatable foods (in large portions) creates an environment where people are more likely to overeat.

Diet: the risk of obesity increases if a person's diet includes foods with high energy density, high fat, sugary drinks, or low fibre. In addition, alcoholic drinks are often high in calories.

Lack of physical activity: changes in transport, technology, and work patterns mean there has been a steady reduction in the energy we expend in our daily lives. Global data indicate that 32% of women and 23% of men do not achieve the recommended level of physical activity: 150 minutes per week of moderate intensity physical activity (Guthold et al., 2018). The proportion of people who are insufficiently physically active is highest in the Americas and the Eastern Mediterranean region, and in areas that are better off in economic terms. Furthermore, a global review of studies of students indicated 81% of adolescents are insufficiently physically active (Guthold et al., 2020).

Work patterns: increased working hours are associated with obesity; and increased income is associated with spending more on take-away food or dining out.

Attitudes and beliefs: patterns of eating and exercising are influenced by attitudes and beliefs (see Chapter 5). Therefore, models of health behaviour can be used to promote more healthy attitudes, beliefs, and eating behaviour.

Economic factors: the cost of food as a proportion of our total expenditure has steadily decreased over the last 50 years. In addition, unhealthy foods that are high in sugar or fat tend to be cheaper than healthy foods such as fruit or vegetables.

Obesogenic environment: a range of social, cultural, and infrastructural factors create an environment where obesity is more likely. These factors include the availability of high-energy foods, the design of buildings and workspaces to minimise physical exertion, effort-saving devices such as escalators, and increases in sedentary entertainment (Masood & Moorthy, 2023).

Case Study 17.2 illustrates how some of these different individual, social, and environmental factors may interact to promote obesity. The relative contribution of different causes of obesity may differ between individuals, so any treatment should be tailored appropriately. A stepped-care approach should be taken to obesity.

Case Study 17.2

Psychosocial Factors and Obesity

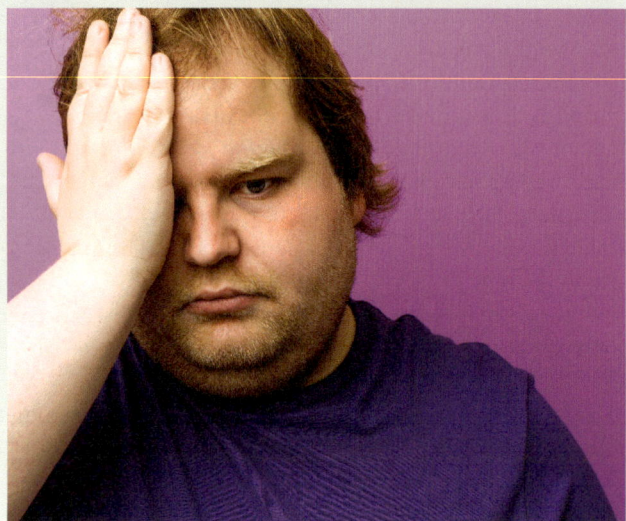

Figure 17.9 Psychosocial factors behind Carl's obesity

Source: © Asier/Adobe Stock

Carl knows that he needs to lose weight, but he finds it difficult to do so. He is morbidly obese at 118 kg (24 stone, BMI = 40.8). Carl is unable to work and is largely confined to the home. He finds it hard to be physically active and has chronic back pain, Type 2 diabetes, and hypertension. He is also being seen by psychiatric services for recurrent depression.

Carl does not seem highly motivated to lose weight. The doctor suspects that there are complex reasons why Carl finds it hard to engage in weight reduction programmes. Carl was sexually abused as a child and started putting on weight during this time. He has not had many relationships but recently got married to someone he met online.

Carl receives government disability benefits and his wife is his full-time carer. Their diet is very poor and includes lots of high-fat and sugar-rich foods. They enjoy take-away food and eat it at least three times a week. His wife says she is supportive of Carl losing weight, but she seems to undermine any attempts at weight loss or changing their diet.

Lifestyle modification, consisting of improving diet and facilitating physical activity as part of broader behavioural therapy, can be effective for reducing weight, with pharmacotherapy a possible supplement if necessary (Tronieri et al., 2019; Wadden et al., 2020). High-intensity behavioural counselling focused on behavioural strategies such as motivational interviewing can be delivered in-person, by phone, or electronically. A programme of 12 or more sessions can result in clinically meaningful weight loss of 4–7 kg. Weight loss is less in lower-intensity programmes, but adding weight loss medication can improve weight loss. Surgery is only used in severe cases, and can lead to dramatic and sustained weight loss (Colquitt et al., 2014; Torbahn et al., 2022). However, treating obesity by focusing on individuals ignores the wide range of environmental and social factors that contribute to the obesity epidemic. Prevention is a priority and must tackle social influences, food production and consumption, psychological factors, individual activity, and environmental barriers to activity.

─Clinical Notes 17.1─

Overweight and Obesity

- Treating overweight and obese people is challenging because weight regain is common.
- Pharmacological treatment results in weight loss but weight is often regained when drugs are stopped.
- Lifestyle changes focused on diet and exercise are more likely to lead to sustained weight loss.
- Combined lifestyle and pharmacological approaches may be more effective.
- Adults and children should be encouraged to build physical activity into their daily lives (e.g. walking instead of driving, taking the stairs instead of the escalator).
- Where possible, families should be involved in weight reduction programmes to address familial influences on eating behaviour.

Summary 17.3

- Obesity is defined as a BMI $\geq$ 30 and is associated with an increased risk of chronic diseases. Its prevalence has increased in recent decades.
- Obesity is caused by a combination of factors, including genetic vulnerability, physiological appetite control, early development, family context, eating behaviour, attitudes and beliefs, a lack of physical activity, and environmental factors.
- Current interventions include behavioural weight loss programmes, pharmacotherapy, and surgery, all of which vary in effectiveness and cost.

17.2.3 Alcohol Use

Alcohol consumption is widespread, and it has an enormous health impact. It is causally linked to over 200 ICD-classified disease and injury conditions, and it is the seventh leading risk factor for the burden of disease worldwide (World Health Organization, 2018), with 5% of deaths and 5% of disability-adjusted life years attributable to alcohol use. Excessive alcohol intake is associated with a wide range of health problems and pathologies, including liver damage, hypertension, stroke, several types of cancer, accidents, sexually transmitted infections, memory loss, anxiety disorders, personality disorders, depression, and drug use. Alcohol-related problems are on the increase worldwide. Whereas a common belief is that moderate alcohol use can have some health benefits, recent analysis shows that any benefits occur only for very low-level drinking. For most adverse health outcomes, any increase in alcohol intake puts people at more risk of harm (Rehm et al., 2021).

Because of these harms, governments in many countries have issued guidelines for lower-risk alcohol consumption for the general population, as well as for subgroups such as drivers of motor vehicles and women who are pregnant or breastfeeding (Furtwängler & de Visser, 2013).

Many people lack the knowledge, motivation, or skills required to adhere to government alcohol intake guidelines, but some interventions that help people to monitor their alcohol intake have been shown to have benefits (de Visser, 2015; de Visser et al., 2017).

Alcohol affects the liver in a number of ways. Alcohol is a toxin so even small amounts put a strain on the liver. Acute alcohol poisoning is caused by heavy episodic drinking (often called 'binge drinking'), and can be fatal. Chronic alcoholic liver disease starts with inflammation (hepatitis), then a fatty liver, both of which are potentially reversible if alcohol use is stopped. The final stage of alcoholic liver disease is cirrhosis, where the scarring of the liver is largely permanent. Symptoms will often only arise when liver disease is advanced. They include abdominal pain, tenderness, thirst, fatigue, jaundice, a loss of appetite, fever, mental confusion, weight gain, and nausea. Alcoholic liver disease is the main reason for liver transplants in many developed countries.

Screening for alcohol use in primary care is important, and simple screening tools such as the AUDIT are available (see Highlight Box 17.2). Such tools may measure alcohol consumption as well as the consequences of consumption. Alcohol *dependence* has physical, psychological, and social components. It usually involves an increased physical tolerance, withdrawal symptoms when intake is stopped, the increasingly dominant role of alcohol in a person's life, difficulty in controlling alcohol intake (e.g. consuming more than intended, unsuccessful attempts to reduce intake), and continued drinking despite the knowledge that it is a problem (Sayette, 2007). Alcohol *abuse* is present when a person has at least one of the following behaviours:

- Continued drinking that interferes with a major role or obligation, such as work.
- Continued drinking despite legal, social, or interpersonal problems related to alcohol use.
- Recurrent drinking in situations where intoxication is dangerous.

─Highlight Box 17.2─

Screening for Alcohol Problems (AUDIT)

Read questions as written. Record answers carefully. Begin AUDIT by saying 'Now I am going to ask you some questions about your use of alcoholic beverages during this past year'. Explain what is meant by 'alcoholic beverages' by using local examples of beer, wine, vodka, etc. Code answers in terms of standard drinks.

Table 17.2 Screening for alcohol problems (AUDIT)

1 How often do you have a drink containing alcohol?	2 How many drinks containing alcohol do you have on a typical day when you are drinking?
(0) Never [Skip to Qs 9–10]	(0) 1 or 2
(1) Monthly or less	(1) 3 or 4
(2) 2 to 4 times a month	(2) 5 or 6
(3) 2 to 3 times a week	(3) 7, 8, or 9
(4) 4 or more times a week	(4) 10 or more

3 How often do you have six or more drinks on one occasion?

(0) Never
(1) Less than monthly
(2) Monthly
(3) Weekly
(4) Daily or almost daily

Skip to Questions 9 and 10 if Total score for Questions 2 and 3 = 0

5 How often during the last year have you failed to do what was normally expected from you because of drinking?

(0) Never
(1) Less than monthly
(2) Monthly
(3) Weekly
(4) Daily or almost daily

7 How often during the last year have you had a feeling of guilt or remorse after drinking?

(0) Never
(1) Less than monthly
(2) Monthly
(3) Weekly
(4) Daily or almost daily

9 Have you or someone else been injured as a result of your drinking?

(0) No
(2) Yes, but not in the last year
(4) Yes, during the last year

4 How often during the last year have you found that you were not able to stop drinking once you had started?

(0) Never
(1) Less than monthly
(2) Monthly
(3) Weekly
(4) Daily or almost daily

6 How often during the last year have you needed a first drink in the morning to get yourself going after a heavy drinking session?

(0) Never
(1) Less than monthly
(2) Monthly
(3) Weekly
(4) Daily or almost daily

8 How often during the last year have you been unable to remember what happened the night before because you had been drinking?

(0) Never
(1) Less than monthly
(2) Monthly
(3) Weekly
(4) Daily or almost daily

10 Has a relative or friend or a doctor or another health worker been concerned about your drinking or suggested you cut down?

(0) No
(2) Yes, but not in the last year
(4) Yes, during the last year

- Total scores of >8 indicate harmful or hazardous drinking (a cut-off score of 10 provides greater specificity, but at the expense of sensitivity).
- Total scores between 8 and 15 suggest a need for simple advice focused on the reduction of hazardous drinking.
- Total scores between 16 and 19 suggest a need for brief counselling and continued monitoring.
- Totals scores of ≥20 indicate possible alcohol dependence and suggest a need for further diagnostic evaluation.

Babor, T.F., Higgins-Biddle, J.C., Saunders, J.B. & Monteiro, M.G. (2007) *AUDIT: The Alcohol Use Disorders Identification Test: Guidelines for Use in Primary Care* (2nd edition). Geneva: World Health Organization.

Activity 17.3

Alcohol Dependence

- How much do you think someone has to drink to become dependent on alcohol?
- Do you think this amount varies between individuals?

Alcoholism is determined by an interaction of genetic, psychological, and cultural factors. Twin and family studies confirm that the children of alcoholics are at greater risk of developing alcohol problems. This may be due to a greater sensitivity to the positive effects of alcohol or a decreased sensitivity to its negative effects (Hägele et al., 2014). Explanations of alcoholism also draw on learning theory (see Chapter 10): alcohol use is reinforced by increasing positive emotions (positive reinforcement) or decreasing negative emotions (negative reinforcement). Alcohol use may become associated with a particular social context or cues, which can make it hard for individuals to abstain when they are exposed to these cues.

Treatments for alcohol disorders should therefore address the physical, psychological, and social aspects of the disorder. Reviews show that the outcome of treatment is also better if the initial alcohol dependence is less severe and if the individual has no comorbid psychopathology, greater self-efficacy, a greater motivation to quit, and a treatment goal. Pharmacotherapy can be used to reduce the positive effects of alcohol, increase negative effects, or reduce cravings, and may be more effective when combined with psychological interventions (Kranzler, 2023; Ray et al., 2020).

Effective psychological interventions include motivational interviewing (see Case Study 2.2), skills training, cognitive behavioural therapy, self-help groups, and couples therapy (Kranzler, 2023; Magill et al., 2019). The importance of addressing social factors is illustrated by the finding that, for married or cohabiting people, couples therapy is more effective than individual therapy in reducing short- and long-term alcohol intake and increasing relationship functioning (O'Farrell & Clements, 2012).

Clinical Notes 17.2

Helping People with Alcohol Problems

- The AUDIT can be used to screen people for alcohol problems (Highlight Box 17.2):

  1. For AUDIT scores of 8–15: give advice on alcohol use, the health risks, and the importance of staying within recommended limits.
  2. For AUDIT scores of 16–19: refer for counselling and monitoring of alcohol use.
  3. For AUDIT scores of 20+: refer to specialist alcohol services for evaluation and treatment.

- Remember that people will often under-report their alcohol use.
- People with a history of alcohol dependence, but who currently have lower AUDIT scores, should still be considered for treatment.
- Use your clinical judgement if what the patient reports is not consistent with other evidence.

Summary 17.4

- Alcohol misuse is associated with a wide range of health problems, including liver damage, hypertension, stroke, cancer, accidents, and psychological disorders.
- Acute alcoholic hepatitis is caused by heavy episodic drinking and can be fatal. Chronic alcoholic liver disease includes inflammation (hepatitis), fatty liver, and cirrhosis.
- Alcohol dependence involves an increased physical tolerance, withdrawal symptoms, and continued drinking despite the knowledge that it is a problem.
- Alcohol abuse occurs when drinking interferes with obligations, causes legal, social or interpersonal problems, or continues despite being dangerous.
- Alcoholism is caused by the interaction between genetic, psychological, and cultural factors.

17.3 GI Disorders

In this section we outline the role of psychosocial factors in three GI conditions.

17.3.1 Irritable Bowel Syndrome

Irritable bowel syndrome (**IBS**) is a functional bowel disorder that is diagnosed when no organic disorder is identified. It is one of the most common GI disorders: it affects around 10% of people globally – more women than men – and often has a remitting and relapsing course (Black & Ford, 2020; Ford et al., 2020). The pathophysiology of irritable bowel syndrome is not fully understood. However, a key component is disordered communication between the gut and the brain, leading to disturbances in gut motility, visceral hypersensitivity, and altered CNS processing of sensory input from the gut. There may also be a role for alterations in gastrointestinal microbiota and disturbances in mucosal and immune function. Although there may be a genetic component, there is no link to food allergies or intolerances (Ford et al., 2020). Symptoms are shown in Highlight Box 17.3.

─Highlight Box 17.3─

Rome-IV Criteria for Irritable Bowel Syndrome

The following elements must have been present for the last three months, with symptom onset at least six months before diagnosis:

- Recurrent abdominal pain, on average, at least one day per week in the last three months, associated with two or more of the following criteria:
  - Related to defecation.
  - Associated with a change in frequency of stool.
  - Associated with a change in form (appearance) of stool.

(*Source*: Lacy et al., 2016)

Irritable bowel syndrome is more likely among people who have experienced traumatic events or ongoing stress (Glynn et al., 2021; Ng et al., 2019; Qin et al., 2014; Schaper & Stengel, 2022). People with IBS have an increased prevalence of depression, generalised anxiety disorder, panic, phobias, and somatisation disorders (Hu et al., 2021; Zamani et al., 2019). They are also hypersensitive to GI symptoms, such as rectal distension. This appears to be due to a greater vigilance for these symptoms and a greater likelihood of labelling such symptoms as negative or painful (Hauser et al., 2014). The suggestion that IBS is best conceptualised as a hyper-reactivity of the brain–gut axis that can be triggered by psychological or biological factors is supported by functional MRI studies showing that, in response to painful stimuli, people with IBS have increased activation in areas of the brain associated with emotional processes such as anxiety and hypervigilance (Hauser et al., 2014).

The role of psychological factors in IBS is illustrated by the fact that it is responsive to placebo and suggestion. One study used a placebo 'analgesia' gel during rectal distention and found that it led to less pain and less cortical activity in the neural pain matrix. This reduced activity was the same as if the rectal distention was smaller (Price et al., 2007). There is inconsistent evidence as to whether intake of probiotics or other dietary modification can alleviate pain and bloating and improve quality of life in IBS (Camilleri & Dilmanghani, 2023; Konstantis et al., 2023). Reviews of the research evidence indicate that effective treatment of the physical symptoms of IBS is provided by antidepressant medication, CBT, hypnotherapy, and other forms of psychotherapy (Black et al., 2020; Ford et al., 2019). Treatment of physical symptoms is clearly important, but so too is the treatment of psychological distress: people with IBS are more likely than people with inflammatory bowel disease or healthy people to consider or attempt suicide: the risk of suicide is positively correlated with more severe or chronic IBS (Spiegel et al., 2007).

17.3.2 Inflammatory Bowel Disorders

The term **inflammatory bowel disorders** (**IBD**) describes a chronic, relapsing immune-mediated inflammatory disease that has a varying and sometimes severe disease course (Bisgaard et al., 2022). It includes Crohn's disease and ulcerative colitis. It has multiple influences, including genes, immune function, psychological and behavioural factors including diet, and the gut microbiome. Rather than there being single or simple causes, there is evidence of interactions between psychological factors, biological factors, and IBD symptoms (Bisgaard et al., 2022; Tavakoli et al., 2021).

The majority of people with IBD think lifestyle and psychological factors such as diet and stress are important for the course of their IBD (Sajadinejad et al., 2012). Although the role of stress in the onset of IBD is yet to be established definitively, there is clear evidence that stress can trigger and exacerbate symptoms of IBD (Labanski et al., 2020; Sajadinejad et al., 2012). The influence of stress on IBD may be due to any of the physical effects of stress on the GI system (see Figure 17.2), but a key pathway appears to be through triggering increased mucosal inflammation in people with IBD.

Lifestyle factors are important, but the precise role they play is unclear. Smoking is associated with an increased risk of Crohn's disease but with a decreased risk of ulcerative colitis. Use of oral contraceptives increases the risk of IBD. Diet is generally thought to be important because food-related antigens in the gut may trigger inflammatory responses: high dietary intake of fats, polyunsaturated fatty acids, omega-6 fatty acids, and meat increase the risk of Crohn's disease and ulcerative colitis. However, there is a need for more evidence to confirm the potential effects of dietary interventions on disease progression (Sasson et al., 2021; Yamamoto et al., 2017).

Various treatments have been developed and applied to IBD, but given the multiple – and interacting – casual factors, there is often no obvious or simple treatment. Pharmacological options include immunomodulators, aminosalicylates, and corticosteroids. The progressive nature of IBD means that 15% or more of people with ulcerative colitis will require surgical interventions (S.M. Adams et al., 2022). Although surgery reduces the severity of symptoms, it can lead to other difficulties, such as faecal incontinence, pouch failure, and female infertility.

There is increasing recognition of the need for psychological assessment and management as part of approaches to treating IBD (Dubinsky et al., 2021; Eugenicos & Ferreira, 2021). This is because IBD is associated with lower quality of life, and has broader social implications through its effects on people's engagement in work and social activities (Dubinsky et al., 2021). Although the precise mechanisms are not known, it is likely that there are reciprocal associations between IBD and depression and anxiety (Gracie et al., 2018).

Adjusting to IBD is a significant challenge. However, comparatively little attention has been paid to this aspect in the psychological literature. One study found that if people blamed themselves for IBD, they were more likely to use avoidant coping (i.e. to avoid thinking or talking about it), which in turn was related to poor adjustment (Voth & Sirois, 2009). In contrast, taking responsibility for IBD resulted in less avoidance and better adjustment. A review of research also found that emotion-focused coping (rather than problem-focused coping) is linked to poorer psychological adjustment to IBD (Jordan et al., 2016). Other important influences on poorer adjustment included perceptions of being under stress, being less able to identify and describe emotions (alexithymia), feeling stigmatised, and believing that the condition will have serious consequences.

Psychological factors are important in the onset and progression of IBD. Around one-third of people with IBD have symptoms of anxiety, and one-quarter have symptoms of depression, with a higher prevalence among women than men (Barberio et al., 2021). There appear to be bi-directional associations between IBD and wellbeing: IBD can increase the likelihood of developing anxiety and depression, anxiety and depression are more common among people with active IBD than among those with inactive disease, anxiety and depression may increase the risk of developing IBD, and increases in anxiety and depression are related to an increased likelihood of worse IBD symptoms and greater treatment needs (Bisgaard et al., 2022; Eugenicos & Ferreira, 2021; Fairbrass et al., 2022). There is some evidence that antidepressant medication may have a beneficial impact on the course of IBD (L. Wang et al., 2023).

Psychological interventions for IBD include cognitive behavioural therapy (CBT), stress management, and support groups. There is evidence that CBT can alleviate anxiety and depression among people with IBD (Dubinsky et al., 2021), and this is likely to affect physical aspects of the condition, but there is less consistent evidence that these interventions affect the physical symptoms of IBD. Physical activity interventions (including aerobic exercise, resistance training, or yoga) can enhance quality of life and reduce IBD-induced stress and anxiety (Eckert et al., 2019). Interventions that combine psychological and physical care may be even more effective, but there is insufficient evidence at present. As for other conditions, there is interest in whether the psychological impact of IBD may be treated using online interventions (see also Research Box 17.1). It is important to determine the efficacy of such interventions because some studies suggest that people with IBD may be more willing to participate in online interventions than face-to-face interventions, perhaps because the former reduce stigmatisation and embarrassment (Guo et al., 2020; McCombie et al., 2014).

17.3.3 Cancer of the GI Tract

Gastrointestinal cancers are common and deadly. Globally, cancer of the lower GI tract (colon and rectum) is the third most common cancer overall, and the second most common cause of death from cancer (Global Cancer Observatory, 2024). Cancer of the upper GI tract (oesophagus, stomach, pancreas) is less common but has high mortality rates because it tends to be asymptomatic in the early stages. Survival rates therefore tend to be low. The symptoms and challenges of cancer in the upper and lower GI tract differ. Cancer of the upper GI tract may lead to problems in eating or swallowing, dysphagia, nausea, and vomiting, whereas cancer of the lower GI tract leads to symptoms associated with bowel function, and treatment may involve an ostomy (a surgically-created opening between the intestines and the abdominal wall).

Cancer of the Upper GI Tract

Cancer of the upper GI tract is associated with being male, being older, *H. pylori* infection, dietary factors, and smoking. In addition, genetic vulnerability may play a role in some stomach and pancreatic cancers. Epidemiological research shows that diets high in salt and processed meat increase the risk of stomach cancer, whereas a high fruit and vegetable intake can reduce the risk (Y. Huang et al., 2021; Hull, 2021). As noted earlier in section 17.2, alcohol consumption increases the risk of oesophageal cancer. There may be important gene–diet interactions that greatly increase some people's risk of cancer of the upper GI tract.

The prognosis is poor because there are very few symptoms in the early stages of upper GI tract cancer, and it is common for the cancer to have metastasised before diagnosis. Survival rates have increased over recent years, but they remain short: for example, less than half of people diagnosed with oesophageal cancer live for another year (Deng et al., 2021). Treatment nearly always involves surgery, such as a partial or total removal of the oesophagus or stomach. These surgical procedures are difficult, and they can have a range of side effects, including pain, difficulty in swallowing, weight loss, malnourishment, acid reflux, and abdominal discomfort. Unfortunately, curative surgery is often not an option for people with gastric cancer. These people are offered palliative care to manage the pain and surgical intervention to manage perforation or obstruction.

Given the poor prognosis, it is understandable that many people experience anxiety and depression (Dengsø et al., 2020). The relationship between depression and cancer is particularly strong in pancreatic cancer, where survival rates are approximately 5% over five years. Many people with pancreatic cancer have severe depression (Parker & Brotchie, 2017). This fact, and the fact that the cancer often progresses without symptoms, means that depression may be listed as a presenting symptom of pancreatic cancer. It is important to screen for and treat depression because life expectancy is shorter among people with depression, but this shortening is attenuated among people who receive mental health treatment (Seoud et al., 2020).

Studies of quality of life show that physical functioning, work, and home life are strongly affected by upper GI tract cancers. Quality of life generally decreases immediately after surgery, but may improve in the long term, especially if treatment is curative. Quality of life is better in people who have less invasive or toxic treatments and who feel involved in decision making about their treatment (Kashaf & McGill, 2015). Psychological wellbeing and coping are important in adjusting to disease and can affect disease outcomes (Calderón et al., 2018; see also Chapter 6) (Y. Zhang et al., 2020). Quality of life is commonly considered an outcome of diagnosis or treatment, but it is notable that in one study, better quality of life predicted survival after chemotherapy among people with advanced gastric cancer (Park et al., 2008). There is a need for better conceptualisation, assessment, and treatment of these dimensions of patient experience (Tzelepis et al., 2014).

Cancer of the Lower GI Tract

Cancer of the lower GI tract is associated with genetic vulnerability, older age, diet, smoking, being sedentary, and being overweight. It is estimated that lifestyle changes, such as being physically active, eating healthily, and maintaining a healthy body weight, could potentially halve the risk of these cancers (Aleksandrova et al., 2014; Veettil et al., 2021).

Exercise and body weight have a dose–response effect on bowel cancer. For example, a review of studies involving nearly a quarter of a million people indicated that the risk of developing early onset colon cancer is significantly greater among overweight people, and even higher among obese people (H. Li et al., 2021). Many studies have shown that physical activity decreases the risk of developing bowel cancer and improves the prognosis in people who have bowel cancer. The underlying mechanisms are unclear, but may involve increased insulin-like growth factor-binding protein and reduced prostaglandins. Exercise in people with bowel cancer is associated with better quality of life, favourable changes in physiological parameters, and reduced mortality from cancer and other causes (Brown, Damjanov et al., 2018; Brown, Troxel et al., 2018; McGettigan et al., 2020).

Much of the literature on quality of life in colorectal cancer focuses on the impact of ostomy surgery. This shows that ostomies can have a significant impact on emotional wellbeing, quality of life, sexuality, and body image (Alenezi et al., 2021). Most people will experience a sharp decline in their body image after surgery, but it then gradually improves over time. People with ostomies are more likely to be depressed and have poorer quality of life than people with the same illness but without ostomies, particularly if they are younger, female, less educated, or have poor support (Alenezi et al., 2021; Kristensen et al., 2019). For many aspects of quality of life, the effect of ostomies appears to be bimodal: people are either not very affected or they are severely affected. This highlights the importance of individual differences in coping and levels of support in helping people to adapt to ostomies and accept changes in their body image (Capilla-Díaz et al., 2019).

Clinical Notes 17.3

Working with GI Disorders

- People with GI disorders, such as IBS or GI cancers, are at a high risk of psychological problems.
- Be alert for people who have psychological and/or social problems because these are associated with poor quality of life and may influence the course of the disease.
- Although IBS is strongly associated with psychological factors, it is not helpful to portray it as 'all in the mind'.
- Explaining the brain–gut axis can help people to understand the impact of psychological, lifestyle, and physical factors.
- It may be helpful to encourage people not to blame themselves or to use avoidant coping, but instead to take responsibility for the course of their illness.
- Encourage lifestyle changes such as increased exercise, healthy diet, and reduced alcohol use: they can improve emotional wellbeing and may improve the prognosis.
- Screen for psychological disorders and offer support or psychological intervention where appropriate.

Summary 17.5

- Irritable bowel syndrome (IBS) is one of the most common GI disorders. It is associated with stress, psychological disorders, and past psychological trauma.
- Psychological intervention and antidepressants can result in some improvement in IBS symptoms.
- Inflammatory bowel disorders (IBD), including Crohn's disease and ulcerative colitis, are caused by an interaction between the environment and a genetic susceptibility that results in immune dysfunction in the GI tract.
- Stress is associated with relapse in IBD. Psychological and social problems predict quality of life and whether symptoms will worsen over time.
- Psychological interventions for IBD reduce symptom-related stress, disease-related worries, depression, anxiety, pain, and the use of anti-inflammatory drugs.
- GI cancers are strongly associated with lifestyle factors, including diet, smoking, physical activity, and weight.
- Anxiety and depression are common in people with GI cancer. This is particularly the case for pancreatic cancer, where depression is a possible presenting symptom.
- Ostomies can have a significant impact on emotional wellbeing, quality of life, sexuality, and body image, but there are large individual differences in how people cope and adjust.

Further Reading

Llewellyn, C.D. et al. (eds) (2019) *Cambridge Handbook of Psychology, Health and Medicine* (3rd edition). Cambridge: Cambridge University Press. Includes short chapters on many relevant topics, including cancers of the digestive tract, obesity, eating disorders, irritable bowel syndrome, inflammatory bowel disorders, and gastric and duodenal ulcers.

Knowles, S.R., Stern, J. & Hebbard,G. (eds) (2018) *Functional Gastrointestinal Disorders: A Biopsychosocial Approach*. London: Routledge. An edited collection that provides an overview of how biology, emotions, beliefs, behaviours, and social factors affect the onset and progression of GI disorders. A series of chapters focuses on various psychological interventions, including psychodynamic therapy, hypnosis, CBT, stress management, and mindfulness.

Levenson, J.L. (ed.) (2019) *The American Psychiatric Publishing Textbook of Psychosomatic Medicine: Psychiatric Care of the Medically Ill* (3rd edition). Arlington, VA: American Psychiatric Association Publishing. Covers many of the topics discussed in this chapter, including gastrointestinal disorders and oncology.

Revision Questions

1   Describe the brain–gut axis.
2   What is the relationship between stress and GI function?
3   Why is a biopsychosocial approach important in GI illness? Illustrate your answer with reference to one specific GI illness.

4   How does diet affect health?
5   What constitutes a healthy diet?
6   Outline three eating disorders and discuss what causes them.
7   How do we define obesity? Outline three different causes of obesity.
8   How does alcohol use affect health?
9   What is the difference between alcohol dependence and alcohol abuse?
10 Discuss the role of psychosocial factors in one GI disorder.

18

REPRODUCTIVE HEALTH

─Learning Objectives─

This chapter is designed to enable you to:

- Outline the psychological changes associated with the menstrual cycle and menopause.
- Discuss the role of psychosocial factors during pregnancy and birth.
- Describe the main psychological problems that can occur during pregnancy and after birth.
- Outline the major links between endocrine disorders and psychosocial wellbeing.
- Consider the ethical issues associated with the use of hormonal treatment.

In this chapter we consider reproduction and endocrinology together, primarily through focusing on reproductive events and disorders. We also consider non-reproductive endocrine disorders. The emphasis of the chapter is on the psychological, behavioural, and social factors that can influence, and are influenced by, the reproductive and endocrine systems.

18.1 Reproduction

Reproductive events include the onset of menstruation (menarche), conception, pregnancy, miscarriage, childbirth, and menopause. Although these events mostly focus on physical changes in women, they also involve issues that affect both men and women, such as sexual dysfunction and infertility. Procedures and treatments associated with reproduction that are particularly common include contraception, cervical smear tests, hysterectomy, and hormone replacement therapy (HRT). Reproductive issues raise unique ethical dilemmas, such as:

- When terminating a pregnancy is morally defensible.
- The rights of donor parents and the children of donors.
- Gender identity.
- The use of assisted reproductive techniques for pregnancy in older women.
- Whether a pregnancy should be used by parents to provide a child with the right genetic make-up to be an organ or tissue donor for a sick older sibling.

These events can be viewed from a biomedical, psychological, social, or cultural perspective. Which perspective we take affects both our understanding and treatment of disorders (see Chapter 1). For example, a biomedical perspective would see premenstrual syndrome (PMS) as caused by fluctuations and imbalances in hormones associated with the menstrual cycle. Treatment would therefore involve pharmacological methods to counteract hormonal imbalances or influence mood. A psychological perspective of PMS might examine how women's patterns of stress and behaviour contribute to worsening mood around menstruation, such as noticing particular triggers and maladaptive responses. Treatment might involve identifying and changing maladaptive thinking or behaviour, and finding coping strategies that help women to respond in a more adaptive way. A social perspective of PMS might examine women's social circumstances and environmental triggers, or cultural beliefs and narratives about premenstrual syndrome. This might lead to interventions such as providing practical support to women during critical times, or public health campaigns to change cultural beliefs and narratives.

It is clear that none of these perspectives on their own provides an adequate explanation for, or treatment of, PMS. Therefore, it is important to take a **biopsychosocial approach** where we consider all the different perspectives outlined above. This in turn will lead to a more informed and holistic approach to consultation and treatment.

In this chapter it is not possible to cover the wide range of reproductive and endocrine events and disorders. We therefore concentrate on menstruation, menopause, pregnancy, and childbirth. We then look at a selection of endocrine disorders. You will also find relevant information in other chapters covering such subjects as puberty (Chapter 8), Cushing's syndrome (Chapter 3), and diabetes (Chapter 15).

18.1.1 Menstruation and Menopause

The age at which girls start menstruating – **menarche** – fell throughout the twentieth century. This change is thought to be due to better health and basic nutrition, but also to increased weight and obesity in young girls (see Chapters 8 and 17). Figure 18.1 shows the biological events and changes that occur during the menstrual cycle.

The effect of the **menstrual cycle** has been examined in relation to a range of behaviours, such as sexual behaviour, diet, and sleep. The so-called 'ovulatory shifts' in motivation and prioritisation of sex or food have been widely studied, with varying results. Studies suggest that motivation for sexual behaviour increases during the fertile phase of the menstrual cycle (Marcinkowska et al., 2023). However, studies comparing women taking hormonal contraceptives with those whose menstrual cycle is naturally cycling suggest that although ovulatory shifts in libido are present, they are observed in both groups of women, regardless of contraception, so they are not necessarily associated with ovulation (Schleifenbaum et al., 2024). The same was found for shifts in motivation towards food intake (Schleifenbaum et al., 2024). Although motivation towards food intake may change during the menstrual cycle, it is not clear whether or how it affects preferences towards different types of food. In contrast, research suggests that changes in food preferences may be more strongly influenced by cultural norms than biological changes. For example, chocolate cravings during the menstrual cycle differ strongly between cultures and do not decrease substantially after menopause when the menstrual cycle has stopped (Hormes & Rozin, 2009).

The menstrual cycle may also affect the duration, pattern, and quality of sleep. There is evidence that the proportion of time spent in different stages of sleep (e.g. REM, slow-wave sleep)

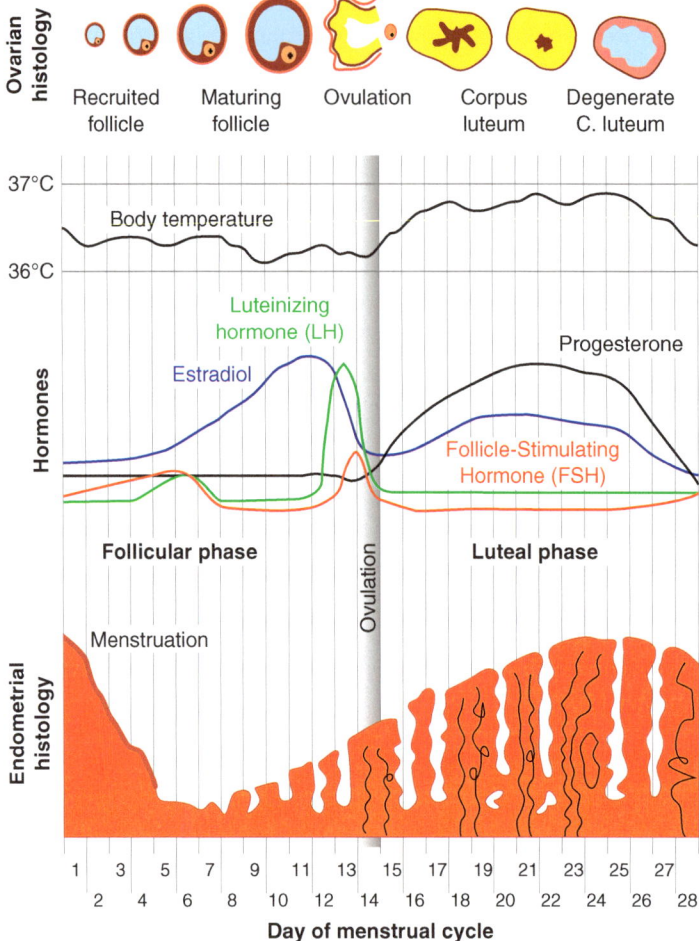

Figure 18.1   Physiological events of the menstrual cycle

Source: © Lyrl/Wikimedia Commons

varies across the menstrual cycle, and reduced quality of sleep is reported by women with PMS or other menstrual symptoms (Alzueta & Baker, 2023; Baker & Lee, 2022). The menstrual cycle may also interact with sleep and circadian rhythms. A review of research found that after ovulation markers of circadian rhythms (cortisol and melatonin) are not as large in amplitude. When circadian rhythms are disrupted, such as when women do shift work, women are also more likely to have irregular, longer, or more painful menstrual cycles (Baker & Driver, 2007; Hu et al., 2023).

Premenstrual Syndrome (PMS)

Psychological symptoms that occur just before menstruation are commonly referred to as **premenstrual tension** (**PMT**) or **premenstrual syndrome** (**PMS**). PMS includes a range of emotional and behavioural symptoms and can have a significant impact on a woman's quality of life. Common symptoms are irritability, depression, anxiety, mood swings, feelings of loss of control, and tiredness. Physical symptoms of abdominal bloating, tender breasts, and muscle aches are also reported (Cary & Simpson, 2024). PMS is estimated to affect around 47% of women globally and is most common among those aged 25–35 (Modzelewski et al., 2024).

Between 3% and 8% of women experience a severe form of PMS, referred to as premenstrual dysphoric disorder (PMDD) (Reilly et al., 2024). Symptoms of PMDD include highly labile emotions, such as anger, depression, or anxiety, and disturbances in home life, social life, and work due to significant changes in sleep, appetite, energy, and concentration, which appear during most of the week prior to menstruation and disappear the week after menstruation (American Psychiatric Association, 2013). PMDD is not simply the exacerbation of an existing mood disorder during the premenstrual period; it is supposed to be 'switched on' during certain days within the menstrual cycle and 'switched off' for the remainder of the cycle. However, women with a past history of depression are more likely to suffer from PMDD. PMS and PMDD have a considerable impact on women's quality of life and functioning (Cary & Simpson, 2024). A review of 44 studies of the menstrual cycle and suicidal behaviour found evidence of higher rates of suicide attempts in the luteal phase (Alnashwan et al., 2023). Women with PMDD may be particularly at risk (Osborn et al., 2021).

The relative contribution of physical, psychological, and cultural factors to PMS and PMDD is unclear, and the diagnosis remains controversial (Naik et al., 2023). The timing of symptoms strongly suggests that fluctuations in hormone levels play a causal role in the psychological symptoms (Modzelewski et al., 2024). However, hormone levels in women with PMDD do not appear to differ from levels in women without PMDD. This finding has led researchers to conclude that 'PMDD is an abnormal brain response to normal menstrual hormonal fluctuations' (Cary & Simpson, 2024: page 8). The increased vulnerability of women with a history of depression suggests that predisposing psychological vulnerability is a factor in PMDD. Other research is examining possible vulnerability factors such as stress, associated inflammation, genetics, and insulin sensitivity. In addition, cultural factors may play a role. A study of 3,856 women from ethnic minority groups in the USA found that women who were born abroad or moved to the USA after the age of six were less likely to have PMDD. The longer a woman had lived in the USA, the more likely she was to suffer from PMDD (Pilver et al., 2011).

Thus, in order to understand PMDD we need to consider physiological, psychological, and cultural factors. One approach that does this is the Material-Discursive-Intrapsychic model (Ussher, 2010), which suggests that PMS and PMDD are due to the interaction between three factors:

- Material factors, such as hormones, physiological arousal, life stresses, relationship, or marital context.
- Intra-psychic factors, such as the mode of evaluating and coping with changes, expectations of self, and defence mechanisms.
- Discursive factors, such as cultural constructions and the discourse of PMS, reproduction, and gender.

This approach suggests that all these factors combine to produce emotions, bodily sensations, and behaviours which are labelled as PMS by the woman, and diagnosed as PMS or PMDD by a clinician (Ussher, 2019).

A range of treatments for PMS and PMDD have been developed. Biomedical interventions, such as antidepressants or hormone treatments, can be effective in reducing symptoms but do not address the other factors involved in PMS and PMDD. Reviews and meta-analyses show that there is good evidence to support the use of antidepressants and gonadotrophin-releasing hormone (GnRH) analogues, but less evidence for oral contraceptives or implants (Cary & Simpson, 2024). Despite this, treatment practices can still vary between countries. A study of patterns of PMS and PMDD in different countries found that women were most commonly treated with medication. Practitioners in the USA, the UK, and Canada favoured antidepressants, French practitioners favoured hormone and analgesic treatment, and German doctors favoured complementary medicine (Weisz & Knaapen, 2009).

Psychological interventions for PMS are effective. Meta-analyses of intervention trials show that education and monitoring are of limited use, but cognitive behavioural therapy (CBT) and CBT-based interventions can result in reduced depression and anxiety, less interference of symptoms on daily functioning, and more positive behaviour changes (Kancheva et al., 2021). There is some evidence that CBT is as effective as antidepressants in reducing distress in the short term and more effective in reducing long-term distress (Hunter et al., 2002). Standard psychological interventions for PMS are now available. Case Study 18.1 gives an example of an eight-session intervention.

—Case Study 18.1—

Therapy for Premenstrual Syndrome

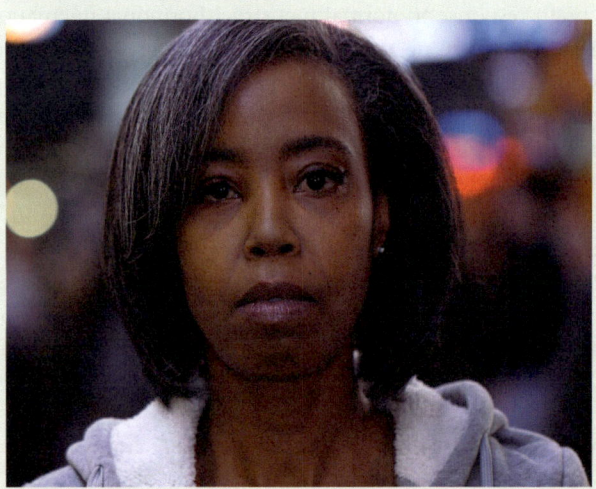

Figure 18.2 Therapy for Margo's PMS symptoms

Source: © blvdone/Adobe Stock

Margo's PMS symptoms are intolerance, impatience, and angry outbursts. Everything annoys her when she has PMS. Anger alternates with feelings of vulnerability, insecurity, depression, and the guilt of knowing she has hurt others. It makes her feel like a Jekyll and Hyde character: she is normally gentle and loving, but PMS makes her angry and aggressive. She is very open about having PMS and uses it to explain her aggressive behaviour. She thinks PMS is due to hormones and diet, but she recognises that the symptoms can be worse if she is stressed or feeling down. Margo had eight sessions of psychotherapy as follows:

Session 1: A history is taken of Margo's PMS and the effect it has on her life. A working model of her PMS is developed that includes physical factors (hormones, diet), psychological factors (mood, stress, relationship issues), and narrative factors (blaming PMS, seeing her PMS-self as someone else).

Session 2: Stress: the influence of stress as a trigger for angry outbursts is examined. Relaxation exercises are given to help Margo cope with stress.

Session 3: Relationships: how relationships are affected by, or contribute to, maladaptive patterns of behaviour is explored. The session looks at how to respond assertively instead of aggressively.

Session 4: Self-care: the session focuses on the importance of expressing needs and doing things she enjoys. Margo develops an activity schedule and discusses the importance of diet and exercise.

Session 5: Thinking positively and 're-writing' her PMS experience so that she feels more in control is the focus of this session.

Sessions 6 and 7: Consolidation: the sessions continue to redefine her PMS, using positive thinking and more adaptive coping.

Session 8: Review of therapy: the session looks at how Margo has changed and what she learned that will help in the future.

After therapy Margo felt more in control, her relationships and self-esteem had improved, and she was more aware of how her behaviour was affecting other people. She also felt more ownership of her PMS: 'I have a lot of relief knowing that it's all under my control really; that it isn't something apart from me.' Her symptoms were also not as intense.

(Adapted from Ussher et al., 2002)

Menopause

Menopause is defined as the end of menstruation. Perimenopause (meaning 'around menopause') is the months or years during which a woman's body is transitioning to menopause, so it is defined as the time from when symptoms start to one year after the final menstrual period. Perimenopause and menopause usually occur between the ages of 45 and 55 but vary between individuals. The physical changes of menopause result in an increased risk of diseases such as osteoporosis and cardiovascular disease (Uddenberg et al., 2024). Perimenopause has been associated with a variety of symptoms that affect between 80% and 90% of women. Symptoms include hot flashes/flushes, night sweats, changes in timing and flow of menstrual periods, vaginal dryness, low libido, problems with skin or hair, disturbed sleep/insomnia, and low or anxious mood (Gatenby & Simpson 2024). There are some geographical and ethnic variations in menopause, with earlier onset of menopause found in women in low- and middle-income countries, and less vasomotor symptoms experienced by Asian women compared to Caucasian women (Talaulikar, 2022). As for PMS, cultural discourses may influence the discussion, interpretation, and management of perimenopause symptoms. For example, reporting of perimenopausal symptoms in Japan increased as cultural awareness of the menopause, or *kônenki*, also increased (Melby et al., 2005). In the UK, prescriptions for **hormone replacement therapy** (HRT) increased by 47% from 2021 to 2022 (NHS Business Services Authority, 2023), which coincided with increased awareness following television documentaries and a government report on menopause (UK Parliament Women and Equalities Committee, 2022).

In terms of mental health, evidence shows that women are at increased risk of depression and anxiety during the perimenopause. Meta-analyses show that worldwide around one-third of women experience depression during menopause, with the highest prevalence in the Middle East and North Africa and the lowest prevalence in the East Asia and Pacific regions (Jia et al., 2024). The risk of depression in perimenopause is greater than the risk before or after perimenopause (Badawy et al., 2024).

Reviews and meta-analyses suggest that a number of interventions can help. Psychosocial interventions, such as CBT and mindfulness-based therapies, are effective at reducing depression and anxiety (Spector et al., 2024). Hormone replacement therapy can improve mood and reduce physical symptoms (Rubinow et al., 2015). However, the use of HRT to treat symptoms of perimenopause is controversial and illustrates the importance of research methods when examining treatment effects. Early studies of HRT were methodologically weak (e.g. they did not control for the baseline health status or have a placebo group as a comparison). Meta-analysis of worldwide evidence suggests that HRT is associated with a small increased risk of breast cancer, which increases with the duration of use of HRT (Collaborative Group on Hormonal Factors in Breast Cancer, 2019). It is thought that this is due to HRT (progestogen) promoting the growth of cancer cells in women who have pre-existing risks for breast cancer (National Institute for Health and Care Excellence (NICE), 2019). Hormone replacement therapy is also associated with a reduced risk of osteoporosis and improved muscle mass and strength (NICE, 2019).

Management of perimenopausal symptoms therefore needs to be considered on an individual basis (NICE, 2019). There are likely to be multiple physical, psychological, and cultural factors associated with symptoms during perimenopause. For example, a meta-analysis of depression in postmenopausal women found that an increased risk was associated with a range of factors, including menopausal symptoms, a history of mental illness, chronic disease, and marital status (J. Li et al., 2024). Similarly, a review of prospective studies concluded that the increased risk of depression during perimenopause is due to subgroups of women with additional vulnerabilities, such as severe menopausal symptoms, stress, or a history of depression (L. Brown, Hunter et al., 2024). In many cultures, it has been found that concurrent stressful events are important predictors of women's wellbeing during menopause. Menopause often coincides with significant role changes, such as children leaving home, or occupational changes. Resilience factors, such as control, optimism, and self-related resilience, are associated with better wellbeing during perimenopause (Süss & Ehlert, 2020). Approaches that empower women during this transition (Hickey et al., 2024) and multidimensional approaches, such as the biopsychosocial or Material-Discursive-Intrapsychic approach (Ussher, 2010), therefore help to provide a better understanding of wellbeing during perimenopause.

Summary 18.1

- The menstrual cycle is associated with changes in behaviours and mood, but these vary between cultures.
- PMS and PMDD are psychological symptoms associated with the luteal phase of the menstrual cycle: PMS affects up to 47% of women and PMDD up to 8% of women.
- Physical, psychological, and cultural factors affect PMS/PMDD, but the specific influence of each is unclear.

- Psychological intervention for PMS/PMDD can be as effective as antidepressants.
- Perimenopause is associated with hot flashes/flushes and a range of other physical and psychological symptoms.
- There is evidence that perimenopause is associated with an increased risk of depression, which is due to a range of physical, psychological, and social risk factors.

18.1.2 Pregnancy and Birth

Pregnancy, birth, and becoming a parent are times of great physical and psychosocial change for women and their partners. Childbirth is a pivotal life event that can be challenging, usually involves pain, and evokes positive and negative emotions. Physiologically, childbirth involves physical systems and hormones that are affected by psychological factors, such as the HPA axis, cortisol, endogenous opioids, and oxytocin. Unpleasant psychosocial factors, such as stress and anxiety in pregnancy are associated with poor outcomes, such as preterm birth and low birth weight (Bergeron et al., 2023). Healthy behaviours during pregnancy are important contributors to the health of women and the developing foetus. Poor health behaviours, such as an unhealthy diet and use of substances, are associated with a range of adverse outcomes for the child (Sebastiani et al., 2018).

Psychological theories and evidence are therefore highly relevant to understanding the experience, behaviour, and outcomes of pregnancy and birth for women and their families. These include theories of health beliefs, health behaviour, assessment, interventions, and implementation. Health-related theories range from broad frameworks for understanding health, such as the biopsychosocial or diathesis-stress models, to specific theories of behavioural and psychological phenomena. Despite this, a lot of research in pregnancy and postpartum (the perinatal period) has been atheoretical. A search of research on postpartum depression found that only 16% of research papers included the word 'theory', and only 3% of papers mentioned 'theory' in the title, abstract, or keywords (Ayers & Olander, 2013). This suggests that very little perinatal research explicitly draws on psychological theory, despite its relevance (Saxby, 2017).

The biopsychosocial approach shows that pregnancy outcomes are influenced by biological, psychological, social, and macro-cultural factors (Suls & Rothman, 2004). At the macro-cultural level, pregnancy and birth are influenced by cultural norms and rituals that affect women's expectations and experiences (Iravani et al., 2015). For example, there is less maternal mortality and morbidity in high-income countries compared to low-income countries. Surgical intervention in the form of caesarean sections has increased the safety of birth, and the World Health Organization (2015) estimates that caesarean sections are necessary in 10–15% of births to prevent mortality and morbidity for women and/or their babies. However, there are large cultural differences in the rates of caesarean section, which range from 5% in sub-Saharan Africa to 42% in Latin America and the Caribbean, with an average rate of 21% worldwide (Betran et al., 2021). Rates of caesarean section are projected to continue rising to around 28% worldwide by 2030 (Betran et al., 2021).

There are many possible reasons for the increase in caesarean sections: changing cultural beliefs and norms, an increase in biological risk factors such as increasing maternal age or obesity, institutional, legal, and economic factors, an increase in maternal requests for caesarean sections, and inequalities in access (World Health Organization, 2021). These findings illustrate how the likelihood of a woman having a caesarean birth may be influenced by macro-cultural, psychological, and social factors, as well as by biological complications and risk.

Pregnancy

Women's physical and psychological health in pregnancy is important for them and their developing foetus. Research on the developmental origins of health and disease shows the association between pregnancy/birth factors and disease in adult offspring. This is most established in terms of physical health. For example, poor nutrition during pregnancy and low birth weight are associated with a greater risk of the infant developing a range of diseases in adulthood, including cardiovascular, respiratory, and chronic renal diseases as an adult (Nobile et al., 2022). Evidence also indicates that psychological factors during pregnancy can affect the developing foetus. The strongest evidence is for links between stress, anxiety, and depression in pregnancy and a greater risk of a range of adverse outcomes for the child (Glover, 2016).

The effect of stress in pregnancy on the infant is probably due to a combination of physiological, epigenetic, and environmental factors. As noted in Chapter 7, the likelihood of a child developing psychological disorders such as schizophrenia may be influenced by a genetic predisposition *and* experiences during pregnancy/birth, early childhood, or later life. Similarly, material presented in Chapter 8 shows how the cognitive potential children inherit in their genes can be optimised or impaired by psychosocial experiences in childhood. The field of **epigenetics** has provided a better understanding of how environmental factors, such as stress in pregnancy, can regulate the activity and expression of genes in the foetus and child (Conradt et al., 2018; see also Chapter 1).

The effect of stress in pregnancy on the infant is thought to occur through epigenetic neurobiological **foetal programming**. The evidence for foetal programming mostly comes from animal and epidemiological research. For example, classic studies of women who were pregnant during the 1998 Quebec ice storm, which cut off power from days to months and shut down many activities, found that exposure to this stress was associated with a range of adverse outcomes for the child, including the baby being more likely to be fussy/difficult, dull, and needing attention (Laplante et al., 2016), poorer child development (Laplante et al., 2008), and greater metabolic changes such as central adiposity and obesity (Cao-Lei, Dancause et al., 2015). The study in Research Box 18.1 shows how both women's exposure to the ice storm (i.e. objective stress) and their appraisal of the ice storm as positive or negative (i.e. subjective stress) were associated with altered patterns of DNA methylation in their children (Cao-Lei, Elgbeili et al., 2015). This is consistent with theories of stress that emphasise the importance of appraisal (see Chapter 3), and it provides an example of epigenetics (see Chapter 1) that illustrates how stress in pregnancy can influence the genome of the unborn child.

─Research Box 18.1─

Stress in Pregnancy and DNA Changes in Offspring

Background

Studies of humans and animals have shown that stress in pregnancy can affect a range of child outcomes that may persist into adulthood. These effects occur through epigenetic changes, such as DNA methylation, in the foetal genome. However, it is not clear whether these effects are due to objective stress (i.e. severity of the stressor) or subjective stress (i.e. a woman's appraisal).

Method and Findings

Project Ice Storm involved 218 women who were pregnant during the 1998 Quebec ice storm and their children. When the children were aged 13,

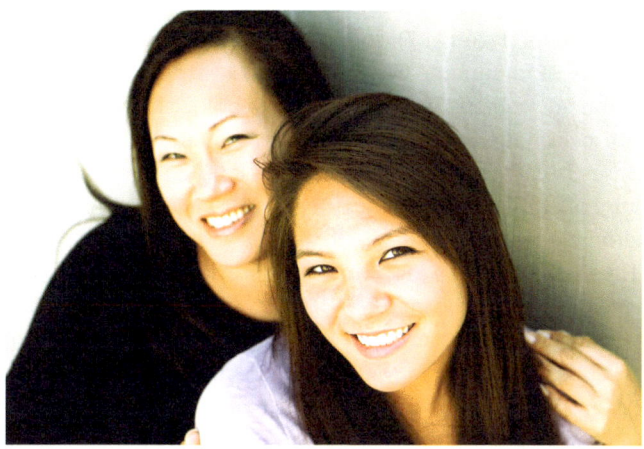

Figure 18.3 Mother and daughter

Source: '00-10' by Emery Co Photo is licensed under CC BY-SA 2.0

this study looked at their DNA methylation and compared children whose mothers rated the storm as negative (n = 12) in 1998 with those whose mothers rated the storm as neutral or positive (n = 22). Significant differences were found in DNA methylation between children whose mothers appraised the storm as positive or negative. Differences were found in the methylation levels of 2,872 child genome sites. These sites are affiliated with 1,564 different genes and 408 biological pathways that prominently feature in immune function.

Significance

This study suggests that pregnant women's experiences and appraisals of stress may have widespread effects on DNA methylation across the entire genome of their unborn children that are detectable during adolescence.

Cao-Lei, L., Elgbeili, G., Massart, R., Laplante, D.P., Szyf, M. & King, S. (2015) Pregnant women's cognitive appraisal of a natural disaster affects DNA methylation in their children 13 years later: Project Ice Storm. *Translational Psychiatry, 24*(5): e515.

There is also evidence from epidemiology and animal research that environmental influences, such as greater adversity or a lack of nurturing, can lead to physiological changes that are then passed from parents to children and grandchildren. This is often referred to as the **intergenerational transmission of vulnerability** (Scorza et al., 2019). It is attributable to both epigenetic transmission (see Chapter 8) and shared aspects of the environment that increase the likelihood of poor child outcomes, such as exposure to domestic violence. However, it is worth highlighting that although stress in pregnancy and the early years is associated with a greater risk of adverse outcomes, most children are not affected. The mechanisms that determine which children are affected, and in which ways, are not yet well understood (Glover, 2016).

Another way in which psychological factors are important in pregnancy is through beliefs and health behaviour. A study of beliefs in late pregnancy, based on the self-regulation model (see Chapter 4, Figure 4.7), found that women's beliefs about personal control, consequences, coherence, and emotional representations of pregnancy explained a large proportion of the variation in women's physical and psychological health in pregnancy (Jessop et al., 2014). Health behaviours such as smoking, alcohol and substance use, exposure to toxins, diet, and exercise also affect the woman and developing foetus in a number of ways. For example, the overuse of alcohol during pregnancy is associated with miscarriage, stillbirth, and foetal alcohol syndrome (Sebastiani et al., 2018).

Theories of health behaviour change can therefore be used to guide health promotion and intervention during pregnancy. The COM-B framework may be particularly useful for perinatal interventions (Olander et al., 2016). This framework was developed from a synthesis of 19 theories of health behaviour change and suggests that change is a function of Capability, Opportunity, and Motivation (Michie et al., 2011; see also Chapter 5). These are likely to fluctuate during pregnancy and after birth because of changes in physical, psychological, and social factors. Therefore, although women may be more motivated to change during pregnancy, they also need the capability and opportunity to change, which can vary across the perinatal period.

Birth

Birth is a significant life event for women and their partners, and women often have detailed expectations of labour and birth. Social norms and women's expectations influence women's choices about where to give birth, how they give birth, and the use of pain relief. The widespread provision of antenatal classes in developed countries is partly based on an assumption that there is a causal relationship between a woman's knowledge/expectations and her experience of birth. Original proponents of natural childbirth, such as Dick-Read (1933, 2004), believed that expectations of pain cause fear, and that fear consequently results in increased tension and pain during labour. They argued that if women are educated so they change their expectations and learn relaxation techniques to combat tension, then pain will be reduced. Although research does not provide unequivocal evidence that attendance at antenatal classes leads to a reduction of pain in labour (Gagnon & Sandall, 2007), the incorporation of antenatal classes is now an accepted part of antenatal care.

The greatest social change in experiences of childbirth has been the context and type of birth. Births have moved from the home to hospital, and the number of caesarean births is increasing. In the UK, caesarean rates have risen from under 5% in the 1950s to 37% in 2022 (NHS Digital, 2022). The suggestion that this increase is partly due to more women wanting caesareans is not supported by the evidence. A review of maternal requests for caesarean section found multiple reasons for this, including fear of pain and childbirth, anxiety about the birth and/or injury to the baby, previous negative birth experiences, time of birth and doctors' suggestion (Jenabi et al., 2020). Most caesareans are performed as emergency births after labour has started, suggesting that the rise in caesarean sections is due to increased complications during labour and/or an increased tendency for clinicians to carry out caesareans rather than continue with non-operative births.

Discourses and ideologies around birth and maternity care are culturally determined, so they vary between and within cultures. Even within a society, different individuals can have contrasting views that birth is risky and care should be highly medicalised, or that birth is a natural process where medical interference is harmful (Benyamini et al., 2017). Maternity services and practitioners may have internalised or embraced a set of ideologies around birth and, for hospital birth, this attitude is likely to be underpinned by a biomedical approach. Differences in beliefs and notions of risk between health professionals and pregnant women may result in conflict and misunderstandings (S. Lee et al., 2019). Giving birth in a hospital may feel reassuring, informed, technologically advanced, and safe to women with a biomedical view of birth, but may feel unsafe and perilous to women with a different view. For example, a study from Australia, where hospital birth is highly medicalised, found that women who chose a home birth against medical advice or without trained health professionals were well educated about the risks of birth, but they perceived hospital care to be riskier than staying at home (Jackson et al., 2020). Women in this study had therefore intensely scrutinised, or personally experienced, the risks inherent in giving birth in a hospital, and decided that the activities of healthcare providers and organisations were riskier than the birth process itself.

Women's expectations of birth are complex and dynamic. Research shows that most women have well-formed expectations of many aspects of childbirth, the baby, being a mother, and their partner's role. Women have positive and negative expectations of different aspects of birth, such as emotions, control, pain, and obstetric events. These expectations can be refined with new information and experiences (Preis et al., 2019). Women's expectations are broadly associated with birth experiences. Positive expectations of birth are associated with experiencing more positive births, such as greater control in birth, greater satisfaction, and emotional wellbeing. Conversely, negative expectations are associated with finding birth less fulfilling, being less satisfied with birth, and reporting less emotional wellbeing after birth (Buyukcan-Tetik et al., 2024). These associations may partly be due to other factors, such as anxiety or self-efficacy.

Fear can have a strong effect on women's expectations and experiences. Severe fear of childbirth (tocophobia) affects 14% of pregnant women (O'Connell et al., 2017). Symptoms include high levels of anxiety about pregnancy and birth, fear of harm or death during birth, poor sleep, and somatic complaints. Fear of childbirth is multifactorial and associated with having a first baby (being nulliparous), poor mental health, younger age, lower education, and low self-efficacy (Laursen et al., 2009; Rouhe et al., 2009; Salomonsson et al., 2013). Although fear of childbirth is more common in nulliparous women, women who have negative or traumatic experiences of birth are five times more likely to report fear of childbirth in a subsequent pregnancy (Størksen et al., 2013). Fear of childbirth increased during the COVID-19 pandemic, presumably exacerbated by the restrictions to maternity care imposed during this time (Kanellopoulos & Gourounti, 2023). Women who fear childbirth are more likely to want interventions such as elective caesarean sections (Kanellopoulos & Gourounti, 2022).

The birth of a baby is usually seen as a positive event. However, evidence shows that around 30% of women in western countries find giving birth traumatic, and 4% develop post-traumatic stress disorder (PTSD) (Heyne et al., 2022). Women who have assisted deliveries or caesarean sections are more likely to develop PTSD, but it is not a straightforward relationship: individual risk factors interact with what happens during birth to determine whether women find it traumatic. A meta-analysis of 55 studies found that the strongest risk factors for PTSD are fear of birth, depression, previous trauma, poor health or complications in pregnancy, negative birth experiences, lack of support during birth, and dissociation (where people feel detached from reality) (Ayers et al., 2016). Symptoms of PTSD following birth include re-experiencing the birth (e.g. flashbacks, intrusive thoughts), avoidance of reminders of the birth, hyperarousal (e.g. hypervigilance, anger, irritability), and negative cognitions and mood (American Psychiatric Association, 2013). Women who have severe complications during pregnancy or birth, such as pre-eclampsia or preterm babies, are at greater risk, with 19% reporting PTSD (Yildiz et al., 2017). An example of cognitive behavioural therapy treatment for a woman with PTSD and depression after birth is given in Chapter 14 (Case Study 14.1).

Support from others during labour and birth has a critical influence on birth outcomes and psychological wellbeing. Women are more likely to have PTSD if they feel poorly informed, not listened to, inadequately cared for, or have poor support from staff or their partner (Horsch et al., 2024). The provision of support for women during labour is not standard in many poorly resourced countries. Experimental studies have been conducted in countries where women are not usually accompanied during birth, so that some women were randomly allocated a lay woman ('doula') to support them during birth. A meta-analysis of the doula studies showed that simply providing a lay person to support a woman during labour resulted in better physical outcomes for both mother and baby, including shorter labours, less analgesia, fewer assisted or operative deliveries, and higher maternal satisfaction with the birth experience (Bohren et al., 2017).

In terms of medical care, the factors outlined above have a number of implications. One is that providing good support during labour may prevent women being traumatised. Another is that reducing fear, stress, and anxiety in pregnancy may improve maternal and infant outcomes. For example, intervention for women with a severe fear of childbirth can reduce fear and caesarean births (Webb et al., 2021).

Another important consideration is the impact of stress on health professionals who are pregnant. As we have seen, stressful and physically demanding jobs are related to adverse pregnancy outcomes. Research shows that pregnant health professionals are at increased risk of pregnancy complications, especially in late pregnancy. During pregnancy, doctors working in hospitals report that the physical demands of the job (e.g. night shifts, standing for long periods) are stressful and there is poor support from colleagues. Institutional support for female healthcare workers during pregnancy is lacking and needs to be properly examined (Ortiz Worthington et al., 2019).

In summary, pregnancy and birth are a time of great change and transition, when biological, psychological, social, and macro-cultural factors all influence outcomes for women and their children. Psychological theories and evidence are highly relevant, as illustrated by the effect of stress and anxiety in pregnancy on the developing foetus, and how expectations and fear of childbirth influence birth.

Clinical Notes 18.1

Antenatal Care

- It is important to identify pregnant women with high levels of distress or anxiety and to offer an appropriate intervention.
- Reducing stress and anxiety in pregnant women potentially benefits the wellbeing of women and their unborn babies.
- Reducing fear of childbirth leads to improved wellbeing in pregnancy and may lead to fewer requests for caesarean sections.
- Referral to perinatal psychology or support services may be appropriate. They can provide psychological support for women and their families during pregnancy and after birth.
- Such services are increasing as healthcare services realise the long-term impact that maternal wellbeing in pregnancy and after birth has on both the mother and the health and development of their child.

18.1.3 High-Risk Pregnancies and Birth

Pregnancy and birth can be high risk for a number of reasons. Pregnancy loss can be particularly difficult and includes miscarriage, termination of pregnancy, and stillbirth. Approximately one in six pregnancies ends in miscarriage. Although often thought of as a lesser event than stillbirth, miscarriage can be distressing for women and is associated with increased risk of anxiety, depression, and PTSD (Quenby et al., 2021).

Worldwide, every year 2.6 million babies are stillborn after 24 weeks of pregnancy. In the majority of cases the reason for death is unexplained. Studies unanimously find that this is an intensely painful loss for parents, with reports of intense grief, marital difficulties, feelings of worthlessness, isolation, shame, and guilt. Around one-third of women report high levels of anxiety, depression, and/or PTSD (Campbell-Jackson & Horsch, 2014). Medical practice in many countries is to offer parents a chance to see and hold their dead infant on the assumption that it will help the grieving process. However, the evidence for this is inconsistent and some research suggests that, although many parents appreciate the opportunity to do this, they may have poorer mental health in the long term (Sun et al., 2023). Stigma and reduced chances to talk about the stillbirth and baby also contribute to poorer mental health in the long term (Crawley et al., 2013).

18.1.4 Mental Health in Pregnancy and after Birth

The transition to parenthood is a time of great change and adjustment, which for some new parents can exacerbate existing mental health problems or lead to the development of new mental health problems. It has been estimated that around 20% of women develop some form of mental health problem in pregnancy or after birth. In addition to affecting women's wellbeing, it has a substantial cost to society. For example, it is estimated that perinatal mental health problems cost the UK £8.1 billion per year. A substantial proportion of this cost (72%) is due to the long-term impact on the child (Bauer et al., 2014). There is also evidence that men can be affected, with up to 10% of fathers having depression in the perinatal period and up to 18% having anxiety disorders (Cameron et al., 2016; Leach et al., 2016).

A range of mental health problems can occur during pregnancy and after birth, such as anxiety, depression, PTSD, postpartum psychosis, and bonding disorders. The most common psychological problems are anxiety and depression, which occur in pregnancy or after birth in approximately 20% of women and 10% of men. Other possible disorders include PTSD, obsessive compulsive disorder (OCD), and stress-related conditions such as adjustment disorder. Mental health conditions are one of the leading indirect causes of maternal death, particularly in the first year after birth (Knight et al., 2023). Most of this is due to drug and alcohol misuse and suicide.

How mental health or illness is conceptualised is important in perinatal mental health (see Chapter 7). It is possible that diagnosis and estimates of prevalence are affected by normal perinatal factors, such as fatigue and anxiety about the baby's wellbeing. Conversely, a focus on psychiatric disorders may mean that many women who have symptoms that do not fit diagnostic criteria will be missed. These symptoms may still be distressing for women and potentially have long-term consequences for them and their child. For example, in a survey of 1,500 women in the UK with self-identified perinatal mental health problems, a wide range of symptoms were reported (see Figure 18.4). These included less commonly recognised symptoms such as anger and changes in appetite. Furthermore, 22% of women in this survey had thought about suicide (Boots Family Trust Alliance, 2013).

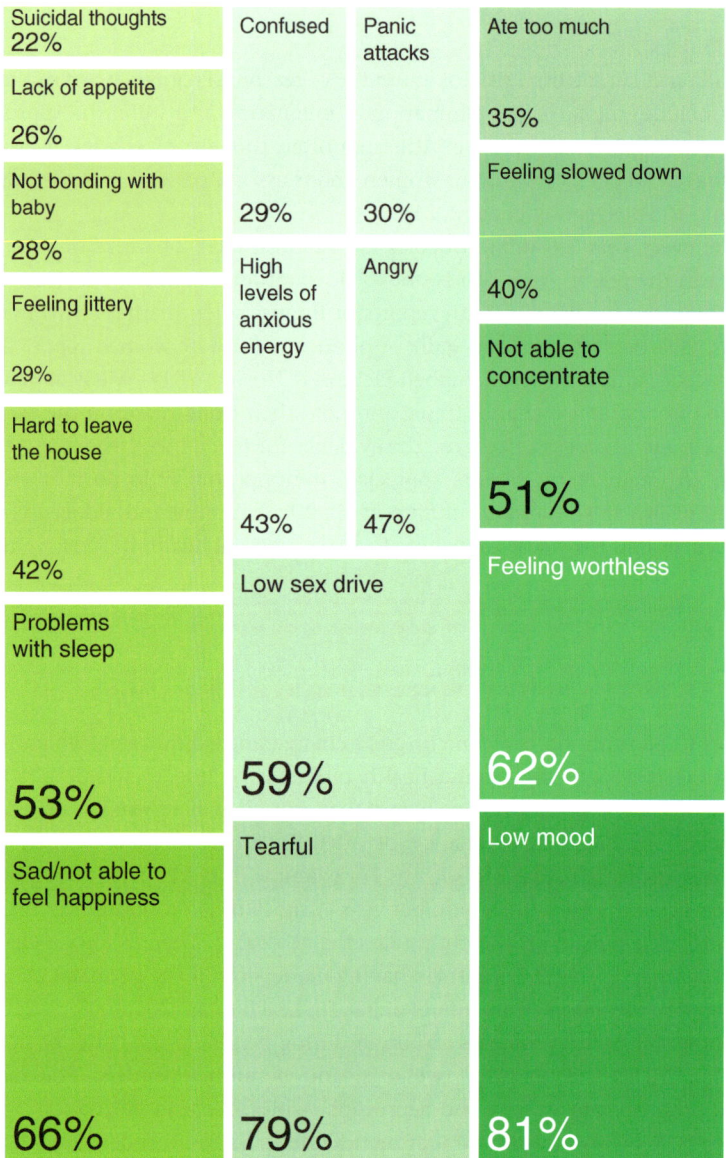

Figure 18.4   Symptoms reported by women with postpartum mental health problems (Boots Family Trust Alliance, 2013)

Source: Reproduced with permission by Tommy's, *Perinatal Mental Health: Experiences of Women and Health Professionals* (Boots Family Trust Alliance, 2013)

One important issue with postpartum mental health problems is determining whether they were present before the birth, as women with anxiety or depression in pregnancy are more likely to have symptoms postpartum. Research also suggests that the prevalence of depression during pregnancy is not significantly different from depression after birth. Thus, some people question whether the notion of 'postpartum' mental health problems is appropriate. It may be that pregnancy, birth, and adjusting to parenthood can exacerbate or initiate a wide range of different mental health problems which are similar to those observed after other stressful events, such as bereavement or divorce.

Risk and Resilience

A number of risk factors make it more likely that women will develop perinatal mental health problems. Some of these risk factors are remarkably consistent across different disorders and cultures. For example, mental health problems are more likely to occur when women live in circumstances of social adversity (e.g. deprivation, low socioeconomic status, domestic violence), have a history of psychological problems or childhood adversity, and/or have poor support available to them. In addition, if women are anxious or depressed during pregnancy, it is likely to continue or worsen postpartum.

Nonetheless, the majority of women are psychologically healthy during pregnancy and after birth, so it is important to look at what characterises health during pregnancy and the factors associated with resilience. Most definitions of resilience see it as a dynamic process which involves activation of coping techniques to manage, adapt to, or recover from adversity, stress, or trauma (Southwick et al., 2014). A study of over 1,300 women in the USA found that women who were resilient were characterised by lower, depression and stress, and higher support and self-efficacy. These women were also less likely to have risky health behaviours in pregnancy and were more likely to have better birth outcomes. In contrast, vulnerable women were characterised by higher depression and stress and poor support and self-efficacy. Vulnerable women were more likely to have an unintended pregnancy, risky health behaviours, or have their baby preterm (Maxson et al., 2016).

The Impact of Perinatal Mental Health Problems

Perinatal mental health problems have a negative impact on women, children, and families. The impact on women and children varies according to the type of mental illness and timing: whether it occurs in the pre- and/or postpartum period, and whether it is acute or chronic. As we have seen, stress and anxiety during pregnancy are associated with an increased risk of a range of adverse outcomes for women and their children, including preterm birth (Ding et al., 2014), which is one of the major causes of morbidity and mortality in children. After birth, mental health problems can have a negative impact on the relationship between the mother and baby, and her partner (Delicate et al., 2018). Women with mental health problems may be less sensitive to their baby's emotional state and display less optimal parenting, such as being withdrawn and unavailable to the baby or over-intrusive (Saharoy et al., 2023). The impact of postpartum mental health problems on the child has been mostly researched in relation to postpartum depression. It shows that depression is associated with poor development and mental health problems in children (Saharoy et al., 2023). Poor parental mental health is also one of many factors associated with child maltreatment (Ayers et al., 2019). However, it must be noted that maltreatment is a rare occurrence, and the majority of parents with mental health problems do *not* maltreat their children. Nevertheless, these are some of the mechanisms through which mental health problems and social adversity can be transmitted from one generation to the next in the intergenerational transmission of vulnerability.

Treatment and interventions during pregnancy and after birth are important to prevent the transmission of social adversity and mental health problems between generations. Progress in this regard is limited for a number of reasons. First, only a small proportion of women with perinatal mental health problems come to the attention of health services, and even fewer of these women receive treatment (Webb et al., 2023b). This is due to a range of factors, which include a lack of screening (or ineffective screening), barriers to women seeking help during this time, clinician barriers to diagnosis and treatment, a lack of perinatal psychology services, and limited evidence on effective treatments (Webb et al., 2023a). In terms of effective treatments, there is most evidence for the treatment of postpartum depression with CBT or interpersonal therapy. Clinical guidelines are available that recommend effective psychotherapies on the basis of current evidence (e.g., National Institute for Clinical Excellence, 2020; Scottish Intercollegiate Guidelines Network, 2023). Despite this, reviews of diagnosis and treatment of perinatal depression by primary care physicians suggest that antidepressants are often the first line of treatment (Ford et al., 2017).

Clinical Notes 18.2

Postpartum Care

- Birth can be experienced as traumatic, and some women develop PTSD following difficult births.
- Watch out for high levels of anxiety and re-experiencing of symptoms, such as nightmares, intrusive thoughts, and flashbacks.
- Postpartum PTSD can be successfully treated if women are referred to psychotherapy in the first few months after birth.
- Be vigilant for signs of postpartum depression. Be aware that many women have depressive symptoms prior to, or during, pregnancy.
- Women may develop a range of anxiety disorders, such as OCD, panic disorders, or social phobia.
- Postpartum psychosis is severe and requires *immediate* inpatient treatment, preferably in a mother–baby unit.
- Make sure you are aware of the availability of psychological interventions for women with postpartum mental health problems, particularly postpartum psychosis, which requires fast action and referral.

Summary 18.2

- Antenatal stress and mental health problems are associated with a range of adverse outcomes for women and their babies.
- The context and type of birth has changed historically, with more women giving birth in hospitals and an increasing number of caesarean births.
- Supporting women well during labour results in better physical outcomes and maternal psychological wellbeing.
- The transition to parenthood is associated with increased risk of depression, anxiety, and psychotic disorders.

- Psychological problems following birth have an adverse impact on women, their relationships, and their baby.
- High-risk pregnancies, miscarriage, and stillbirth are associated with high levels of distress, such as depression and PTSD.

18.2 Endocrine Function and Psychosocial Wellbeing

Psychoneuroendocrinology is the study of how psychological states are related to changes in hormone secretion. It has an increasing role in the diagnosis and treatment of affective disorders and anxiety disorders. One of the most obvious reasons for this change is the observation that people with primary endocrine disorders are more likely than the general population to experience psychiatric morbidity. Another reason is better understanding of the synergies between the neural and endocrine systems and the differing roles of hormonal and neuronal control of the function of the pituitary (which is often referred to as the 'master gland') by the hypothalamus. Dysfunction in the hypothalamus or other brain regions can affect the functioning of the endocrine system, which is in turn associated with psychiatric symptoms.

The notion of the 'psychopharmacological bridge' has also guided work in this area. If a drug produces a therapeutic effect (e.g. relieving symptoms) and has specific biochemical actions (e.g. modifying hormone secretion), then it suggests a causal link between the therapeutic effects, the biochemical changes, and the cause of the syndrome. For example, if a drug known to treat cortisol hypersecretion also reduces the psychiatric symptoms of depression, then it suggests that cortisol hypersecretion is a casual factor in the onset and progression of the depression.

18.2.1 Hypothalamic-Pituitary-Adrenal Axis (HPA)

There is a wealth of research evidence documenting HPA axis hyperactivity in people with depression who are not taking medication. Changes in the HPA axis in depressed people include elevated corticotrophin releasing hormone (CRH) in cerebrospinal fluid, enlarged pituitary and/or adrenal glands, and increased production of adrenocorticotropic hormone (ACTH) and/or cortisol during periods of depression. It is not completely clear whether these HPA axis changes are a cause or symptom of depression. For example, dysregulation of the HPA axis can occur after periods of chronic or severe stress. It is also observed in other stress-related conditions, such as PTSD, where, conversely, there is a reduced cortisol response (see Chapter 3).

Cortisol Hypersecretion (Cushing's Syndrome)

Common psychiatric aspects of cortisol hypersecretion include depression and irritability. In the initial description of his eponymous syndrome, Cushing (1932) described a relationship between cortisol hypersecretion and psychological symptoms. People with Cushing's syndrome often have a consistent constellation of psychological symptoms, predominantly impaired affect (Piasecka et al., 2020). Depression and irritability are very common. Fatigue is universal and may be explained by common insomnia. Many people also report decreased libido. Cognitive symptoms include decreased concentration and poor problem solving and memory. These factors combine to influence social withdrawal, which may also be affected by changes in physical appearance, such as truncal obesity, a round face, and a 'buffalo hump'.

There may be problems of **differential diagnosis** in people with cortisol hypersecretion. Without thorough investigation, it may be difficult to determine whether a person with hyper-cortisolaemia has primary depression or early Cushing's syndrome.

Cortisol Hyposecretion (Addison's Disease)

The major behavioural manifestations of cortisol hyposecretion are lethargy and apathy. Other behavioural manifestations include irritability, crying, and impaired sleep. People may also have problems with memory and concentration, and report tachycardia (Ramos-Levi et al., 2023). There may be problems of differential diagnosis in people with cortisol hyposecretion because the person may show non-specific symptoms that wax and wane. In addition, periods of stress exacerbate symptoms – because the adrenal glands are called on to increase secretion (see Chapter 3) – and these symptoms decrease when the stress abates. These presenting symptoms mean hypocortisolism can be misdiagnosed as a primary psychiatric condition. For example, tachycardia, dizziness, and complaints of lethargy may be misdiagnosed as anxiety disorders or chronic fatigue syndrome.

For both of the cortisol-related syndromes just described, there is evidence that changes in cortisol levels produce the original psychiatric symptoms (Gan & Pearce, 2017; Piasecka et al., 2020; Ramos-Levi et al., 2023). Effective treatment of cortisol hypersecretion is associated with improvements in mood and cognitive function. Effective treatment of cortisol hyposecretion alleviates psychological and behavioural symptoms.

Activity 18.1

Differential Diagnosis

- What is meant by differential diagnosis?
- Why may differential diagnosis be difficult in people with cortisol hyposecretion or hypersecretion?

18.2.2 Hypothalamic-Pituitary-Thyroid Axis (HPT)

The link between thyroid function and behaviour was first documented 200 years ago. Parry (1825) noted that hyperfunction of the thyroid was associated with 'various nervous affecta-tions' and symptoms, such as restlessness, hyperactivity, and impaired concentration. A causative role of hypothyroidism in psychopathology was demonstrated by Asher (1949), who conducted a case series showing that administration of desiccated thyroid alleviated psycholog-ical symptoms of depression and psychotic symptoms. Abnormal thyroid function is more common among people with psychiatric illnesses than in the general population. However, part of this difference is iatrogenic: various psychotropic medications (e.g. lithium, neuroleptics, and antidepressants) will disturb HPT axis function to varying degrees.

In recent decades there has been an increase in understanding of the links between thyroid function and psychological wellbeing. Most people with thyroid disorders complain of a psychological disturbance that is alleviated on correction of the thyroid illness. This indicates the involvement of the HPT system in psychological states.

Hyperthyroidism

The behavioural states observed in hyperthyroidism include intense dysphoria, usually with pronounced anxiety. Other common complaints include nervousness, emotional lability, restlessness, and impaired concentration. Insomnia and fatigue are common, and people may feel too weak and tired to carry out planned activities. Decreased concentration and impaired memory are correlated with thyrotoxicosis.

Hypothyroidism

Hypothyroidism is the most common clinical disorder of thyroid function. The most prevalent psychological symptoms can be grouped into cognitive dysfunction (impaired memory, inattentiveness, slower and poorer problem solving) and mood changes (predominantly depressed mood, but also anxiety, insomnia, irritability, and confusion). Psychosis may be present in severe hypothyroidism.

For both of the thyroid-related syndromes just described, there is evidence that psychological symptoms are more pronounced in clinical hyperthyroidism or hypothyroidism, and may abate following effective treatments of the hormonal abnormality (Bode et al., 2022; Samuels, 2014). This suggests that the hormonal imbalance causes the psychological symptoms. In hyperthyroidism, scores on measures of mood, anxiety, and cognitive function often return to normal after a return to euthyroid status. Similarly, in hypothyroidism, psychiatric symptoms are alleviated following effective treatment of the thyroid disorder. However, it is important to note that many people have impaired quality of life even after thyroid hormone levels have returned to within the normal range, often because of an altered relationship with their body (Nexø et al., 2015).

18.2.3 Growth Hormone

Excess secretion of growth hormone (GH) results in gigantism in children and acromegaly in adults. The most common cause of GH hypersecretion is pituitary adenoma. Physical symptoms are usually obvious, such as abnormal growth of the hands and feet, and changes in bony and soft tissue, including an altered facial appearance. Psychiatric symptoms are rare, although depression may occasionally occur. Although clinical psychiatric symptoms are rare, people with acromegaly have lower scores on measures of quality of life and self-esteem, which appear to be related to differences in body image (Crespo et al., 2017) (see Research Box 18.2). These changes can lead to social withdrawal, disruption in interpersonal relations, mood swings, and a loss of initiative and spontaneity. In addition to medical or surgical treatment to address the cause of GH hypersecretion, there may be benefits from exercise therapy to improve quality of life and self-esteem (Hatipoglu et al., 2014). Treatment of excessive secretion of GH to cure acromegaly can lead to improvements to quality of life (Broersen et al., 2021), as can cognitive behavioural therapy (Kunzler et al., 2018). However, many people still have impaired quality of life even when the disease has been controlled in biochemical terms (Kimball et al., 2022). The remainder of this section examines the psychosocial impact of GH deficiency.

GH deficiency causes an absence or delay in the lengthening and widening of the skeletal bones. In some cases, the onset of the disorder occurs antenatally and in others the condition occurs months or years later. However, it has clear impacts on self-esteem and distorted body image. Children with GH deficiency have higher rates of anxiety, depression, social phobia, and attentional dysfunction than their peers. In adults, quality of life is lower in those with growth hormone deficiencies (Hull & Harvey, 2003). This may be displayed as social phobia, fear of negative evaluation, decreased interest or pleasure in activities, depression, fatigue, and irritability.

—Research Box 18.2—

Psychological Aspects of Treated Endocrine Disorders

Background

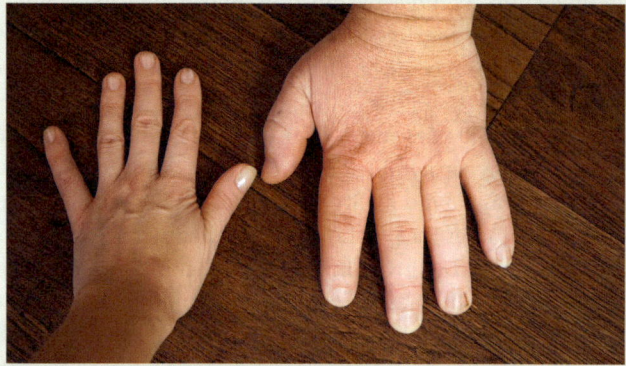

Many people with endocrine disorders complain of disturbances to psychological wellbeing and quality of life. The close links between psychological wellbeing and endocrine function mean that it is important to consider psychosocial issues in the concept of recovery in endocrine disorders such as acromegaly.

Figure 18.5 Acromegaly

Source: © Magorzata/Adobe stock

Method and Findings

The study participants were 223 people aged 18–85 years with acromegaly who were recruited from five referral centres in Italy: 165 were under medical treatment and 58 were in surgical remission. Psychosocial difficulties were common, and included depression and anxiety, cognitive impairment, impaired body image, sleep disorders, and sexual dysfunction. Longer disease duration, greater patient age, and female age were strong determinants of these conditions. However, acromegaly was found to be associated with impairments to psychosocial wellbeing that persisted despite remission and long-term medical treatment.

Significance

This study shows that a purely biomedical approach to treating endocrine disorders is not sufficient. It highlights the need for ongoing attention to the psychological wellbeing of people who have been treated for the physiological aspects of endocrine disorders.

Pivonello, R., Auriemma, R.S., Delli Veneri, A. et al. (2022) Global psychological assessment with the evaluation of life and sleep quality and sexual and cognitive function in a large number of patients with acromegaly: A cross-sectional study. *European Journal of Endocrinology, 187*: 823–845. doi:10.1530/EJE-22-0263.

Some of the psychological impacts of GH deficiency are height-related, especially for men. However, the observed differences cannot be explained solely on the basis of short stature. Comparisons among adults of a very short stature show that people who are short but do not have a GH deficiency have fewer psychosocial problems than people who have GH deficiencies (Hull & Harvey, 2003). Although treatment of a GH deficiency in adults does not increase height, there is some evidence that it may reduce premature mortality and improve quality of life, but it may increase the risk of neoplasms and diabetes (Díez et al., 2018; He & Barkan, 2020; van Bunderen & Olsson, 2023). Further research is required.

The close links between psychological wellbeing and endocrine function have prompted some to suggest that the concept of recovery in endocrine disorders should be expanded to give greater consideration to psychosocial issues (Sonino & Fava, 2012).

Clinical Notes 18.3

Endocrine Disorders

- Given the common occurrence of psychological symptoms in endocrine disorders, it is important to make an accurate diagnosis.
- Do not assume that psychological symptoms are 'just psychological'. They may be the result of endocrine disorders.
- Differential diagnosis is important for ensuring that appropriate treatment is administered.
- Even when physiological aspects of endocrine disorders are successfully treated, there may be a need for ongoing psychosocial support.

18.2.4 Sex Hormones and Psychosocial Wellbeing

Testosterone has two effects on the body: androgen effects (the development and maintenance of secondary male sexual characteristics) and anabolic effects (the promotion of muscle growth). **Anabolic androgenic steroids** (AAS) are synthetic compounds that are structurally related to testosterone. Bodybuilders and athletes may use AAS to develop a more muscular physique. The practice is generally banned in competitive sports because of concerns that competition should be fair and based on natural ability.

Long-term AAS use can have serious consequences for physical and psychological wellbeing. It can lead to irreversible toxicity in the cardiovascular system and organ systems, including the liver (Linhares et al., 2022). The misuse of AAS also appears to be associated with psychosocial problems such as dependence syndromes, mood disorders, psychotic syndromes, and progression to other forms of substance abuse (Chegeni et al., 2021; Goldman et al., 2019). Although psychological problems may be a contributor to AAS misuse, it should be noted that people who have low self-esteem or mood disturbances, or those who have experienced negative or adverse events during childhood, may be more likely to misuse AAS. Most research has focused on young men, but attention is also being given to AAS use among women (Onakomaiya & Henderson, 2016).

In men, use of AAS has unwanted physical side effects, such as testicular atrophy, reduced sperm production, acne, and the development of abnormally large mammary glands (Linhares et al., 2022). There is also concern about the psychological side effects of using androgenic anabolic steroids, particularly the phenomenon colloquially known as 'roid rage'. Reviews of research provide some evidence of increased rates of hypomania and increased aggressiveness and violence among steroid users (Linhares et al., 2022; Lundholm et al., 2015). However, it is important to note that underlying personality traits of aggression and hostility may be relevant, because not all AAS users display these behaviours. Furthermore, as noted in Chapter 9 (section 9.4.1 on aggression), there is no simple explanation for all aggressive or violent behaviour. Research in this area is hampered by the fact that, because non-prescribed steroid use is illegal, it is difficult to estimate the size of the population at risk, or to recruit large numbers of steroid users into controlled trials. There is also concern about the use of unsafe fake products available on the black market (Magnolini et al., 2022).

18.2.5 Ethical Issues in Hormone Therapy

The sections above highlight how the treatment of hormonal abnormalities can improve psychological wellbeing. However, it is also true that hormonal treatment can be used to treat problems that do not have a hormonal cause. Such use of hormones is often accompanied by ethical and moral concerns. One example of this is an Australian study of girls who had been treated with oestrogen in order to reduce their adult height. The treatment was found to reduce adult height, and it was administered to reduce the supposed negative psychosocial impacts of being 'too tall'. The study revealed that the assessment and treatment procedures carried out during the sensitive period of adolescence were a negative experience for many of the girls involved (Pyett et al., 2005). Furthermore, hormonal treatment increased the likelihood of fertility problems in adulthood (Venn et al., 2004), and it did not lead to better psychosocial wellbeing (Bruinsma et al., 2006).

The use of hormonal treatment raises a range of other ethical issues. For example, in our society, tallness is usually desirable and the treatment of growth hormone deficiencies can be used to increase final adult height. However, its potential use by people without growth hormone deficiencies raises important questions about where we draw the line between medical therapy and psychosocial enhancement.

More recently, other uses of hormonal therapy have been the subject of public debate. Increasing awareness of the experiences of people who are transgender or gender non-binary has drawn attention to the use of hormone blockers in young people who experience gender dysphoria. Gender dysphoria is an experience of unease or dissatisfaction that can arise when a person experiences a mismatch between their biological sex and their gender identity. Intense dysphoria can lead to depression and anxiety, and have a harmful impact on daily life.

Most treatments offered for gender dysphoria are psychological rather than medical. For many children, gender dysphoria may disappear as they reach puberty. However, if the dysphoria is intense and persistent, and the children meet eligibility criteria, then they may also undergo treatment with hormone blockers. These blockers pause the physiological changes of puberty, such as the growth of facial hair in boys or breast development in girls. Later in puberty, young people may be given 'cross-sex' hormones – that is, people who are biologically female but who identify as male may be given testosterone, and people who are biologically male but who identify as female may be given oestrogen to promote breast development. Various concerns have been raised about denying or providing such hormone therapy. For example, some argue that chidlren's concerns and distress should be responded to with treatment. Others are concerned about children's capacity to make decisions about what may be irreversible changes. The timing of pubertal changes means that many young people may not be recognised legally as having capacity to give consent for treatment. There is also concern about the known (and unknown) side effects and risks of such treatment. Case Study 18.2 illustrates some of these concerns and debates.

An additional domain in which endocrinology and hormonal treatment raises ethical issues is fertility control. Many people have concerns about the use (or the timing of the use) of hormonal contraception, emergency post-coital contraception (often called the 'morning-after pill'), and hormonal methods to terminate unwanted pregnancy.

Case Study 18.2

Medical, Legal, and Ethical Aspects of Gender Re-assignment

Puberty blockers and cross-sex hormones can be used by young people who experience gender dysphoria and wish to change gender. However, there is debate about whether such intervention is appropriate, when it should occur, and who should be involved in decision making. The history of use of puberty blockers in England illustrates the complex debates that are likely to continue. In 2014, the Gender Identity Development Service (GIDS) at London's Tavistock Clinic was allowed to offer puberty blockers to children aged 12 and older, rather than only to those aged 16, who have

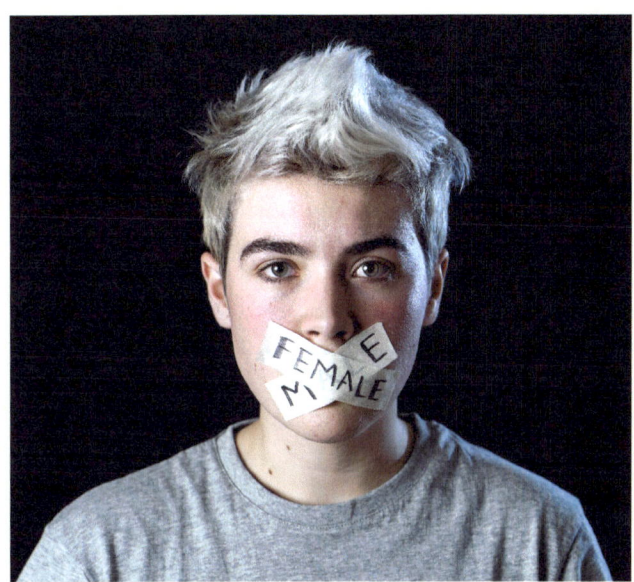

Figure 18.6   The debate about puberty blockers in England

Source: © samuel/Adobe Stock

legal capacity for consent. The change was influenced by legal recognition that children aged under 16 may be recognised as having legal capacity for consent 'if and when the child achieves sufficient understanding and intelligence to fully understand what is proposed'.

However, a landmark legal case in the High Court in January 2020 pitted lawyers representing the GIDS against lawyers representing a former psychiatric nurse at the GIDS, a former patient dissatisfied with their treatment, and the mother of a 15-year-old on the treatment waiting list. The former patient, who now identifies as female, said that she regretted being allowed to transition to male at age 16, and did not believe that children are able to give consent to treatments whose effects may be irreversible and whose long-term side effects may be unknown. The High Court ruled that children below age 16 could not give consent in this context. That decision was overturned following a hearing in the Court of Appeal. However, the debate continues.

In March 2024, NHS England decided that children (up to the age of 16) experiencing gender dysphoria will no longer be able to use puberty blockers. The decision was informed by an evidence review and a public consultation, which led to the conclusion that there is insufficient evidence about the safety and clinical efficacy of puberty blockers. Currently, children are only able to use puberty blockers if they are taking part in a clinical trial.

18.2.6 Stress and Endocrine Function

In addition to considering how changes in endocrine function can affect psychological wellbeing, it is important to note that psychological states can affect endocrine function. A key focus of research in this domain is the study of responses to stress. All stressors – be they physical threats or psychological stress – produce a two-phase pattern of endocrine response (Pinel & Barnes, 2021). In the first phase, stress prompts adaptive changes in the endocrine system to help the person (or other animal) to deal with physical threats, for example, the mobilisation of energy resources, the inhibition of inflammatory responses, and increased resistance to infections. However, where stress is prolonged or repeated, it can produce maladaptive changes in the endocrine system, such as enlarged adrenal glands.

Prolonged stress can lead to the dysregulation of endocrine function and increased strain on systems regulated by the endocrine system, labelled allostatic load. Prolonged stress can also lead to impaired immune function because of interactions between the endocrine and immune systems: cortisol inhibits the production of pro-inflammatory molecules by macrophages and other immune cells, and adrenalin and noradrenalin can modulate the production of cytokines by immune cells (Kovacs & Ojeda, 2011). The influence of stress on immunity is covered in detail in Chapter 3.

Summary 18.3

- Psychoneuroendocrinology is the study of how psychological states are influenced by changes in hormone secretion.
- Disorders of the HPA axis, thyroid function, and sex hormones all have associated psychological symptoms, suggesting some biological basis for these symptoms. Growth hormone disorders are less associated with psychological symptoms.
- The use of hormonal treatment for HPA axis disorders reduces psychological symptoms, suggesting there is a biological basis.
- The use of hormonal treatment for social problems, such as height or gender dysphoria, raises a range of ethical issues, especially if it does not improve psychological wellbeing.
- Endocrine function is affected by stress, which can result in dysregulated responses, such as those observed in depression and PTSD.

Further Reading

Llewellyn, C.D. et al. (eds) (2019) *Cambridge Handbook of Psychology, Health and Medicine* (3rd edition). Cambridge: Cambridge University Press. Includes short chapters on many topics discussed in this chapter, including HRT, antenatal screening, pregnancy and birth, birth complications, perinatal mental health, endocrine disorders, growth retardation, and hyperthyroidism.

Martin, C. (ed.) (2010) *Perinatal Mental Health*. Keswick: M&K. A comprehensive, up-to-date book that covers a wide range of psychological disorders in pregnancy and after birth.

Schatzberg, A.F. & Nemeroff, C.B. (eds) (2017) *American Psychiatric Association Publishing Textbook of Psychopharmacology* (5th edition). Arlington, VA: American Psychiatric Association Publishing. A textbook that has broad coverage of many topics and includes a chapter on psychoneuroendocrinology.

Revision Questions

1   Describe the psychological and cultural factors that affect symptoms of menstruation, premenstrual syndrome (PMS), and premenstrual dysphoric disorder (PMDD).
2   What strategies can be used to help women to manage PMS or PMDD?
3   Describe the psychosocial impact of perimenopause.
4   Discuss the psychosocial factors that are important in pregnancy outcomes.
5   Discuss which factors are important in women's experiences of birth.
6   Outline women's psychological responses to miscarriage and stillbirth. Why do these responses occur?
7   Describe the main psychological problems that can arise during pregnancy and after birth.
8   Choose one endocrine disorder. Outline its common psychosocial symptoms.
9   Outline the arguments for and against hormonal treatment to delay or alter puberty in children who experience gender dysphoria.
10 How might prolonged stress lead to the development of endocrine disorders?

19

GENITOURINARY MEDICINE

───Learning Objectives───────────────────────────────────

This chapter is designed to enable you to:

- Understand sexual health from a biopsychosocial perspective.
- Outline psychological approaches to limiting the spread of sexually transmitted infections.
- Appreciate how concerns about reputation, embarrassment, and gender identity can affect the experience of illness and help-seeking behaviour.
- Outline patient experiences and concerns in kidney disease.

───

Genitourinary medicine is an umbrella term that covers aspects of andrology (men's reproductive health), gynaecology (women's reproductive health), and urology. Genitourinary medicine is primarily related to diagnosing and treating **sexually transmitted infections** (**STIs**). Thus, much of this chapter focuses on STIs. First, however, we consider broader issues related to sexual health. The closing section of this chapter looks at problems in the urinary and renal systems.

19.1 Sexual Health

People commonly equate **sexual health** with **reproductive health** (see Chapter 18). However, sexual health is much broader. If we were to equate 'sexual health' with 'reproductive health', we would exclude a consideration of the sexual health needs of people who (1) are infertile, (2) choose not to reproduce, (3) are post-reproductive, or (4) are not heterosexual. The World Health Organization definition of health (see Chapter 1) has therefore been adapted for a working definition that describes sexual health as:

> A state of physical, emotional, mental and social well-being in relation to sexuality; it is not merely the absence of disease, dysfunction or infirmity. Sexual health requires a positive and respectful approach to sexuality and sexual relationships, as well as the possibility of having pleasurable and safe sexual experiences, free of coercion, discrimination and violence. (World Health Organization, 2006: 4)

This is a broad, biopsychosocial conceptualisation of sexual health that includes a consideration of the three domains of sexual freedom, sexual pleasure, and sexual safety. These three domains are outlined below.

Within this chapter, most attention is given to sexual behaviour, and some attention is given to sexual identity. It is important to note that behaviour, identity, and attraction/desire do not always match. For example, although less than 5% of the population identify as gay, lesbian, or bisexual, over 10% have had some same-sex experience, and around 10% report some current same-sex attraction (Richters et al., 2014). It is also important not to assume that people are heterosexual (i.e. avoid heteronormative assumptions) or to assume that all gay men, lesbians, or bisexual people have the same patterns of sexual desire or behaviour.

19.1.1 Sexual Freedom

Following on from the definition of sexual health given above, sexual freedom can be conceptualised as having pleasurable and safe sexual experiences that are free of coercion, discrimination, or violence. Unfortunately, **sexual coercion** and abuse are widespread: over 20% of women and 5% of men report that they have had unwanted sexual activity because of actual or threatened force (Dworkin et al., 2021). Experience of sexual coercion is related to a range of subsequent difficulties. People who have been coerced have poorer psychological wellbeing, poorer physical health, greater health anxiety, and use health services more. They are more likely to engage in health-compromising behaviours, such as smoking, heavy drinking, and illicit drug use, and are more likely to have been diagnosed with an STI. They are also more likely to experience sexual problems such as a fear of intimacy, a lack of sexual pleasure, and anxiety about sexual performance. Research reveals that any sexual coercion – not just early, repeated, or more severe coercion – leads to poorer health and less healthy patterns of behaviour (de Visser et al., 2007). It is clear that there is a need for support services for people who experience sexual coercion in order to minimise its impact.

Treating the aftermath of sexual coercion or abuse requires sensitivity and excellent communication skills (see Chapter 13). More broadly, health professionals need to be aware that people's understandings of sex and related issues may vary (see Highlight Box 19.1). People may report a diverse array of sexual orientations and sexual behaviours. As long as these behaviours are consensual and legal, any judgemental attitudes or discrimination from health professionals are inappropriate and may be a barrier to promoting sexual health.

Highlight Box 19.1

What is Sex?

Although people will usually assume that 'sex' means 'vaginal intercourse', it is important when taking a medical history to be very clear about what people mean when they talk about sex.

During his presidency, Bill Clinton was questioned several times about whether he had had a sexual relationship with White House intern Monica Lewinsky. Clinton publicly stated 'I did not have sexual relations with that woman', but later revealed that his use of the term 'sexual relations' excluded him receiving oral sex. It is interesting to note that many people agree with Bill Clinton that oral sex does not count as sex (Rissel et al., 2003; Sanders & Reinisch, 1999).

Activity 19.1

How Do We Talk about Sex?

- Take a few minutes to write different colloquial or 'slang' terms for different sexual behaviours.
- Now write down the terms that you would use if you were talking to a medical professional about your own sexual behaviour.

It is important to be aware of the terms that people may use to refer to sexual behaviour. Some may prefer slang terms. Others may prefer euphemisms or will refer indirectly to their sexual behaviour.

19.1.2 Sexual Pleasure and Sexual Problems

The vast majority of adults believe that an active sex life is important for their overall wellbeing and relationships (de Visser et al., 2014b). Unfortunately, **sexual problems** or **sexual dysfunctions** are remarkably common, and many become more common with age. Large population-based studies indicate that the majority of women and men report at least one sexual problem in the previous year (Koops et al., 2023; Richters et al., 2022). Some sexual problems have an organic cause, while others are primarily psychological in nature: most have both physical and psychological components. Whatever their causes, sexual problems can impair quality of life. For example, many people report that they feel anxious about their sexual performance or do not find sex pleasurable. It has been noted that the avoidance of sex or reporting dissatisfying sex can be valuable diagnostic indicators for the presence of sexual dysfunction (Koops et al., 2023).

Many men report that they achieve orgasm too quickly and many experience problems in achieving or maintaining an erection. Rapid ejaculation has a strong psychological component, and psychological interventions can therefore be effective treatments. In contrast, erectile dysfunction commonly has an organic cause. The likelihood of erectile dysfunction is significantly greater in older men, particularly if they have cardiovascular disease, diabetes, or undiagnosed hyperglycaemia (Kessler et al., 2019). Notably, erectile dysfunction and cardiovascular disease are two presentations of the same physiological phenomenon, but because erectile dysfunction typically precedes symptomatic cardiovascular disease, better screening of sexual function could help prevent cardiovascular morbidity and mortality (Mostafaei et al., 2021). It is notable that after treatments for erectile problems became available in the late 1990s, increasing numbers of men reported erectile difficulties (Kaye & Jick, 2003). This was likely to be due to both pharmaceutical companies' marketing of drugs designed to treat erectile problems as 'lifestyle' drugs for all men (Lexchin, 2006), and changes in social norms related to discussing erectile difficulties. Such findings indicate that a biopsychosocial approach (see Chapter 1) is just as important in genitourinary medicine as in other medical domains.

Activity 19.2

How Young is Too Young? How Old is Too Old?

- What would you think – and what would you say – if a 15-year-old asked you for a prescription for oral contraception?
- What would you think – and what would you say – if an 80-year-old asked you for a prescription for medication to treat erectile dysfunction?

Common sexual problems among women include vaginal dryness and pain during intercourse or an inability to orgasm (de Visser et al., 2017a; Moreau et al., 2016; Richters et al., 2022). Some of these problems are more common among older women, particularly vaginal dryness, which is influenced by hormonal changes associated with menopause (see Chapter 18). However, other problems, such as painful intercourse, are more common in younger women.

When treating sexual problems, it is often useful to distinguish between Desire for sex, Arousal once sex is initiated, and obtaining Orgasm (DAO). Dysfunction is often limited to one of these stages, so it is important to make an accurate diagnosis to allow the appropriate targeting of interventions. Sexual difficulties are an important focus of treatment because they are related to less satisfaction with physical and emotional aspects of relationships and a lower level of general happiness (Richters et al., 2022). However, it is important to note that many people do not seek treatment, even for long-lasting problems that they report have a major impact on their lives, often because people find it difficult to discuss sex and sexual wellbeing (Richters et al., 2022). Health professionals may also find such discussions difficult or feel under-prepared for them (Kelder et al., 2022; Manninen et al., 2021).

Chronic Pelvic Pain

Chronic pelvic pain (**CPP**) is not a diagnosis of a single disease; rather, it is a symptom which may be the result of underlying processes in one or more different organ systems. Chronic pelvic pain is defined as constant or intermittent pain in the pelvis or lower abdomen not associated with menstruation, pregnancy, or sexual intercourse. It affects around 15–20% of women (Lamvu et al., 2021). However, the actual prevalence may be higher because many women accept the symptoms as part of being female, and when they do seek medical help, the lack of a clear cause of CPP means that it may be diagnosed in different ways. Numerous potential causes of CPP in different organ systems have been proposed:

- Gynaecological (e.g. endometriosis, chronic pelvic inflammatory disease).
- Gastrointestinal (e.g. irritable bowel syndrome, inflammatory bowel disorder).
- Urological (e.g. interstitial cystitis).
- Musculoskeletal (e.g. fibromyalgia, pelvic floor abnormalities).
- Psychoneurological (e.g. nerve entrapment).

Rather than thinking of CPP as a single disease with a single cause, it may be better to conceptualise it as series of symptoms that may have more than one cause (Lamvu et al., 2021). Nevertheless, women who experience CPP usually want a diagnosis or explanation of their symptoms, even though it may not always be possible. Because of the complex nature of CPP and the large number of different causes with similar or overlapping symptoms, it is important to conduct a thorough patient history, which will allow a differential diagnosis and the selection of the appropriate treatment. The history should include psychological factors because women with CPP are more likely than other women to have experienced sexual abuse. They are also more likely to experience depression, anxiety, and catastrophic thinking. These psychological phenomena could be implicated in CPP as causes or consequences (or both). Whatever their role is in CPP, it should be noted that such negative states influence the perception of pain (see Chapter 4), and that they should be addressed by suitably qualified professionals.

Treatment for CPP is directed more toward managing symptoms than curing the disease. There is a lack of solid evidence about the efficacy of different treatments for CPP (Leonardi et al., 2021). Systematic reviews have revealed support for the efficacy of progestogen and psychological interventions for improving wellbeing (Brooks et al., 2020). Pain has been shown to be alleviated among women who undergo reassurance ultrasound scans accompanied by counselling (compared to women treated with a standard 'wait and see' approach), and among women who undertake disclosure writing therapy (compared to a non-disclosure group).

Although much of the research into CPP has focused on women, men may also experience chronic pelvic pain, and this is often a symptom of prostate cancer (see section 19.3.1) (Suskind et al., 2013).

19.1.3 Sexual Safety

Sexual safety is important: it protects against unwanted pregnancy and STIs. Teenage birth rates in many developed countries are high: they are higher in high-income countries (e.g. Western Europe and North America) than they are in low- and middle-income (or 'developing') countries (United Nations Department of Economic and Social Affairs, 2020). Although some teenagers are happy to become parents, most teenage pregnancies are unplanned. Teenage motherhood is associated with fewer educational qualifications and poor employment prospects (World Health Organization Human Reproduction Programme, 2019). When teenage birth rates are combined with the high rates of termination of pregnancy in teenagers, it is evident that many young people do not take adequate precautions to avoid an unintended pregnancy. A failure to practise **safer sex** consistently also explains why STIs are widespread. This is the focus of the following section.

Summary 19.1

- Sexual health is broader than reproductive health and includes sexual freedom, sexual pleasure, and sexual safety.
- A substantial minority of women and men have experienced sexual coercion or abuse. It is associated with poor psychological and physical wellbeing, increased health anxiety, increased health service use, and more health-compromising behaviours.
- Sexual problems are remarkably common, with the majority of adult women and men reporting at least one sexual problem in the previous year.

- Chronic pelvic pain may arise from dysfunction in several different organ systems. Because its underlying causes may be difficult to determine, it may not be possible to give people the accurate diagnosis or effective treatment they are seeking.
- Sexual risks include unwanted pregnancies and contracting STIs, both of which can be avoided by practising safer sex.

19.2 Sexually Transmissible Infections

In this section, we outline the role of psychosocial factors in three aspects of sexually transmissible infections.

19.2.1 HIV/AIDS

Human Immunodeficiency Virus (HIV) is a retrovirus that causes **Acquired Immune Deficiency Syndrome (AIDS)**. The predominant mode of transmission is unprotected sexual activity. It is estimated that approximately 39 million people worldwide are infected with HIV, with over 2 million new infections per year, the vast majority of which are in sub-Saharan Africa (UNAIDS, 2024). The prevalence of HIV infection varies widely between regions, and is markedly higher in sub-Saharan Africa than elsewhere.

In most regions of the world, sex between men and women is the primary route of transmission. Heterosexual transmission is an important contributor to the spread of HIV, even in areas where sex between men and injection drug use have been, or continue to be, the major transmission routes. For example, in Western Europe, approximately 30% of new infections every year are attributed to heterosexual activity (European Centre for Disease Prevention and Control, 2018, 2021).

Although the virus was identified in the early 1980s, no vaccine or cure has been developed. Since the mid-1990s highly-active antiretroviral therapies (HAART) that suppress viral replication have been available. Suppression of viral replication significantly slows disease progression and significantly reduces the risk of onward transmission. As a consequence, for many people, HIV/AIDS is now a chronic illness rather than a terminal illness. However, these medications are expensive and are not available in all contexts. The result is large global discrepancies in the proportion of people with HIV who are virally suppressed: from over 70% in Europe, North America, and Southern Africa to less than 50% in Eastern Europe and the Middle East (UNAIDS, 2024).

Although HAART is effective for prolonging life, the treatment regimens can be quite complicated and burdensome in terms of the timing of doses and changes to food and fluid intake. This means that adherence is often a problem, but fortunately, people who obtain viral suppression may switch to a simpler two-drug regimen (Cahn et al., 2020). Evidence reviews indicate that interventions can improve adherence and produce lower viral loads (Whiteley et al., 2021). Effective programme components include: adherence counselling, web-based or face-to-face cognitive behavioural intervention, home visits by nurses, text-message reminders, contingency management, modified directly observed therapy, and a once-daily (rather than twice-daily) drug regimen. It is also crucial to provide information about the importance of adherence, and to discuss people's beliefs, motivations, and expectations about treatment so that support can be tailored to individual needs and circumstances (see Chapter 12).

The complexity of HAART regimens, together with impaired health, stigma, and uncertainty about the future, often combine in ways that worsen quality of life in people living with HIV (Andersson et al., 2020; Ghiasvand et al., 2019). The psychological impacts of HIV infection are addressed in Chapter 15 and include higher rates of depression than in the general population (Hoare et al., 2021). Interventions designed to treat psychological distress among people with HIV/AIDS are effective at both reducing depression and improving immune function (Dianatinasab et al., 2020; Jiang et al., 2021; Scott-Sheldon et al., 2019; Zhang, L. et al., 2023).

Until recently, safer sexual behaviour was the only way to contain the further spread of the epidemic because there is no vaccine or cure for HIV infection. However, the development of HAART and its application mean that viral load can be reduced to such an extent that the risk of transmission is virtually eliminated. As a result, rates of mother-to-child transmission have reduced (Yang et al., 2023), as have transmission rates in serodiscordant couples where one partner has HIV and the other does not (Anglemyer et al., 2013). HAART can also be used to prevent sexual transmission of HIV either through post-exposure prophylaxis (PEP) immediately after high-risk events or pre-exposure prophylaxis (PrEP) for people who engage in recurrent high-risk behaviours (Krakower et al., 2015). The World Health Organization has also recommended the dapivirine vaginal ring for women at high risk of contracting HIV: it is inserted in the vagina and releases an antiviral drug over a 28-day period, after which it can be replaced (Velloza et al., 2023). Although such medical interventions are effective at preventing HIV, it is important to note that they do not protect against other STIs, so there is a need for the continued encouragement of condom use to prevent other STIs (J.J. Ong et al., 2021). Figure 19.1 highlights the need for multifaceted approaches to prevention.

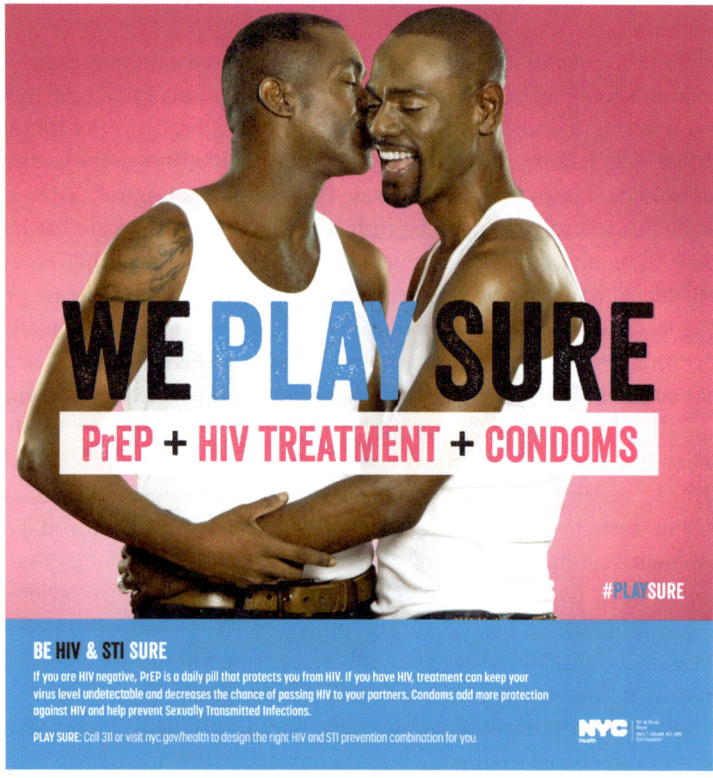

Figure 19.1 Multifaceted approaches to STI prevention

Source: Reproduced with permission from the New York City Department of Health

Behavioural means for preventing the sexual transmission of HIV are the same as those for other STIs. The epidemiology, psychosocial impacts, and prevention of STIs are addressed in the following section.

19.2.2 Sexually Transmitted Infections

The terms sexually transmitted infection (STI) and **sexually transmitted disease** (**STD**) are used interchangeably, but it is important to note that the two acronyms can refer to quite different things. The term STD refers to disease and physical manifestations of infection. An STD-focused sexual health programme would only target those people who have physical manifestations of disease. In contrast, all people infected or at risk of infection are the targets of an STI-focused programme. This distinction is important because asymptomatic STIs may still damage the reproductive organs.

After notable declines during the late 1980s and early 1990s as a result of people's responses to the promotion of safer sex, the prevalence and incidence of numerous sexually transmitted infections (STIs) have risen in many countries and continue to rise or show no signs of marked decline (European Centre for Disease Prevention and Control, 2018, 2019, 2023; World Health Organization, 2019b). However, these increases have not been observed in all countries. The large cross-national differences cannot be explained by differences in rates of sexual behaviour *per se*, but instead reflect differences in patterns of preventative behaviours, cultural attitudes toward sex, and the provision of sexual health services.

In population-representative samples, around 15% of adults report ever having been diagnosed with an STI, and 2–3% test positive for STIs or were diagnosed with an STI in the previous year (Grulich et al., 2014; Sonnenberg et al., 2013). However, many more people have STIs that are undiagnosed because of a lack of knowledge or consultation with health professionals. Young people are particularly likely to have diagnosed or undiagnosed STIs. Many STIs can be prevented by the consistent and correct use of condoms. However, as noted in the next section, rates of condom use are not as high as is desired by health professionals.

Although young people are a key focus of STI prevention activities, the sexual health of older people should not be overlooked. Older people are now more likely than in past generations to be single or undergoing relationship change, and changes to dating and relationships facilitated by social media and mobile technologies mean that their sexual networks may be broader than those of previous generations. The availability of drugs to treat erectile dysfunction may also contribute to greater levels of sexual activity and a corresponding increase in the likelihood of STI transmission. However, health professionals and older people often find it embarrassing to talk about sexual issues (Kelder et al., 2022; Manninen et al., 2021).

Treatment with antibiotics is available for many bacterial STIs (e.g. chlamydia, gonorrhoea). However, cures for viral STIs are not available, although symptomatic treatment is available (e.g. relief from sores due to genital herpes). Untreated STIs can lead to serious complications, including infertility in women. Many STIs can be asymptomatic for some time. This explains why the proportion of people treated for STIs is often lower than the prevalence rates found in population-based screening. Furthermore, people may delay seeking treatment because of embarrassment about talking to others about their sexual behaviour (Baigry et al., 2023; Onukwugha et al., 2019).

19.2.3 Promoting Condom Use

In the absence of vaccines or cures for HIV and many other STIs, it is vital to encourage behaviours that limit the spread of STIs between people. These are sometimes split into the **'ABC' of STI prevention**: Abstaining, Being faithful, and using Condoms (see Table 19.1).

Table 19.1   The ABC of safe sex

A	Abstain from sex	If you don't have sex, then you cannot get an STI
B	Be faithful	If you are in a monogamous relationship with a partner who has no STIs, you cannot get an STI
C	Use condoms	If you use condoms, the risk of acquiring an STI is reduced

Most attention within public health and health promotion has been given to Part C (using condoms), because A and B require more fundamental changes in sexual behaviour. Indeed, research into abstinence-based sexual health programmes indicates that they have no overall impact on the delay of initiating sex, limiting sexual partners, or increasing the use of condoms or other contraception. Indeed, there is concern that abstinence-only programmes may be counterproductive in the long run because such programmes do not teach people how to have safer sex if they cease to abstain from sex (see Research Box 19.1).

Although the vast majority of people do use condoms sometimes, rates of consistent condom use are low. For example, when people are asked about their most recent sexual experiences, fewer than 25% report that they used a condom (de Visser et al., 2014a). Furthermore, among people who do use condoms, around one in seven do not put the condom on before genital contact, thereby exposing themselves to infection with a range of STIs. It is therefore necessary to promote correct and consistent condom use.

─Research Box 19.1─

Does Promoting Sexual Abstinence Work?

Background

Over the past two decades, school-based sexuality education in the USA has moved away from more comprehensive programmes in favour of abstinence-based curricula that stress the importance of monogamous sexual relationships. Several States require programmes to promote the message that abstinence is the only certain way to avoid pregnancy and STIs, and do not educate young people about the use of contraception.

Method and Findings

This study aimed to determine whether abstinence-only programmes had the intended positive effects on young people's sexual health. Data covering a 12-year period from 2000 to 2011 were collected from five States that had abstinence-only education, and 21 States that delivered comprehensive sex and relationships education. Analyses focused on changes over time of rates of pregnancy, termination of pregnancy, and STI diagnoses. There was no evidence that the abstinence-only programmes had better outcomes related to the risks of teenage pregnancy, termination of pregnancy, or STI infection.

Significance

Abstinence-only education programmes produce outcomes that are no better or

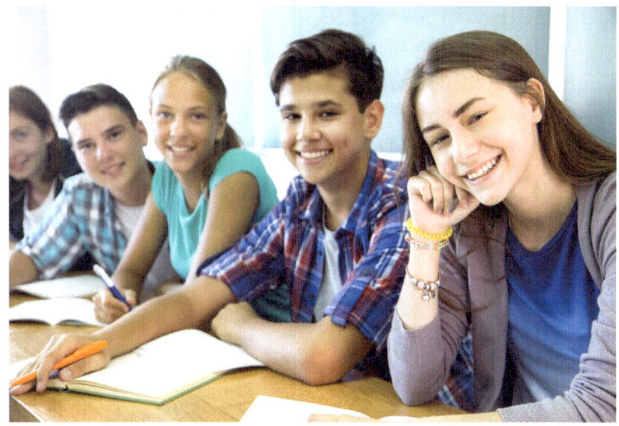

Figure 19.2   School-based sexuality education in the USA

Source: © yanlev/Adobe Stock

worse than conventional sex and relationships education. However, given the high levels of STIs and unplanned pregnancies among teenagers and young adults, comprehensive education programmes aimed at improving knowledge and skills may be more likely to provide the best long-term outcomes. It is also important to note that in addition to formal education, peers and media provide an informal curriculum that may differ in terms of its content and impact.

Carr, J.B. & Packham, A. (2017) The effects of state-mandated abstinence-based sex education on teen health outcomes. *Health Economics*, *26*: 403–420.

Impact of Behavioural Interventions

Research based on social cognitive models of behaviour (see Chapter 5) shows that people's condom use may be predicted from their attitudes, subjective norms, self-efficacy, and intentions to use condoms (Albarracín et al., 2001; Teye-Kwadjo et al., 2017). Condom use tends not to be influenced by knowledge about HIV/STIs, perceived susceptibility to infection, or the perceived severity of infection. Thus, scare campaigns are likely to be ineffective in promoting condom use (Kirby, 2006; Ruiter et al., 2014). It is better to focus on attitudes, beliefs, skills, and confidence. Indeed, because condom use involves more than one person, it is important that people develop the skills to communicate about condom use with their sexual partners (Isaacs et al., 2021). Interventions to promote condom use are more effective when they focus on the skills required to negotiate safer sex rather than only focusing on changing individuals' knowledge and attitudes (Albarracín et al., 2003; Gause et al., 2018). Systematic reviews of the literature indicate that significant reductions in HIV/STI risk behaviours and HIV/STI transmission can be achieved via interventions focused on individuals, couples, small groups, or the community (Fu et al., 2023; Henderson et al., 2020; Shangase et al., 2021).

The observed low rates of condom use among heterosexual people are influenced by the availability of hormonal contraception. People tend to be more concerned about unplanned pregnancy than STIs and will often make a trade-off between condoms and other contraception (Eeckhaut & Fitzpatrick, 2022). This means that if people are using hormonal contraception to prevent pregnancy, they tend not to use condoms. Condom use is much less common between regular partners than between new partners or in 'one-night stands'. Reasons for condom use differ in these different contexts – people tend to be less worried about HIV/STIs with regular partners (Senn et al., 2014; Skakoon-Sparling & Cramer, 2021). However, the decision not to use condoms in regular relationships is not always based on an accurate knowledge of partners' STI status.

Clinical Notes 19.1

Sexual Behaviour and Contraception

- Many people feel embarrassed talking about sexual behaviour and sexual problems. Let people know that you are comfortable talking about these issues in a non-judgemental way.
- When prescribing oral contraception, ensure that people are aware that non-barrier methods do not offer protection against STIs. Encourage individuals and their sexual partners to be tested (and treated) for STIs.
- People are more likely to use condoms if you address their attitudes and beliefs. However, it is also important to help people to develop the skills needed to negotiate condom use with sexual partners.

Rates of condom use may continue to decline in response to the increasing availability and use of the oral contraceptive pill, long-lasting hormonal contraception implants, and post-coital contraception (the 'morning-after pill'). Because hormonal contraception offers no barrier to STI transmission, it can be argued that it is irresponsible to prescribe the pill without also encouraging people to use condoms to protect against STI transmission. Communication research suggests that promotion of dual use requires multiple and diverse messaging strategies to address the various concerns of different users (Wilkinson et al., 2022).

Case Study 19.1

A Sexually Transmitted Infection

Lucy is a student who recently attended a specialist sexual health service for the first time. Several months ago, she met someone through a dating app and they ended up having intercourse. They did not use a condom. Lucy was using oral contraception, and she didn't want to spoil the moment by asking him to use a condom. She was worried he would think she was suggesting he might have an STI.

A few weeks later, Lucy noticed discharge from her vagina and soreness/itchiness when urinating. She was embarrassed about this and even more embarrassed about seeing her usual doctor, so she waited for days, hoping that the symptoms would clear up. When they didn't, she decided to visit a specialist STI clinic.

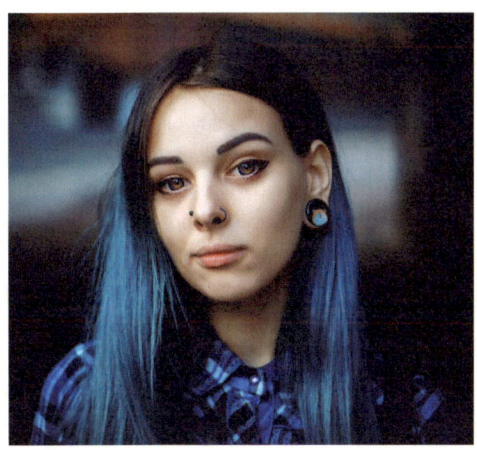

Figure 19.3   Lucy visits an STI clinic

Source: © kohanova1991/Adobe Stock

> I was a bit embarrassed going in to get tested … I was worried that there would be real matron-type nurses telling me off for being stupid … or dirty old men in the waiting room. I didn't want to see anyone I knew, because it wouldn't be good for my reputation. So I didn't make eye contact with anyone in the waiting room. I think most other people there felt the same way.

She said that it was very reassuring to be treated by staff who did not judge her, but simply addressed the facts and offered reassurance. Lucy was diagnosed with gonorrhea and treated with a single dose of antibiotics.

Lucy was relieved that treatment was so quick and effective, but the information she was given by the clinic staff made her more concerned about other STIs and the impact they could have on her reproductive capacity:

> It did get me thinking about condoms, but it's hard when you're getting carried away. I know that I need to get better at asking guys to use condoms. One tip a friend gave me was to say that you aren't on the pill even if you are. That way you can get a guy to use a condom without saying anything about diseases.

Given that unplanned pregnancy and STIs are both attributable to sexual activity without adequate precautions, it makes sense to address both outcomes together. However, reviews of research reveal that there is a need for better integration of sexual health and family planning services. Different domains for the integration of services have been identified:

- Provider level: health professionals offering both family planning and STI services.
- Facility level: internal referral between family planning specialists and STI specialists.
- Referral services: external referrals from family planning to STI services and vice versa.

Within primary care, brief interventions can be an efficient way of addressing sexual health issues in people who may not otherwise attend specialist sexual health services.

Summary 19.2

- In addition to its physical effects, HIV has detrimental effects on psychological wellbeing and quality of life. Quality of life can also be affected by complex treatment regimens which can suppress viral replication but do not offer a cure.
- Rates of STIs have increased in recent years in many countries. This increase has not been limited to young people, but has also occurred among older adults.
- Although condoms offer effective protection against HIV, other STIs, and unwanted pregnancy, few people regularly use condoms.
- Among heterosexual people, there is often a trade-off between condom use and oral contraceptives.
- Condom use can be increased by targeting people's knowledge and attitudes. However, it is also important to equip people with the necessary skills to negotiate and use condoms.

19.3 Prostate and Testicular Cancer

Cancers of the prostate and testicles are common and may affect, and be affected by, men's views of masculinity or sexuality. Many men endorse and embody traditional definitions of masculinity, according to which men are supposed to be 'strong silent types'. Such beliefs help to explain why men are less likely to use healthcare services (de Visser & McDonnell, 2013; McGraw et al., 2021). Men's reluctance to seek screening and treatment may be particularly marked for health conditions that affect sexual potency, because sexual potency is a central aspect of many people's definitions of strong masculinity.

19.3.1 Prostate Cancer

Prostate cancer is the second most common cancer in men, accounting for about one-seventh of all diagnosed cancers among men (Bray et al., 2024). Although the causal mechanisms involved in prostate cancer are not precisely known, risk factors include greater age, African heritage, and a family history of prostate cancer or breast cancer. Specific concerns related to prostate cancer include its potential impact on masculinity and sexuality (de Sousa et al., 2012; McAteer & Gillanders, 2019).

Epidemiology and Screening

The prostate gland surrounds part of the urethra of men and produces a fluid component of semen. At the time of diagnosis with prostate cancer, many men are asymptomatic. Symptoms become more prominent when the cancer is advanced. A common symptom is urinary incontinence. Pain in the lower back, hips, or thighs may be experienced if the cancer has metastasised. Diagnosis of prostate cancer may lead to anxiety or depression that may arise from an unmet desire for information about the prognosis, uncertainty about treatment options and their potential side effects, and concern about the impacts on masculine identity (Groarke et al., 2020; Larkin et al., 2022). However, anxiety and depression often go unnoticed, and many men feel that their psychological needs are not met by the services available to them.

Health professionals must be aware of the psychological aspects of screening, diagnosis, and treatment for prostate cancer. **Prostate specific antigen** (**PSA**) levels are a widely used marker for prostate cancer. However, PSA screening has been somewhat controversial because of concerns about the accuracy of testing and possibility that false positives may increase anxiety and lead to over-treatment (Tsodikov et al., 2017). There is interest in developing more targeted screening that is informed by knowledge of the greater susceptibility among some ethnic groups (McHugh et al., 2022). Digital rectal examination is another form of screening where a physician feels for abnormalities that may indicate prostate cancer. However, many men find rectal examinations involving the insertion of a finger more difficult than the insertion of a piece of equipment (Christy et al., 2014).

Treatment

Treatment options vary depending on whether the cancer is restricted to the prostate or has metastasised. Men with low-risk localised tumours may be offered active monitoring or 'watchful waiting' rather than treatment. Higher-risk localised cancers may be treated by a radical prostatectomy – surgery to remove the prostate gland – external radiotherapy, or internal radiotherapy.

Surgery, radiation, and hormone treatment commonly have side effects which reduce quality of life. Radical prostatectomy and radiotherapy often lead to transient or permanent urinary incontinence and impotence (Nolsøe et al., 2021). Urinary incontinence is experienced by the majority of men post-surgery and can lead to embarrassment, a loss of a sense of control, depression, and reduced social interactions (see also section 19.4.1). The impact of impotence is influenced by men's pre-surgery levels of sexual activity and their partners' levels of concern about impotence. Nerve-sparing surgery can reduce the likelihood and severity of urinary incontinence and impotence. Furthermore, research suggests that after prostatectomy, psychoeducational interventions can improve urinary incontinence and sexual difficulties (Johnson, 2023; Rogers et al., 2022).

It is important to discuss concerns about urinary incontinence and sexual function when decisions are made about surgery, radiation therapy, or watchful waiting. The choice of therapy is not simple because there is a lack of conclusive evidence that any single approach consistently offers better long-term prospects (Vernooij et al., 2020; Wallis et al., 2018). This means that it may be particularly important to consider the impact of different treatments on quality of life, especially because complications are quite common. For example, men's willingness to undergo a radical prostatectomy may be influenced by the extent to which they are concerned about potential impairments to urinary continence or sexual function. The adverse psychosocial impacts of diagnosis and treatment for prostate cancer can be reduced via various kinds of individual-focused, couple-focused, or group interventions (see Case Study 19.2) (W. Chen et al., 2022; Mundle et al., 2021; Pyle et al., 2021). Counselling and providing erectile aids or medication may be beneficial.

If a tumour has spread beyond the capsule surrounding the prostate, then surgery or radiotherapy may be combined with a course of hormone treatment – the growth and function of the prostate is affected by testosterone, so some treatments work by reducing the testosterone levels. However, interventions to lower testosterone levels are related to cognitive impairments, so there is some concern about this potential side effect (Sari Motlagh et al., 2021).

Case Study 19.2

Prostate Cancer Diagnosis and Treatment

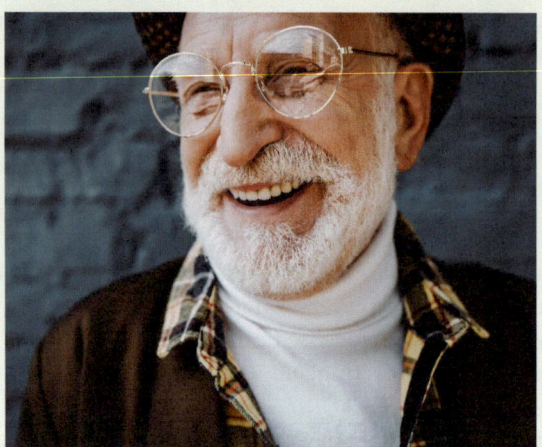

Figure 19.4   Vince's diagnosis of prostate cancer

Source: © Yakobchuk Olena/Adobe Stock

Vince is a retired teacher who was diagnosed with prostate cancer two years ago. His experiences highlight a number of important psychosocial issues related to the care and treatment of men with prostate cancer.

Vince found some of the screening processes and tests difficult. This was partly due to the uncertainty of some of the test results. It was also because some of the tests were challenging, particularly when the doctor inserted a gloved finger into Vince's rectum to feel for lumps, hardness, or other abnormalities in the prostate gland:

> Some parts of the whole diagnosis process were pretty strange. I mean, having another man put his finger up your back passage is not something that had happened to me before … and I won't be rushing back to do it again!

The experience of diagnosis was made worse by the insensitivity of some staff. There were times when unknown staff walked in and out of the room without introducing themselves or having any apparent reason to come in when he was (and felt) so exposed.

Once the diagnosis had been made, Vince found it hard to decide about treatment – surgery, radiotherapy, or 'watchful waiting'. The outcomes and side effects associated with each option were quite varied. Furthermore, he felt he was having to deal with probabilities rather than certainties:

> A friend of mine is hyper-logical and he suggested I draw up a table of different pros and cons and give each treatment option a score and decide that way … but I mean, how can you really weigh up the different options? What's more important – living, having sex, or not wetting myself? I was tempted to take the 'wait and see' approach just to avoid having to decide.

Vince found it useful to attend a group support network. Although he was apprehensive about talking to other men about his concerns, he appreciated the benefits after attending a few sessions:

> It was great because all the people there had prostate cancer, and some were worse off than me, but they were all very genuine. They weren't so concerned any more about how much money they earned, or what car they drove, or those kinds of things. Everyone was on a very genuine level. This made it easier to join the group. It gave me a lot of support and helped me decide on which treatment to undertake.

19.3.2 Testicular Cancer

Testicular cancer is relatively rare, accounting for around 1% of cancers in men. However, it is most common among men in their 20s and 30s, and it is the most common cancer among young adult men. It is more common in Caucasian men than men with Asian or African ethnic backgrounds.

Epidemiology and Screening

The testicles produce sperm, so are vital for men's reproductive capacity. They also produce testosterone, which is the principal male sex hormone. **Testicular self-examination** (**TSE**) is an important element of diagnosing and treating testicular cancer because (as for other cancers) early detection and treatment are associated with better outcomes. Because it is unusual to develop cancer in both testicles at the same time, men can compare one testicle to the other to identify any lumps or swellings which should be checked by a medical professional. Although TSE may be an important part of monitoring, very few men practise the behaviour and many are unaware of the importance of TSE (Rovito et al., 2015; Saab et al., 2016).

There is a clear need to increase awareness of the importance of TSE, and to identify effective strategies to increase rates of TSE. A review of the research in this area indicated that the Health Belief Model and Theory of Planned Behaviour (see Chapter 5) are effective frameworks for TSE-promotion interventions, but that not all interventions have a strong theoretical foundation (Rovito et al., 2015). Studies indicate that rates of TSE can be improved significantly by helping young men to develop the requisite skills, and encouraging them to form goals and **implementation intentions** specifying 'when', 'where', and 'how' they would perform TSE (Jones et al., 2015; Robertson et al., 2008).

Treatment

It is sometimes possible surgically to remove small tumours from a testicle. However, the most common surgical response is removal of the affected testicle (an orchidectomy or orchiectomy). This procedure reduces the risk that pre-cancerous cells may remain in the testis, and is possible because men with only one testicle can maintain their fertility and hormone production. Treatments can cure around 90% of people with testicular cancer, and may involve an orchidectomy with or without radiotherapy or chemotherapy.

However, treatment side effects include impairments to sexual function and fertility, and impairments to quality of life (Dax et al., 2022). These issues are important to consider given the epidemiology of testicular cancer – that diagnosis and treatment often occur before men have become fathers and at an age when sexual activity is important to them. Men may be concerned that the removal of a testicle will make them impotent (i.e. unable to get or maintain an erection) and infertile (i.e. unable to produce children). However, a man with one healthy testicle can still have normal erections and produce healthy sperm. Nevertheless, problems with impotence and fertility do often occur in men post-orchidectomy.

Studies of the psychosocial outcomes of testicular cancer treatment have found that the prevalence of sexual problems varies widely, but may include ejaculatory dysfunction (related to surgery in the retroperitoneal region), erectile problems, and decreases in sexual desire, sexual activity, orgasm intensity, or sexual satisfaction (Alexis et al., 2020; Kerie et al., 2021). Many men also report concerns about their reproductive capacity, and impairments to their body image and masculine identity (Alexis et al., 2020; Dax et al., 2022).

It is important to note that not all of the observed impairments can be attributed to disease or treatment factors. Psychosocial factors are also important (Smith et al., 2018). The symbolic importance given to men's genitals means that removal of a testicle can be a challenge to their perceived masculinity.

In addition to the impact of testicular cancer on men, it is important to consider its impact on relationships, and to consider how supportive relationships may affect men's adjustment to testicular cancer. Being in a stable relationship appears to reduce the likelihood that men will experience sexual problems, and sexual and emotional satisfaction among men and their partners are mutually correlated (Jankowska, 2011).

Clinical Notes 19.2

Prostate and Testicular Health

- Encouraging men to say exactly how, when, and where they will perform testicular self-examination is a simple way to increase self-screening behaviour.
- When diagnosing and treating cancers of the prostate and testicles, be aware of how men's beliefs about their masculinity may be affected by the cancer itself and the symptoms and side effects, such as urinary incontinence and impaired sexual functioning.

Summary 19.3

- Prostate cancer is one of the most common cancers in men.
- Treatment options for prostate cancer depend on how advanced the cancer is and men's evaluations of the side effects of treatment.
- Many men experience transient or permanent urinary incontinence and erectile problems following surgery or radiotherapy. The importance of maintaining normal functioning in these domains may influence men's decision to be treated or to undertake 'watchful waiting'.
- Testicular cancer is not as common as prostate cancer. However, it is more common among younger men than older men.
- Treatment of testicular cancer often involves the removal of the affected testicle. Although this need not affect men's sexual or reproductive capacity, men often experience impairments in these domains after treatment: psychological factors are important.
- Psychological interventions can be effective in treating the psychological distress arising from the diagnosis and treatment for cancers of the prostate and testicles.

19.4 Urinary Incontinence and Renal Failure

This section outlines two common disorders of the renal and urinary systems. The first (urinary incontinence) is not life-threatening, whereas the second (renal failure) often is. In both cases, psychosocial factors must be considered in treatment and management plans.

19.4.1 Urinary Incontinence

Urinary incontinence (**UI**) is the involuntary leakage of urine, which can have different causes. The population prevalence of any form of UI is around 15% (Sadri et al., 2024). It is more common among women than men. The prevalence and severity of urinary incontinence tends to increase with age. UI is the result of bladder dysfunction (urge incontinence) or sphincter dysfunction (stress incontinence). It is not possible to determine accurately whether people have urge-, stress-, or mixed-incontinence simply by studying the symptoms.

Urge incontinence is the involuntary loss of urine occurring for no apparent reason while suddenly feeling the need or urge to urinate. It occurs when bladder muscles inappropriately contract to expel urine, often regardless of the amount of urine that is in the bladder. It may be called 'reflex incontinence' if it results from overactive nerves controlling the bladder. People with urge incontinence may be described as having an 'unstable' or 'overactive' bladder. In addition to surgical and medical treatments, there is a role for psychological and behavioural therapies. These include exercises to strengthen the pelvic floor muscles and 'bladder training', whereby people are taught to 'hold on' to their urine for increasingly longer times and to empty their bladders at regular, scheduled intervals so that they can increase their capacity to resist the urge to void their bladders (Dumoulin et al., 2018).

Stress incontinence arises when the pelvic floor muscles have insufficient strength. It involves the loss of small amounts of urine when people cough, laugh, sneeze, exercise, or perform other movements that increase pressure on the bladder. Among women, stress incontinence is more common during pregnancy, because of greater pressure on the bladder. During the premenstrual period and during menopause, lowered oestrogen levels can lead to lower muscular pressure around the urethra. Among men, stress incontinence is a common side effect of prostatectomy. Because stress incontinence arises from muscle weakness, it can be treated via psychological and behavioural means, such as pelvic floor muscle training and bladder training (Dumoulin et al., 2018). There is evidence that these approaches can be effectively delivered using mobile digital technology (Hou et al., 2022).

Urinary incontinence may cause embarrassment, distress, and discomfort. It has measurable detrimental effects on psychological wellbeing and quality of life (Cheng et al., 2020). Many people with UI report that it limits their ability to engage in activities which either increase the strain on the bladder (e.g. physical exercise) or where the availability of toilets may be uncertain, intermittent, or restricted (e.g. long-distance travel, vacations, theatre/cinema, etc.). Useful aids for people in this situation include toilet maps, which are designed to help people with urinary incontinence to engage in social activities with less concern about being unable to find a toilet (www.toiletmap.gov.au; www.toiletmap.org.uk).

Discussions of the problems related to urinary function can be difficult and embarrassing for many people, including health professionals. Clinical Notes 19.3 outlines some important points to bear in mind when carrying out intimate examinations. Legal, cultural, and religious factors may influence what people believe to be appropriate behaviour from health professionals.

—Clinical Notes 19.3—

Carrying out Intimate Examinations

- Embarrassment and anxiety tend to be 'contagious'. The calmer and more professional you are, the easier the examination will be for you and the patient.
- Guidelines for intimate examinations include:

  - Explain why the examination is necessary.
  - Explain exactly what it involves and what you will be doing.
  - Get the person's consent.
  - Offer a chaperone, if appropriate.
  - Make sure the room is private and that other people will not interrupt.
  - Treat the person with respect and dignity (e.g. cover exposed parts of the body when you have finished).
  - Keep all discussion *relevant*. Avoid unnecessary personal comments.
  - Be prepared to stop the examination at any time if the patient asks you to.

19.4.2 Renal Failure and Dialysis

Chronic kidney disease (**CKD**) is the gradual loss of kidney function over time. The early stages of CKD may be asymptomatic, but symptoms do appear as the capacity of the kidneys to remove toxins, wastes, and excess water from the body becomes more impaired. Chronic kidney disease often develops into **end-stage renal disease** (**ESRD**), which is when the kidneys no longer function. People with ESRD require a kidney transplant or must undergo **dialysis** to remove wastes and excess water from the body.

Kidney disease is becoming more common and is a major public health problem, with a global prevalence in adults of just under 10% (Ying et al., 2024). This prevalence increases with age, and can be explained in large part by the increasing prevalence of diabetes and hypertension, which are important CKD risk factors (Jha et al., 2013). Obesity also increases the risk of CKD, in part because of its links to Type 2 diabetes and hypertension.

Psychosocial Aspects of Kidney Disease and Treatment

People with CKD and ESRD often have impaired quality of life, especially emotional wellbeing, but often too little attention is given to these important experiences (Mclaren et al., 2021). Particular challenges for people with kidney disease include depression and anxiety arising from their current poor health and the prospect of further declines in health (Fletcher et al., 2022; C.W. Huang et al., 2021; Palmer et al., 2013). Depression and other psychosocial impacts are more common among people with CKD and ESRD than the general population, and are more common or severe when illness interferes with important aspects of people's lives, such as work or family life (Fletcher et al., 2022; Teasdale et al., 2017). Depression and impaired quality of life are important because they are independent predictors of adverse outcomes and mortality (Porter et al., 2016; Shirazian et al., 2016).

People with ESRD who experience depression may benefit from antidepressant medication, but many patients dislike initiating or continuing such treatment (Mehrotra et al., 2019; Pena-Polanco et al., 2017). In this context, psychological interventions are important, and they are effective for reducing the symptoms of depression in people undergoing dialysis. A review of psychosocial interventions found evidence that cognitive behavioural therapy is effective for reducing symptoms of depression and improving quality of life, and that exercise and relaxation can also reduce depressive symptoms (Natale et al., 2019).

Treatment of kidney disease entails restrictions to the diet and fluid intake. People with ESRD undergoing dialysis must regulate their fluid intake in order to avoid fluid overload, which can lead to congestive heart failure, hypertension, pulmonary oedema, and a shortened life span. The demands of intensive treatment regimens can induce fatigue and impair quality of life (Jacobson et al., 2019). Time demands are particularly marked for people undergoing clinic-based dialysis, which entails three- to four-hour sessions three times per week. For these reasons, home dialysis or peritoneal dialysis (involving the use of a catheter and portable bags of dialysis fluids) may be more appealing. All people undergoing dialysis must also adjust to their dependence on artificial means for survival and a lack of control over their health (Reid et al., 2016). For these reasons, kidney transplantation may appear more appealing than ongoing dialysis. **Kidney transplantation** should not be thought of as a cure for ESRD, but a new phase of treatment, because although transplant recipients are free from the dietary restrictions of dialysis, they must adhere to strict regimens of immunosuppressant drugs and be alert to any physical changes that may indicate infection or the rejection of the organ.

Reviews of the evidence indicate that quality of life tends to be better among transplant recipients than among people undergoing dialysis (Schoot et al., 2022). However, when looking at different aspects of quality of life, transplant recipients tend to have more pain and discomfort and poorer body image. There is a need to consider and address the ways in which different treatments affect overall quality of life as well different domains of life, such as family, work, and friendships.

In addition to being of concern in their own right, impaired affect and quality of life are important because they may affect adherence to treatment pre-dialysis, during dialysis, or after organ transplantation (Ghimire et al., 2015; Seng et al., 2020). Other factors linked to lower adherence include younger age, minority ethnicity, experiencing more effects of illness on family life, not having a partner, being a smoker, a longer duration of treatment, comorbidities like diabetes and hypertension, more demanding medication regimens, low self-efficacy, an external (rather than an internal) locus of control, and less social support (Christensen & Ehlers, 2002; Ghimire et al., 2015; Seng et al., 2020). Intervention research indicates that adherence can be improved by cognitive behavioural strategies such as self-monitoring, forming behavioural contracts, and positive reinforcement reward systems (Murali et al., 2019). As for other conditions, increasing use is being made of mobile technology to improve adherence (see Research Box 19.2 and Chapter 12), but there is a need to be aware of how to ensure equality of access (Graham-Brown et al., 2022).

─Research Box 19.2─

Digital Intervention to Promote Healthy Lifestyles among People with Chronic Kidney Disease

Background

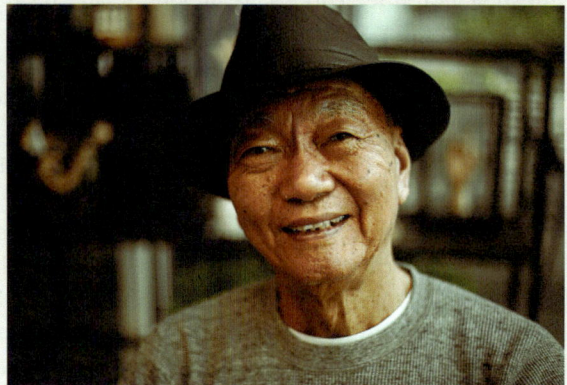

Figure 19.5   Managing chronic kidney disease

Source: © Chevanon Photography/Pexels

In kidney disease, adherence to treatment, lifestyle advice, and dietary requirements are important predictors of outcomes. However, poor adherence is common, so there is a need to develop and assess effective interventions. The increasing availability of wearable digital technology provides a possible way to promote and monitor adherence.

Method and Findings

This trial was conducted in Taiwan, where CKD incidence and prevalence are among the highest in the world. Sixty people with CKD were provided with a wearable device that collected exercise-related data and were given access to a smartphone app to record dietary diaries. They were then allocated to the intervention group or the control group (with an equal chance of being in either group), and followed up over three months. During that time, the intervention group received diet and exercise advice, and mutual support from a social media group. Use of the intervention was associated with significant improvements in self-efficacy, self-management, quality of life, and levels of physical activity. The intervention group also showed better renal function, and slower declines in renal function.

Significance

An intervention based on wearable devices and digital health advice and social media led to a heightened sense of control among people with CKD, improved quality of life, healthier lifestyles, and better health outcomes. Although the authors argued that their results establish a new self-management model for health promotion among people with CKD, we must be aware of how to ensure equality of access, especially among people with lower levels of digital literacy.

Li, W.Y., Chiu, F.C., Zeng, J.K., Li, Y.W., Huang, S.-H., Yeh, H.C., Cheng, B.W. & Yang, F.J. (2020) Mobile health app with social media to support self-management for patients with chronic kidney disease: Prospective randomized controlled study. *Journal of Medical Internet Research, 22*(12): e19452. doi:10.2196/19452.

Summary 19.4

- Urinary incontinence (UI) may be caused by muscle weakness or a lack of control over an inappropriate urge to urinate.
- The prevalence and severity of UI increase with age. Urinary incontinence is often a cause of embarrassment and can lead people to restrict their social activities.
- Psychological and behavioural factors are important in treating UI. Treatment may involve muscle-strengthening exercises and bladder training designed to improve people's control over their urge to urinate.
- Chronic kidney disease (CKD) and end-stage renal disease (ESRD) are becoming increasingly common. The increase in cases can be partially explained by increases in diseases that are risk factors for CKD, such as diabetes and hypertension.
- People with ESRD rely on kidney transplants or dialysis. Transplantation is associated with a better quality of life.
- Dialysis places large demands on people's lifestyles and is associated with depression and impaired quality of life.
- Psychological interventions are effective for alleviating impairments to psychological wellbeing among people with ESRD. They are also effective for improving people's adherence to the recommended lifestyle changes.

─Further Reading─

Llewellyn, C.D. et al. (eds) (2019) *Cambridge Handbook of Psychology, Health and Medicine* (3rd edition). Cambridge: Cambridge University Press. Includes short chapters on prostate cancer, contraception, HIV/AIDS, pelvic pain, sexual assault, sexual dysfunction, sexually transmitted infections, and urinary tract symptoms.

National Institute for Health and Care Excellence (2021) *Chronic Kidney Disease: Assessment and Management*. NICE Guideline NG203. London: NICE. Available at: www.nice.org.uk/guidance/ng203. Addresses the care and treatment of people with, or at risk of, CKD. It covers how to prevent or delay the progression of the disease, and how to reduce the risk of complications of CKD.

Wylie, K. (ed.) (2015) *ABC of Sexual Health* (3rd edition). London: Wiley. Developed specifically for doctors, this book covers a wide range of topics. It addresses a range of physical and psychological aspects of sexual health and sexual relationships, and includes a useful chapter on taking a sexual history.

─Revision Questions─

1   What is sexual health? Describe three components of sexual health.
2   What impact – according to the evidence – does sexual coercion or abuse have on people?
3   How might the increasing use of pre- and post-exposure prophylaxis for HIV affect rates of other STIs?

4   What are the possible causes of chronic pelvic pain? What impact does chronic pelvic pain have on women?

5   What psychological interventions are effective for promoting safer sex?

6   How has the prevalence of STIs changed over time? What factors may contribute to this?

7   Discuss the specific psychological challenges that may be experienced by men with prostate or testicular cancer.

8   Outline the psychological interventions that may be effective in the treatment of urinary incontinence.

9   What is the psychological impact of chronic kidney disease and end-stage renal disease?

10   Which psychological interventions are effective additional treatments for chronic kidney disease and end-stage renal disease? What aspects of patient wellbeing and behaviour do they affect?

REFERENCES

Abbass, A.A., Kisely, S.R., Town, J.M., Leichsenring, F., Driessen, E., De Maat, S., et al. (2014) Short-term psychodynamic psychotherapies for common mental disorders. *Cochrane Database Systematic Reviews*, 7 (Art. CD004687). doi: 10.1002/14651858.CD004687.pub4.

Abbey, G., Thompson, S.B.N., Hickish, T. & Heathcote, D. (2015) A meta-analysis of prevalence rates and moderating factors for cancer-related post-traumatic stress disorder. *Psycho-Oncology*, 24(4): 371–381.

Abdullah, N., Defaye, M. & Altier, C. (2020) Neural control of gut homeostasis. *American Journal of Physiology: Gastrointestal and Liver Physiology*, 319(6): G718–732. doi:10.1152/ajpgi.00293.2020.

Abraham, C. & Michie, S. (2008) A taxonomy of behavior change techniques used in interventions. *Health Psychology*, 27(3): 379–387.

Abrahams, H.J.G., Gielissen, M.F.M., Braamse, A.M.J., Bleijenberg, G., Buffart, L.M. & Knoop, H. (2019) Graded activity is an important component in cognitive behavioral therapy to reduce severe fatigue: Results of a pragmatic crossover trial in cancer survivors. *Acta Oncology*, 58(12): 1692–1698. doi: 10.1080/0284186X.2019.1659513.

Abrahams, H.J.G., Gielissen, M.F.M., Donders, R.R.T., Goedendorp, M.M., van der Wouw, A.J., et al. (2017) The efficacy of internet-based cognitive behavioral therapy for severely fatigued survivors of breast cancer compared with care as usual: A randomized controlled trial. *Cancer*, 123(19): 3825–3834. doi: 10.1002/cncr.30815.

Adamczyk, W.M., Buglewicz, E., Szikszay, T.M., Luedtke, K. & Bąbel, P. (2019) Reward for Pain: Hyperalgesia and allodynia induced by operant conditioning: Systematic review and meta-analysis. *Journal of Pain*, 20(8): 861–875. doi: 10.1016/j.jpain.2019.01.009.

Adams, C., Gringart, E., & Strobel, N. (2022). Explaining adults' mental health help-seeking through the lens of the theory of planned behavior: a scoping review. *Systematic Reviews*, 11(1): 160. doi:10.1186/s13643-022-02034-y.

Adams, J.A. (1971) A closed loop theory of motor learning. *Journal of Motor Behaviour*, 3(2): 111–150.

Adams, S.M., Close, E.D. & Shreenath, A.P. (2022) Ulcerative colitis: Rapid evidence review. *American Family Physician*, 105: 406–411.

Adejumo, O.A., Edeki, I.R., Sunday Oyedepo, D., Falade, J., Yisau, O. E., et al. (2024). Global prevalence of depression in chronic kidney disease: A systematic review and meta-analysis. *Journal of Nephrology*, 37(9): 2455–2472. doi:10.1007/s40620-024-01998-5.

Ader, R. (2003) Conditioned immunomodulation: Research needs and directions. *Brain, Behavior, and Immunity*, 17(Suppl. 1): s51–s57.

Adler, H.M. (2002) The sociophysiology of caring in the doctor–patient relationship. *Journal of General Internal Medicine*, 17(11): 874–881. doi: 10.1046/j.1525-1497.2002.10640.x.

Agishtein, P. & Brumbaugh, C. (2013) Cultural variation in adult attachment: The impact of ethnicity, collectivism, and country of origin. *Journal of Social, Evolutionary, and Cultural Psychology*, 7(4): 384–405. doi: 10.1037/h0099181.

Ahinkorah, B.O. (2020) Individual and contextual factors associated with mistimed and unwanted pregnancies among adolescent girls and young women in selected high fertility countries in sub-Saharan Africa: A multilevel mixed effects analysis. *PLoS One*, *15*(10): e0241050. doi:10.1371/journal.pone.0241050.

Ahmadi, M. & Lanphear, B. (2022) The impact of clinical and population strategies on coronary heart disease mortality: An assessment of Rose's big idea. *BMC Public Health*, *22*(1): 14. doi:10.1186/s12889-021-12421-0.

Ahn, D.H., Lee, Y.J., Jeong, J.H., Kim, Y.R. & Park, J.B. (2015) The effect of post-stroke depression on rehabilitation outcome and the impact of caregiver type as a factor of post-stroke depression. *Annals of Rehabilation Medicine*, *39*(1): 74–80.

Ainiwaer, A., Zhang, S., Ainiwaer, X. & Ma, F. (2021) Effects of message framing on cancer prevention and detection behaviors, intentions, and attitudes: Systematic review and meta-analysis. *Journal of Medical Internet Research*, *23*(9): e27634 doi:10.2196/27634.

Ainsworth, M.D.S., Blehar, M.C., Waters, E. & Wall, S. (1978) *Patterns of Attachment: A Psychological Study of the Strange Situation*. Hillsdale, NJ: Erlbaum.

Ajzen, I. (1988) *Attitudes, Personality, and Behaviour*. Buckingham: Open University Press.

Akinade, T., Kheyfets, A., Piverger, N., Layne, T.M., Howell, E.A. & Janevic, T. (2023) The influence of racial-ethnic discrimination on women's health care outcomes: A mixed methods systematic review. *Social Science & Medicine*, *316*, 114983. doi:10.1016/j.socscimed.2022.114983.

Albarracín, D., Johnson, B.T., Fishbein, M. & Muellerleile, P.A. (2001) Theories of reasoned action and planned behavior as models of condom use. *Psychological Bulletin*, *127*(1): 142–161.

Albarracín, D., McNatt, P.S., Klein, C.T.F., Ho, R.M., Mitchell, A.L. & Kumkale, G.T. (2003) Persuasive communications to change actions: An analysis of behavioral and cognitive impact in HIV prevention. *Health Psychology*, *22*(2): 166–177.

Aleksandrova, K., Pischon, T., Jenab, M., Bueno-de-Mesquita, H.B., Fedirko, V., Norat, T., et al. (2014) Combined impact of healthy lifestyle factors on colorectal cancer: A large European cohort study. *BMC Medicine*, *12*: 168. doi: 10.1186/s12916-014-0168-4.

Alelwani, S.M. & Ahmed, Y.A. (2014) Medical training for communication of bad news: A literature review. *Journal of Education and Health Promotion*, *3*: 51.

Alenezi, A., McGrath, I., Kimpton, A., & Livesay, K. (2021) Quality of life among ostomy patients: A narrative literature review. *Journal of Clinical Nursing*, *30*(21–22): 3111–3123. doi:10.1111/jocn.15840.

Alexander, M. & Turnbaugh, P.J. (2020) Deconstructing mechanisms of diet-microbiome-immune interactions. *Immunity*, *53*: 264–276. doi:10.1016/j.immuni.2020.07.015.

Alexandrova-Karamanova, A., Todorova, I., Montgomery, A., Panagopoulou, E., Costa, P., Baban, A., et al. (2016) Burnout and health behaviors in health professionals from seven European countries. *International Archive of Occupational and Environmental Health*, *89*(7): 1059–1075.

Alexis, O., Adeleye, A.O., & Worsley, A.J. (2020) Men's experiences of surviving testicular cancer: An integrated literature review. *Journal of Cancer Survivorship: Research and Practice*, *14*(3): 284–293. doi:10.1007/s11764-019-00841-2.

Ali, S.A., Mathur, N., Malhotra, A.K. & Braga, R.J. (2019) Electroconvulsive therapy and schizophrenia: A systematic review. *Molecular Neuropsychiatry*, *5*(2): 75–83. doi: 10.1159/000497376.

Allen, J., Balfour, R., Bell, R., & Marmot, M. (2014) Social determinants of mental health. *International Review of Psychiatry*, *26*(4): 392–407. doi:10.3109/09540261.2014.928270.

Allida, S.M., Hsieh, C.F., Cox, K.L., et al. (2023) Pharmacological, non-invasive brain stimulation and psychological interventions, and their combination, for treating depression after stroke. *Cochrane Database of Systematic Reviews*, 7(7): Art. CD003437. doi:10.1002/14651858. CD003437.pub5

Alm, S. & Låftman, S.B. (2018) The gendered mirror on the wall: Satisfaction with physical appearance and its relationship to global self-esteem and psychosomatic complaints among adolescent boys and girls. *Young*, 26(2): 525–541. doi: 10.1177/1103308817739733.

Alnashwan, Y.A., Rashid, A.M., Javaid, S.S., Kharoshah, M.A., Arun, M., Dsouza, H.L., et al. (2023) Incidence and comparison of suicide in various phases of the menstrual cycle: A systematic review and meta-analysis. *Acta Informatica Medica*, 31(1): 76–83. doi: 10.5455/aim.2023.31.76-83.

Alsbrooks, K. & Hoerauf, K. (2022) Prevalence, causes, impacts, and management of needle phobia: An international survey of a general adult population. *PLoS One*, 17(11): e0276814. doi:10.1371/journal. pone.0276814.

Althaus, D., Stefanek, J., Hasford, J. & Hegerl, U. (2002) Knowledge and attitude of the general public regarding symptoms, etiology and possible treatments of depressive illnesses. *Der Nervenarzt*, 73(7): 659–664.

Alzueta, E. & Baker, F.C. (2023) The menstrual cycle and sleep. *Sleep Medicine Clinics*, 18(4): 399–413. doi: 10.1016/j.jsmc. 2023.06.003.

Amare, A.T., Vaez, A., Hsu, Y.H., et al. (2020) Bivariate genome-wide association analyses of the broad depression phenotype combined with major depressive disorder, bipolar disorder or schizophrenia reveal eight novel genetic loci for depression. *Molecular Psychiatry*, 25(7): 1420–1429. doi:10.1038/s41380-018-0336-6.

Ambady, N., LaPlante, D., Nguyen, T., Rosenthal, R., Chaumeton, N. & Levinson, W. (2002) Surgeons' tone of voice: A clue to malpractice history. *Surgery*, 132(1): 5–9.

American Psychiatric Association (1994) *Diagnostic and Statistical Manual of Mental Disorders* (3rd edition). Washington, DC: APA.

American Psychiatric Association (2013) *Diagnostic and Statistical Manual of Mental Disorders* (5th edition) (DSM-5). Washington, DC: APA.

American Psychiatric Association (2022) *Diagnostic and Statistical Manual of Mental Disorders* (5th edition, text revision, DSM-5-TR). Washington, DC: APA.

Amonoo, H.L., Celano, C.M., Sadlonova, M. & Huffman, J. (2021) Is optimism a protective factor for cardiovascular disease? *Current Cardiology Reports*, 23(11): 158. doi:10.1007/s11886-021-01590-4.

Anderson, L. & Taylor, R.S. (2014) Cardiac rehabilitation for people with heart disease: An overview of Cochrane systematic reviews. *Cochrane Database of Systematic Reviews*, 12(12): Art. CD011273.

Anderson, L.J., Nuckols, T.K., Coles, C., Le, M.M., Schnipper, J.L., Shane, R., et al. (2020) A systematic overview of systematic reviews evaluating medication adherence interventions. *American Journal of Health-System Pharmacy*, 77(5): 138–147. doi: 10.1093/ajhp/zxz284.

Andersson, G.Z., Reinius, M., Eriksson, L.E., Svedhem, V., Esfahani, F.M., Deuba, K., et al. (2020) Stigma reduction interventions in people living with HIV to improve health-related quality of life. *Lancet HIV*, 7(2): e129–e140. doi: 10.1016/S2352-3018(19)30343-1.

Anenberg, S.C., Mohegh, A., Goldberg, D.L., Kerr, G.H., Brauer, M., Burkart, K., et al. (2022) Long-term trends in urban NO_2 concentrations and associated paediatric asthma incidence: Estimates from global datasets. *Lancet Planetary Health*, 6(1): e49–e58. doi:10.1016/S2542-5196(21)00255-2.

Anger, W.K., Dimoff, J.K. & Alley, L. (2024) Addressing health care workers' mental health: A systematic review of evidence-based interventions and current resources. *American Journal of Public Health*, 114(S2): 213–226. doi:10.2105/AJPH.2023.307556.

Anglemyer, A., Rutherford, G.W., Horvath, T., Baggaley, R.C., Egger, M. & Siegfried, N. (2013) Antiretroviral therapy for prevention of HIV transmission in HIV-discordant couples. *Cochrane Database of Systematic Reviews*, *4*(4): Art. CD009153. doi: 10.1002/14651858.CD009153.pub3.

Anik, E., West, R.M., Cardno, A.G. & Mir, G. (2021) Culturally adapted psychotherapies for depressed adults: A systematic review and meta-analysis. *Journal of Affective Disorders*, *278*: 296–310.

Antoni, M.H. & Dhabhar, F.S. (2019) The impact of psychosocial stress and stress management on immune responses in patients with cancer. *Cancer, 125*(9): 1417–1431. doi: 10.1002/cncr.31943.

Antoni, M. H., Moreno, P. I., & Penedo, F. J. (2023) Stress management interventions to facilitate psychological and physiological adaptation and optimal health outcomes in cancer patients and survivors. *Annual Review of Psychology*, *74*: 423–455. doi:10.1146/annurev-psych-030122-124119.

Antonopoulos, C.R., Sugden, N. & Saliba, A. (2023) Implicit bias toward people with disability: A systematic review and meta-analysis. *Rehabilitation Psychology*, *68*(2): 121–134. doi:10.1037/rep0000493.

Antonovsky, A. (1987) *Unraveling the Mystery of Health: How People Manage Stress and Stay Well*. San Francisco, CA: Jossey-Bass.

Antypas, K. & Wangberg, S.C. (2014) Combining users' needs with health behavior models in designing an internet- and mobile-based intervention for physical activity in cardiac rehabilitation. *Journal of Medical Internet Research: Research Protocols*, *3*(1): e4. doi: 10.2196/resprot.2725.

Arbuthnott, A. & Sharpe, D. (2009) The effect of physician–patient collaboration on patient adherence in non-psychiatric medicine. *Patient Education and Counseling*, *77*(1): 60–67.

Arendt, J. (2018) Approaches to the pharmacological management of jet lag. *Drugs*, *78*(14): 1419–1431. doi: 10.1007/s40265-018-0973-8.

Arık, A., Dodd, E., Cairns, A. & Streftaris, G. (2021) Socioeconomic disparities in cancer incidence and mortality in England and the impact of age-at-diagnosis on cancer mortality. *PloS One*, *16*(7): e0253854. doi:10.1371/journal.pone.0253854.

Arnett, J.J. (2004) *Emerging Adulthood: The Winding Road from Late Teens through the Twenties*. Oxford: Oxford University Press.

Arrebola-Moreno, M., Petrova, D., Garcia-Retamero, R., Rivera-López, R., Jordan-Martínez, L., Arrebola, J.P., Ramírez-Hernández, J.A. & Catena, A. (2020) Psychological and cognitive factors related to prehospital delay in acute coronary syndrome: A systematic review. *International Journal of Nursing Studies*, *108*: 103613. doi: 10.1016/j.ijnurstu.2020.103613.

Arsandaux, J., Montagni, I., Macalli, M., Bouteloup, V., Tzourio, C. & Galéra, C. (2020) Health risk behaviors and self-esteem among college students: Systematic review of quantitative studies. *International Journal of Behavioral Medicine*, *27*(2): 142–159. doi:10.1007/s12529-020-09857-w

Asada, K., Tojo, Y., Osanai, H., Saito, A., Hasegawa, T. & Kumagaya, S. (2016) Reduced personal space in individuals with autism spectrum disorder. *PLoS One*, *11*(1): e0146306.

Asch, S.E. (1956) Studies of independence and conformity: A minority of one against a unanimous majority. *Psychological Monographs: General and Applied*, *70*(9): 1–70.

Asghari, E., Gholizadeh, L., Kazami, L., Taban Sadeghi, M., Separham, A. & Khezerloy-Aghdam, N. (2022) Symptom recognition and treatment-seeking behaviors in women experiencing acute coronary syndrome for the first time: A qualitative study. *BMC Cardiovascular Disorders*, *22*(1): 508. doi:10.1186/s12872-022-02892-3.

Asher, R. (1949) Myxoedematous madness. *British Medical Journal*, *2*(4627): 555–562.

Ashford, M.T., Olander, E.K. & Ayers, S. (2016) Finding web-based anxiety interventions on the World Wide Web: A scoping review. *JMIR Mental Health*, *3*(2): e14.

Ashworth, M., Godfrey, E., Harvey, K. & Darbishire, L. (2003) Perceptions of psychological content in the GP consultation: The role of practice, personal and prescribing attributes. *Family Practice*, *20*(4): 373–375.

Ask, H., Cheesman, R., Jami, E.S., Levey, D.F., Purves, K.L. & Weber, H. (2021) Genetic contributions to anxiety disorders: Where we are and where we are heading. *Psychological Medicine*, *51*(13): 2231–2246. doi:10.1017/S0033291720005486.

Asmer, M.S., Kirkham, J., Newton, H., Ismail, Z., Elbayoumi, H., Leung, R.H. & Seitz, D.P. (2018) Meta-analysis of the prevalence of major depressive disorder among older adults with dementia. *Journal of Clinical Psychiatry*, *79*(5): 17r11772. doi: 10.4088/JCP.17r11772.

Astramskaitė, I., Poškevičius, L. & Juodžbalys, G. (2016) Factors determining tooth extraction anxiety and fear in adult dental patients: A systematic review. *International Journal of Oral Maxillofacial Surgery*, *45*(12): 1630–1643.

Atchison, A.E. & Zickgraf, H.F. (2022) Orthorexia nervosa and eating disorder behaviors: A systematic review of the literature. *Appetite*, *177*: 106134. doi:10.1016/j.appet.2022.106134.

Atlas, L. Y. (2023) How instructions, learning, and expectations shape pain and neurobiological responses. *Annual Review of Neuroscience*, *46*, 167–189. doi:10.1146/annurev-neuro-101822-122427.

Atlas, L.Y. & Wager, T.D. (2014) A meta-analysis of brain mechanisms of placebo analgesia: Consistent findings and unanswered questions. *Handbook of Experimental Pharmacology*, *225*: 37–69.

Atoui, S., Chevance, G., Romain, A.J., Kingsbury, C., Lachance, J.P. & Bernard, P. (2021) Daily associations between sleep and physical activity: A systematic review and meta-analysis. *Sleep Medicine Reviews*, *57*(1): 101426. doi:10.1016/j.smrv.2021.101426.

Atwood, M.E. & Friedman, A. (2020) A systematic review of enhanced cognitive behavioral therapy (CBT-E) for eating disorders. *International Journal of Eating Disorders*, *53*(3): 311–330. doi:10.1002/eat.23206.

Aust, J. & Bradshaw, T. (2017) Mindfulness interventions for psychosis: A systematic review of the literature. *Journal of Psychiatric and Mental Health Nursing*, *24*(1): 69–83.

Austin, A., Flynn, M., Richards, K., Hodsoll, J., Duarte, T.A., Robinson, P., Kelly, J. & Schmidt, U. (2021) Duration of untreated eating disorder and relationship to outcomes: A systematic review of the literature. *European Eating Disorders Review*, *29*: 329–345. doi: 10.1002/erv.2745.

Australian Bureau of Statistics (2023) *Aboriginal and Torres Strait Islander Life Expectancy*. Canberra: ABS. Available from www.abs.gov.au/statistics/people/aboriginal-and-torres-strait-islander-peoples/aboriginal-and-torres-strait-islander-life-expectancy/latest-release (accessed 2 February 2024).

Australian Institute of Health and Welfare (AIHW) (2023) *Chronic Health Conditions among Culturally and Linguistically Diverse Australians, 2021*. Canberra: AIHW. Last updated 8 February 2023. Available from www.aihw.gov.au/reports/cald-australians/chronic-conditions-cald-2021 (accessed 6 March 2024).

Australian Institute of Health and Welfare (AIHW) (2024) *Health across Socioeconomic Groups*. Canberra: AIHW. Available from www.aihw.gov.au/reports/australias-health/health-across-socioeconomic-groups (accessed 17 January 2024).

Avishai, E., Yeghiazaryan, K. & Golubnitschaja, O. (2017) Impaired wound healing: Facts and hypotheses for multi-professional considerations in predictive, preventive and personalised medicine. *EPMA Journal*, *8*(11): 23–33. doi: 10.1007/s13167-017-0081-y.

Aw, P.Y., Pang, X.Z., Wee, C.F., Tan, N.H.W. et al. (2023) Co-prevalence and incidence of myocardial infarction and/or stroke in patients with depression and/or anxiety: A systematic review and meta-analysis. *Journal of Psychosomatic Research*, *165*: 111141. doi:10.1016/j.jpsychores.2022.111141.

Ayers, S., Bond, R., Bertullies, S. & Wijma, K. (2016) The aetiology of post-traumatic stress following childbirth: A meta-analysis and theoretical framework. *Psychological Medicine*, *46*(6): 1121–1134.

Ayers, S., Bond, R., Webb, R., Miller, P. & Bateson, K. (2019) Perinatal mental health and risk of child maltreatment: A systematic review and meta-analysis. *Child Abuse & Neglect*, *98*: 104172. doi: 10.1016/j.chiabu.2019.104172.

Ayers, S., Copland, C. & Dunmore, E. (2009) A preliminary study of negative appraisals and dysfunctional coping associated with post-traumatic stress disorder symptoms following myocardial infarction. *British Journal of Health Psychology*, *14*(3): 459–471.

Ayers, S., McKenzie-McHarg, K. & Eagle, A. (2007) Cognitive behaviour therapy for postnatal post-traumatic stress disorder: Case studies. *Journal of Psychosomatic Obstetrics & Gynaecology*, *28*(3): 177–184.

Ayers, S. & Olander, E.K. (2013) What are we measuring and why? Using theory to guide perinatal research and measurement. *Journal of Reproductive and Infant Psychology*, *31*(5): 439–448.

Ayling, K., Fairclough, L., Tighe, P., Todd, I., Halliday, V. et al. (2018) Positive mood on the day of influenza vaccination predicts vaccine effectiveness: A prospective observational cohort study. *Brain, Behavior, and Immunity*, *67*: 314–323. doi:10.1016/j.bbi.2017.09.008.

Ayling, K., Sunger, K. & Vedhara, K. (2020) Effects of brief mood-improving interventions on immunity: A systematic review and meta-analysis. *Psychosomatic Medicine*, *82*(1): 10–28. doi: 10.1097/PSY.0000000000000760.

Aziz, R. & Steffens, D.C. (2013) What are the causes of late-life depression? *Psychiatric Clinics of North America*, *36*(4): 497–516.

Babor, T.F., Higgins-Biddle, J.C., Saunders, J.B. & Monteiro, M.G. (2007) *AUDIT: The Alcohol Use Disorders Identification Test: Guidelines for Use in Primary Care* (2nd edition). Geneva: World Health Organization.

Babygeetha, A. & Devineni, D. (2024) Social support and adherence to self-care behavior among patients with coronary heart disease and heart failure: A systematic review. *European Journal of Psychology*, *20*(1): 63–77. doi: 10.5964/ejop.12131.

Badawy, Y., Spector, A., Li, Z. & Desai, R. (2024) The risk of depression in the menopausal stages: A systematic review and meta-analysis. *Journal of Affective Disorders*, *357*: 126–133. doi: 10.1016/j.jad.2024.04.041.

Badenes-Ribera, L., Rubio-Aparicio, M., Sánchez-Meca, J., Fabris, M.A. & Longobardi, C. (2019) The association between muscle dysmorphia and eating disorder symptomatology: A systematic review and meta-analysis. *Journal of Behavioral Addictions*, *8*(3): 351–371. doi: 10.1556/2006.8.2019.44.

Baigry, M.I., Ray, R., Lindsay, D., Kelly-Hanku, A. & Redman-MacLaren, M. (2023) Barriers and enablers to young people accessing sexual and reproductive health services in Pacific Island Countries and Territories: A scoping review. *PloS One*, *18*(1): e0280667. doi:10.1371/journal.pone.0280667.

Baile, W.F., Buckman, R., Lenzi, R., Glober, G., Beale, E.A. & Kudelka, A.P. (2000) SPIKES – a six-step protocol for delivering bad news: Application to the patient with cancer. *The Oncologist*, *5*(4): 302–311.

Baker, F.C. & Driver, H.S. (2007) Circadian rhythms, sleep, and the menstrual cycle. *Sleep Medicine*, *8*(6): 613–622.

Baker, F.C. & Lee, K.A. (2022) Menstrual cycle effects on sleep. *Sleep Medicine Clinics*, *17*(2): 283–294. doi: 10.1016/j.jsmc.2022.02.004.

Baker, N. & Billick, S.B. (2022) Psychiatric consequences of skin conditions: Multiple case study analysis with literature review. *Psychiatric Quarterly*, *93*(1): 841–847. doi:10.1007/s11126-022-09991-6.

Balantekin, K.N. (2019) The influence of parental dieting behavior on child dieting behavior and weight status. *Current Obesity*

Reports, *8*(2): 137–144. doi: 10.1007/s13679-019-00338-0.

Baldridge, S. & Symes, L. (2018) Just between us: An integrative review of confidential care for adolescents. *Journal of Pediatric Health Care*, *32*(2): e45–e58. doi: 10.1016/j.pedhc.2017.09.009.

Balendran, B., Bath, M.F., Awopetu, A.I. & Kreckler, S.M. (2021) Burnout within UK surgical specialties: A systematic review. *The Annals of The Royal College of Surgeons of England*, *103*(7): 464–470. doi:10.1308/rcsann.2020.7058.

Ballering, A.V., Olde Hartman, T.C., Verheij, R. & Rosmalen, J.G.M. (2023) Sex and gender differences in primary care help-seeking for common somatic symptoms: A longitudinal study. *Scandinavian Journal of Primary Health Care*, *41*: 132–139. doi:10.1080/02813432.2023.2191653.

Ballesio, A., Zagaria, A., Violani, C. & Lombardo, C. (2023) Psychosocial and behavioural predictors of immune response to influenza vaccination: A systematic review and meta-analysis. *Health Psychology Review*, *18*(2): 255–284. doi:10.1080/17437199.2023.2208652.

Bandura, A., Ross, D. & Ross, S.A. (1961) Transmission of aggression through imitation of aggressive models. *Journal of Abnormal and Social Psychology*, *63*(3): 575–582.

Baniaghil, A.S., Ghasemi, S., Rezaei-Aval, M. & Behnampour, N. (2022) Effect of communication skills training using the Calgary-Cambridge model on interviewing skills among midwifery students: A randomized controlled trial. *Iranian Journal of Nursing and Midwifery Research*, *27*(1): 24–29. doi: 10.4103/ijnmr.IJNMR_42_20.

Bar-Haim, Y., Lamy, D., Pergamin, L., Bakerman-Kranenburg, M.J. & van Ijzendoorn, M.H. (2007) Threat-related attentional bias in anxious and non-anxious individuals: A meta-analytic study. *Psychological Bulletin*, *133*(1): 1–24.

Barakou, I., Hackett, K.L., Finch, T. & Hettinga, F.J. (2023) Self-regulation of effort for a better health-related quality of life: A multidimensional activity pacing model for chronic pain and fatigue management. *Annals of Medicine*, *55*(2): 2270688. doi:10.1080/07853890.2023.2270688.

Barber, S. & Moreno-Leguizamon, C.J. (2017) Can narrative medicine education contribute to the delivery of compassionate care? A review of the literature. *Medical Humanities*, *43*: 199–203. doi:10.1136/medhum-2017-011242.

Barberio, B., Zamani, M., Black, C.J., Savarino, E.V. & Ford, A.C. (2021) Prevalence of symptoms of anxiety and depression in patients with inflammatory bowel disease: A systematic review and meta-analysis. *Lancet Gastroenterology & hepatology*, *6*(5): 359–370. doi:10.1016/S2468-1253(21)00014-5.

Barrett, L.F. (2017) *How Emotions are Made: The Secret Life of the Brain*. Boston, MA: Houghton Mifflin Harcourt.

Barry, V., Stout, M.E., Lynch, M.E., Mattis, S., Tran, D.Q., Antun, A., Ribiero, M.J.A., Stein, S.F. & Kempton, C.L. (2020) The effect of psychological distress on health outcomes: A systematic review and meta-analysis of prospective studies. *Journal of Health Psychology*, *25*(2): 227–239. doi: 10.1177/1359105319842931.

Barsness, J.G., Regnier, C.R., Hook, C.C. & Mueller, P.S. (2020) US medical and surgical society position statements on physician-assisted suicide and euthanasia: A review. *BMC Medical Ethics*, *21*(1): 111. doi:10.1186/s12910-020-00556-5.

Bas-Sarmiento, P., Fernández-Gutiérrez, M., Díaz-Rodríguez, M. & iCARE Team (2019) Teaching empathy to nursing students: A randomised controlled trial. *Nurse Education Today*, *80*: 40–51. doi: 10.1016/j.nedt.2019.06.002.

Batty, G.D., Russ, T.C., Stamatakis, E. & Kivimäki, M. (2017) Psychological distress in relation to site specific cancer mortality: Pooling of unpublished data from 16 prospective cohort studies. *British Medical Journal*, *356*: j108. doi: 10.1136/bmj.j108.

Bauer, A., Parsonage, M., Knapp, M., Iemmi, V. & Adelaja, B. (2014) *Costs of Perinatal Mental Health Problems: The Costs of Perinatal Mental Health Problems.* London: Centre for Mental Health.

Baumeister, H., Haschke, A., Munzinger, M., Hutter, N. & Tully, P.J. (2015) Inpatient and outpatient costs in patients with coronary artery disease and mental disorders: A systematic review. *Biopsychosocial Medicine*, 9(1): 11. doi: 10.1186/s13030-015-0039-z.

Baumeister, R.F., Campbell, J.D., Krueger, J.I. & Vohs, K.D. (2003) Does high self-esteem cause better performance, interpersonal success, happiness, or healthier lifestyles? *Psychological Science in the Public Interest*, 4(1): 1–44.

Bayne, M., Fairey, M., Silarova, B., Griffin, S.J., Sharp, S.J., Klein, W.M.P., Sutton, S. & Usher-Smith, J.A. (2020) Effect of interventions including provision of personalised cancer risk information on accuracy of risk perception and psychological responses: A systematic review and meta-analysis. *Patient Education and Counseling*, 103(1): 83–95. doi: 10.1016/j.pec.2019.08.010.

Beatty, L. & Binnion, C. (2016) A systematic review of predictors of, and reasons for, adherence to online psychological interventions. *International Journal of Behavioral Medicine*, 23(6): 776–794.

Bechthold, A., Boeing, H., Schwedhelm, C., Hoffmann, G., Knüppel, S., Iqbal, K., De Henauw, S., Michels, N., Devleesschauwer, B., Schlesinger, S. & Schwingshackl, L. (2019) Food groups and risk of coronary heart disease, stroke and heart failure: A systematic review and dose-response meta-analysis of prospective studies. *Critical Reviews in Food Science & Nutrition*, 59(7): 1071–1090. doi: 10.1080/10408398.2017.1392288.

Beck, A.T. (1967) *Depression: Clinical, Experimental and Theoretical Aspects.* New York: Harper & Row.

Beckie, T.M. (2012) A systematic review of allostatic load, health, and health disparities. *Biological Research for Nursing*, 14(4): 311–346.

Bedrov, A. & Gable, S.L. (2023) Thriving together: The benefits of women's social ties for physical, psychological and relationship health. *Philosophical Transactions of the Royal Society of London B: Biological Sciences*, 378(1868): 20210441. doi:10.1098/rstb.2021.0441.

Belbasis, L., Köhler, C.A., Stefanis, N., Stubbs, B., van Os, J., Vieta, E., Seeman, M.V., Arango, C., Carvalho, A.F. & Evangelou, E. (2018) Risk factors and peripheral biomarkers for schizophrenia spectrum disorders: An umbrella review of meta-analyses. *Acta Psychiatrica Scandinavica*, 137(2): 88–97. doi: 10.1111/acps.12847.

Benedetti, F., Maggi, G., Lopiano, L., Lanotte, M., Rainero, I., Vighetti, S. & Pollo, A. (2003) Open versus hidden medical treatments: The patient's knowledge about a therapy affects the therapy outcome. *Prevention & Treatment*, 6(1): Article 1.

Bennett, P. (2007) Coronary heart disease: Impact. In S. Ayers et al. (eds), *Cambridge Handbook of Psychology, Health & Medicine* (2nd edition). Cambridge: Cambridge University Press (pp. 644–647).

Bensing, J.M., Roter, D.L. & Hulsman, R.L. (2003) Communication patterns of primary care physicians in the United States and the Netherlands. *Journal of General Internal Medicine*, 18(5): 335–342.

Benyamini, Y., Molcho, M.L., Dan, U., Gozlan, M. & Preis, H. (2017) Women's attitudes towards the medicalization of childbirth and their associations with planned and actual modes of birth. *Women and Birth*, 30(5): 424–430. doi: 10.1016/j.wombi.2017.03.007.

Bergeron, J., Cederkvist, L., Fortier, I., Rod, N.H., Andersen, P.K. & Andersen, A.N. (2023) Maternal stress during pregnancy and gestational duration: A cohort study from the Danish National Birth Cohort. *Paediatric and Perinatal Epidemiology*, 37(1): 45–56. doi: 10.1111/ppe.12918.

Berkowitz, L. (1989) Frustration-aggression hypothesis: Examination and reformulation. *Psychological Bulletin*, *106*(1): 59–73.

Bernal, G., Bonilla, J., & Bellido, C. (1995). Ecological validity and cultural sensitivity for outcome research: issues for the cultural adaptation and development of psychosocial treatments with Hispanics. *Journal of Abnormal Child Psychology*, *23*(1): 67–82. doi:10.1007/BF01447045.

Bernal, M., Haro, J.M., Bernert, S., Brugha, T., de Graaf, R., Bruffaerts, R., Lépine, J.P., de Girolamo, G., Vilagut, G., Gasquet, I., Torres, J.V., Kovess, V., Heider, D., Neeleman, J., Kessler, R., Alonso, J. & ESEMED/MHEDEA Investigators (2007) Risk factors for suicidality in Europe: Results from the ESEMED study. *Journal of Affective Disorders*, *101*(1–3): 27–34.

Bernard, L.C., Mills, M., Swenson, L. & Walsh, R.P. (2005) An evolutionary theory of human motivation. *Genetic, Social, and General Psychology Monographs*, *131*(2): 129–184. doi: 10.3200/MONO.131.2.129-184.

Besedovsky, L., Lange, T. & Haack, M. (2019) The sleep-immune crosstalk in health and disease. *Physiological Reviews*, *99*(3): 1325–1380. doi:10.1152/physrev.00010.2018.

Betran, A.P., Ye, J., Moller, A.B., Souza, J.P. & Zhang, J. (2021) Trends and projections of caesarean section rates: Global and regional estimates. *BMJ Global Health*, *6*(6): e005671. doi: 10.1136/bmjgh-2021-005671.

Bibace, R. & Walsh, M.E. (1980) Development of children's concepts of illness. *Pediatrics*, *66*(6): 912–917.

Bienvenu, L.A., Noonan, J., Wang, X. & Peter, K. (2020) Higher mortality of COVID-19 in males: Sex differences in immune response and cardiovascular comorbidities. *Cardiovascular Research*, *116*(14): 2197–2206. doi:10.1093/cvr/cvaa284.

Bierstetel, S.J., Jiang, Y., Slatcher, R.B. & Zilioli, S. (2021) Parent–child conflict and physical health trajectories among youth with asthma. *Journal of Psychosomatic Research*, *150*: 110606. doi:10.1016/j.jpsychores.2021.110606.

Bilman, E., van Kleef, E. & van Trijp, H. (2017) External cues challenging the internal appetite control system: Overview and practical implications. *Critical Reviews in Food Science and Nutrition*, *57*(13): 2825–2834. doi: 10.1080/10408398.2015.1073140.

Birk, J.L., Kronish, I.M., Moise, N., Falzon, L., Yoon, S. & Davidson, K.W. (2019) Depression and multimorbidity: Considering temporal characteristics of the associations between depression and multiple chronic diseases. *Health Psychology*, *38*(9): 802–811. https://doi.org/10.1037/hea0000737

Birmingham, E. & Kingstone, A. (2009) Human social attention: A new look at past, present, and future investigations. *Annals of the New York Academy of Sciences*, *1156*(1): 118–140. doi: 10.1111/j.1749-6632.2009.04468.x.

Birnie, K.A., Noel, M., Chambers, C.T., Uman, L.S. & Parker, J.A. (2018) Psychological interventions for needle-related procedural pain and distress in children and adolescents. *Cochrane Database of Systematic Reviews*, *10*(10): Art. CD005179. doi: 10.1002/14651858.CD005179.pub4.

Bischof, G., Bischof, A. & Rumpf, H. J. (2021) Motivational interviewing: An evidence-based approach for use in medical practice. *Deutsches Arzteblatt International*, *118*(7): 109–115. doi:10.3238/arztebl.m2021.0014.

Bisgaard, T.H., Allin, K.H., Keefer, L., Ananthakrishnan, A.N. & Jess, T. (2022) Depression and anxiety in inflammatory bowel disease: Epidemiology, mechanisms and treatment. *Nature Reviews. Gastroenterology & Hepatology*, *19*(11): 717–726. doi:10.1038/s41575-022-00634-6.

Bjerregaard, L.G., Adelborg, K. & Baker, J.L. (2020) Change in body mass index from childhood onwards and risk of adult cardiovascular disease. *Trends in Cardiovascular Medicine*, *30*(1): 39–45. doi:10.1016/j.tcm.2019.01.011.

Black, C.J. & Ford, A.C. (2020) Global burden of irritable bowel syndrome: Trends, predictions and risk factors. *Nature Reviews Gastroenterology & Hepatology*, *17*: 473–486. doi: 10.1038/s41575-020-0286-8.

Black, C.J., Thakur, E.R., Houghton, L.A., Quigley, E.M.M., Moayyedi, P. & Ford, A.C. (2020) Efficacy of psychological therapies for irritable bowel syndrome: Systematic review and network meta-analysis. *Gut*, *69*(8): 1441–1451. doi:10.1136/gutjnl-2020-321191.

Blakeman, J.R. & Prasun, M.A. (2022) Perceived personal risk and vulnerability in recognizing and responding to symptoms of acute coronary syndrome: An integrative review. *European Journal of Cardiovascular Nursing*, *21*: 405–413. doi:10.1093/eurjcn/zvab112.

Blaxter, M. (1990) *Health and Lifestyles*. London: Routledge.

Blom, T., Fieten, K.B., Kemperman, P.M.J.H., Spillekom-van Koulil, S. & Dikmans, R.E.G. (2023) Skin distress screening: Validation of an efficient one-question tool. *Acta Dermato-Venereologica*, *103*: adv4590. doi:10.2340/actadv.v103.4590.

Bode, H., Ivens, B., Bschor, T., Schwarzer, G., Henssler, J. & Baethge, C. (2022) Hyperthyroidism and clinical depression: A systematic review and meta-analysis. *Translational Psychiatry*, *12*(1): 362. doi:10.1038/s41398-022-02121-7.

Boerebach, B.C., Scheepers, R.A., van der Leeuw, R.M., Heineman, M.J., Arah, O.A. & Lombarts, K.M. (2014) The impact of clinicians' personality and their interpersonal behaviors on the quality of patient care: A systematic review. *International Journal for Quality in Health Care*, *26*(4): 426–481.

Bogart, L.M., Bird, S.T., Walt, L.C., Delahanty, D.L. & Figler, J.L. (2004) Association of stereotypes about physicians to health care satisfaction, help-seeking behavior, and adherence to treatment. *Social Science & Medicine*, *58*(6): 1049–1058.

Böhnlein, J., Altegoer, L., Muck, N.K., Roesmann, K., Redlich, R., Dannlowski, U. & Leehr, E.J. (2020) Factors influencing the success of

exposure therapy for specific phobia: A systematic review. *Neuroscience & Biobehavioral Reviews*, *108*: 796–820. doi: 10.1016/j.neubiorev.2019.12.009.

Bohren, M.A., Hofmeyr, G., Sakala, C., Fukuzawa, R.K. & Cuthbert, A. (2017) Continuous support for women during childbirth. *Cochrane Database of Systematic Reviews*, *7*: Art. CD003766. doi: 10.1002/14651858.CD003766.pub6.

Bonanno, G.A. & Kaltman, S. (2001) The varieties of grief experience. *Clinical Psychology Review*, *21*(5): 705–734.

Bonini, L., Rotunno, C., Arcuri, E. & Gallese, V. (2022) Mirror neurons 30 years later: Implications and applications. *Trends in Cognitive Sciences*, *26*(9): 767–781. doi:10.1016/j.tics.2022.06.003.

Bonn, G.B. (2013) Re-conceptualizing free will for the 21st century: Acting independently with a limited role for consciousness. *Frontiers in Psychology*, *4*: 920.

Booth, J., Connelly, L., Lawrence, M., Chalmers, C., Joice, S., Becker, C. & Dougall, N. (2015) Evidence of perceived psychosocial stress as a risk factor for stroke in adults: A meta-analysis. *BMC Neurology*, *15*: 233. doi: 10.1186/s12883-015-0456-4.

Boots Family Trust Alliance (2013) *Perinatal Mental Health: Experiences of Women and Health Professionals*. London: Boots Family Trust. Available at: https://www.tommys.org/sites/default/files/legacy/Perinatal_Mental_Health_Experiences%20of%20women.pdf (accessed 29 November 2020).

Bor, R. & Eriksen, C. (2019) Counselling. In C.D. Llewellyn, S. Ayers, C. McManus, S. Newman, K.J. Petrie, T.A. Revenson & J. Weinman (eds), *The Cambridge Handbook of Psychology, Health and Medicine* (3rd edition). Cambridge: Cambridge University Press.

Bora, E. (2021) A meta-analysis of theory of mind and 'mentalization' in borderline personality disorder: A true neuro-social-cognitive or meta-social-cognitive impairment? *Psychological Medicine*, *51*(15): 2541–2551. doi: 10.1017/S0033291721003718.

Borowski, S., Groh, A.M., Bakermans-Kranenburg, M., Pasco Fearon, R.M., Roisman, G.I., van IJzendoorn, M.H. & Vaughn, B.E. (2021) The significance of early temperamental reactivity for children's social competence with peers: A meta-analytic review and comparison with the role of early attachment. *Psychological Bulletin*, *147*(11): 1125–1158. doi:10.1037/bul0000346.

Borrell-Carrio, F., Suchman, A.L. & Epstein, R.M. (2004) The biopsychosocial model 25 years later: Principles, practice and scientific enquiry. *Annals of Family Medicine*, *2*(6): 576–582.

Bortolato, B., Hyphantis, T.N., Valpione, S., Perini, G., Maes, M., Morris, G., Kubera, M., Köhler, C.A., Fernandes, B.S., Stubbs, B., Pavlidis, N. & Carvalho, A.F. (2017) Depression in cancer: The many biobehavioral pathways driving tumor progression. *Cancer Treatment Reviews*, *52*: 58–70. doi: 10.1016/j.ctrv.2016.11.004.

Bortolotti, L. & Antrobus, M. (2015) Costs and benefits of realism and optimism. *Current Opinion in Psychiatry*, *28*(2): 194–198.

Bostrom, J., Sweeney, G., Whiteson, J. & Dodson, J.A. (2020) Mobile health and cardiac rehabilitation in older adults. *Clinical Cardiology*, *43*(2): 118–126. doi:10.1002/clc.23306.

Bottera, A.R., Thiel, A.M. & De Young, K.P. (2018) Negative affect and past month binge eating may drive perceptions of loss of control. *Appetite*, *128*: 116–119. doi: 10.1016/j.appet.2018.06.008.

Boucher, V.G., Gemme, C., Dragomir, A.I., Bacon, S.L., Larue, F. & Lavoie, K.L. (2020) Evaluation of communication skills among physicians: A systematic review of existing assessment tools. *Psychosomatic Medicine*, *82*(4): 440–451. doi: 10.1097/PSY.0000000000000794.

Bower, P., Knowles, S., Coventry, P.A. & Rowland, N. (2011) Counselling for mental health and psychosocial problems in primary care. *Cochrane Database of Systematic Reviews*, 9: Art. CD001025.

Bowlby, J. (1969) *Attachment and Loss*: *Vol. 1. Attachment*. New York: Basic Books.

Bowlby, J. (1973) *Attachment and Loss*: *Vol. 2. Separation: Anxiety and Anger*. New York: Basic Books.

Bowleg, L. (2012) The problem with the phrase women and minorities: Intersectionality – an important theoretical framework for public health. *American Journal of Public Health*, *102*: 1267–1273.

Boyce, W.T., Chesney, M., Alkon, A., Tschann, J.M., Adams, S., Chesterman, B., Cohen, F., Kaiser, P., Folkman, S. & Wara, D. (1995) Psychobiologic reactivity to stress and childhood respiratory illnesses: Results of two prospective studies. *Psychosomatic Medine*, *57*(5): 411–422.

Boylan, J.M., Cundiff, J.M. & Matthews, K.A. (2018) Socioeconomic status and cardiovascular responses to standardized stressors: A systematic review and meta-analysis. *Psychosomatic Medicine*, 80(3): 278–293. doi:10.1097/PSY.0000000000000561.

Bradt, J., Dileo, C., Magill, L. & Teague, A. (2016) Music interventions for improving psychological and physical outcomes in cancer patients. *Cochrane Database of Systematic Reviews*, 8: Art. CD006911. doi: 10.1002/14651858.CD006911.pub3.

Bradt, J., Dileo, C., Myers-Coffman, K. & Biondo, J. (2021) Music interventions for improving psychological and physical outcomes in people with cancer. *Cochrane Database of Systematic Reviews*, *10*(10): Art. CD006911. doi:10.1002/14651858.CD006911.pub4.

Bramley, N. & Eatough, V. (2005) The experience of living with Parkinson's disease: An interpretative phenomenological analysis case study. *Psychology & Health*, *20*(2): 223–235.

Bräscher, A.K., Raymaekers, K., Van den Bergh, O. & Witthöft, M. (2017) Are media reports able to cause somatic symptoms attributed to WiFi radiation? An experimental test of the negative expectation hypothesis. *Environmental Research*, *31*(156): 265–271.

Braveman, P. & Gottlieb, L. (2014) The social determinants of health: It's time to consider the causes of the causes. *Public Health Reports*, 29(Suppl. 2): 19–31.

Bray, F., Laversanne, M., Sung, H., Ferlay, J., Siegel, R.L., Soerjomataram, I. & Jemal, A. (2024) Global cancer statistics 2022: GLOBOCAN estimates of incidence and mortality worldwide for 36 cancers in 185 countries. *CA: A Cancer Journal for Clinicians*, 74(3): 229–263. doi:10.3322/caac.21834.

Breedvelt, J.J.F., Warren, F.C., Segal, Z., Kuyken, W. & Bockting, C.L. (2021) Continuation of antidepressants vs sequential psychological interventions to prevent relapse in depression: An individual participant data meta-analysis. *JAMA Psychiatry*, 78: 868–875. doi:10.1001/jamapsychiatry.2021.0823.

Breiding, M.J., Smith, S.G., Basile, K.C., Walters, M.L., Chen, J. & Merrick, M.T. (2014) Prevalence and characteristics of sexual violence, stalking, and intimate partner violence victimization: National intimate partner and sexual violence survey, United States, 2011. *Morbidity and Mortality Weekly Report. Surveillance Summaries*, 63(8): 1–18.

Brewin, C.R. & Holmes, E.A. (2003) Psychological theories of posttraumatic stress disorder. *Clinical Psychology Review*, 23(3): 339–376.

British Association for Counselling and Psychotherapy (2020) *A Guide to the BACP Counselling Skills Competence Framework*. Lutterworth: BACP. Available from www.bacp.co.uk/media/8889/bacp-counselling-skills-framework-user-guide-may20.pdf (accessed 30 July 2024).

British Medical Association (2019) *Caring, Supportive, Collaborative: Doctors' Vision for Change in the NHS*. London: BMA.

Broadbent, E. & Petrie, K.J. (2019) Symptom perception. In C.D. Llewellyn, S. Ayers, C. McManus, S. Newman, K.J. Petrie, T.A. Revenson & J. Weinman (eds), *The Cambridge Handbook of Psychology, Health and Medicine* (3rd edition). Cambridge: Cambridge University Press.

Broersen, L.H.A., Zamanipoor Najafabadi, A.H., Pereira, A.M., Dekkers, O.M. van Furth, W.R. & Biermasz, N.R. (2021) Improvement in symptoms and health-related quality of life in acromegaly patients: A systematic review and meta-analysis. *Journal of Clinical Endocrinology and Metabolism*, 106(2): 577–587. doi:10.1210/clinem/dgaa868.

Brooks, H., Llewellyn, C.D., Nadarzynski, T., et al. (2018) Sexual orientation disclosure in health care: A systematic review. *British Journal of General Practice*, 68(668): e187–e196. doi: doi:10.3399/bjgp18X694841.

Brooks, T., Sharp, R., Evans, S., Baranoff, J. & Esterman, A. (2020) Predictors of psychological outcomes and the effectiveness and experience of psychological interventions for adult women with chronic pelvic pain: A scoping review. *Journal of Pain Research*, 13: 1081–1102. doi: 10.2147/JPR.S245723.

Brown, C.E.B., Richardson, K., Halil-Pizzirani, B., Atkins, L., Yücel, M. & Seagrave, R.A. (2024) Key influences on university students' physical activity: A systematic review using the Theoretical Domains Framework and the COM-B model of human behaviour. *BMC Public Health*, 24(1): 418. doi:10.1186/s12889-023-17621-4.

Brown, H.M., Waszczuk, M.A., Zavos, H.M., Trzaskowski, M., Gregory, A.M. & Eley, T.C. (2014) Cognitive content specificity in anxiety and depressive disorder symptoms: A twin study of cross-sectional associations with anxiety sensitivity dimensions across development. *Psychological Medicine*, 44(16): 3469–3480.

Brown, J., Kotz, D., Michie, S., Stapleton, J., Walmsley, M. & West, R. (2014) How effective and cost-effective was the national mass media smoking cessation campaign Stoptober? *Drug & Alcohol Dependence*, 135(100): 52–58. doi: 10.1016/j.drugalcdep.2013.11.003.

Brown, J.C., Damjanov, N., Courneya, K.S., Troxel, A.B., Zemel, B.S., Rickels, M.R., Ky, B., Rhim, A.D., Rustgi, A.K. & Schmitz, K.H. (2018) A randomized dose-response trial of aerobic exercise and health-related quality of life in colon cancer survivors. *Psycho-Oncology*, *27*(4): 1221–1228. doi: 10.1002/pon.4655.

Brown, J.C., Troxel, A.B., Ky, B., Damjanov, N., Zemel, B.S., Rickels, M.R., Rhim, A.D., Rustgi, A.K., Courneya, K.S. & Schmitz, K.H. (2018) Dose–response effects of aerobic exercise among colon cancer survivors: A randomized phase II trial. *Clinical Colorectal Cancer*, *17*(1): 32–40. doi: 10.1016/j.clcc.2017.06.001.

Brown, L., Hunter, M.S., Chen, R., Crandall, C.J., Gordon, J.L., Mishra, G.D., Rother, V., Joffe, H. & Hickey M. (2024) Promoting good mental health over the menopause transition. *Lancet*, *403*(10430): 969–983. doi: 10.1016/S0140-6736(23)02801-5.

Brown, L.C., Murphy, A.R., Lalonde, C.S., Subhedar, P.D., Miller, A.H. & Stevens, J.S. (2020) Posttraumatic stress disorder and breast cancer: Risk factors and the role of inflammation and endocrine function. *Cancer*, *126*: 3181–3191. doi:10.1002/cncr.32934.

Brown, L.G., Hoover, E.R., Besrat, B.N. et al. (2022) Application of the Capability, Opportunity, Motivation and Behavior (COM-B) model to identify predictors of two self-reported hand hygiene behaviors (handwashing and hand sanitizer use) to prevent COVID-19 infection among U.S. adults, Fall 2020. *BMC Public Health*, *22*(1): 2360. doi:10.1186/s12889-022-14809-y.

Brown, R., Dunn, S., Byrnes, K., Morris, R., Heinrich, P. & Shaw, J. (2009) Doctors' stress responses and poor communication performance in simulated bad-news consultations. *Academic Medicine*, *84*(11): 1595–602.

Brown, T.A., Forney, K.J., Klein, K.M., Grillot, C. & Keel, P.K. (2020) A 30-year longitudinal study of body weight, dieting, and eating pathology across women and men from late adolescence to later midlife. *Journal of Abnormal Psychology*, *129*: 376–386. doi:10.1037/abn0000519.

Brown, V.M., Price, R. & Dombrovski, A.Y. (2023) Anxiety as a disorder of uncertainty: Implications for understanding maladaptive anxiety, anxious avoidance, and exposure therapy. *Cognitive, Affective, & Behavioral Neuroscience*, *23*(3): 844–868. doi: 10.3758/s13415-023-01080-w.

Bruinsma, F., Venn, A.J., Patton, G.C., Rayner, J.A., Pyett, P., Werther, G., Jones, P. & Lumley, J.M. (2006) Concern about tall stature during adolescence and depression in later life. *Journal of Affective Disorders*, *91*(2–3): 145–152.

Brummett, B.H., Barefoot, J.C., Siegler, I.C., Clapp-Channing, N.E., Lytle, B.L., Bosworth Jr, H.B., Williams, R.B. & Mark, D.B. (2001) Characteristics of socially isolated patients with coronary artery disease who are at elevated risk for mortality. *Psychosomatic Medicine*, *63*(2): 267–272.

Bruno, D. & Schurmann Vignaga, S. (2019) Addenbrooke's cognitive examination III in the diagnosis of dementia: A critical review. *Neuropsychiatric Disease & Treatment*, *15*: 441–447. doi: 10.2147/NDT.S151253.

Bryant, E.J., Rehman, J., Pepper, L.B. & Walters, E.R. (2019) Obesity and eating disturbance: The role of TFEQ restraint and disinhibition. *Current Obesity Reports*, *8*(4): 363–372. doi: 10.1007/s13679-019-00365-x.

Bryere, J., Dejardin, O., Launay, L., Colonna, M., Grosclaude, P. & Launoy, G. (2018) Socioeconomic status and site-specific cancer incidence, a Bayesian approach in a French Cancer Registries Network study. *European Journal of Cancer Prevention*, *27*(4): 391–398. doi:10.1097/CEJ.0000000000000326.

Buchanan, H., Newton, J.T., Baker, S.R. & Asimakopoulou, K. (2021) Adopting the COM-B model and TDF framework in oral and dental research: A narrative review. *Community Dentistry and Oral Epidemiology*, *49*(5): 385–393. doi:10.1111/cdoe.12677.

Buglass, E. (2010) Grief and bereavement theories. *Nursing Standard*, *24*(41): 44–47.

Bunda, K. & Busseri, M.A. (2019) Lay theories of health, self-rated health, and health behavior intentions. *Journal of Health*

Psychology, 24(7): 979–988. doi: 10.1177/13591053 16689143.

Burger, J.M. (1999) The foot-in-the-door compliance procedure: A multiple-process analysis and review. *Personality and Social Psychology Review, 3*(4): 303–325.

Burns, J.W., Gerhart, J.I., Post, K.M., Smith, D.A. et al. (2015) The communal coping model of pain catastrophizing in daily life: A within-couples daily diary study. *Journal of Pain, 16*(11): 1163–1175. doi:10.1016/j.jpain.2015.08.005.

Burton, C., Fink, P., Henningsen, P., Löwe, B., Rief, W. & EURONET-SOMA Group (2020) Functional somatic disorders: Discussion paper for a new common classification for research and clinical use. *BMC Medicine, 18*(1): 34. doi:10.1186/s12916-020-1505-4.

Buske-Kirschbaum, A., von Auer, K., Kreiger, S., Weis, S., Rauh, W. & Hellhammer, D. (2003) Blunted cortisol responses to psychosocial stress in asthmatic children: A general feature of atopic disease? *Psychosomatic Medicine, 65*(5): 806–810.

Buss, M.K., Rock, L.K. & McCarthy, E.P. (2017) Understanding palliative care and hospice: A review for primary care providers. *Mayo Clinic Proceedings, 92*(2): 280–286. doi:10.1016/j.mayocp.2016.11.007.

Butler, A.C., Chapman, J.E., Forman, E.M. & Beck, A.T. (2006) The empirical status of cognitive-behavioral therapy: A review of meta-analyses. *Clinical Psychology Review, 26*(1): 17–31.

Buyukcan-Tetik, A., Seefeld, L., Bergunde, L., Ergun, T.D., Dikmen-Yildiz, P., Horsch, A., Garthus-Niegel, S., Oosterman, M., Lalor, J., Weigl, T., Bogaerts, A., Van Haeken, S., Downe, S. & Ayers, S. (2024) Birth expectations, birth experiences and childbirth-related post-traumatic stress symptoms in mothers and birth companions: Dyadic investigation using response surface analysis. *British Journal of Health Psychology*, 26 June. doi: 10.1111/bjhp.12738. Epub ahead of print.

Cabral, R.R. & Smith, T.B. (2011) Racial/ethnic matching of clients and therapists in mental health services: A meta-analytic review of preferences, perceptions, and outcomes. *Journal of Counseling Psychology, 58*(4): 537–554. doi:10.1037/a0025266.

Cahn, P., Madero, J.S., Arribas, J.R., Antinori, A. et al. (2020) Durable efficacy of dolutegravir plus lamivudine in antiretroviral treatment-naive adults with HIV-1 infection: 96-week results from the GEMINI-1 and GEMINI-2 randomized clinical trials. *Journal of Acquired Immune Deficiency Syndrome, 83*: 310–318. doi:10.1097/QAI.0000000000002275.

Cai, J., Zhang, J. & Sun, X. (2020) Influence of subliminal stimuli on interpersonal trust: A possible mechanism. *PsyCh Journal, 9*(11): 644–650. doi:10.1002/pchj.364.

Cai, W., Mueller, C., Li, Y.-J., Shen, W.-D. & Stewart, R. (2019) Post stroke depression and risk of stroke recurrence and mortality: A systematic review and meta-analysis. *Ageing Research Reviews, 50*: 102–109. doi:10.1016/j.arr.2019.01.013.

Cai, W., Ma, W., Mueller, C., Stewart, R., Ji, J. & Shen, W. D. (2023) Association between late-life depression or depressive symptoms and stroke morbidity in elders: A systematic review and meta-analysis of cohort studies. *Acta Psychiatrica Scandinavica, 148*(5): 405–415. doi:10.1111/acps.13613.

Caini, S., Del Riccio, M., Vettori, V., Scotti, V., Martinoli, C., Raimondi, S., et al. (2022) Quitting smoking at or around diagnosis improves the overall survival of lung cancer patients: A systematic review and meta-analysis. *Journal of Thoracic Oncology, 17*(5): 623–636. doi:10.1016/j.jtho.2021.12.005.

Calcedo-Barba, A., Fructuoso, A., Martinez-Raga, J., et al. (2020) A meta-review of literature reviews assessing the capacity of patients with severe mental disorders to make decisions about their healthcare. *BMC Psychiatry, 20*: 339. doi:10.1186/s12888-020-02756-0.

Calderón, C., Jimenez-Fonseca, P., Jara, C., Hernández, R., Martínez de Castro, E., Varma, S., Ghanem, I. & Carmona-Bayonas,

A. (2018) Comparison of coping, psychological distress, and level of functioning in patients with gastric and colorectal cancer before adjuvant chemotherapy. *Journal of Pain and Symptom Management, 56*(3): 399–405. doi: 10.1016/j.jpainsymman.2018.05.010.

Cameron, D.S., Bertenshaw, E.J. & Sheeran, P. (2015) The impact of positive affect on health cognitions and behaviours: A meta-analysis of the experimental evidence. *Health Psychology Review, 9*(3): 345–365.

Cameron, E.E., Sedov, I.D. & Tomfohr-Madsen, L.M. (2016) Prevalence of paternal depression in pregnancy and the postpartum: An updated meta-analysis. *Journal of Affective Disorders, 206*: 189–203.

Cameron, L.D. & Moss-Morris, R. (2004) Illness-related cognition and behaviour. In A.A. Kaptein & J.A. Weinman (eds), *Health Psychology: An Introduction*. Oxford: Blackwell (pp. 84–110).

Camilleri, M. & Dilmaghani, S. (2023) Update on treatment of abdominal pain in irritable bowel syndrome: A narrative review. *Pharmacology & Therapeutics, 245*: 108400. doi:10.1016/j.pharmthera.2023.108400.

Campaign for Dignity in Dying (2019) Largest ever poll on assisted dying finds increase in support to 84% of Britons. *Campaign for Dignity in Dying*, 2 April. Available from www.dignityindying.org.uk/news/poll-assisted-dying-support-84-britons/ (accessed 29 July 2024).

Campbell-Jackson, L. & Horsch, A. (2014) The psychological impact of stillbirth on women: A systematic review. *Illness, Crisis & Loss, 22*(3): 237–256.

Campos-Rodríguez, R., Godínez-Victoria, M., Abarca-Rojano, E., Pacheco-Yépez, J., Reyna-Garfias, H., Barbosa-Cabrera, R. E., & Drago-Serrano, M. E. (2013) Stress modulates intestinal secretory immunoglobulin A, *Frontiers in Integrative Neuroscience, 7*(86): 1–10. https://doi.org/10.3389/fnint.2013.00086

Cane, J., O'Connor, D. & Michie, S. (2012) Validation of the theoretical domains framework for use in behaviour change and implementation research. *Implementation Science, 7*: 37. doi:10.1186/1748-5908-7-37.

Cañigueral, R. & Hamilton, A.F.C. (2019) The role of eye gaze during natural social interactions in typical and autistic people. *Frontiers in Psychology, 10*: 560. doi: 10.3389/fpsyg.2019.00560.

Cao-Lei, L., Dancause, K.N., Elgbeili, G., Massart, R., Szyf, M., Liu, A., Laplante, D.P. & King, S. (2015) DNA methylation mediates the impact of exposure to prenatal maternal stress on BMI and central adiposity in children at age 13½ years: Project Ice. *Storm Epigenetics, 10*(8): 749–761.

Cao-Lei, L., Elgbeili, G., Massart, R., Laplante, D.P., Szyf, M. & King, S. (2015) Pregnant women's cognitive appraisal of a natural disaster affects DNA methylation in their children 13 years later: Project Ice Storm. *Translational Psychiatry, 24*(5): e515.

Capers, Q., Clinchot, D., McDougle, L. & Greenwald, A. (2017) Implicit racial bias in medical school admissions. *Academic Medicine, 92*(3): 365–369 doi: 10.1097/ACM.0000000000001388.

Capilla-Díaz, C., Bonill-de Las Nieves, C., Hernández-Zambrano, S.M., Montoya-Juárez, R., Morales-Asencio, J.M., Pérez-Marfil, M.N. & Hueso-Montoro, C. (2019) Living with an intestinal stoma: A qualitative systematic review. *Qualitative Health Research, 29*(9): 1255–1265. doi: 10.1177/1049732318820933.

Caraballo, C., Ndumele, C.D., Roy, B., et al. (2022) Trends in racial and ethnic disparities in barriers to timely medical care among adults in the US, 1999 to 2018. *JAMA Health Forum, 3*(10): e223856. doi:10.1001/jamahealthforum.2022.3856.

Care Quality Commission (2013) *Dignity and Nutrition for Older People*. Newcastle upon Tyne: CQC. Available from www.cqc.org.uk/content/dignity-and-nutrition-older-people-2 (accessed 1 August 2017).

Carlisle, M., Uchino, B.N., Sanbonmatsu, D.M., Smith, T.W., Cribbet, M.R., Birmingham, W., Light, K.C. & Vaughn, A.A. (2012) Subliminal activation of social ties moderates cardiovascular reactivity during acute stress. *Health Psychology, 31*(2): 217–225.

Carlson, N.R. & Birkett, M.A. (2021) *Physiology of Behavior* (13th edition). Boston, MA: Allyn & Bacon.

Carlyle, J. (2007) Psychodynamic psychotherapy. In S. Ayers, A. Baum, C. McManus, S. Newman, K. Wallston, J. Weinman & R. West (eds), *Cambridge Handbook of Psychology, Health and Medicine* (2nd edition). Cambridge: Cambridge University Press (pp. 379–383).

Caro, P., Turner, W., Caldwell, D.M. & Macdonald, G. (2023) Comparative effectiveness of psychological interventions for treating the psychological consequences of sexual abuse in children and adolescents: A network meta-analysis. *Cochrane Database of Systematic Reviews, 6*(6): Art. CD013361. doi: 10.1002/14651858.CD013361.pub2.

Carr, J.B. & Packham, A. (2017) The effects of state-mandated abstinence-based sex education on teen health outcomes. *Health Economics, 26*: 403–420.

Carr, M.M., Wiedemann, A.A., Macdonald-Gagnon, G. & Potenza, M.N. (2021) Impulsivity and compulsivity in binge eating disorder: A systematic review of behavioral studies. *Progress in Neuropsychopharmacology & Biological Psychiatry, 110*: 110318. doi:10.1016/j.pnpbp.2021.110318.

Carr, R.M., Prestwich, A., Kwasnicka, D., Thøgersen-Ntoumani, C., Gucciardi, D.F., et al. (2019) Dyadic interventions to promote physical activity and reduce sedentary behaviour: Systematic review and meta-analysis. *Health Psychology Review, 13*(1): 91–109. doi: 10.1080/17437199.2018.1532312.

Carriedo-Diez, B., Tosoratto-Venturi, J.L., Cantón-Manzano, C., Wanden-Berghe, C. & Sanz-Valero, J. (2022) The effects of the exogenous melatonin on shift work sleep disorder in health personnel: A systematic review. *International Journal of Environmental Research and Public Health, 19*(16): 10199. doi:10.3390/ijerph191610199.

Carter, C.S. (2021) Oxytocin and love: Myths, metaphors and mysteries. *Comprehensive Psychoneuroendocrinology, 9*(2): 100107. doi:10.1016/j.cpnec.2021.100107.

Carvalho, C., Caetano, J.M., Cunha, L., Rebouta, P., Kaptchuk, T.J. & Kirsch, I. (2016) Open-label placebo treatment in chronic low back pain: A randomized controlled trial. *Pain, 157*(12): 2766–2772.

Carvalho, C., Pais, M., Cunha, L., Rebouta, P., Kaptchuk, T.J. & Kirsch, I. (2021) Open-label placebo for chronic low back pain: A 5-year follow-up. *Pain, 162*(5): 1521–1527. doi: 10.1097/j.pain.0000000000002162.

Cary, E. & Simpson, P. (2024) Premenstrual disorders and PMDD – a review. *Best Practice and Research Clinical Endocrinology & Metabolism, 38*(1): 101858. doi: 10.1016/j.beem.2023.101858.

Castro, F.G., Barrera Jr, M. & Holleran Steiker, L.K. (2010) Issues and challenges in the design of culturally adapted evidence-based interventions. *Annual Review of Clinical Psychology, 6*: 213–239. doi:10.1146/annurev-clinpsy-033109-132032.

Catanzano, M., Bennett, S.D., Sanderson, C., Patel, M., Manzotti, G., et al. (2020) Brief psychological interventions for psychiatric disorders in young people with long term physical health conditions: A systematic review and meta-analysis. *Journal of Psychosomatic Research, 136*: 110187. doi: 10.1016/j.jpsychores.2020.110187.

Catarino, A. (2015) Failing to forget: Inhibitory-control deficits compromise memory suppression in posttraumatic stress disorder. *Psychological Science, 26*(5): 604–616.

Celeghin, A., Diano, M., Bagnis, A., Viola, M. & Tamietto, M. (2017) Basic emotions in human neuroscience: Neuroimaging and beyond. *Frontiers in Psychology, 8*: 1432. doi: 10.3389/fpsyg.2017.01432.

Cené, C.W., Beckie, T.M., Sims, M., Suglia, S.F., Aggarwal, B., et al. (2022) Effects of objective and perceived social isolation on cardiovascular and brain health: A scientific statement from the American Heart Association. *Journal of the American Heart Association, 11*(16): e026493. doi:10.1161/JAHA.122.026493.

Centifanti, L.C.M., Modecki, K.L., MacLellan, S. & Gowling, H. (2016) Driving under the influence of risky peers: An experimental study of adolescent risk taking. *Journal of Research on Adolescence, 26*(1): 207–222. doi: 10.1111/jora.12187.

Cepoiu, M., McCusker, J., Cole, M.G., Sewitch, M., Belzile, E. & Ciampi, A. (2008) Recognition of depression by non-psychiatric physicians: A systematic literature review and meta-analysis. *Journal of General Internal Medicine, 23*(1): 25–36.

Cerolini, S., Zagaria, A., Franchini, C., Maniaci, V.G., Fortunato, A., et al. (2023) Psychological counseling among university students worldwide: A systematic review. *European Journal of Investigation in Health, Psychology and Education, 13*(9): 1831–1849. doi: 10.3390/ejihpe13090133.

Chalder, T. & Willis, C. (2019) Medically unexplained symptoms. In C.D. Llewellyn, S. Ayers, C. McManus, S. Newman, K.J. Petrie, T.A. Revenson & J. Weinman (eds), *Cambridge Handbook of Psychology, Health and Medicine* (3rd edition). Cambridge: Cambridge University Press (pp.78–83).

Champagne, F. & Meaney, M.J. (2001) Like mother, like daughter: Evidence for non-genomic transmission of parental behaviour and stress responsivity. *Progress in Brain Research, 133*: 287–302.

Chan, A., De Simoni, A., Wileman, V., Holliday, L., Newby, C. J., et al. (2022) Digital interventions to improve adherence to maintenance medication in asthma. *Cochrane Database of Systematic Reviews, 6*(6): CD013030. doi:10.1002/14651858.CD013030.pub2

Chan, A.O., Cheng, C., Hui, W.M., Hu, W.H., Wong, N.Y., Lam, K.F., Wong, W.M., Lai, K.C., Lam, S.K. & Wong, B.C. (2005) Differing coping mechanisms,

stress level and anorectal physiology in patients with functional constipation. *World Journal of Gastroenterology, 11*(34): 5362–5366.

Chan, J.K.N., Correll, C.U., Wong, C.S.M., et al. (2023) Life expectancy and years of potential life lost in people with mental disorders: A systematic review and meta-analysis. *eClinicalMedicine, 65*: 102294. doi:10.1016/j.eclinm.2023.102294.

Chan, K.L., Poller, W.C., Swirski, F.K. & Russo, S.J. (2023) Central regulation of stress-evoked peripheral immune responses. *Nature Reviews. Neuroscience, 24*(10): 591–604. doi:10.1038/s41583-023-00729-2.

Chang, H.C., Huang, Y.C., Lien, Y.J. & Chang, Y.S. (2022) Association of rosacea with depression and anxiety: A systematic review and meta-analysis. *Journal of Affective Disorders, 299*: 239–245. doi:10.1016/j.jad.2021.12.008.

Charles, C., Gafni, A. & Whelan, T. (1997) Shared decision-making in the medical encounter: What does it mean? (Or it takes at least two to tango). *Social Science & Medicine, 44*(5): 681–692.

Chartrand, T.L. & Lakin, J.L. (2013) The antecedents and consequences of human behavioral mimicry. *Annual Review of Psychology, 64*: 285–308. doi:10.1146/annurev-psych-113011-143754.

Chartrand, T.L., Van Baaren, R.B. & Bargh, J.A. (2006) Linking automatic evaluation to mood and information processing style: Consequences for experienced affect, impression formation, and stereotyping. *Journal of Experimental Psychology: General, 135*(1): 70–77.

Charuvastra, A. & Cloitre, M. (2008) Social bonds and posttraumatic stress disorder. *Annual Review of Psychology, 59*: 301–328.

Chase, W.G. & Ericsson, K.A. (1982) Skill and working memory. In G.H. Bower (ed.), *The Psychology of Learning and Motivation* (*Vol. 16*). New York: Academic Press (pp. 1–58).

Chayadi, E., Baes, N. & Kiropoulos, L. (2022) The effects of mindfulness-based interventions on symptoms of depression, anxiety, and cancer-related fatigue in oncology patients: A systematic review and meta-analysis. *PLoS One, 17*(7): e0269519. doi:10.1371/journal.pone.0269519.

Chegeni, R., Pallesen, S., McVeigh, J. & Sagoe, D. (2021) Anabolic-androgenic steroid administration increases self-reported aggression in healthy males: A systematic review and meta-analysis of experimental studies. *Psychopharmacology, 238*: 1911–1922. doi:10.1007/s00213-021-05818-7.

Chen, A., Murphy, D., Brabec, J.A. & Bjork, R.A. (2024) The effects of lecture speed and note-taking on memory for educational material. *Applied Cognitive Psychology, 38*(1): e4166. doi:10.1002/acp.4166.

Chen, B., Yang, T., Xiao, L., Xu, C. & Zhu, C. (2023) Effects of mobile mindfulness meditation on the mental health of university students: Systematic review and meta-analysis. *Journal of Medical Internet Research*, 25: e39128. https://doi.org/10.2196/39128.

Chen, F.T., Etnier, J.L., Chan, K.H., Chiu, P.K., Hung, T.M. & Chang, Y.K. (2020) Effects of exercise training interventions on executive function in older adults: A systematic review and meta-analysis. *Sports Medicine*, 50(8): 1451–1467. doi:10.1007/s40279-020-01292-x.

Chen, H., Zhang, B., Xue, W., Li, J., Li, Y., Fu, K., Chen, X., Sun, M., Shi, H., Tian, L. & Teng, W. (2019) Anger, hostility and risk of stroke: A meta-analysis of cohort studies. *Journal of Neurology, 266*(4): 1016–1026. doi: 10.1007/s00415-019-09231-1.

Chen, W., Li, H., Qin, N., Zhou, J., Ou-Yang, J., & Wang, K.Y. (2022) Effectiveness of couple-based interventions for prostate cancer patients and their spouses on their quality of life: A systematic review and meta-analysis. *Supportive Care in Cancer, 31*(1): 34. doi:10.1007/s00520-022-07532-2.

Chen, Z., Song, X., Lee, T.M.C. & Zhang, R. (2023) The robust reciprocal relationship between loneliness and depressive symptoms among the general population: Evidence from a quantitative analysis of 37 studies. *Journal of Affective Disorders, 343*: 119–128. doi:10.1016/j.jad.2023.09.035.

Cheng, H. & Furnham, A. (2019) Teenage locus of control, psychological distress, educational qualifications and occupational prestige as well as gender as independent predictors of adult binge drinking. *Alcohol, 76*: 103–109. doi: 10.1016/j.alcohol.2018.08.008.

Cheng, S., Lin, D., Hu, T., Cao, L., Liao, H., et al. (2020) Association of urinary incontinence and depression or anxiety: A meta-analysis. *Journal of International Medical Research, 48*(6), 300060520931348. doi:10.1177/0300060520931348.

Cheng, Z., Hao, H., Tsofliou, F., Katz, M.D. & Zhang, Y. (2023) Effects of online support and social media communities on gestational diabetes: A systematic review. *International Journal of Medical Informatics, 180*: 105263. doi: 10.1016/j.ijmedinf.2023.105263.

Chesnut, M., Harati, S., Paredes, P. et al. (2021) Stress markers for mental states and biotypes of depression and anxiety: A scoping review and preliminary illustrative analysis. *Chronic Stress, 5*: 24705470211000338. doi:10.1177/24705 470211000338.

Chida, Y. & Steptoe, A. (2009) The association of anger and hostility with future coronary heart disease. *Journal of the American College of Cardiology, 53*(11): 936–946.

Chinnaiyan, K.M. (2019) Role of stress management for cardiovascular disease prevention. *Current Opinion in Cardiology, 34*(5): 531–535. doi: 10.1097/HCO.0000000000000649.

Chipojola, R., Khwepeya, M., Gondwe, K.W., Rias, Y.A. & Huda, M.H. (2022) The influence of breastfeeding promotion programs on exclusive breastfeeding rates in Sub-Saharan Africa: A systematic review and meta-analysis. *Journal of Human Lactation, 38*(3): 466–476. doi:10.1177/08903344221097689.

Chiu, M., Austin, P.C., Manuel, D.G., Shah, B.R. & Tu, J.V. (2011) Deriving ethnic-specific BMI cutoff points for assessing diabetes risk. *Diabetes Care, 34*(8): 1741–1748.

Chomsky, N. (1965) *Aspects of the Theory of Syntax.* Cambridge, MA: MIT Press.

Christensen, A.J. & Ehlers, S.L. (2002) Psychological factors in end-stage renal disease: An emerging context for behavioral medicine research. *Journal of Consulting & Clinical Psychology, 70*(3): 712–724.

Christy, S.M., Mosher, C.E. & Rawl, S.M. (2014) Integrating men's health and masculinity theories to explain colorectal cancer screening behavior. *American Journal of Men's Health, 8*(1): 54–65.

Chu, D. J., Al Rifai, M., Virani, S. S., Brawner, C. A., Nasir, K., & Al-Mallah, M. H. (2020). The relationship between cardiorespiratory fitness, cardiovascular risk factors and atherosclerosis. *Atherosclerosis, 304*, 44–52. doi:10.1016/j.atherosclerosis.2020.04.019

Chu, D.K., Akl, E.A., Duda, S., Solo, K., Yaacoub, S., et al. (2020) Physical distancing, face masks, and eye protection to prevent person-to-person transmission of SARS-CoV-2 and COVID-19: A systematic review and meta-analysis. *Lancet, 395*(10242): 1973–1987. doi:10.1016/S0140-6736(20)31142-9.

Cialdini, R.B., Schaller, M., Houlihan, D., Arps, K., Fultz, J. & Beaman, A.L. (1987) Empathy-based helping: Is it selflessly or selfishly motivated? *Journal of Personality & Social Psychology, 52*(4): 749–758.

Cillessen, L., Johannsen, M., Speckens, A.E.M. & Zachariae, R. (2019) Mindfulness-based interventions for psychological and physical health outcomes in cancer patients and survivors: A systematic review and meta-analysis of randomized controlled trials. *Psychooncology, 28*(12): 2257–2269. doi: 10.1002/pon.5214.

Cipriani, A., Furukawa, T.A., Salanti, G., Chaimani, A., Atkinson, L.Z., et al. (2018) Comparative efficacy and acceptability of 21 antidepressant drugs for the acute treatment of adults with major depressive disorder: A systematic review and network meta-analysis. *Lancet, 391*(10128): 1357–1366. doi:10.1016/S0140-6736(17)32802-7.

Claar, R.L., Simons, L.E. & Logan, D.E. (2008) Parental response to children's pain: The moderating impact of children's emotional distress on symptoms and disability. *Pain, 138*(1): 172–179.

Clark, J.E. (2015) Diet, exercise or diet with exercise: Comparing the effectiveness of treatment options for weight-loss and changes in fitness for adults (18–65 years old) who are overfat, or obese: Systematic review and meta-analysis. *Journal of Diabetes and Metabollic Disorders, 14*: 31.

Clark, M., Kelly, T. & Deighan, C. (2011) A systematic review of the Heart Manual literature. *European Journal of Cardiovascular Nursing, 10*(1): 3–13.

Clark, M.L., Abimanyi-Ochom, J., Le, H., Long, B., Orr, C. & Khanh-Dao Le, L. (2023) A systematic review and meta-analysis of depression and apathy frequency in adult-onset Huntington's disease. *Neuroscience and Biobehavioral Reviews, 149*: 105166. https://doi.org/10.1016/j.neubiorev.2023.105166.

Cohen, S., Alper, C.M., Doyle, W.J., Adler, N., Treanor, J.J. & Turner, R.B. (2008) Objective and subjective socioeconomic status and susceptibility to the common cold. *Health Psychology, 27*(2): 268–274. doi: 10.1037/0278-6133.27.2.268.

Cohen, S., Chiang, J.J., Janicki-Deverts, D. & Miller, G.E. (2020) Good relationships with parents during childhood as buffers of the association between childhood disadvantage and adult susceptibility to the common cold. *Psychosomatic Medicine, 82*(6): 538–547. doi:10.1097/PSY.0000000000000818.

Cohen, S., Chin, B. & Zajdel, M. (2019) Cold, common. In C.D. Llewellyn, S. Ayers, C. McManus, S. Newman, K.J. Petrie, T.A. Revenson & J. Weinman (eds), *Cambridge Handbook of Psychology, Health and Medicine* (3rd edition). Cambridge: Cambridge University Press. pp. 466–467.

Cohen, S., Kamarck, T. & Mermelstein, R. (1983) A global measure of perceived stress. *Journal of Health and Social Behavior, 24*(4): 385–396.

Cohn, L.D., Macfralane, S., Yanez, C. & Imai, W.K. (1995) Risk-perception: Differences between adolescents and adults. *Health Psychology, 14*(3): 217–222.

Cojocaru, C.M., Popa, C.O., Schenk, A., Suciu, B.A. & Szasz, S. (2024) Cognitive-behavioral therapy and acceptance and commitment therapy for anxiety and depression in patients with fibromyalgia: A systematic review and meta-analysis. *Medicine and Pharmacy Reports, 97*(1): 26–34. https://doi.org/10.15386/mpr-2661

Colagiuri, B., Schenk, L.A., Kessler, M.D., Dorsey, S.G. & Colloca, L. (2015) The placebo effect: From concepts to genes. *Neuroscience, 307*: 171–190.

Cole, S.A. & Bird, J. (2014) *The Medical Interview: The Three Function Approach* (3rd edition). Philadelphia, PA: Elsevier Saunders.

Coles, N.A., Larsen, J.T. & Lench, H.C. (2019) A meta-analysis of the facial feedback literature: Effects of facial feedback on emotional experience are small and variable. *Psychological Bulletin, 145*(6): 610–651. doi: 10.1037/bul0000194.

Collaborative Group on Hormonal Factors in Breast Cancer (2019) Type and timing of menopausal hormone therapy and breast cancer risk: Individual participant meta-analysis of the worldwide epidemiological evidence. *Lancet, 394*(10204): 1159–1168. doi: 10.1016/S0140-6736(19)31709-X.

Colloca, L., Lopiano, L., Lanotte, M. & Benedetti, F. (2004) Overt versus covert treatment for pain, anxiety, and Parkinson's disease. *Lancet Neurology, 3*(11): 679–684.

Colloca, L. & Miller, F.G. (2011) The nocebo effect and its relevance for clinical practice. *Psychosomatic Medicine, 73*(7): 598–603.

Colquitt, J.L., Pickett, K., Loveman, E. & Frampton, G.K. (2014) Surgery for weight loss in adults. *Cochrane Database of Systematic Reviews, 8*: Art. CD003641. doi: 10.1002/14651858.CD003641.pub4.

Conn, V.S., Enriquez, M., Ruppar, T.M. & Chan, K.C. (2016) Meta-analyses of theory use in medication adherence intervention research. *American Journal of Health Behavior, 40*(2): 155–171.

Connell, N.B., Prathivadi, P., Lorenz, K.A., Zupanc, S.N., Singer, S.J., Krebs, E.E., et al. (2022) Teaming in interdisciplinary chronic pain management interventions in primary care: A systematic review of randomized controlled trials. *Journal of General Internal Medicine, 37*(6): 1501–1512. doi:10.1007/s11606-021-07255-w.

Conner, M. (2019) Models of health behaviour, in C.D. Llewellyn et al. (eds), *Cambridge Handbook of Psychology, Health and Medicine* (3rd edition). Cambridge: Cambridge University Press (pp. 55–60).

Conner, M., Povey, R., Sparks, P., James, R. & Shepherd, R. (2003) Moderating role of attitudinal ambivalence within the theory of planned behaviour. *British Journal of Social Psychology, 42*(Pt 1): 75–94.

Conner, M., Wilding, S., van Harreveld, F. & Dalege, J. (2021) Cognitive-affective inconsistency and ambivalence: Impact on the overall attitude–behavior relationship. *Personality and Social Psychology Bulletin, 47*(4): 673–687. doi:10.1177/0146167220945900.

Connor, J. (2017) Alcohol consumption as a cause of cancer. *Addiction, 112*(2): 222–228.

Conradt, E., Adkins, D.E., Crowell, S.E., Raby, K.L., Diamond, L.M. & Ellis, B. (2018) Incorporating epigenetic mechanisms to advance fetal programming theories. *Developmental Psychopathology, 30*(3): 807–824. doi: 10.1017/S0954579418000469.

Contrada, R.J. & Goyal, T.M. (2005) Individual differences, health and illness: The role of emotional traits and generalized expectancies. In S. Sutton, A. Baum & M. Johnston (eds), *SAGE Handbook of Health Psychology*. London: Sage. pp. 143–168.

Cook, C.C.H. (2019) *Hearing Voices, Demonic and Divine: Scientific and Theological Perspectives*. Oxford: Routledge.

Cooke, R., McEwan, H. & Norman, P. (2023) The effect of forming implementation intentions on alcohol consumption: A systematic review and meta-analysis. *Drug and Alcohol Review*, *42*(1): 68–80. doi:10.1111/dar.13553.

Cooper, S., Schmidt, B.-M., Sambala, E.Z., Swartz, A., Colvin, C.J., Leon, N. & Wiysonge, C.S. (2021) Factors that influence parents' and informal caregivers' views and practices regarding routine childhood vaccination: A qualitative evidence synthesis. *Cochrane Database of Systematic Reviews*, *10*(10): Art. CD013265. doi:10.1002/14651858.CD013265.pub2.

Copeland, J.L., Currie, C.L. & Moon-Riley, K.C. et al. (2021) Physical activity buffers the adverse impacts of racial discrimination on allostatic load among Indigenous adults. *Annals of Behavioral Medicine*, *55*: 520–529. doi:10.1093/abm/kaaa068.

Coughlin, S.S. (2020) Social determinants of colorectal cancer risk, stage, and survival: A systematic review. *International Journal of Colorectal Diseases*, *35*: 985–995. doi:10.1007/s00384-020-03585-z

Courtenay, W. (2000) Constructions of masculinity and their influence on men's well-being: A theory of gender and health. *Social Science & Medicine*, *50*(10): 1385–1401.

Coustaury, C., Jeannot, E., Moreau, A., Nietge, C., Maharani, A., et al. (2023) Subjective socioeconomic status and self-rated health in the English Longitudinal Study of Aging. *Social Science & Medicine*, *336*: 116235. doi:10.1016/j.socscimed.2023.116235.

Cowdery, S.P., Bjerkeset, O., Sund, E.R., Mohebbi, M., Pasco, J.A., et al. (2022) Depressive symptomology and cancer incidence in men and women: Longitudinal evidence from the HUNT study. *Journal of Affective Disorders*, *316*: 1–9. doi:10.1016/j.jad.2022.08.002.

Coyle, A.C., Yen, R.W. & Elwyn, G. (2022) Interrupted opening statements in clinical encounters: A scoping review. *Patient Education and Counseling*, *105*(8): 2653–2663. doi: 10.1016/j.pec.2022.03.026.

Crawley, R., Lomax, S. & Ayers, S. (2013) Recovering from stillbirth: The effects of making and sharing memories on maternal mental health. *Journal of Reproductive and Infant Psychology*, *31*(2): 195–207.

Cream, P. (2019) Intimate examinations. In C.D. Llewellyn, S. Ayers, C. McManus, S. Newman, K.J. Petrie, T.A. Revenson & J. Weinman (eds), *The Cambridge Handbook of Psychology, Health and Medicine* (3rd edition). Cambridge: Cambridge University Press.

Crenshaw, K.W. (1991) Mapping the margins: Intersectionality, identity politics, and violence against women of color. *Stanford Law Review*, *43*(6): 1241–1299.

Crespo, I., Valassi, E. & Webb, S.M. (2017) Update on quality of life in patients with acromegaly. *Pituitary*, *20*(1): 185–188. doi: 10.1007/s11102-016-0761-y.

Crombez, G., Eccleston, C., Van Damme, S., Vlaeyen, J.W. & Karoly, P. (2012) Fear-avoidance model of chronic pain: The next generation. *Clinical Journal of Pain*, *28*(6): 475–483.

Crosby, E.S., Spitzer, E.G. & Kavookjian, J. (2023) Motivational interviewing effects on Positive Airway Pressure therapy (PAP) adherence: A systematic review and meta-analysis of randomized controlled trials. *Behavioral Sleep Medicine*, *21*(4): 460–487. doi: 10.1080/15402002.2022.2108033.

Cross, H., Bremner, S., Meads, C., Pollard, A. & Llewellyn, C. (2023) Bisexual people experience worse health outcomes in England: Evidence from a cross-sectional survey in primary care. *Journal of Sex Research*, *61*(9): 1342–1350. doi:10.1080/00224499.2023.2220680.

Cross, M.P., Acevedo, A.M., Leger, K.A. & Pressman, S.D. (2023) How and why could smiling influence physical health? A conceptual review. *Health Psychology Review*, *17*(2): 321–343. https://doi.org/10.1080/17437199.2022.2052740.

Crow, S.J. (2019) Pharmacologic treatment of eating disorders. *Psychiatric Clinics of North America*, *42*(2): 253–262. doi: 10.1016/j.psc.2019.01.007.

Crowley, D., Cullen, W. & Van Hout, M.C. (2021) Transgender health care in primary care. *British Journal of General Practice*,

71(709): 377–378. doi:10.3399/bjgp21X716753.

Cruwys, T., Brossard, B., Zhou, H., Helleren-Simpson, G., Klik, K.A., Van Rooy, D., et al. (2023) Disciplinary differences in the study of the relationship between social variables and mental health: A systematic mapping review. *Health*, *27*(5): 810–828. doi:10.1177/13634593211063049.

Cruz-Pereira, J.S., Rea, K., Nolan, Y.M., O'Leary, O.F., Dinan, T.G. & Cryan, J.F. (2020) Depression's unholy trinity: Dysregulated stress, immunity, and the microbiome. *Annual Review of Psychology*, *71*, 49–78.

Cunningham, A.J. & Watson, K. (2004) How psychological therapy may prolong survival in cancer patients: New evidence and a simple theory. *Integrative Cancer Therapies*, *3*(3): 214–229.

Currier, J.M., Neimeyer, R.A. & Berman, J.S. (2008) The effectiveness of psychotherapeutic interventions for bereaved persons: A comprehensive quantitative review. *Psychological Bulletin*, *134*(5): 648–661.

Cushing, H.W. (1932) The basophil adenomas of the pituitary body and their clinical manifestations. *Bulletin of Johns Hopkins Hospital*, *50*: 137–195.

D'Agostino, T.A., Atkinson, T.M., Latella, L.E., Rogers, M., Morrissey, D., DeRosa, A.P. & Parker, P.A. (2017) Promoting patient participation in healthcare interactions through communication skills training: A systematic review. *Patient Education and Counselling*, *100*(7): 1247–1257. doi:10.1016/j.pec.2017.02.016.

Dahy, A., El-Qushayri, A.E., Mahmoud, A.R., Al-Kelany, T.A. & Salman, S. (2020) Telemedicine approach for psoriasis management, time for application? A systematic review of published studies. *Dermatologic Therapy*, *33*(6): e13908. doi:10.1111/dth.13908.

Dalgard, F.J., Gieler, U., Tomas-Aragones, L., Lien, L., Poot, F., et al. (2015) The psychological burden of skin diseases: A cross-sectional multicenter study among dermatological out-patients in 13 European countries. *Journal of Investigative Dermatology*, *135*(4): 984–991.

Dalgleish, T., Black, M., Johnston, D. & Bevan, A. (2020) Transdiagnostic approaches to mental health problems: Current status and future directions. *Journal of Consulting and Clinical Psychology*, *88*(3): 179–195. doi:10.1037/ccp0000482.

Danhauer, S.C., Crawford, S.L., Farmer, D.F. & Avis, N.E. (2009) A longitudinal investigation of coping strategies and quality of life among younger women with breast cancer. *Journal of Behavioral Medicine*, *32*(4): 371–379.

Daniel, T. (2023) The stubborn persistence of grief stage theory. *Omega – Journal of Death and Dying*, 4 September (online first). doi:10.1177/00302228221149801.

Daniels, H (ed.) (2017) *Introduction to Vygotsky* (3rd edition). London: Routledge.

Dannemiller, J.L. & Stephens, B.R. (1988) A critical test of infant pattern preference models. *Child Development*, *59*(1): 210–216.

Dante, G., Pedrielli, G., Annessi, E. & Facchinetti, F. (2013) Herb remedies during pregnancy: A systematic review of controlled clinical trials. *Journal of Maternal-Fetal & Neonatal Medicine*, *26*(3): 306–312.

Datta, N., Matheson, B.E., Citron, K., Van Wye, E.M. & Lock, J.D. (2023) Evidence based update on psychosocial treatments for eating disorders in children and adolescents. *Journal of Clinical Child & Adolescent Psychology*, *52*(2): 159–170. doi:10.1080/15374416.2022.2109650.

Davies, J.M., Sleeman, K.E., Leniz, J., Wilson, R., Higginson, I.J., et al. (2019) Socioeconomic position and use of healthcare in the last year of life: A systematic review and meta-analysis. *PLoS Medicine*, *16*(4): e1002782. doi:10.1371/journal.pmed.1002782.

Davis, S., Serfaty, M., Low, J., Armstrong, M., Kupeli, N. & Lanceley, A. (2023) Experiential avoidance in advanced cancer: A mixed-methods systematic review. *International Journal of Behavioral Medicine*,

30: 585–604. doi:10.1007/s12529-022-10131-4.

Davison, G.C. & Garcia, L.M. (2019) Behaviour therapy. In C.D. Llewellyn, S. Ayers, C. McManus, S. Newman, K.J. Petrie, T.A. Revenson & J. Weinman (eds), *The Cambridge Handbook of Psychology, Health and Medicine* (3rd edition). Cambridge: Cambridge University Press.

Davison, K., Queen, R., Lau, F. & Antonio, M. (2021) Culturally competent gender, sex, and sexual orientation information practices and electronic health records: Rapid review. *JMIR Medical Informatics, 9*(2): e25467. doi: 10.2196/25467.

Dawes, M., Summerskill, W., Glasziou, P., Cartabellotta, A., Martin, J., Hopayian, K., Porzsolt, F., Burls, A. & Osborne, J. (2005) Second International Conference of Evidence-Based Health Care Teachers and Developers: Sicily statement on evidence-based practice. *BMC Medical Education, 5*(1): 1–7.

Dax, V., Ftanou, M., Tran, B., Lewin, J., Wallace, R., Seidler, Z. & Wiley, J.F. (2022) The impact of testicular cancer and its treatment on masculinity: A systematic review. *Psycho-oncology, 31*(9): 1459–1473. doi:10.1002/pon.5994.

de Brouwer, S.J., Kraaimaat, F.W., Sweep, F.C., Creemers, M.C., Radstake, T.R., et al. (2010) Experimental stress in inflammatory rheumatic diseases: A review of psychophysiological stress responses. *Arthritis Research & Therapy, 12*(3): r89.

de Oliveira, P.B.F., Dornelles, T.M., Gosmann, N.P. & Camozzato, A. (2023) Efficacy of telemedicine interventions for depression and anxiety in older people: Systematic review and meta-analysis. *International Journal of Geriatric Psychiatry, 38*(5): e5920. doi:10.1002/gps.5920.

de Sousa, A., Sonavane, S. & Mehta, J. (2012) Psychological aspects of prostate cancer: A clinical review. *Prostate Cancer and Prostatic Diseases, 15*(2): 120–127.

de Visser, R.O. (2015) Personalized feedback based on a drink-pouring exercise may improve knowledge of, and adherence to, government guidelines for alcohol consumption. *Alcoholism: Clinical & Experimental Research, 39*(2): 317–323. doi: 10.1111/acer.12623.

de Visser, R.O., Badcock, P.B., Rissel, C., Richters, J., Smith, A.M., Grulich, A.E. & Simpson, J.M. (2014a) Safer sex and condom use: Findings from the Second Australian Study of Health and Relationships. *Sex Health, 11*(5): 495–504.

de Visser, R.O., Badcock, P.B., Simpson, J.M., Grulich, A.E., Smith, A.M., Richters, J. & Rissel, C. (2014b) Attitudes toward sex and relationships: The Second Australian Study of Health and Relationships. *Sex Health, 11*(5): 397–405.

de Visser, R.O., Barnard, S., Benham, D. & Morse, R. (2021) Beyond 'Meat Free Monday': A mixed method study of giving up eating meat. *Appetite, 166*: 105463. doi:10.1016/j.appet.2021.105463.

de Visser, R.O., Brown, C.E., Cooke, R., Cooper, G. & Memon, A. (2017) Using alcohol unit-marked glasses enhances capacity to monitor intake: Evidence from a mixed-method intervention trial. *Alcohol and Alcoholism, 52*(2): 206–212.

de Visser, R.O. & McDonnell, E.J. (2013) 'Man points': Masculine capital and men's health behaviour. *Health Psychology, 32*: 5–14.

de Visser, R.O. & Nicholls J. (2020) Temporary abstinence during Dry January: Predictors of success; impact on well-being and self-efficacy. *Psychology & Health, 35*(11): 1293–1305. doi:10.1080/08870446.2020.1743840.

de Visser, R.O. & Piper, R. (2020) Short- and longer-term benefits of temporary alcohol abstinence during 'Dry January' are not also observed among adult drinkers in the general population: Prospective cohort study. *Alcohol & Alcoholism, 55*(4): 433–438. doi: 10.1093/alcalc/agaa025.

de Visser, R.O., Rissel, C., Richters, J. & Smith, A. (2007) The impact of sexual coercion on psychological, physical, and sexual well-being in a representative sample of

Australian women. *Archives of Sexual Behavior, 36*(5): 676–686.

De Vries, A.M., de Roten, Y., Meystre, C., Passchier, J., Despland, J.N. & Stiefel, F. (2014) Clinician characteristics, communication, and patient outcome in oncology: A systematic review. *Psychooncology, 23*(4): 375–381.

Deasy, C., Coughlan, B., Pironom, J., Jourdan, D. & Mcnamara, P.M. (2015) Psychological distress and lifestyle of students: Implications for health promotion. *Health Promotion International, 30*(1): 77–87. doi: 10.1093/heapro/dau086.

Debiec, J. & Sullivan, R.M. (2017) The neurobiology of safety and threat learning in infancy. *Neurobiology of Learning and Memory, 143*: 49–58. doi: 10.1016/j.nlm.2016.10.015.

Del Giudice, M., Ellis, B.J. & Shirtcliff, E.A. (2011) The adaptive calibration model of stress responsivity. *Neuroscience and Biobehavioral Review, 35*(7): 1562–1592.

Deleemans, J.M., Mather, H., Spiropoulos, A., Toivonen, K., Baydoun, M. & Carlson, L.E. (2023) Recent progress in mind-body therapies in cancer care. *Current Oncology Reports, 25*(4): 293–307. doi:10.1007/s11912-023-01373-w.

Delicate, A., Ayers, S., Easter, A. & McMullen, S. (2018) The impact of childbirth-related post-traumatic stress on a couple's relationship: A systematic review and meta-synthesis. *Journal of Reproductive and Infant Psychology, 36*(1): 102–115.

Dell'Osso, B., Albert, U., Carrà, G. Pompili, M. et al. (2020) How to improve adherence to antidepressant treatments in patients with major depression: A psychoeducational consensus checklist. *Annals of General Psychiatry, 19*(61). doi:10.1186/s12991-020-00306-2

Delvaux, N., Razavi, D., Marchal, S., Bredart, A., Farvacques, C. & Slachmuylder, J.L. (2004) Effects of a 105-hour psychological training program on attitudes, communication skills and occupational stress in oncology: A randomised study. *British Journal of Cancer, 90*(1): 106–114.

Dempster, M., Howell, D. & McCorry, N.K. (2015) Illness perceptions and coping in physical health conditions: A meta-analysis. *Journal of Psychosomatic Research, 79*(6): 506–513.

Deng, W., Yu, R., Yang, Z., Dong, X. & Wang, W. (2021) Trends in conditional overall survival of esophageal cancer: A population-based study. *Annals of Translational Medicine, 9*(2): 102. doi:10.21037/atm-20-2798.

Dengsø, K.E., Andersen, E.W., Thomsen, T., Hansen, C.P., Christensen, B.M. Hillingsø, J. & Dalton, S.O. (2020) Increased psychological symptom burden in patients with pancreatic cancer: A population-based cohort study. *Pancreatology, 20*(3): 511–521. doi:10.1016/j.pan.2020.01.001.

Dennis, J.A., Khan, O., Ferriter, M., Huband, N., Powney, M.J. & Duggan, C. (2012) Psychological interventions for adults who have sexually offended or are at risk of offending. *Cochrane Database of Systematic Reviews, 12*: Art. CD007507. doi: 10.1002/14651858.CD007507.pub2.

Dent, E., Davinson, N. & Wilkie, S. (2022) The impact of gastrointestinal conditions on psychosocial factors associated with the biopsychosocial model of health: A scoping review. *Applied Psychology. Health and Well-being, 14*(2): 626–644. doi:10.1111/aphw.12323.

Department of Health (2001) *Treatment Choice in Psychological Therapies and Counselling: Evidence Based Clinical Practice Guidelines.* London: Department of Health.

Descartes, R. (1637) *Discours de la Méthode.* Leiden, NL: Elsevier.

Devonport, T.J., Nicholls, W. & Fullerton, C. (2019) A systematic review of the association between emotions and eating behaviour in normal and overweight adult populations. *Journal of Health Psychology, 24*(1): 3–24. doi: 10.1177/1359105317697813.

Dhindsa, D.S., Khambhati, J., Schultz, W.M., Tahhan, A.S. & Quyyumi, A.A. (2020) Marital status and outcomes in patients with cardiovascular disease. *Trends in*

Cardiovascular Medicine, 30(4): 215–220. doi:10.1016/j.tcm.2019.05.012.

Dianatinasab, M., Ghahri, S., Dianatinasab, A., Amanat, S. & Fararouei, M. (2020). Effects of exercise on the immune function, quality of life, and mental health in HIV/AIDS individuals. *Advances in Experimental Medicine and Biology, 1228*: 411–421. doi:10.1007/978-981-15-1792-1_28.

Díaz Crescitelli, M.E., Ghirotto, L., Sisson, H., et al. (2020) A meta-synthesis study of the key elements involved in childhood vaccine hesitancy. *Public Health, 180*: 38–45. doi:10.1016/j.puhe.2019.10.027.

Díaz-Vázquez, B., López-Romero, L. & Romero, E. (2024) Emotion recognition deficits in children and adolescents with psychopathic traits: A systematic review. *Clinical Child and Family Psychology Review, 27*(1): 165–219. doi:10.1007/s10567-023-00466-z.

Dibben, G., Faulkner, J., Oldridge, N., Rees, K., Thompson, D. R., et al. (2021) Exercise-based cardiac rehabilitation for coronary heart disease. *Cochrane Database of Systematic Reviews, 11*(11): Art. CD001800. doi:10.1002/14651858.CD001800.pub4.

Dick-Read, G. (1933) *Natural Childbirth.* London: Pinter & Martin.

Dick-Read, G. (2004) *Childbirth without Fear: The Principles and Practice of Natural Childbirth.* London: Pinter & Martin.

Dieckmann, L. & Czamara, D. (2024) Epigenetics of prenatal stress in humans: The current research landscape. *Clinical Epigenetics, 16*: 20. doi:10.1186/s13148-024-01635-9.

Díez, J.J., Sangiao-Alvarellos, S. & Cordido, F. (2018) Treatment with growth hormone for adults with growth hormone deficiency syndrome: Benefits and risks. *International Journal of Molecular Science, 19*(3): 893. doi:10.3390/ijms19030893.

DiLorenzo-Klas, M.G., Waxman, J.A., Flora, D.B., Schmidt, L.A., Garfield, H., et al. (2023) Caregiver and child distress as predictors of dyadic physiological attunement during vaccination. *Clinical Journal of Pain, 39*(7): 340–348. doi:10.1097/AJP.0000000000001125.

DiMatteo, M.R., Giordani, P.J., Lepper, H.S. & Croghan, T.W. (2002) Patient adherence and medical treatment outcomes: A meta-analysis. *Medical Care, 40*(9): 794–811.

Dimidjian, S., Arch, J.J., Schneider, R.L., Desormeau, P., Felder, J.N. & Segal, Z.V. (2016) Considering meta-analysis, meaning, and metaphor: A systematic review and critical examination of 'third wave' cognitive and behavioral therapies. *Behavior Therapy, 47*(6): 886–905.

Dimova, E.D., Ward, A., Swanson, V. & Evans, J.M.M. (2019) Patients' illness perceptions of Type 2 diabetes: A scoping review. *Current Diabetes Reviews, 15*(1): 15–30. doi: 10.2174/1573399814666171227214845.

Ding, X.X., Wu, Y.L., Xu, S.J., Zhu, R.P., Jia, X.M., et al. (2014) Maternal anxiety during pregnancy and adverse birth outcomes: A systematic review and meta-analysis of prospective cohort studies. *Journal of Affective Disorders, 159*: 103–110.

Dixon, M.L., Thiruchselvam, R., Todd, R. & Christoff, K. (2017) Emotion and the prefrontal cortex: An integrative review. *Psychological Bulletin, 143*(10): 1033–1081. doi: 10.1037/bul0000096.

Dixon, R.P., Roberts, L.M., Lawrie, S., Jones, L.A. & Humphreys, M.S. (2008) Medical students' attitudes to psychiatric illness in primary care. *Medical Education, 42*(11): 1080–1087.

Dobrina, R., Vianello, C., Tenze, M. & Palese, A. (2016) Mutual needs and wishes of cancer patients and their family caregivers during the last week of life: A descriptive phenomenological study. *Journal of Holistic Nursing, 34*(1), 24–34. doi:10.1177/0898010115581936.

Dokucu, M.E. & Cloninger, C.R. (2019) Personality disorders and physical comorbidities: A complex relationship. *Current Opinion in Psychiatry, 32*(5): 435–441. doi: 10.1097/YCO.0000000000000536.

Dolan, S.C., Khindri, R., Franko, D.L., Thomas, J.J., Reilly, E.E. & Eddy, K.T. (2022) Anhedonia in eating disorders: A meta-analysis and systematic review. *International Journal of Eating Disorders, 55*(2): 161–175. doi:10.1002/eat.23645.

Domino, J., McGovern, C., Chang, K.W., Carlozzi, N.E., Yang, L.J. (2014) Lack of physician–patient communication as a key factor associated with malpractice litigation in neonatal brachial plexus palsy. *Journal of Neurosurgery. Pediatrics*, *13*(2): 238–242. doi: 10.3171/2013.11.PEDS13268.

Dommershuijsen, L.J., Dedding, C.W.M. & Van Bruchem-Visser, R.L. (2019) Consultation recording: What is the added value for patients aged 50 years and over? A systematic review. *Health Communication*, *36*(2): 168–178. doi: 10.1080/10410236.2019.1669270.

Doucet, M.H., Guzzo, M.F. & Groleau, D. (2018) Brief report: A qualitative evidence synthesis of the psychological processes of school-based expressive writing interventions with adolescents. *Journal of Adolescence*, *69*(1): 113–117. doi:10.1016/j. adolescence.2018.09.010.

Douglas, R.M., Hemilä, H., Chalker, E. & Treacy, B. (2007) Vitamin C for preventing and treating the common cold. *Cochrane Database of Systematic Reviews*, *3*: Art. CD000980.

Doyle, C., Lennox, L. & Bell, D. (2013) A systematic review of evidence on the links between patient experience and clinical safety and effectiveness. *BMJ Open*, *3*(1): pii: e001570.

Drabish, K. & Theeke, L.A. (2022) Health impact of stigma, discrimination, prejudice, and bias experienced by transgender people: A systematic review of quantitative studies. *Issues in Mental Health Nursing*, *43*(2): 111–118. doi:10.1080/01612840. 2021.1961330.

Dragioti, E., Karathanos, V., Gerdle, B. & Evangelou, E. (2017) Does psychotherapy work? An umbrella review of meta-analyses of randomized controlled trials. *Acta Psychiatrica Scandinavica*, *136*(3): 236–246. doi: 10.1111/acps.12713.

Dreyer, R.P., Pavlo, A.J., Hersey, D., Horne, A., Dunn, R., Norris, C.M. & Davidson, L. (2021) 'Is my heart healing?' A meta-synthesis of patients' experiences after acute myocardial infarction. *Journal of*

Cardiovascular Nursing, *36*(5): 517–530. doi:10.1097/JCN.0000000000000732.

D'Souza, D.C., DiForti, M., Ganesh, S., et al. (2022) Consensus paper of the WFSBP task force on cannabis, cannabinoids and psychosis. *World Journal of Biological Psychiatry*, *23*(10): 719–742. doi:10.1080/15 622975.2022.2038797.

Du, X., Witthöft, M., Zhang, T., Shi, C. & Ren, Z. (2023) Interpretation bias in health anxiety: A systematic review and meta-analysis. *Psychological Medicine*, *53*(1): 34–45. doi:10.1017/S0033291722003427.

Duan, H., Zhu, L., Li, M., Zhang, X., Zhang, B. & Fang, S. (2022) Comparative efficacy and acceptability of selective serotonin reuptake inhibitor antidepressants for binge eating disorder: A network meta-analysis. *Frontiers in Pharmacology*, *13*: 949823. doi:10.3389/ fphar.2022.949823.

Dubinsky, M.C., Dotan, I., Rubin, D.T., Bernauer, M., Patel, D., et al. (2021) Burden of comorbid anxiety and depression in patients with inflammatory bowel disease: A systematic literature review. *Expert Review of Gastroenterology & Hepatology*, *15*(9): 985–997. doi:10.1080/17474124.2021.1911644.

Dufresne, L., Bussières, E.L., Bédard, A., Gingras, N., Blanchette-Sarrasin, A. & Bégin, C. (2020) Personality traits in adolescents with eating disorder: A meta-analytic review. *The International Journal of Eating Disorders*, *53*(2): 157–173. doi:10.1002/eat.23183.

Dumoulin, C., Cacciari, L.P. & Hay-Smith, E.J.C. (2018) Pelvic floor muscle training versus no treatment, or inactive control treatments, for urinary incontinence in women. *Cochrane Database of Systematic Reviews*, *10*(10): Art. CD005654. doi: 10.1002/14651858.CD005654.pub4.

Duncan, R.E., Vandeleur, M., Derks, A. & Sawyer, S. (2011) Confidentiality with adolescents in the medical setting: What do parents think? *Journal of Adolescent Health*, *49*(4): 428–430.

Dworkin, E.R., Krahé, B. & Zinzow, H. (2021) The global prevalence of sexual assault: A systematic review of international research since 2010. *Psychology of Violence, 11*(5): 497–508. doi:10.1037/vio0000374.

Dyrbye, L.N., Power, D.V., Massie, F.S., Eacker, A., Harper, W., et al. (2010) Factors associated with resilience to and recovery from burnout: A prospective, multi-institutional study of US medical students. *Medical Education, 44*(10): 1016–1026. doi: 10.1111/j.1365-2923.2010.03754.x.

Dzierzanowski, T. & Kozlowski, M. (2019) Personal fear of their own death and determination of philosophy of life affects the breaking of bad news by internal medicine and palliative care clinicians. *Archives of Medical Science, 18*(6): 1505–1512. doi: 10.5114/aoms.2019.85944.

Eagle, A. & Worrell, M. (2019) Cognitive behaviour therapy. In C.D. Llewellyn, S. Ayers, C. McManus, S. Newman, K.J. Petrie, T.A. Revenson & J. Weinman (eds), *The Cambridge Handbook of Psychology, Health and Medicine* (3rd edition). Cambridge: Cambridge University Press.

Eagley, A. & Chaiken, S. (1993) *The Psychology of Attitudes.* Fort Worth, TX: Harcourt Brace.

Eccles, R. & Wilkinson, J.E. (2015) Exposure to cold and acute upper respiratory tract infection. *Rhinology, 53*(2): 99–106. doi: 10.4193/Rhin14.239.

Eckerling, A., Ricon-Becker, I., Sorski, L., Sandbank, E. & Ben-Eliyahu, S. (2021) Stress and cancer: Mechanisms, significance and future directions. *Nature Reviews. Cancer, 21*(12), 767–785. doi:10.1038/s41568-021-00395-5.

Eckert, K.G., Abbasi-Neureither, I., Köppel, M. & Huber, G. (2019) Structured physical activity interventions as a complementary therapy for patients with inflammatory bowel disease: A scoping review and practical implications. *BMC Gastroenterology, 19*(1): 115. doi: 10.1186/s12876-019-1034-9.

Eeckhaut, M.C.W. & Fitzpatrick, K. (2022) Are LARC users less likely to use condoms? An analysis of US women initiating LARC in 2008–2018. *Womens Health Issues, 32*: 431–439. doi:10.1016/j.whi.2022.05.002.

Ehlers, D. K., DuBois, K. & Salerno, E. A. (2020) The effects of exercise on cancer-related fatigue in breast cancer patients during primary treatment: A meta-analysis and systematic review. *Expert Review of Anticancer Therapy, 20*(10): 865–877. doi:10.1080/14737140.2020.1813028

Eilert, N., Wogan, R., Leen, A. & Richards, D. (2022) Internet-delivered interventions for depression and anxiety symptoms in children and young people: Systematic review and meta-analysis. *JMIR Pediatrics & Parenting, 5*(2): e33551. doi:10.2196/33551.

Eken, H.N., Dee, E.C., Powers, A.R. III & Jordan, A. (2021) Racial and ethnic differences in perception of provider cultural competence among patients with depression and anxiety symptoms: A retrospective, population-based, cross-sectional analysis. *Lancet Psychiatry, 8*: 957–968. doi:10.1016/S2215-0366(21)00285-6.

Ekholm, O., Diasso, P.D.K, Davidsen, M., Kurita, G.P. & Sjøgren, P. (2022) Increasing prevalence of chronic non-cancer pain in Denmark from 2000 to 2017: A population-based survey. *European Journal of Pain, 26*(3): 624–633. doi:10.1002/ejp.1886.

Ekman, P. (1999) Basic emotions. In T. Dalgleish & T. Power (eds), *Handbook of Cognition and Emotion.* Chichester: Wiley. pp. 45–60.

El Boghdady, M. & Ewalds-Kvist, B.M. (2020) The influence of music on the surgical task performance: A systematic review. *International Journal of Surgery, 73*: 101–112. doi: 10.1016/j.ijsu.2019.11.012.

Elias, A., Phutane, V.H., Clarke, S. & Prudic, J. (2018) Electroconvulsive therapy in the continuation and maintenance treatment of depression: Systematic review and meta-analyses. *Australian & New Zealand Journal of Psychiatry, 52*(5): 415–424. doi: 10.1177/0004867417743343.

Elkind, D. (1967) Egocentrism in adolescence. *Child Development, 38*(4): 1025–1034.

Ellis, B.J. & Del Giudice, M. (2019) Developmental adaptation to stress: An evolutionary perspective. *Annual Review of Psychology*, *70*: 111–1139. doi:10.1146/annurev-psych-122216-011732.

Emanuel, E.J., Onwuteaka-Philipsen, B.D., Urwin, J.W. & Cohen, J. (2016) Attitudes and practices of euthanasia and physician-assisted suicide in the United States, Canada, and Europe. *JAMA*, *316*(1): 79–90. doi:10.1001/jama.2016.8499.

Emdin, C.A., Odutayo, A., Wong, C.X., Tran, J., Hsiao, A.J. & Hunn, B.H. (2016) Meta-analysis of anxiety as a risk factor for cardiovascular disease. *American Journal of Cardiology*, *118*(4): 511–519.

Emery, C.F., Kiecolt-Glaser, J.K., Glaser, R., Malarkey, W.B. & Frid, D.J. (2005) Exercise accelerates wound healing among healthy older adults: A preliminary investigation. *Journals of Gerontology, Series A*, *60*(11): 1432–1436.

Enck, P. & Zipfel, S. (2019) Placebo effects in psychotherapy: A framework. *Frontiers in Psychiatry*, *10*: 456. doi: 10.3389/fpsyt.2019.00456.

Engel, G. (1977) The need for a new medical model: The challenge for biomedicine. *Science*, *196*(4286): 129–136.

Ensaff, H. (2021) A nudge in the right direction: The role of food choice architecture in changing populations' diets. *Proceedings of the Nutrition Society*, *80*(2): 195–206. doi:10.1017/S0029665120007983.

Ericsson, K.A. (2015) Acquisition and maintenance of medical expertise: A perspective from the expert-performance approach with deliberate practice. *Academic Medicine*, *90*(11): 1471–1486. doi: 10.1097/ACM.0000000000000939.

Ericsson, K.A. (2020) Towards a science of the acquisition of expert performance in sports: Clarifying the differences between deliberate practice and other types of practice. *Journal of Sports Sciences*, *38*(2): 159–176. doi:10.1080/02640414.2019.1688618.

Erikson, E.H. (1950) *Childhood and Society*. New York: W.W. Norton.

Erikson, E.H. (1968) *Identity: Youth and Crisis*. New York: W.W. Norton.

Eugenicos, M.P. & Ferreira, N.B. (2021) Psychological factors associated with inflammatory bowel disease. *British Medical Bulletin*, *138*: 16–28. doi:10.1093/bmb/ldab010.

European Centre for Disease Prevention and Control (2018) *Chlamydia Infection: Annual Epidemiological Report for 2017*. Stockholm: European CDPC.

European Centre for Disease Prevention and Control (2019) *Gonorrhoea: Annual Epidemiological Report for 2018*. Stockholm: European CDPC.

European Centre for Disease Prevention and Control & WHO Regional Office for Europe (2021) *HIV/AIDS Surveillance in Europe 2021–2020 Data*. Stockholm: ECDC.

European Centre for Disease Prevention and Control (2023) *STI Cases on the Rise across Europe*. 8 December [website]. Available from www.ecdc.europa.eu/en/news-events/rising-rates-sexually-transmitted-infections-across-europe (accessed 11 May 2024).

Evans, G.W., Wener, R.E. & Phillips, D. (2002) The morning rush hour: Predictability and commuter stress. *Environment and Behavior*, *34*: 521–530.

Evans, J.R. & Lawrenson, J.G. (2017) Antioxidant vitamin and mineral supplements for slowing the progression of age-related macular degeneration. *Cochrane Database of Systematic Reviews*, *7*: Art. CD000254. doi: 10.1002/14651858.CD000254.pub4.

Evidence Development and Standards Branch, Health Quality Ontario (2014) Arthroscopic debridement of the knee: An evidence update. *Ontario Health Technology Assessment Series*, *14*(13): 1–43.

Eysenck, M.W. (2000) *Psychology: A Student's Handbook*. Hove: Psychology Press.

Fagan, J., Galea, S., Ahern, J., Bonner, S. & Vlahov, D. (2003) Relationship of self-reported asthma severity and urgent health care utilization to psychological sequelae of the September 11, 2001 terrorist attacks on the World Trade Center among New York

City area residents. *Psychosomatic Medicine*, 65(6): 993–996.

Fairbrass, K.M., Lovatt, J., Barberio, B., Yuan, Y., Gracie, D.J. & Ford, A.C. (2022) Bidirectional brain-gut axis effects influence mood and prognosis in IBD: A systematic review and meta-analysis. *Gut*, 71(9): 1773–1780. doi:10.1136/gutjnl-2021-325985.

Fallowfield, L. & Jenkins, V. (2004) Communicating sad, bad, and difficult news in medicine. *Lancet*, 363(9405): 312–319.

Fantin, R., Ulloa, C.S. & Solís, C.B. (2020) Social gradient in cancer incidence in Costa Rica: Findings from a national population-based cancer registry. *Cancer Epidemiology*, 68: 101789. doi:10.1016/j.canep.2020.101789.

Faraclas, E. (2023) Interventions to improve quality of life in multiple sclerosis: New opportunities and key talking points. *Degenerative Neurological and Neuromuscular Disease*, 13: 55–68. doi:10.2147/DNND.S395733.

Farley, J.P. & Kim-Spoon, J. (2014) The development of adolescent self-regulation: Reviewing the role of parent, peer, friend, and romantic relationships. *Journal of Adolescence*, 37: 433–440. doi:10.1016/j.adolescence.2014.03.009.

Fässler, M., Meissner, K., Schneider, A. & Linde, K. (2010) Frequency and circumstances of placebo use in clinical practice: A systematic review of empirical studies. *BMC Medicine*, 8: 15.

Favaro, A., Busetto, P., Collantoni, E. & Santonastaso, P. (2019) The age of onset of eating disorders. In G. de Girolamo, P. McGorry & N. Sartorius (eds), *Age of Onset of Mental Disorders*. Cham, Switzerland: Springer.

Feinstein, R.E., Blumenfield, M., Orlowski, B., Frishman, W.H. & Ovanessian, S. (2006) A national survey of cardiovascular physicians' beliefs and clinical care practices when diagnosing and treating depression in patients with cardiovascular disease. *Cardiology in Review*, 14(4): 164–169.

Feldman, J.M., Becker, J., Arora, A., DeLeon, J. et al. (2021) Depressive symptoms and overperception of airflow obstruction in older adults with asthma. *Psychosomatic Medicine*, 83: 787–794. doi:10.1097/PSY.0000000000000951.

Feldman, J.M. Kutner, H., Matte, L., Lupkin, M., Steinberg, D., et al. (2012) Prediction of peak flow values followed by feedback improves perception of lung function and adherence to inhaled corticosteroids in children with asthma. *Thorax*, 67(12): 1040–1045. doi:10.1136/thoraxjnl-2012- 201789.

Feldman, J. M., Arcoleo, K., Greenfield, N., et al. (2023). Under-perception of airflow limitation, self-efficacy, and beliefs in older adults with asthma. *Journal of Psychosomatic Research*, 170, 111353. doi:10.1016/j.jpsychores.2023.111353.

Felez-Nobrega, M. & Koyanagi, A. (2023) Health status and quality of life in comorbid physical multimorbidity and depression among adults aged >50 years from low- and middle-income countries. *International Journal of Social Psychiatry*, 69(5): 1250–1259. doi:10.1177/00207640231157253.

Feng, L., Li, L., Liu, W., Yang, J., Wang, Q., Shi, L. & Luo, M. (2019) Prevalence of depression in myocardial infarction: A PRISMA-compliant meta-analysis. *Medicine*, 98(8): e14596. doi:10.1097/MD.0000000000014596.

Ferdousi, M. & Finn, D.P. (2018) Stress-induced modulation of pain: Role of the endogenous opioid system. *Progress in Brain Research*, 239: 121–177. doi: 10.1016/bs.pbr.2018.07.002.

Ferjan Ramírez, N., Weiss, Y., Sheth, K.K. & Kuhl, P.K. (2024) Parentese in infancy predicts 5-year language complexity and conversational turns. *Journal of Child Language*, 51: 359–384. doi:10.1017/S0305000923000077.

Ferner, R.E. & McDowell, S.E. (2006) Doctors charged with manslaughter in the course of medical practice, 1795–2005: A literature review. *Journal of the Royal Society of Medicine*, 99(6): 309–314.

Festinger, L. (1957) *A Theory of Cognitive Dissonance*. Evanston, IL: Row, Peterson.

Fiedorowicz, J.G. (2014) Depression and cardiovascular disease: An update on how course of illness may influence risk. *Current Psychiatry Reports*, 16(10): 492.

Fink, G. (2017) Selye's general adaptation syndrome: Stress-induced gastro-duodenal ulceration and inflammatory bowel disease. *Journal of Endocrinology*, 232(5): F1–F5. doi: 10.1530/JOE-16-0547.

Fink, H.A., Hemmy, L.S., Linskens, E.J., Silverman, P.C., MacDonald, R., McCarten, J.R., Talley, K.M.C., Desai, P.J., Forte, M.L., Miller, M.A., Brasure, M., Nelson, V.A., Taylor, B.C., Ng, W., Ouellette, J.M., Greer, N.L., Sheets, K.M., Wilt, T.J. & Butler, M. (2020) *Diagnosis and Treatment of Clinical Alzheimer's-Type Dementia: A Systematic Review*. Rockville, MD: Agency for Healthcare Research and Quality.

Fink, M., Klein, K., Sayers, K., Valentino, J. et al. (2020) Objective data reveals gender preferences for patients' primary care physician. *Journal of Primary Care & Community Health*, 11. doi:10.1177/2150132720967221.

Fiscella, K., Epstein, R. M., Griggs, J. J., Marshall, M.M. & Shields, C.G. (2021) Is physician implicit bias associated with differences in care by patient race for metastatic cancer-related pain?. *PloS one*, 16(10), e0257794. doi:10.1371/journal.pone.0257794.

Fischer, P., Krueger, J.I., Greitemeyer, T., Vogrincic, C., Kastenmüller, A., Frey, D., Heene, M., Wicher, M. & Kainbacher, M. (2011) The bystander-effect: A meta-analytic review on bystander intervention in dangerous and non-dangerous emergencies. *Psychological Bulletin*, 137(4): 517–537.

Fish, J.N. & Exten, C. (2020) Sexual orientation differences in alcohol use disorder across the adult life course. *American Journal of Preventive Medicine*, 59(3): 428–436. doi:10.1016/j.amepre.2020.04.012

Fisher, J.D. & Fisher, W.A. (1992) Changing AIDS-risk behavior. *Psychological Bulletin*, 111(3): 455–474. doi: 10.1037/0033-2909.111.3.455.

Fisher, V., Li, W.W. & Malabu, U. (2023) The effectiveness of mindfulness-based stress reduction (MBSR) on the mental health, HbA1C, and mindfulness of diabetes patients: A systematic review and meta-analysis of randomised controlled trials. *Applied Psychology: Health and Well-Being*, 15(4): 1733–1749. doi: 10.1111/aphw.12441.

FitzGerald, C. & Hurst, S. (2017) Implicit bias in healthcare professionals: A systematic review. *BMC Medical Ethics*, 18(1): 19. doi: 10.1186/s12910-017-0179-8.

FitzGerald, C., Mumenthaler, C., Berner, D., Schindler, M., Brosch, T., & Hurst, S. (2022) How is physicians' implicit prejudice against the obese and mentally ill moderated by specialty and experience? *BMC Medical Ethics*, 23(1): 86. doi:10.1186/s12910-022-00815-7.

Fletcher, A., Crowe, M., Manuel, J. & Foulds, J. (2021) Comparison of patients' and staff's perspectives on the causes of violence and aggression in psychiatric inpatient settings: An integrative review. *Journal of Psychiatric and Mental Health Nursing*, 28(5): 924–939. doi:10.1111/jpm.12758.

Fletcher, B.R., Damery, S., Aiyegbusi, O.L., Anderson, N., Calvert, M., et al. (2022) Symptom burden and health-related quality of life in chronic kidney disease: A global systematic review and meta-analysis. *PLoS Medicine*, 19(4): e1003954. doi:10.1371/journal.pmed.1003954.

Floyd, D.L., Prentice-Dunn, S. & Rogers, R.W. (2006) A meta-analysis of research on protection motivation theory. *Journal of Applied Social Psychology*, 30(2): 407–429.

Flygare, O., Boberg, J., Rück, C., Hofmann, R., Leosdottir, M., et al. (2023) Association of anxiety or depression with risk of recurrent cardiovascular events and death after myocardial infarction: A nationwide registry study. *International Journal of Cardiology*, 381: 120–127. doi:10.1016/j.ijcard.2023.04.023.

Folstein, M.F., Folstein, S.E. & McHugh, P.R. (1975) 'Mini-mental state': A practical method for grading the cognitive state of patients for the clinician. *Journal of Psychiatric Research, 12*(3): 189–198.

Fontil, V., Pacca, L., Bellows, B.K. et al. (2022) Association of differences in treatment intensification, missed visits, and scheduled follow-up interval with racial or ethnic disparities in blood pressure control. *JAMA Cardiology, 7*: 204–212. doi:10.1001/jamacardio.2021.4996.

Ford, A.C., Lacy, B.E., Harris, L.A. & Quigley, E.M.M. (2019) Effect of antidepressants and psychological therapies in irritable bowel syndrome: An updated systematic review and meta-analysis. *American Journal of Gastroenterology, 114*(Suppl 1): 21–39. doi:10.1038/s41395-018-0222-5.

Ford, A.C., Sperber, A.D., Corsetti, M. & Camilleri, M. (2020) Irritable bowel syndrome. *Lancet, 396*(10263): 1675–1688. doi:10.1016/S0140-6736(20)31548-8.

Ford, E., Shakespeare, J., Elias, F. & Ayers, S. (2017) Recognition and management of perinatal depression and anxiety by general practitioners: A systematic review. *Family Practice, 34*(1): 11–19.

Fornaro, M., Daray, F. M., Hunter, F., Anastasia, A., Stubbs, B., et al. (2021) The prevalence, odds and predictors of lifespan comorbid eating disorder among people with a primary diagnosis of bipolar disorders, and vice-versa: Systematic review and meta-analysis. *Journal of Affective Disorders, 280*(A): 409–431. doi:10.1016/j.jad.2020.11.015.

Foroushani, P.S., Schneider, J. & Assareh, N. (2011) Meta-review of the effectiveness of computerised CBT in treating depression. *BMC Psychiatry, 11*: 131.

Forte, A.J., Guliyeva, G., McLeod, H. et al. (2022) The impact of optimism on cancer-related and postsurgical cancer pain: A systematic review. *Journal of Pain and Symptom Management, 63*(2): e203–e11. doi:10.1016/j.jpainsymman.2021.09.008

França, K. & Jafferany, M. (eds) (2017) *Stress and Skin Disorders: Basic and Clinical Aspects.* New York: Springer.

Frankel, R.M. & Sherman, H.B. (2015) The secret of the care of the patient is in knowing and applying the evidence about effective clinical communication. *Oral Diseases, 21*(8): 919–926.

Frankel, R.M. & Stein, T. (2001) Getting the most out of the clinical encounter: The four habits model. *Journal of Medical Practice Management, 16*(4): 184–191.

Frankum, S. & Ogden, J. (2005) Estimation of blood glucose levels by people with diabetes: A cross-sectional study. *The British Journal of General Practice: Journal of the Royal College of General Practitioners, 55*(521): 944–948.

Frattaroli, J. (2006) Experimental disclosure and its moderators: A meta-analysis. *Psychological Bulletin, 132*(6): 823–865.

Fredrickson, B.L. (2004) The broaden-and-build theory of positive emotions. *Philosophical Transactions Royal Society of London Series B. Biological Sciences, 359*(1449): 1367–1378.

French, D.P., Cooper, A. & Weinman, J. (2006) Illness perceptions predict attendance at cardiac rehabilitation following acute myocardial infarction: A systematic review with meta-analysis. *Journal of Psychosomatic Research, 61*(6): 757–767.

Friedman, H.S. (2019) Neuroticism and health as individuals age. *Personality Disorders: Theory, Research, and Treatment, 10*(1): 25–32. doi:10.1037/per0000274.

Fries, J.F., Green, L.W. & Levine, S. (1989) Health promotion and the compression of morbidity. *Lancet, 333*(8636): 481–483.

Fryt, J., Szczygieł, M. & Duell, N. (2022) Positive and negative risk-taking: Age patterns and relations to domain-specific risk-taking. *Advances in Life Course Research, 54*: 100515. doi:10.1016/j.alcr.2022.100515.

Fu, R., Hou, J., Gu, Y. & Yu, N.X. (2023) Do couple-based interventions show larger effects in promoting HIV preventive behaviors than individualized interventions in couples? A systematic review and meta-analysis of 11 randomized controlled trials. *AIDS and Behavior, 27*(1): 314–334. doi:10.1007/s10461-022-03768-5

Furtwängler, N.A. & de Visser, R.O. (2013) Lack of international consensus in low-risk drinking guidelines. *Drug and Alcohol Review, 32*(1): 11–18. doi: 10.1111/j.1465-3362.2012.00475.x.

Gaertner, J., Siemens, W., Meerpohl, J. J., Antes, G., Meffert, C., et al. (2017) Effect of specialist palliative care services on quality of life in adults with advanced incurable illness in hospital, hospice, or community settings: Systematic review and meta-analysis. *BMJ (Clinical Research Ed.), 357*: j2925. doi:10.1136/bmj.j2925.

Gagnon, A.J. & Sandall, J. (2007) Individual or group antenatal education for childbirth or parenthood, or both. *Cochrane Database of Systematic Reviews, 3*: Art. CD002869.

Gajdos, P., Chrisztó, Z. & Rigó, A. (2021) The association of different interoceptive dimensions with functional gastrointestinal symptoms. *Journal of Health Psychology, 26*: 2801–2810. doi: 10.1177/1359105320929426.

Gál, É., Ştefan, S. & Cristea, I.A. (2021) The efficacy of mindfulness meditation apps in enhancing users' well-being and mental health related outcomes: A meta-analysis of randomized controlled trials. *Journal of Affective Disorders, 279*: 131–142. doi: 10.1016/j.jad.2020.09.134.

Galanti, M., Birger, R., Ud-Dean, M., Filip, I., Morita, H., et al. (2019) Rates of asymptomatic respiratory virus infection across age groups. *Epidemiology and Infection, 147*: e176. doi:10.1017/S0950268819000505.

Gale, C.R., Batty, G.D. & Deary, I.J. (2008) Locus of control at age 10 years and health outcomes and behaviors at age 30 years: The 1970 British cohort study. *Psychosomatic Medicine, 70*(4): 397–403.

Gallagher, M.W., Long, L.J. & Phillips, C.A. (2020) Hope, optimism, self-efficacy, and posttraumatic stress disorder: A meta-analytic review of the protective effects of positive expectancies. *Journal of Clinical Psychology, 76*(3): 329–355. doi:10.1002/jclp.22882.

Gallagher, S., Creaven, A.M., Hackett, R.A., O'Connor, D.B. & Howard, S. (2024) Social network size moderates the association between loneliness and cardiovascular reactivity to acute stress. *Physiology & Behavior, 275*: 114452. doi:10.1016/j.physbeh.2023.114452.

Gan, E.H. & Pearce, S.H. (2017) Management of endocrine disease: Regenerative therapies in autoimmune Addison's disease. *European Journal of Endocrinology, 176*(3): R123–R135. doi: 10.1530/EJE-16-0581.

Gandhi, S., Goodman, S.G., Greenlaw, N., Ford, I., McSkimming, P., et al. (2019) Living alone and cardiovascular disease outcomes. *Heart, 105*(14): 1087–1095. doi: 10.1136/heartjnl-2018-313844.

Gao, W., Ho, Y.K., Verne, J., Gordon, E. & Higginson, I.J. (2014) Geographical and temporal understanding in place of death in England (1984–2010): Analysis of trends and associated factors to improve end-of-life care (GUIDE_Care) – primary research. *Health Services and Delivery Research*, 2.42. Southampton: NIHR Journals Library.

Garbarino, S., Lanteri, P., Bragazzi, N.L., Magnavita, N. & Scoditti, E. (2021) Role of sleep deprivation in immune-related disease risk and outcomes. *Communications Biology, 4*(1): 1304. doi:10.1038/s42003-021-02825-4.

Garssen, B. (2004) Psychological factors and cancer development: Evidence after 30 years of research. *Clinical Psychology Review, 24*(3): 315–338.

Gatenby, C. & Simpson, P. (2024) Menopause: Physiology, definitions, and symptoms. *Best Practice & Research Clininical Endocrinology & Metabolism, 38*(1): 101855. doi: 10.1016/j.beem.2023.101855.

Gathright, E.C., Goldstein, C.M., Josephson, R.A. & Hughes, J.W. (2017) Depression increases the risk of mortality in patients with heart failure: A meta-analysis. *Journal of Psychosomatic Research, 94*: 82–89.

Gaube, S., Fischer, P., Windl, V. & Lermer, E. (2020) The effect of persuasive messages on hospital visitors' hand hygiene behavior. *Health Psychology*, *39*(6): 471–481. doi: 10.1037/hea0000854.

Gause, N.K., Brown, J.L., Welge, J. & Northern, N. (2018) Meta-analyses of HIV prevention interventions targeting improved partner communication: Effects on partner communication and condom use frequency outcomes. *Journal of Behavioral Medicine*, *41*(4): 423–440. doi: 10.1007/s10865-018-9916-9.

GBD 2017 Diet Collaborators (2019) Health effects of dietary risks in 195 countries, 1990–2017: A systematic analysis for the Global Burden of Disease Study 2017. *Lancet*, *393*(10184): 1958–1972. doi:10.1016/S0140-6736(19)30041-8.

GBD 2019 Dementia Forecasting Collaborators (2022) Estimation of the global prevalence of dementia in 2019 and forecasted prevalence in 2050: An analysis for the Global Burden of Disease Study 2019. *Lancet Public Health*, *7*(2): e105–e125. doi:10.1016/S2468-2667(21)00249-8.

GBD 2019 Mental Disorders Collaborators (2022) Global, regional, and national burden of 12 mental disorders in 204 countries and territories, 1990–2019: A systematic analysis for the Global Burden of Disease Study 2019. *Lancet Psychiatry*, *9*(2): 137–150. doi:10.1016/S2215-0366(21)00395-3.

GBD 2019 Risk Factors Collaborators (2020) Global burden of 87 risk factors in 204 countries and territories, 1990–2019: A systematic analysis for the Global Burden of Disease Study 2019. *Lancet*, *396*(10258): 1223–1249. doi:10.1016/S0140-6736(20)30752-2.

GBD 2021 Demographics Collaborators (2021) Global age-sex-specific mortality, life expectancy, and population estimates in 204 countries and territories and 811 subnational locations, 1950–2021, and the impact of the COVID-19 pandemic: A comprehensive demographic analysis for the Global Burden of Disease Study 2021. *Lancet*, *403*(10440): 1989–2056. doi:10.1016/S0140-6736(24)00476-8.

GBD 2021 Fertility and Forecasting Collaborators (2024) Global fertility in 204 countries and territories, 1950–2021, with forecasts to 2100: A comprehensive demographic analysis for the Global Burden of Disease Study 2021. *Lancet*, *403*(10440): 2057–2099. doi:10.1016/S0140-6736(24)00550-6.

Geen, R.G. & O'Neal, E.C. (1969) Activation of cue-elicited aggression by general arousal. *Journal of Personality and Social Psychology*, *11*(3): 289–292.

Geeraerts, B., Vandenberghe, J., Van Oudenhove, L., Gregory, L.J., Aziz, Q., Dupont, P., Demyttenaere, K., Janssens, J. & Tack, J. (2005) Influence of experimentally induced anxiety on gastric sensorimotor function in humans. *Gastroenterology*, *129*(5): 1437–1444.

Gelis, A., Cervello, S., Rey, R., Llorca, G., Lambert, P., Franck, N., Dupeyron, A., Delpont, M. & Rolland, B. (2020) Peer role-play for training communication skills in medical students: A systematic review. *Simulation in Healthcare*, *15*(2): 106–111. doi: 10.1097/SIH.0000000000000412.

Georgescu, A.L., Kuzmanovic, B., Roth, D., Bente, G. & Vogeley, K. (2014) The use of virtual characters to assess and train non-verbal communication in high-functioning autism. *Frontiers in Human Neuroscience*, *15*(8): 807.

Georgopoulou, S., Prothero, L. & D'Cruz, D.P. (2018) Physician–patient communication in rheumatology: A systematic review. *Rheumatology International*, *38*(5): 763–775. doi: 10.1007/s00296-018-4016-2.

Gerstberger, L., Blanke, E.S., Keller, J., & Brose, A. (2023) Stress buffering after physical activity engagement: An experience sampling study. *British Journal of Health Psychology*, *28*(3): 876–892. doi:10.1111/bjhp.12659.

Ghiasvand, H., Waye, K.M., Noroozi, M., Harouni, G.G., Armoon, B. & Bayani, A. (2019) Clinical determinants associated with quality of life for people who live with

HIV/AIDS: A meta-analysis. *BMC Health Services Research*, *19*(1): 768. doi: 10.1186/s12913-019-4659-z.

Ghielen, I., Rutten, S., Boeschoten, R.E., Houniet-de Gier, M., van Wegen, E.E.H., et al. (2019) The effects of cognitive behavioral and mindfulness-based therapies on psychological distress in patients with multiple sclerosis, Parkinson's disease and Huntington's disease: Two meta-analyses. *Journal of Psychosomatic Research*, *122*: 43–51. doi: 10.1016/j.jpsychores.2019.05.001.

Ghimire, S., Castelino, R.L., Lioufas, N.M., Peterson, G.M. & Zaidi, S.T. (2015) Nonadherence to medication therapy in haemodialysis patients: A systematic review. *PLoS One*, *10*(12): e0144119. doi:10.1371/journal.pone.0144119.

Gigerenzer, G., Gaissmaier, W., Kurz-Milcke, E., Schwartz, L.M. & Woloshin, S. (2008) Helping doctors and patients to make sense of health statistics. *Psychological Science in the Public Interest*, 8(2): 53–96.

Gil, K., Jones, M., Mouw, T., Al-Kasspooles, M., Brahmbhatt, T. & DiPasco, P.J. (2020) Satisfaction or distraction: Exposure to nonpreferred music may alter the learning curve for surgical trainees. *Journal of Surgical Education*, *77*(6): 1370–1376. doi: 10.1016/j.jsurg.2020.04.019.

Gil-González, I., Martín-Rodríguez, A., Conrad, R. & Pérez-San-Gregorio, M.Á. (2020) Quality of life in adults with multiple sclerosis: A systematic review. *BMJ Open*, *10*(11): e041249. doi:10.1136/bmjopen-2020-041249.

Gilmore-Bykovskyi, A., Block, L., Johnson, R. & Goris, E.D. (2019) Symptoms of apathy and passivity in dementia: A simultaneous concept analysis. *Journal of Clinical Nursing*, *28*(3–4): 410–419. doi: 10.1111/jocn.14663.

Glaser, B. & Strauss, A. (1966) *Awareness of Dying*. Chicago, IL: Aldine.

Glaser, J., Nouri, S., Fernandez, A., Sudore, R.L., Schillinger, D., Klein-Fedyshin, M. & Schenker, Y. (2020) Interventions to improve patient comprehension in informed consent for medical and surgical procedures: An updated systematic review. *Medical Decision Making*, *40*(2): 119–143. doi: 10.1177/0272989X19896348.

Glaser, R., Kennedy, S., Lafuse, W.P., Bonneau, R.H., Speicher, C., Hillhouse, J. & Kiecolt-Glaser, J.K. (1990) Psychological stress-induced modulation of interleukin 2 receptor gene expression and interleukin 2 production in peripheral blood leukocytes. *Archives of General Psychiatry*, *47*(8): 707–712. doi: 10.1001/archpsyc.1990.01810200015002.

Gleicher, S.T., Chalmiers, M.A., Aiyanyor, B., Jain, R., Kotha, N., Scott, K., Song, R.S., Tram, J., Vuong, C.L. & Kesselheim, J. (2022) Confronting implicit bias toward patients: A scoping review of post-graduate physician curricula. *BMC Medical Education*, *22*(1): 696. doi:10.1186/s12909-022-03720-0.

Global Breastfeeding Collective, UNICEF & WHO (2023) *Global Breastfeeding Scorecard 2023*. Available from www.who.int/publications/i/item/WHO-HEP-NFS-23.17 (accessed 6 May 2023).

Global Cancer Observatory (2024) *Cancer Today*. Lyon, France: International Agency for Research on Cancer. Available from https://gco.iarc.who.int/today (accessed 23 April 2024).

Global Initiative for Asthma (GINA) (2018) *Global Strategy for Asthma Management and Prevention, 2018*. Available from www.ginasthma.org/ (accessed 19 June 2020).

Glover, V. (2016) Maternal stress during pregnancy and infant and child outcomes. In A. Wenzel (ed.), *The Oxford Handbook of Perinatal Psychology*. New York and Oxford: Oxford University Press.

Gluyas, H. (2015) Patient-centred care: Improving healthcare outcomes. *Nursing Standards*, *30*(4): 50–57. doi: 10.7748/ns.30.4.50.e10186.

Glynn, H., Möller, S.P., Wilding, H., Apputhurai, P., Moore, G. & Knowles, S.R. (2021) Prevalence and impact of posttraumatic stress disorder in gastrointestinal conditions: A systematic review. *Digestive Diseases and Sciences*,

66(12): 4109–4119. doi:10.1007/s10620-020-06798-y

Goebel, M.U., Neykadeh, N., Kou, W., Schedlowski, M. & Hengge, U.R. (2008) Behavioral conditioning of antihistamine effects in patients with allergic rhinitis. *Psychotherapy & Psychosomatics*, *77*(4): 227–234.

Goffman, E. (1959) *The Presentation of Self in Everyday Life*. New York: Doubleday.

Goffman, E. (1972) *Relations in Public: Microstudies of the Public Order*. Ringwood, Vic.: Penguin.

Goldman, A.L., Pope, H.G. & Bhasin, S. (2019) The health threat posed by the hidden epidemic of anabolic steroid use and body image disorders among young men. *Journal of Clinical Endocrinology and Metabolism*, *104*(4): 1069–1074. doi: 10.1210/jc.2018-01706.

Gollwitzer, P.M. & Sheeran, P. (2006) Implementation intentions and goal achievement: A meta-analysis of effects and processes. *Advances in Experimental Social Psychology*, *38*: 69–119. doi: 10.1016/S0065-2601(06)38002-1.

Golonka, K., Piątek, E. & Stach, R. (2023) Study directions and development of cognitive theory of depression. *Psychiatria Polska*, *58*(4): 669–680. English, Polish. doi: 10.12740/PP/OnlineFirst/161676.

Gonzalez, J.S. (2008) Depression and diabetes treatment nonadherence: A meta-analysis. *Diabetes Care*, *31*(12): 2398–2403.

Gonzalez, J.S., Batchelder, A.W., Psaros, C. & Safren, S.A. (2011) Depression and HIV/AIDS treatment nonadherence: A review and meta-analysis. *Journal of Acquired Immune Deficiency Syndromes*, *58*(2): 181–187.

Gonzalez, J.S., Tanenbaum, M.L. & Commissariat, P.V. (2016) Psychosocial factors in medication adherence and diabetes self-management: Implications for research and practice. *American Psychologist*, *71*(7): 539–551. doi:10.1037/a0040388.

Gorbeña, S., Govillard, L. & Iraurgi, I. (2021) A taxonomy of groups at risk based on reported and desired body mass index and its relationships with health. *Psychology,*

Health & Medicine, *26*(sup1): 49–61. doi:10.1080/13548506.2021.1966699.

Gordon, C.S., Jarman, H.K., Rodgers, R.F. et al. (2021) Outcomes of a cluster randomized controlled trial of the SoMe social media literacy program for improving body image-related outcomes in adolescent boys and girls. *Nutrients*, *13*(11): 3825. doi:10.3390/nu13113825.

Gorrell, S., Reilly, E.E., Schaumberg, K., Anderson, L.M. & Donahue, J.M. (2019) Weight suppression and its relation to eating disorder and weight outcomes: A narrative review. *Eating Disorders*, *27*(1): 52–81. doi: 10.1080/10640266.2018.1499297.

Gottlieb, B. (2007) Social support interventions. In S. Ayers, A. Baum, C. McManus, S. Newman, K. Wallston, J. Weinman & R. West (eds), *Cambridge Handbook of Psychology, Health and Medicine* (2nd edition). Cambridge: Cambridge University Press (pp. 397–402).

Gouin, J.P., Kiecolt-Glaser, J.K., Malarky, W.B. & Glaser, R. (2008) The influence of anger expression on wound healing. *Brain, Behaviour and Immunity*, *22*(5): 699–708.

Goyal, M., Singh, S., Sibinga, E.M., Gould, N.F., Rowland-Seymour, A., et al. (2014) Meditation programs for psychological stress and well-being: A systematic review and meta-analysis. *JAMA Internal Medicine*, *174*(3): 357–368.

Goyal, R.K. & Hirano, I. (1996) The enteric nervous system. *New England Journal of Medicine*, *334*(17): 1106–1115.

Gracely, R.H., Geisser, M.E., Giesecke, T., Grant, M.A., Petzke, F., Williams, D.A. & Clauw, D.J. (2004) Pain catastrophizing and neural responses to pain among persons with fibromyalgia. *Brain*, *127*(Pt 4): 835–843.

Gracie, D.J., Guthrie, E.A., Hamlin, P.J. & Ford, A.C. (2018) Bi-directionality of brain-gut interactions in patients with inflammatory bowel disease. *Gastroenterology*, *154*(6): 1635–1646.e3. doi:10.1053/j.gastro.2018.01.027.

Gragnano, A., Negrini, A., Miglioretti, M. & Corbière, M. (2018) Common psychosocial factors predicting return to work after common mental disorders, cardiovascular diseases, and cancers: A review of reviews supporting a cross-disease approach. *Journal of Occupational Rehabilitation*, *28*(2): 215–231. doi: 10.1007/s10926-017-9714-1.

Graham-Brown, M.P.M., Smith, A.C. & Greenwood, S. A. (2022) Digital health interventions in chronic kidney disease: Levelling the playing field? *Clinical Kidney Journal*, *16*(5): 763–767. doi:10.1093/ckj/sfac259.

Grande, A.J., Keogh, J., Hoffmann, T.C., Beller, E.M. & Del Mar, C.B. (2015) Exercise versus no exercise for the occurrence, severity and duration of acute respiratory infections. *Cochrane Database of Systematic Reviews*, (6): CD010596. doi:10.1002/14651858. CD010596.pub2.

Grant, B.F., Hasin, D.S., Stinson, F.S., Dawson, D.A., Goldstein, R.B., et al. (2006) The epidemiology of DSM-IV panic disorder and agoraphobia in the United States: Results from the national epidemiologic survey on alcohol and related conditions. *Journal of Clinical Psychiatry*, *67*(3): 363–374.

Grave, J., Soares, S.C., Morais, S., Rodrigues, P. & Madeira, N. (2017) The effects of perceptual load in processing emotional facial expression in psychotic disorders. *Psychiatry Research*, *250*: 121–128.

Gravely-Witte, S., Stewart, D.E., Suskin, N., Higginson, L., Alter, D.A. & Grace, S.L. (2008) Cardiologists' charting varied by risk factor, and was often discordant with patient report. *Journal of Clinical Epidemiology*, *61*(10): 1073–1079.

Green, L. (2017) The trouble with touch? New insights and observations on touch for social work and social care. *British Journal of Social Work*, *47*, 773–792.

Greenhalgh, T. (2016) *Cultural Contexts of Health: The Use of Narrative Research in the Health Sector*. Copenhagen: WHO Regional Office for Europe. Available from www.ncbi. nlm.nih.gov/books/NBK391066/.

Greenhalgh, T. (2019) *How to Read a Paper: The Basics of Evidence-Based Medicine and Healthcare* (6th edition). Oxford: Blackwell.

Gregório, M., Teixeira, A., Henriques, T., Páscoa, R., Baptista, S., Carvalho, R. & Martins, C. (2021) What role do patients prefer in medical decision-making? A population-based nationwide cross-sectional study. *BMJ Open*, *11*(10): e048488. doi: 10.1136/bmjopen-2020-048488.

Greitemeyer, T. (2022) The dark and bright side of video game consumption: Effects of violent and prosocial video games. *Current Opinion in Psychology*, *46*: 101326. doi:10.1016/j.copsyc.2022.101326.

Griffith, D.M., Cornish, E.K., Bergner, E.M., Bruce, M.A. & Beech, B.M. (2018) 'Health is the ability to manage yourself without help': How older African American men define health and successful aging. *The Journals of Gerontology: Series B*, *73*(2): 240–247. doi:10.1093/geronb/gbx075.

Griffith, R. (2015) Intimate examinations and treatments. *British Journal of Nursing*, *24*(3): 178–179. doi: 10.12968/bjon.2015.24.3.178.

Grimley, C.E., Kato, P.M. & Grunfeld, E.A. (2020) Health and health belief factors associated with screening and help-seeking behaviours for breast cancer: A systematic review and meta-analysis of the European evidence. *British Journal of Health Psychology*, *25*(1): 107–128. doi:10.1111/bjhp.12397.

Groarke, A., Curtis, R., Skelton, J. & Groake, J.M. (2020) Quality of life and adjustment in men with prostate cancer: Interplay of stress, threat and resilience. *PLoS One*, *15*(9): e0239469. doi:10.1371/journal. pone.0239469.

Groome, D. & Eysenck, M. (2016) *An Introduction to Applied Cognitive Psychology* (2nd edition). Hove: Psychology Press.

Grootens-Wiegers, P., Hein, I.M., van den Broek, J.M. & de Vries, M.C. (2017) Medical decision-making in children and adolescents: Developmental and neuroscientific aspects. *BMC Pediatrics*, *17*(1): 120. doi:10.1186/s12887-017-0869-x.

Groß, M., Herr, A., Hower, M., Kuhlmann, A., Mahlich, J. & Stoll, M. (2016) Unemployment, health, and education of HIV-infected males in Germany. *International Journal of Public Health*, *61*(5): 593–602.

Grover, A.K. & Samson, S.E. (2014) Antioxidants and vision health: Facts and fiction. *Molecular and Cellular Biochemistry*, *388*(1–2): 173–183.

Groves, P.S., Bunch, J.L. & Sabin, J.A. (2021) Nurse bias and nursing care disparities related to patient characteristics: A scoping review of the quantitative and qualitative evidence. *Journal of Clinical Nursing*, *30*: 3385–3397. doi:10.1111/jocn.15861.

Grulich, A.E., de Visser, R.O., Badcock, P.B., Smith, A.M., Richters, J., Rissel, C. & Simpson, J.M. (2014) Knowledge about and experience of sexually transmissible infections in a representative sample of adults: The Second Australian Study of Health and Relationships. *Sexual Health*, *11*(5): 481–494.

Guaiana, G., Abbatecola, M., Aali, G. et al. (2022) Cognitive behavioural therapy (group) for schizophrenia. *Cochrane Database of Systematic Reviews*, *7*(7): Art. CD009608. doi:10.1002/14651858. CD009608.pub2.

Guéguen, N., Silone, F. & David, M. (2016) The effect of the two feet-in-the-door technique on tobacco deprivation. *Psychology & Health*, *31*(6): 768–775.

Guellaï, B., Hausberger, M., Chopin, A. & Streri, A. (2020) Premises of social cognition: Newborns are sensitive to a direct versus a faraway gaze. *Scientific Reports*, *10*(1): 9796. doi:10.1038/s41598-020-66576-8.

Guidi, J. & Fava, G.A. (2021) Sequential combination of pharmacotherapy and psychotherapy in major depressive disorder: A systematic review and meta-analysis. *JAMA Psychiatry*, *78*(3): 261–299. doi:10.1001/jamapsychiatry.2020.3650.

Guidi, J., Lucente, M., Sonino, N. & Fava, G.A. (2021) Allostatic load and its impact on health: A systematic review. *Psychotherapy and Psychosomatics*, *90*(1): 11–27. doi:10.1159/000510696.

Guillaumie, L., Boiral, O. & Champagne, J. (2016) A mixed-methods systematic review of the effects of mindfulness on nurses. *Journal of Advanced Nursing*, *73*(5): 1017–1034.

Guo, L. (2023) The delayed, durable effect of expressive writing on depression, anxiety and stress: A meta-analytic review of studies with long-term follow-ups. *British Journal of Clinical Psychology*, *62*: 272–297. doi:10.1111/bjc.12408.

Guo, L., Rohde, J. & Farraye, F.A. (2020) Stigma and disclosure in patients with inflammatory bowel disease. *Inflammatory Bowel Disease*, *26*(7): 1010–1016. doi:10.1093/ibd/izz260.

Gurková, E., Štureková, L., Mandysová, P. & Šaňák, D. (2023) Factors affecting the quality of life after ischemic stroke in young adults: A scoping review. *Health and Quality of Life Outcomes*, *21*(1): 4. doi:10.1186/s12955-023-02090-5.

Guthold, R., Stevens, G.A., Riley, L.M. & Bull, F.C. (2018) Worldwide trends in insufficient physical activity from 2001 to 2016: A pooled analysis of 358 population-based surveys with 1.9 million participants. *Lancet Global Health*, *6*(10): e1077–e1086. doi:10.1016/S2214-109X(18)30357-7.

Guthold, R., Stevens, G.A., Riley, L.M. & Bull, F.C. (2020) Global trends in insufficient physical activity among adolescents: A pooled analysis of 298 population-based surveys with 1·6 million participants. *Lancet Child & Adolescent Health*, *4*(1): 23–35. doi:10.1016/S2352-4642(19)30323-2.

Habib, S., Sangaraju, S.L., Yepez, D., Grandes, X.A. & Talanki Manjunatha, R. (2022) The nexus between diabetes and depression: A narrative review. *Cureus*, *14*(6): e25611. doi:10.7759/cureus.25611.

Hackshaw, A., Morris, J.K., Boniface, S., Tang, J.L. & Milenković, D. (2018) Low cigarette consumption and risk of coronary heart disease and stroke: Meta-analysis of 141 cohort studies in 55 study reports.

British Medical Journal, 360: j5855. doi: 10.1136/bmj.j5855.

HaGani, N., Yagil, D. & Cohen, M. (2022) Burnout among oncologists and oncology nurses: A systematic review and meta-analysis. *Health Psychology, 41*(1): 53–64. doi:10.1037/hea0001155.

Hägele, C., Friedel, E., Kienast, T. & Kiefer, F. (2014) How do we 'learn' addiction? Risk factors and mechanisms getting addicted to alcohol. *Neuropsychobiology, 70*(2): 67–76.

Hagger, M.S., Cheung, M.W.-L., Ajzen, I. & Hamilton, K. (2022) Perceived behavioral control moderating effects in the theory of planned behavior: A meta-analysis. *Health Psychology, 41*(2): 155–167. doi:10.1037/hea0001153.

Hagger, M.S., Poletb, J. & Lintunen, T. (2018) The reasoned action approach applied to health behavior: Role of past behavior and tests of some key moderators using meta-analytic structural equation modeling. *Social Science & Medicine, 213*: 85–94. doi: 10.1016/j.socscimed.2018.07.038.

Hajek, A., Kretzler, B. & König, H.-H. (2020) Personality and the use of cancer screenings: A systematic review. *PLoS One, 15*(12): e0244655. doi:10.1371/journal.pone.0244655.

Hajek, A., Kretzler, B. & König, H.-H. (2021) Relationship between personality factors and frailty: A systematic review. *Archives of Gerontology and Geriatrics, 97*: 104508. doi:10.1016/j.archger.2021.104508.

Hall, C. (2014) Bereavement theory: Recent developments in our understanding of grief and bereavement. *Bereavement Care, 33*(1): 7–12. doi: 10.1080/02682621.2014.902610.

Hall, E.T. (1966) *The Hidden Dimension.* Garden City, NY: Doubleday.

Hall, W.J., Chapman, M.V., Lee, K.M., Merino, Y.M., Thomas, T.W., Payne, B.K., Eng, E., Day, S.H. & Coyne-Beasley, T. (2015) Implicit racial/ethnic bias among health care professionals and its influence on health care outcomes: A systematic review. *American Journal of Public Health, 105*(12): e60–e76. doi: 10.2105/AJPH.2015.302903.

Haller, H., Cramer, H., Lauche, R. & Dobos, G. (2015) Somatoform disorders and medically unexplained symptoms in primary care: A systematic review and meta-analysis of prevalence. *Deutsches Ärzteblatt International, 112*(16): 279–287. doi: 10.3238/arztebl.2015.0279.

Hamer, M., Chida, Y. & Molloy, G.J. (2009) Psychological distress and cancer mortality. *Journal of Psychosomatic Research, 66*(3): 255–258.

Hamilton, K., van Dongen, A. & Hagger, M.S. (2020) An extended theory of planned behavior for parent-for-child health behaviors: A meta-analysis. *Health Psychology, 39*(10): 863–878. doi:10.1037/hea0000940.

Han, A. & Kim, T.H. (2022) Efficacy of internet-based acceptance and commitment therapy for depressive symptoms, anxiety, stress, psychological distress, and quality of life: Systematic review and meta-analysis. *Journal of Medical Internet Research, 24*(12): e39727. doi: 10.2196/39727.

Hankivsky, O. & Christoffersen, A. (2008) Intersectionality and the determinants of health: A Canadian perspective. *Critical Public Health, 18*: 271–283.

Hansford, M. & Jobson, L. (2022) Sociocultural context and the posttraumatic psychological response: Considering culture, social support, and posttraumatic stress disorder. *Psychological Trauma: Theory, Research, Practice, and Policy, 14*(4): 669–679. doi:10.1037/tra0001009.

Hao, J., Huang, B., Remis, A. & He, Z. (2024) The application of virtual reality to home-based rehabilitation for children and adolescents with cerebral palsy: A systematic review and meta-analysis. *Physiotherapy: Theory and Practice, 40*(7): 1588–1608. doi: 10.1080/09593985.2023.2184220.

Harcourt, D. (2017) Disfigurement. In C.D. Llewellyn, S. Ayers, C. McManus, S. Newman, K.J. Petrie, T.A. Revenson & J. Weinman (eds), *Cambridge Handbook of*

Psychology, Health and Medicine (3rd edition). Cambridge: Cambridge University Press.

Hare, D.L., Stewart, A.G.O., Driscoll, A., Mathews, S. & Toukhsati, S.R. (2020) Screening, referral and treatment of depression by Australian cardiologists. *Heart, Lung & Circulation, 29*(3): 401–404. doi:10.1016/j.hlc.2019.03.009.

Harlow, H.F. (1958) The nature of love. *American Psychologist, 13*: 673–685.

Harrison, J.A., Mullen, P.D. & Green, L.W. (1992) A meta-analysis of studies of the health belief model with adults. *Health Education Research, 7*(1): 107–116.

Harrison, S.L., Lee, A., Janaudis-Ferreira, T., Goldstein, R.S. & Brooks, D. (2016) Mindfulness in people with a respiratory diagnosis: A systematic review. *Patient Education and Counselling, 99*(3): 348–355.

Harrop, E., Morgan, F., Longo, M., Semedo, L., Fitzgibbon, J., et al. (2020) The impacts and effectiveness of support for people bereaved through advanced illness: A systematic review and thematic synthesis. *Palliative Medicine, 34*(7): 871–888. doi: 10.1177/0269216320920533.

Hashim, M.J. (2024) Verbal probability terms for communicating clinical risk – a systematic review. *Ulster Medical Journal, 93*(1): 18–23. PMID: 38707974.

Haslam, N., Loughnan, S. & Perry, G. (2014) Meta-Milgram: An empirical synthesis of the obedience experiments. *PLoS One, 9*(4): e93927.

Hatipoglu, E., Topsakal, N., Atilgan, O.E., Alcalar, N., Camliguney, A.F., et al. (2014) Impact of exercise on quality of life and body-self perception of patients with acromegaly. *Pituitary, 17*(1): 38–43.

Hatoum, A.H. & Burton, A.L. (2024) Applications and efficacy of radically open dialectical behavior therapy (RO DBT): A systematic review of the literature. *Journal of Clinical Psychology*, 26 July. doi: 10.1002/jclp.23735. Epub ahead of print.

Hauser, G., Pletikosic, S. & Tkalcic, M. (2014) Cognitive behavioral approach to understanding irritable bowel syndrome.

World Journal of Gastroenterology, 20(22): 6744–6758.

Hay, K., McDougal, L., Percival, V. et al. (2019) Disrupting gender norms in health systems: Making the case for change. *Lancet, 393*: 2535–2549. doi:10.1016/S0140-6736(19)30648-8.

Hayes, S.C. (2004) Acceptance and commitment therapy and the new behaviour therapies: Mindfulness, acceptance, and relationship. In S.C. Hayes, V.M. Follette & M.M. Linehan (eds), *Mindfulness and Acceptance: Expanding the Cognitive Behavioural Tradition*. New York: Guilford Press (pp. 1–29).

Hayes, S.C., Levin, M.E., Plumb-Vilardaga, J., Villatte, J.L. & Pistorello, J. (2013) Acceptance and commitment therapy and contextual behavioral science: Examining the progress of a distinctive model of behavioral and cognitive therapy. *Behavioral Therapy, 44*(2): 180–198. doi: 10.1016/j.beth.2009.08.002.

Haykin, H. & Rolls, A. (2021) The neuroimmune response during stress: A physiological perspective. *Immunity, 54*: 1933–1947. doi:10.1016/j.immuni.2021.08.023.

Haynos, A.F., Wall, M.M., Chen, C., Wang, S.B., Loth, K. & Neumark-Sztainer, D. (2018) Patterns of weight control behavior persisting beyond young adulthood: Results from a 15-year longitudinal study. *International Journal of Eating Disorders, 51*(9), 1090–1097. doi: 10.1002/eat.22963.

He, X. & Barkan, A.L. (2020) Growth hormone therapy in adults with growth hormone deficiency: A critical assessment of the literature. *Pituitary, 23*: 294–306. doi:10.1007/s11102-020-01031-5.

Healthline (2022) What is gender-affirming healthcare and why is it important? *Healthline*, 28 April. Available from www.healthline.com/health/transgender/gender-affirming-healthcare-importance (accessed 13 March 2024).

Hegarty, G., Storey, L., Dempster, M. & Rogers, D. (2021) Correlates of post-traumatic growth following a myocardial infarction: A systematic review. *Journal of Clinical Psychology in Medical Settings*, 28(2): 394–404. doi:10.1007/s10880-020-09727-3

Heilmayr, D., & Friedman, H. S. (2020) Cultivating healthy trajectories: An experimental study of community gardening and health. *Journal of Health Psychology*, 25(13–14): 2418–2427. https://doi.org/10.1177/1359105318800784

Heim, E., Kohrt, B., Koschorke, M., Milenova, M. & Thornicroft, G. (2020) Reducing mental health-related stigma in primary health care settings in low- and middle-income countries: A systematic review. *Epidemiology and Psychiatric Sciences*, 29: e3. doi: 10.1017/S2045796018000458.

Hemilä, H. & Chalker, E. (2013) Vitamin C for preventing and treating the common cold. *Cochrane Database of Systematic Reviews*, 1: Art. CD000980. doi: 10.1002/14651858. CD000980.pub4.

Henderson, J.T., Henninger, M., Bean, S.I., Senger, C.A., Redmond, N. & O'Connor, E. A. (2020) *Behavioral Counseling Interventions to Prevent Sexually Transmitted Infections: A Systematic Evidence Review for the U.S. Preventive Services Task Force.* Rockville, MD: Agency for Healthcare Research and Quality.

Henn, A.T., Larsen, B., Frahm, L., Xu, A., Adebimpe, A., et al. (2023). Structural imaging studies of patients with chronic pain: An anatomical likelihood estimate meta-analysis. *Pain*, 164(1): e10–e24. doi:10.1097/j.pain.0000000000002681.

Hennessy, M.B., Kaiser, S. & Sachser, N. (2009) Social buffering of the stress response: Diversity, mechanisms, and functions. *Frontiers in Neuroendocrinology*, 30(4): 470–482.

Henry, S.G., Fuhrel-Forbis, A., Rogers, M.A.M. & Eggly, S. (2012) Association between nonverbal communication during clinical interactions and outcomes: A systematic review and meta-analysis. *Patient Education and Counselling*, 86(3): 297–315.

Herbert, T.B. & Cohen, S. (1993) Depression and immunity: A meta-analytic review. *Psychological Bulletin*, 113(3): 472–486.

Hernandez-Bustamante, M., Cjuno, J., Hernández, R.M. & Ponce-Meza, J.C. (2024) Efficacy of Dialectical Behavior Therapy in the treatment of borderline personality disorder: A systematic review of randomized controlled trials. *Iranian Journal of Psychiatry*, 19(1): 119–129. doi: 10.18502/ijps.v19i1.14347.

Hettema, J., Steele, J. & Miller, W.R. (2005) Motivational interviewing. *Annual Review of Clinical Psychology*, 1: 91–111.

Heyne, C.S., Kazmierczak, M., Souday, R., Horesh, D., Lambregtse-van den Berg, M., Weigl, T., Horsch, A., Oosterman, M., Dikmen-Yildiz, P. & Garthus-Niegel, S. (2022) Prevalence and risk factors of birth-related posttraumatic stress among parents: A comparative systematic review and meta-analysis. *Clinical Psychology Review*, 94: 102157. doi: 10.1016/j.cpr.2022.102157.

Hickey, M., LaCroix, A.Z., Doust, J., Mishra, G.D., Sivakami, M., Garlick, D. & Hunter, M.S. (2024) An empowerment model for managing menopause. *Lancet*, 403(10430): 947–957. doi: 10.1016/S0140-6736(23) 02799-X.

Hides, L., Dingle, G., Quinn, C., Stoyanov, S.R., Zelenko, O., Tjondronegoro, D., Johnson, D., Cockshaw, W. & Kavanagh, D.J. (2019) Efficacy and outcomes of a music-based emotion regulation mobile app in distressed young people: Randomized controlled trial. *JMIR mHealth and uHealth*, 7(1): e11482.

Higgins, E.T. (1987) Self-discrepancy: A theory relating self and affect. *Psychological Review*, 94(3): 319–340.

Hilderink, P.H., Collard, R., Rosmalen, J.G.M. & Oude Voshaar, R.C. (2013) Prevalence of somatoform disorders and medically unexplained symptoms in old age populations in comparison with younger age groups: A systematic review. *Ageing Research Reviews*, 12(1): 151–156. doi: 10.1016/j.arr.2012.04.004.

Hill, D., Conner, M., Clancy, F., Moss, R., Wilding, S., Bristow, M., & O'Connor, D.B. (2022) Stress and eating behaviours in healthy adults: A systematic review and meta-analysis. *Health*

Psychology Review, 16(2): 280–304. doi:10.1080/17437199.2021.1923406

Hirsch, C.R., Krahé, C., Whyte, J., Bridge, L., Loizou, S., Norton, S. & Mathews, A. (2020) Effects of modifying interpretation bias on transdiagnostic repetitive negative thinking. *Journal of Consulting and Clinical Psychology*, 88(3): 226–239. doi: 10.1037/ccp0000455.

Hitchcock, J.L., Munroe, R.L. & Munroe, R.H. (1976) Coins and countries: The value-size hypothesis. *Journal of Social Psychology*, 100(2): 307–308.

Ho, C.Y., Kow, C.S., Chia, C.H.J., Low, J.Y., Lai, Y.H., et al. (2020) The impact of death and dying on the personhood of medical students: A systematic scoping review. *BMC Medical Education*, 20(1): 516. doi:10.1186/s12909-020-02411-y.

Hoare, J., Sevenoaks, T., Mtukushe, B., Williams, T., Heany, S. & Phillips, N. (2021) Global systematic review of common mental health disorders in adults living with HIV. *Current HIV/AIDS Reports*, 18(6): 569–580. doi:10.1007/s11904-021-00583-w.

Hoare, S., Morris, Z.S., Kelly, M.P., Kuhn, I. & Barclay, S. (2015) Do patients want to die at home? A systematic review of the UK literature, focused on missing preferences for place of death. *PloS One*, 10(11): e0142723. doi:10.1371/journal.pone.0142723.

Hofling, C.K., Brotzman, E., Dalrymple, S., Graves, N. & Pierce, C.M. (1966) An experimental study of nurse–physician relationships. *Journal of Nervous and Mental Disease*, 143(2): 171–180.

Hofmann, M., Dack, C., Barker, C. & Murray, E. (2016) The impact of an internet-based self-management intervention (HeLP-Diabetes) on the psychological well-being of adults with Type 2 diabetes: A mixed-method cohort study. *Journal of Diabetes Research*, 2016: 1476384. doi: 10.1155/2016/1476384.

Hofmann, W., De Houwer, J., Perugini, M., Baeyens, F. & Crombez, G. (2010) Evaluative conditioning in humans: A meta-analysis. *Psychological Bulletin*, 136(3): 390–421. doi: 10.1037/a0018916.

Hofmann, W., Friese, M. & Wiers, R.W. (2008) Impulsive versus reflective influences on health behavior: A theoretical framework and empirical review. *Health Psychology Review*, 2(2): 111–137. doi: 10.1080/17437190802617668.

Hogg, M.A. & Vaughan, G.M. (2008) *Social Psychology* (5th edition). Harlow: Pearson Prentice-Hall.

Hohman, Z.P., Crano, W.D. & Niedbala, E.M. (2016) Attitude ambivalence, social norms, and behavioral intentions: Developing effective antitobacco persuasive communications. *Psychology of Addictive Behaviors*, 30(2): 209–219. doi: 10.1037/adb0000126.

Hohman, Z.P., Crano, W.D., Siegel, J.T. & Alvaro, E.M. (2014) Attitude ambivalence, friend norms, and adolescent drug use. *Prevention Science*, 15(1): 65–74.

Höhn, A., Gampe, J., Lindahl-Jacobsen, R., Christensen, K. & Oksuyzan, A. (2020) Do men avoid seeking medical advice? A register-based analysis of gender-specific changes in primary healthcare use after first hospitalisation at ages 60+ in Denmark. *Journal of Epidemiology and Community Health*, 74(7): 573–579. doi:10.1136/jech-2019-213435.

Hole, B. & Salem, J. (2016) How long do patients with chronic disease expect to live? A systematic review of the literature. *Clinical Medicine*, 16(Suppl. 3): s32. doi:10.7861/clinmedicine.16-3-s32.

Holliday, R., Hong, B., McColl, E., Livingstone-Banks, J. & Preshaw, P.M. (2021) Interventions for tobacco cessation delivered by dental professionals. *Cochrane Database of Systematic Reviews*, 2(2): CD005084. doi:10.1002/14651858.CD005084.pub4.

Holman, E.A., Silver, R.C., Poulin, M., Andersen, J., Gil-Rivas, V. & McIntosh, D.N. (2008) Terrorism, acute stress, and cardiovascular health: A 3-year national study following the September 11th attacks. *Archives of General Psychiatry*, 65(1): 73–80.

Holt-Lunstad, J., Smith, T.B. & Layton, J.B. (2010) Social relationships and mortality risk: A meta-analytic review. *PLoS Medicine, 7*(7): e1000316.

Holt-Lunstad, J., Smith, T.B., Baker, M., Harris, T. & Stephenson, D. (2015) Loneliness and social isolation as risk factors for mortality: A meta-analytic review. *Perspectives on Psychological Science, 10*(2): 227–237.

Hong, Y., Peña-Purcell, N.C. & Ory, M.G. (2012) Outcomes of online support and resources for cancer survivors: A systematic literature review. *Patient Education and Counselling, 86*(3): 288–296.

Horesh, A., Tsur, A.M., Bardugo, A. & Twig, G. (2021) Adolescent and childhood obesity and excess morbidity and mortality in young adulthood: A systematic review. *Current Obesity Reports, 10*(3): 301–310. doi:10.1007/s13679-021-00439-9.

Hormes, J.M. & Rozin, P. (2009) Perimenstrual chocolate craving: What happens after menopause. *Appetite, 53*(2): 256–259.

Horn, A., Jírů-Hillmann, S., Widmann, J. Montellano, F.A., Salmen, J., et al. (2023) Systematic review on the effectiveness of mobile health applications on mental health of breast cancer survivors. *Journal of Cancer Survivorship*, 31 October. doi:10.1007/s11764-023-01470-6.

Horn, A., Stangl, S. Parisi, S., et al. (2023) Systematic review with meta-analysis: Stress-management interventions for patients with irritable bowel syndrome. *Stress Health, 39*(4): 694–707. doi:10.1002/smi.3226.

Horn, D.J. & Johnston, C.B. (2020) Burnout and self care for palliative care practitioners. *Medical Clinics of North America, 104*: 561–572. doi:10.1016/j.mcna.2019.12.007.

Horn, S.R., Charney, D.S. & Feder, A. (2016) Understanding resilience: New approaches for preventing and treating PTSD. *Experimental Neurology, 284*(Pt B): 119–132.

Horne, R., Chapman, S.C., Parham, R., Freemantle, N., Forbes, A. & Cooper, V. (2013) Understanding patients' adherence-related beliefs about medicines prescribed for long-term conditions: A meta-analytic review of the necessity-concerns framework. *PLoS One, 8*(12): e80633.

Horsch, A., Garthus-Niegel, S., Ayers, S., Chandra, P., Hartmann, K., Vaisbuch, E. & Lalor, J. (2024) Childbirth-related posttraumatic stress disorder: Definition, risk factors, pathophysiology, diagnosis, prevention, and treatment. *American Journal of Obstetrics & Gynecology, 230*(3S): S1116–S1127. doi: 10.1016/j.ajog.2023.09.089.

Hort, J., Duning, T., & Hoerr, R. (2023) Ginkgo biloba Extract EGb 761 in the Treatment of Patients with Mild Neurocognitive Impairment: A Systematic Review. *Neuropsychiatric Disease and Treatment, 19*: 647–660. doi:10.2147/NDT.S401231

Horta, B.L., Loret de Mola, C. & Victora, C.G. (2015) Breastfeeding and intelligence: A systematic review and meta-analysis. *Acta Paediatrica, 104*(467): 14–19.

Hossain, S.N., Jaglal, S.B., Shepherd, J., Perrier, L., Tomasone, J.R., et al. (2021) Web-based peer support interventions for adults living with chronic conditions: Scoping review. *JMIR Rehabilitation and Assistive Technologies, 8*(2): e14321. doi:10.2196/14321.

Hou, Y., Feng, S., Tong, B., Lu, S. & Jin, Y. (2022) Effect of pelvic floor muscle training using mobile health applications for stress urinary incontinence in women: A systematic review. *BMC Women's Health, 22*(1): 400. doi:10.1186/s12905-022-01985-7.

Hovenkamp-Hermelink, J.H.M., Jeronimus, B.F., van der Veen, D.C., Spinhoven, P., Penninx, B.W.J.H., et al. (2019) Differential associations of locus of control with anxiety, depression and life-events: A five-wave, nine-year study to test stability and change. *Journal of Affective Disorders, 253*: 26–34. doi: 10.1016/j.jad.2019.04.005.

Howard, S. (2023) Old ideas, new directions: Re-examining the predictive utility of the hemodynamic profile of the stress response in healthy populations. *Health Psychology Review, 17*(1): 104–120. doi:10.1080/17437199.2022.2067210.

Howarth, A., Smith, J.G., Perkins-Porras, L. & Ussher, M. (2019) Effects of brief mindfulness-based interventions on health-related outcomes: A systematic review. *Mindfulness*, 10: 1957–1968. doi: 10.1007/s12671-019-01163-1.

Hu, F., Wu, C., Jia, Y., Zhen, H., Cheng, H., et al. (2023) Shift work and menstruation: A meta-analysis study. *SSM – Population Health*, 24: 101542. doi: 10.1016/j.ssmph.2023.101542.

Hu, Z., Li, M., Yao, L., Wang, Y., Wang, E., et al. (2021) The level and prevalence of depression and anxiety among patients with different subtypes of irritable bowel syndrome: A network meta-analysis. *BMC Gastroenterology*, 21(1): 23. doi:10.1186/s12876-020-01593-5.

Hua, T., Kim, L.S., Yousaf, M., Gwillim, E.C., Yew, Y.W., et al. (2023) Psychological interventions are more effective than educational interventions at improving atopic dermatitis severity: A systematic review. *Dermatitis: Contact, Atopic, Occupational, Drug*, 34(4): 301–307. doi:10.1097/DER.0000000000000868.

Huang, C.W., Wee, P.H., Low, L.L., Koong, Y.L.A., Htay, H., et al. (2021) Prevalence and risk factors for elevated anxiety symptoms and anxiety disorders in chronic kidney disease: A systematic review and meta-analysis. *General Hospital Psychiatry*, 69: 27–40. doi:10.1016/j.genhosppsych.2020.12.003.

Huang, X., Xu, N., Wang, Y., Sun, Y. & Guo, A. (2023) The effects of motivational interviewing on hypertension management: A systematic review and meta-analysis. *Patient Education and Counseling*, 112: 107760. doi: 10.1016/j.pec.2023.107760.

Huang, Y., Cao, D., Chen, Z., Chen, B., Li, J., et al. (2021) Red and processed meat consumption and cancer outcomes: Umbrella review. *Food Chemistry*, 356: 129697. doi:10.1016/j.foodchem.2021.129697.

Huang, Y., Li, Q., Zhou, F. & Song, J. (2022) Effectiveness of internet-based support interventions on patients with breast cancer: A systematic review and narrative synthesis. *BMJ Open*, 12(5): e057664. doi: 10.1136/bmjopen-2021-057664.

Huang, Y.Y., Gan, Y.H., Yang, L., Cheng, W. & Yu, J.T. (2023) Depression in Alzheimer's disease: Epidemiology, mechanisms, and treatment. *Biological Psychiatry*, 95(11): 992–1005. doi:10.1016/j.biopsych.2023.10.008s.

Huber, J.P., Milton, A., Brewer, M.C., Norrie, L.M., Hartog, S.M. & Glozier, N. (2024) The effectiveness of brief non-pharmacological interventions in emergency departments and psychiatric inpatient units for people in crisis: A systematic review and narrative synthesis. *Australian and New Zealand Journal of Psychiatry*, 58(3): 207–226. doi: 10.1177/00048674231216348.

Hudson, J.L., Bundy, C., Coventry, P.A. & Dickens, C. (2014) Exploring the relationship between cognitive illness representations and poor emotional health and their combined association with diabetes self-care: A systematic review with meta-analysis. *Journal of Psychosomatic Research*, 76(4): 265–274.

Hughes, D.J., Kratsiotis, I.K., Niven, K. & Holman, D. (2020) Personality traits and emotion regulation: A targeted review and recommendations. *Emotion*, 20(1): 63–67. doi:10.1037/emo0000644

Hughes, T.L. (2016) The influence of gender and sexual orientation on alcohol use and alcohol-related problems: Toward a global perspective. *Alcohol Research*, 38(1): 121–132.

Hull, K.L. & Harvey, S. (2003) Growth hormone therapy and quality of life: Possibilities, pitfalls and mechanisms. *Journal of Endocrinology*, 179(3): 311–333.

Hull, M.A. (2021) Nutritional prevention of colorectal cancer. *Proceedings of the Nutrition Society*, 80(1): 59–64. doi:10.1017/S0029665120000051.

Hunt, M., Miguez, S., Dukas, B., Onwude, O. & White, S. (2021) Efficacy of Zemedy, a mobile digital therapeutic for the self-management of irritable bowel syndrome:

A cross-over randomized controlled trial. *JMIR mHealth and uHealth*, 9(5): e26152. doi:10.2196/26152.

Hunter, M., Ussher, J., Cariss, M., Browne, S. & Jelly, R. (2002) A randomised comparison of psychological (cognitive behaviour therapy, CBT), medical (fluoxetine) and combined treatment for women with premenstrual dysphoric disorder. *Journal of Psychosomatic Obstetrics and Gynaecology*, 23(3): 193–199.

Hurst, J.R, Skolnik, N., Hansen, G.J., Anzueto, A., Donaldson, G.C., et al. (2020) Understanding the impact of chronic obstructive pulmonary disease exacerbations on patient health and quality of life. *European Journal of Internal Medicine*, 73: 1–6. doi:10.1016/j.ejim.2019.12.014.

Hwang, W.C. (2006) The psychotherapy adaptation and modification framework: Application to Asian Americans. *American Psychology*, 61: 702–715.

Hwang W.C. (2009) The Formative Method for Adapting Psychotherapy (FMAP): A community-based developmental approach to culturally adapting therapy. *Professional Psychology, Research and Practice*, 40(4): 369–377. doi:10.1037/a0016240.

Icenogle, G. & Cauffman, E. (2021) Adolescent decision making: A decade in review. *Journal of Research on Adolescence*, 31(4): 1006–1022. doi:10.1111/jora.12608.

Ihrig, A., Karschuck, P., Haun, M.W., Thomas, C. & Huber, J. (2020) Online peer-to-peer support for persons affected by prostate cancer: A systematic review. *Patient Education and Counseling*, 103(10): 2107–2115. doi:10.1016/j.pec.2020.05.009.

Imeri, H., Toth, J., Arnold, A. & Barnard, M. (2022) Use of the transtheoretical model in medication adherence: A systematic review. *Research in Social & Administrative Pharmacy*, 18(5): 2778–2785. doi:10.1016/j.sapharm.2021.07.008.

Ince, B., Schlatter, J., Max, S., Plewnia, C., Zipfel, S., Giel, K.E. & Schag, K. (2021) Can we change binge eating behaviour by interventions addressing food-related impulsivity? A systematic review. *Journal of Eating Disorders*, 9(1): 38. doi:10.1186/s40337-021-00384-x.

International Committee of Medical Journal Editors (2024) *Recommendations for the Conduct, Reporting, Editing, and Publication of Scholarly Work in Medical Journals*. Available from www.icmje.org/recommendations/ (accessed 31 July 2024).

Iravani, M., Zarean, E., Janghorbani, M. & Bahrami, M. (2015) Women's needs and expectations during normal labor and delivery. *Journal of Education and Health Promotion*, 4: 6.

Isaacs, C., Skakoon-Sparling, S., Kohut, T. & Fisher, W.A. (2021) A dyadic approach to understanding safer sex behavior in intimate heterosexual relationships. *Journal of Health Psychology*, 26(9): 1364–1376. doi:10.1177/1359105319873958.

Ishigami, T. (1919) The influence of psychic acts on the progress of pulmonary tuberculosis. *American Review of Tuberculosis*, 2(8): 470–484.

Jackson, J.L., Passamonti, M. & Kroenke, K. (2007) Outcome and impact of mental disorders in primary care at 5 years. *Psychosomatic Medicine*, 69(3): 270–276. doi:10.1097/PSY.0b013e3180314b59.

Jackson, M.K., Schmied, V. & Dahlen, H.G. (2020) Birthing outside the system: The motivation behind the choice to freebirth or have a homebirth with risk factors in Australia. *BMC Pregnancy Childbirth*, 20(1): 254. doi: 10.1186/s12884-020-02944-6.

Jackson, T., Wang, Y. & Fan, H. (2014) Associations between pain appraisals and pain outcomes: Meta-analyses of laboratory pain and chronic pain literatures. *Journal of Pain*, 15(6): 586–601.

Jacobson, J., Ju, A., Baumgart, A., Unruh, M., O'Donoghue, D., et al. (2019) Patient perspectives on the meaning and impact of fatigue in hemodialysis: A systematic review and thematic analysis of qualitative studies. *American Journal of*

Kidney Diseases, 74(2): 179–192. doi:10.1053/j.ajkd.2019.01.034.

Jadhakhan, F., Romeu, D., Lindner, O., Blakemore, A. & Guthrie, E. (2022) Prevalence of medically unexplained symptoms in adults who are high users of healthcare services and magnitude of associated costs: A systematic review. *BMJ Open, 12*(10): e059971. doi:10.1136/bmjopen-2021-059971.

Janis, I.L. & Mann, L. (1977) *Decision Making: A Psychological Analysis of Conflict, Choice, and Commitment.* New York: Free Press.

Jankowska, M. (2011) Sexual functioning of testicular cancer survivors and their partners: A review of literature. *Reports of Practical Oncology and Radiotherapy, 17*(1): 54–62.

Jansingh, A., Danner, U.N., Hoek, H.W. & van Elburg, A.A. (2020) Developments in the psychological treatment of anorexia nervosa and their implications for daily practice. *Current Opinion in Psychiatry, 33*(6): 534–541. doi:10.1097/YCO.0000000000000642.

Janssens, T., Verleden, G., De Peuter, S., Van Diest, I. & Van den Bergh, O. (2009) Inaccurate perception of asthma symptoms: A cognitive-affective framework and implications for asthma treatment. *Clinical Psychology Review, 29*(4): 317–327. doi:10.1016/j.cpr.2009.02.006.

Jarbøl, D.E., Larsen, P.V., Gyrd-Hansen, D., Søndergaard, J., Brandt, C., et al. (2017) Determinants of preferences for lifestyle changes versus medication and beliefs in ability to maintain lifestyle changes: A population-based survey. *Preventive Medicine Reports, 6*: 66–73. doi: 10.1016/j.pmedr.2017.02.010.

Jayes, M., Palmer, R. & Enderby, P. (2020) Evaluation of the MCAST, a multidisciplinary toolkit to improve mental capacity assessment. *Disability & Rehabilitation, 44*(2): 323–330. doi:10.1080/09638288.2020.1765030.

Jefferson, L., Bloor, K., Birks, Y., Hewitt, C. & Bland, M. (2013) Effect of physicians' gender on communication and consultation length: A systematic review and meta-analysis. *Journal of Health Services Research & Policy, 18*(4): 242–248.

Jefferson, T., Del Mar, C.B., Dooley, L., Ferroni, E., Al-Ansary, L.A., et al. (2011) Physical interventions to interrupt or reduce the spread of respiratory viruses. *Cochrane Database of Systematic Reviews, 7*: Art. CD006207. doi: 10.1002/14651858.CD006207.pub4.

Jefferson, T., Dooley, L., Ferroni, E., Al-Ansary, L.A. et al. (2023) Physical interventions to interrupt or reduce the spread of respiratory viruses. *Cochrane Database of Systematic Reviews, 1*(1): Art. CD006207. doi:10.1002/14651858.CD006207.pub6.

Jeffrey, D. (2016) Empathy, sympathy and compassion in healthcare: Is there a problem? Is there a difference? Does it matter? *Journal of the Royal Society of Medicine, 109*(12): 446–452. doi: 10.1177/0141076816680120.

Jenabi, E., Khazaei, S., Bashirian, S., Aghababaei, S. & Matinnia, N. (2020) Reasons for elective cesarean section on maternal request: A systematic review. *Journal of Maternal-Fetal & Neonatal Medicine, 33*(22): 3867–3872. doi: 10.1080/14767058.2019.1587407.

Jennings, E.M., Okine, B.N., Roche, M. & Finn, D.P. (2014) Stress-induced hyperalgesia. *Progress in Neurobiology, 121*: 1–18. doi:10.1016/j.pneurobio.2014.06.003.

Jensen, P.M., Trollope-Kumar, K., Waters, H. & Everson, J. (2008) Building physician resilience. *Canadian Family Physician, 54*(5): 722–729.

Jessop, D.C., Craig, L. & Ayers, S. (2014) Applying Leventhal's self-regulatory model to pregnancy: Evidence that pregnancy-related beliefs and emotional responses are associated with maternal health outcomes. *Journal of Health Psychology, 19*(9): 1091–1102.

Jetter, M., Laudage, S. & Stadelmann, D. (2019) The intimate link between income levels and life expectancy: Global evidence from 213 years. *Social Science Quarterly, 100*(4): 1387–1403. doi:10.1111/ssqu.12638.

Jha, V., Garcia-Garcia, G., Iseki, K., Li, Z., Naicker, S., et al. (2013) Chronic kidney disease: Global dimension and perspectives. *Lancet*, *382*(9888): 260–272.

Jia, Y., Zhou, Z., Xiang, F., Hu, W. & Cao, X. (2024) Global prevalence of depression in menopausal women: A systematic review and meta-analysis. *Journal of Affective Disorders*, *358*: 474–482. doi: 10.1016/j.jad.2024.05.051.

Jiang, M.Y.W., Upton, E. & Newby, J.M. (2020) A randomised wait-list controlled pilot trial of one-session virtual reality exposure therapy for blood-injection-injury phobias. *Journal of Affective Disorders*, *276*: 636–645. doi:10.1016/j.jad.2020.07.076.

Jiang, T., Hou, J., Sun, R., Dai, L., Wang, W., et al. (2021) Immunological and psychological efficacy of meditation/yoga intervention among people living with HIV (PLWH): A systematic review and meta-analyses of 19 randomized controlled trials. *Annals of Behavioral Medicine*, *55*(6): 505–519. doi:10.1093/abm/kaaa084.

Jiang, Y., Zou, D., Li, Y., et al. (2022) Monoamine neurotransmitters control basic emotions and affect major depressive disorders. *Pharmaceuticals*, *15*(10): 1203. doi:10.3390/ph15101203.

Joekes, K. (2019) Breaking bad news. In C.D. Llewellyn, S. Ayers, C. McManus, S. Newman, K.J. Petrie, T.A. Revenson & J. Weinman (eds), *The Cambridge Handbook of Psychology, Health and Medicine* (3rd edition). Cambridge: Cambridge University Press.

Johansen, M.L. & Risor, M.B. (2017) What is the problem with medically unexplained symptoms for GPs? A meta-synthesis of qualitative studies. *Patient Education and Counselling*, *100*(4): 647–654.

Johnson, A.L., Jung, L., Song, Y., Brown, K.C., Weaver, M.T. & Richards, K.C. (2014). Sleep deprivation and error in nurses who work the night shift. *Journal of Nursing Administration*, *44*: 17–22.

Johnson, E.E. (2023) Conservative interventions for managing urinary incontinence after prostate surgery. *Cochrane Database of Systematic Reviews*, *4*(4): Art. CD014799. doi:10.1002/14651858.CD014799.pub2.

Jolliffe, D.A., Camargo, C.A., Sluyter, J.D., Aglipay, M., Aloia, J.F., et al. (2021) Vitamin D supplementation to prevent acute respiratory infections: A systematic review and meta-analysis of aggregate data from randomised controlled trials. *Lancet. Diabetes & Endocrinology*, *9*(5): 276–292. doi:10.1016/S2213-8587(21)00051-6.

Jonas, A. (2022) Impact of vaping on respiratory health. *BMJ*, *378*: e065997. doi:10.1136/bmj-2021-065997.

Jones, C.J., Smith, H. & Llewellyn, C. (2014) Evaluating the effectiveness of health belief model interventions in improving adherence: A systematic review. *Health Psychology Review*, *8*(3): 253–269. doi: 10.1080/17437199.2013.802623.

Jones, R.M., Wallace, I.J., Westerberg, A., Hoy, K.N., Quillin, J.M. & Danish, S.J. (2015) Getting youth to Check it Out!®: A new approach to teaching self-screening. *American Journal of Health Behavior*, *39*(2): 197–204. doi: 10.5993/AJHB.39.2.6.

Jonker, F.A., Jonker, C., Scheltens, P. & Scherder, E.J. (2015) The role of the orbitofrontal cortex in cognition and behavior. *Reviews in the Neurosciences*, *26*(1): 1–11. https://doi.org/10.1515/revneuro-2014-0043.

Jonker, N.C., Bennik, E.C., de Lang, T.A., & de Jong, P.J. (2020) Influence of hunger on attentional engagement with and disengagement from pictorial food cues in women with a healthy weight. *Appetite*, *151*: 104686. doi:10.1016/j.appet.2020.104686.

Jordan, C., Sin, J., Fear, N.T. & Chalderd, T. (2016) A systematic review of the psychological correlates of adjustment outcomes in adults with inflammatory bowel disease. *Clinical Psychology Review*, *47*: 28–40. doi: 10.1016/j.cpr.2016.06.001.

Jordan, J.R. & Neimeyer, R.A. (2003) Does grief counseling work? *Death Studies*, *27*(9): 765–786.

Juruena, M.F., Eror, F., Cleare, A.J. & Young, A.H. (2020) The role of early life stress in HPA axis and anxiety. *Advances in Experimental Medicine and Biology,* 1191: 141–153. https://doi.org/10.1007/978-981-32-9705-0_9.

Juvonen, K., Lapveteläinen, A., Närväinen, J., Absetz, P., Kantanen, T., et al. (2020) Effect of metabolic state on implicit and explicit responses to food in young healthy females. *Appetite, 148*: 104593. doi:10.1016/j.appet.2020.104593.

Kabat-Zinn, J. (1990) *Full Catastrophe Living.* New York: Delacorte.

Kabir, A., Conway, D.P., Ansari, S., Tran, A., Rhee, J.J. & Barr, M. (2024) Impact of multimorbidity and complex multimorbidity on healthcare utilisation in older Australian adults aged 45 years or more: A large population-based cross-sectional data linkage study. *BMJ Open, 14*(1): e078762. doi:10.1136/bmjopen-2023-078762.

Kader, S.B., Shakurun, N., Janzen, B. & Pahwa, P. (2024) Impaired sleep, multimorbidity, and self-rated health among Canadians: Findings from a nationally representative survey. *Journal of Multimorbidity and Comorbidity, 14*: 26335565241228549. doi:10.1177/26335565241228549.

Kahneman, D. (2003) A perspective on judgment and choice: Mapping bounded rationality. *American Psychologist, 58*(9): 697–720. doi: 10.1037/0003-066x.58.9.697.

Kaidesoja, M., Cooper, Z. & Fordham, B. (2023) Cognitive behavioral therapy for eating disorders: A map of the systematic review evidence base. *International Journal of Eating Disorders, 56*(2): 295–313. doi:10.1002/eat.23831.

Kalichman, S.C. & Eaton, L.A. (2023) The emergence and persistence of the anti-vaccination movement. *Health Psychology, 42*: 516–520. doi:10.1037/hea0001273.

Kamen, C., Tejani, M.A., Chandwani, K., Janelsins, M., Peoples, A.R., Roscoe, J.A. & Morrow, G.R. (2014) Anticipatory nausea and vomiting due to chemotherapy.

European Journal of Pharmacology, 722: 172–179.

Kamiński, M. & Hrycaj, P. (2024) Celebrities influence on rheumatic diseases interest: A Google Trends analysis. *Rheumatology International, 44*(3): 517–521. doi:10.1007/s00296-023-05361-y.

Kan, C., Eid, L., Treasure, J. & Himmerich, H. (2020) A meta-analysis of dropout and metabolic effects of antipsychotics in anorexia nervosa. *Frontiers in Psychiatry, 11*: 208. doi: 10.3389/fpsyt.2020.00208.

Kancheva Landolt, N. & Ivanov, K. (2021) Short report: Cognitive behavioral therapy – a primary mode for premenstrual syndrome management: Systematic literature review. *Psychology, Health & Medicine, 26*(10): 1282–1293. doi: 10.1080/13548506.2020.1810718.

Kandola, A., Edwards, K., Straatmen, J., Dührkoop, B., Hein, B. & Hayes, J. (2024) Digital self-management platform for adult asthma: Randomized attention-placebo controlled trial. *Journal of Medical Internet Research, 26*: e50855. doi:10.2196/50855.

Kanellopoulos, D. & Gourounti, K. (2022) Tocophobia and women's desire for a caesarean section: A systematic review. *MAEDICA – A Journal of Clinical Medicine, 17*(1): 186–193. doi: 10.26574/maedica.2022.17.1.186.

Kanellopoulos, D. & Gourounti, K. (2023) A systematic review of tocophobia rate before and during the COVID-19 pandemic. *MAEDICA – A Journal of Clinical Medicine, 18*(3): 455–462. doi: 10.26574/maedica.2023.18.3.455.

Kang, W., Steffens, F., Pineda, S. et al. (2023) Personality traits and dimensions of mental health. *Science Reports, 13*: 7091. doi: 10.1038/s41598-023-33996-1.

Kanters, S., Park, J.J.H., Chan, K., Socias, M.E., Ford, N., Forrest, J.I., Thorlund, K., Nachega, J.B. & Mills, E.J. (2017) Interventions to improve adherence to antiretroviral therapy: A systematic review and network meta-analysis. *Lancet HIV, 4*(1): e31–e40.

Kao, T.A., Ling, J., Vu, C., Hawn, R. & Christodoulos, H. (2023) Motivational interviewing in pediatric obesity: A meta-analysis of the effects on behavioral outcomes. *Annals of Behavioral Medicine*, *57*(8): 605–619. doi: 10.1093/abm/kaad006.

Karo, M., Simorangkir, L., Daryanti Saragih, I., Suarilah, I. & Tzeng, H.M. (2024) Effects of mindfulness-based interventions on reducing psychological distress among nurses: A systematic review and meta-analysis of randomized controlled trials. *Journal of Nursing Scholarship*, 56(2): 319–330. doi:10.1111/jnu.12941.

Kashaf, M.S. & McGill, E. (2015) Does shared decision making in cancer treatment improve quality of life? A systematic literature review. *Medical Decision Making*, 35(8): 1037–1048. doi:10.1177/02729 89X15598529.

Kassianos, A.P., Ward, E., Rojas-Garcia, A., Kurti, A., Mitchell, F.C., et al. (2019) A systematic review and meta-analysis of interventions incorporating behaviour change techniques to promote breastfeeding among postpartum women. *Health Psychology Review*, *13*(3): 344–372. doi: 10.1080/17437199.2019.1618724.

Katelaris, P., Hunt, R., Bazzoli, F., Cohen, H., Fock, K.M., et al. (2023) Helicobacter pylori World Gastroenterology Organization Global Guideline. *Journal of Clinical Gastroenterology*, 57(2): 111–126. doi:10.1097/MCG.0000000000001719.

Kato, P.M. & Mann, T. (1999) A synthesis of psychological interventions for the bereaved. *Clinical Psychology Review*, 19(3): 275–296.

Katz, M.L., Broder-Oldach, B., Fisher, J.L., King, J., Eubanks, K., Fleming, K. & Paskett, E.D. (2012) Patient–provider discussions about colorectal cancer screening: Who initiates elements of informed decision making? *Journal of General Internal Medicine*, 27(9): 1135–1141.

Kaur, T., Ranjan, P., Sarkar, S., Kaloiya, G.S., Khan, M., et al. (2022) Psychological interventions for medically unexplained physical symptoms: A systematic review and meta-analysis. *General Hospital Psychiatry*, 77: 92–101. doi:10.1016/j.genhosppsych.2022.04.006.

Kaye, J.A. & Jick, H. (2003) Incidence of erectile dysfunction and characteristics of patients before and after the introduction of sildenafil in the United Kingdom: Cross sectional study with comparison patients. *British Medical Journal*, 326(7386): 424–425.

Kecklund, G. & Axelsson, J. (2016) Health consequences of shift work and insufficient sleep. *British Medical Journal*, *355*: i5210. doi:10.1136/bmj.i5210.

Keightley, P.C., Koloski, N.A. & Talley, N.J. (2015) Pathways in gut-brain communication: Evidence for distinct gut-to-brain and brain-to-gut syndromes. *Australian and New Zealand Journal of Psychiatry*, 49(3): 207–214.

Keith, F., Krantz, D.S., Chen, R., Harris, K.M., Ware, C.M., Lee, A.K., Bellini, P.G. & Gottlieb, S.S. (2017) Anger, hostility, and hospitalizations in patients with heart failure. *Health Psychology*, 36(9): 829–838. doi: 10.1037/hea0000519.

Kelder, I., Sneijder, P., Klarenbeek, A. & Laan, E. (2022) Communication practices in conversations about sexual health in medical healthcare settings: A systematic review. *Patient Education and Counseling*, 105(4): 858–868. doi:10.1016/j.pec.2021.07.049.

Keller, V.F. & Caroll, J.G. (1994) A new model for physician-patient communication. *Patient Education and Counseling*, 23(2): 131–140.

Kenny, D.T. (2007) Stress management. In S. Ayers, A. Baum, C. McManus, S. Newman, K. Wallston, J. Weinman & R. West (eds), *Cambridge Handbook of Psychology, Health and Medicine* (2nd edition). Cambridge: Cambridge University Press. (pp. 403–407).

Kerie, S., Workineh, Y., Kasa, A.S., Ayalew, E. & Menberu, M. (2021) Erectile dysfunction among testicular cancer survivors: A systematic review and meta-analysis. *Heliyon*, 7(7): e07479. doi:10.1016/j.heliyon.2021.e07479.

Kerr, A., Kelleher, C., Pawlikowska, T. & Strawbridge, J. (2021) How can pharmacists develop patient–pharmacist communication skills? A realist synthesis. *Patient Education and Counseling*, *104*(10): 2467–2479. doi: 10.1016/j.pec.2021.03.010.

Kesavayuth, D., Binh Tran, D. & Zikos, V. (2022) Locus of control and subjective well-being: Panel evidence from Australia. *PloS One*, *17*(8): e0272714. doi:10.1371/journal.pone.0272714.

Keski-Rahkonen, A. (2021) Epidemiology of binge eating disorder: Prevalence, course, comorbidity, and risk factors. *Current Opinion in Psychiatry*, *34*: 525–531. doi:10.1097/YCO.0000000000000750.

Kessels, R.P.C. (2003) Patients' memory for medical information. *Journal of the Royal Society of Medicine*, *96*(5): 219–222.

Kessler, A., Sollie, S., Challacombe, B., Briggs, K. & Van Hemelrijck, M. (2019) The global prevalence of erectile dysfunction: A review. *BJU International*, *124*(4): 587–599. doi: 10.1111/bju.14813.

Kew, K.M., Nashed, M., Dulay, V. & Yorke, J. (2016) Cognitive behavioural therapy (CBT) for adults and adolescents with asthma. *Cochrane Database of Systematic Reviews*, *9*(9): Art. CD011818.

Khakbazan, Z., Taghipour, A., Latifnejad Roudsari, R. & Mohammadi, E. (2014) Help seeking behavior of women with self-discovered breast cancer symptoms: A meta-ethnographic synthesis of patient delay. *PLoS One*, *9*(12): e110262.

Khalil, M.I.M., Ashour, A., Shaala, R.S., Allam, R.M., Abdelaziz, T.M. & Mousa, E.F.S. (2024) Effect of health belief model-based educational intervention on prostate cancer prevention; knowledge, practices, and intentions. *BMC Cancer*, *24*(1): 289. doi:10.1186/s12885-024-12044-9.

Khan, L. (2015). *Falling Through the Gaps: Perinatal Mental Health and General Practice*. London: Royal College of General Practitioners and Centre for Mental Health.

Khan, S., Sebastian, S.A., Parmar, M.P., Ghadge, N., Padda, I., et al. (2024) Factors influencing the quality of life in inflammatory bowel disease: A comprehensive review. *Disease-a-month*, *70*(1S): 101672. doi:10.1016/j.disamonth.2023.101672.

Kharawala, S., Kaur, G., Shukla, H., Scott, D. A., Hawkins, N., et al. (2022) Health-related quality of life, fatigue and health utilities in lupus nephritis: A systematic literature review. *Lupus*, *31*(9): 1029–1044. doi:10.1177/09612033221100910.

Khaw, K.T., Wareham, N., Bingham, S., Welch, A., Luben, R. & Day, N. (2008) Combined impact of health behaviours and mortality in men and women: The EPIC-Norfolk prospective population study. *PLoS Medicine*, *5*(1): e12.

Kiecolt-Glaser, J.K. & Glaser, R. (2002) Depression and immune function: Central pathways to morbidity and mortality. *Journal of Psychosomatic Research*, *53*(4): 873–876.

Killian, M.O., Schuman, D.L., Mayersohn, G.S. & Triplett, K.N. (2018) Psychosocial predictors of medication non-adherence in pediatric organ transplantation: A systematic review. *Pediatriatic Transplant*, *22*(4): e13188. doi:10.1111/petr.13188.

Kim, B. & White, K. (2018) How can health professionals enhance interpersonal communication with adolescents and young adults to improve health care outcomes? Systematic literature review. *International Journal of Adolescence & Youth*, *23*(2): 198–218. doi: 10.1080/02673 843.2017.1330696.

Kim, M.C., Fricchione, G.L. & Akeju, O. (2021) Accidental awareness under general anaesthesia: Incidence, risk factors, and psychological management. *BJA Education*, *21*: 154–161. doi:10.1016/j.bjae.2020.12.001.

Kim, S. & Kim, E. (2020) The use of virtual reality in psychiatry: A review. *Soa Chongsonyon Chongsin Uihak*, *31*(1): 26–32. doi:10.5765/jkacap.190037.

Kim, S.H. & Lee, A. (2016) Health-literacy-sensitive diabetes self-management interventions: A systematic review and meta-analysis. *Worldviews on Evidence-Based Nursing*, *13*(4): 324–333.

Kim, Y.K. & Yoon, H.K. (2018) Common and distinct brain networks underlying panic and social anxiety disorders. *Progress in Neuropsychopharmacology & Biological Psychiatry*, *80*(Pt B): 115–122. doi: 10.1016/j.pnpbp.2017.06.017.

Kimball, A., Dichtel, L.E., Yuen, K.C.J., et al. (2022) Quality of life after long-term biochemical control of acromegaly. *Pituitary*, *25*: 531–539. doi:10.1007/s11102-022-01224-0.

King, K., McGuinness, S., Watson, N., Norton, C., Chalder, T. & Czuber-Dochan, W. (2023) What do we know about medication adherence interventions in inflammatory bowel disease, multiple sclerosis and rheumatoid arthritis? A scoping review of randomised controlled trials. *Patient Preference and Adherence*, *17*: 3265–3303. doi:10.2147/PPA.S424024.

Kino, S., Bernabé, E. & Sabbah, W. (2017) Socioeconomic inequality in clusters of health-related behaviours in Europe: Latent class analysis of a cross-sectional European survey. *BMC Public Health*, *17*(1): 497. doi: 10.1186/s12889-017-4440-3.

Kirby, D. (2006) Can fear arousal in public health campaigns contribute to the decline of HIV prevalence? *Journal of Health Communication*, *11*(3): 262–266.

Kirsch, I. (2019) Placebo and nocebo. In C.D. Llewellyn, S. Ayers, C. McManus, S. Newman, K.J. Petrie, T.A. Revenson & J. Weinman (eds), *The Cambridge Handbook of Psychology, Health and Medicine* (3rd edition). Cambridge: Cambridge University Press.

Kirsch, I., Deacon, B.J., Huedo-Medina, T.B., Scoboria, A., Moore, T.J. & Johnson, B.T. (2008) Initial severity and antidepressant benefits: A meta-analysis of data submitted to the Food and Drug Administration. *PLoS Medicine*, *5*(2): e45.

Kis, H., Endres, K., Karwowska, A., Harrison, M., Lau, S., et al. (2022) 'Teddy Bear Hospital Project' school visits improve pre-clerkship students' comfort explaining medical concepts to children. *Canadian Medical Education Journal*, *13*(3): 70–74. doi:10.36834/cmej.73167.

Kitselaar, W.M., van der Vaart, R., Perschl, J., Numans, M.E. & Evers, A.W.M. (2023) Predictors of persistent somatic symptoms in the general population: A systematic review of cohort studies. *Psychosomatic Medicine*, *85*: 71–78. doi:10.1097/PSY.0000000000001145.

Kjeldbjerg, M.L. & Clausen, L. (2023) Prevalence of binge-eating disorder among children and adolescents: A systematic review and meta-analysis. *European Child & Adolescent Psychiatry*, *32*(2): 549–574. doi:10.1007/s00787-021-01850-2.

Knapp, P., Dunn-Roberts, A., Sahib, N., Cook, L., Astin, F., et al. (2020) Frequency of anxiety after stroke: An updated systematic review and meta-analysis of observational studies. *International Journal of Stroke*, *15*(3): 244–255. doi:10.1177/1747493019896958.

Knauer, K., Bach, A., Schäffeler, N., Stengel, A. & Graf, J. (2022) Personality traits and coping strategies relevant to posttraumatic growth in patients with cancer and survivors: A systematic literature review. *Current Oncology*, *29*(12): 9593–9612. doi:10.3390/curroncol29120754.

Knight, A., Palermo, C., Reedy, G. & Whelan, K. (2024) Teaching and assessment of communication skills in dietetics: A scoping review. *Journal of Human Nutrition and Dietetics*, *37*(2): 524–537. doi: 10.1111/jhn.13276.

Knight, M., Bunch, K., Felker, A., Patel, R., Kotnis, R., et al (2023) *Saving Lives, Improving Mothers' Care Core Report – Lessons Learned to Inform Maternity Care from the UK and Ireland Confidential Enquiries into Maternal Deaths and Morbidity 2019–21*. Oxford: National Perinatal Epidemiology Unit, University of Oxford.

Knoll, L.J., Leung, J.T., Foulkes, L. & Blakemore, S.-J. (2017) Age-related differences in social influence on risk perception depend on the direction of influence. *Journal of Adolescence*, *60*: 53–63. doi:10.1016/j.adolescence.2017.07.002.

Knoll, L.J., Magis-Weinberg, L., Speekenbrink, M. & Blakemore, S.J. (2015) Social influence on risk perception during adolescence. *Psychological Science*, 26(5): 583–592. doi: 10.1177/0956797615569578.

Knowles, S.R., Austin, D.W., Sivanesan, S., Tye-Din, J., Leung, C., et al. (2017) Relations between symptom severity, illness perceptions, visceral sensitivity, coping strategies and well-being in irritable bowel syndrome guided by the common sense model of illness. *Psychology, Health & Medicine*, 22(5): 524–534. doi:10.1080/13548506.2016.1168932.

Koehly, L.M., Persky, S., Philip Shaw, Bonham, V.L., Marcum, C.S., Sudre, G.P., et al. (2021) Social and behavioral science at the forefront of genomics: Discovery, translation, and health equity. *Social Science & Medicine*, 271: 112450. doi:10.1016/j.socscimed.2019.112450.

Kohler, M.J., Hendrickx, M.D., Powell-Jones, A. & Bryan-Hancock, C. (2020) A systematic review of cognitive functioning after traumatic brain injury in individuals aged 10–30 years. *Cognitive and Behavioral Neurology: Official Journal of the Society for Behavioral and Cognitive Neurology*, 33(4): 233–252. doi:10.1097/WNN.0000000000000236.

Kok, G. (2007) Health promotion. In S. Ayers, A. Baum, C. McManus, S. Newman, K. Wallston, J. Weinman & R. West (eds), *Cambridge Handbook of Psychology, Health and Medicine* (2nd edition). Cambridge: Cambridge University Press (pp. 355–359).

Kok, G., Peters, G.Y., Kessels, L.T.E., Ten Hoor, G.A. & Ruiter, R.A.C. (2018) Ignoring theory and misinterpreting evidence: The false belief in fear appeals. *Health Psychology Review*, 12(2): 111–125. doi: 10.1080/17437199.2017.1415767.

Koncz, A., Demetrovics, Z. & Takacs, Z.K. (2021) Meditation interventions efficiently reduce cortisol levels of at-risk samples: A meta-analysis. *Health Psychology Review*, 15(1): 56–84. doi:10.1080/17437199.2020.1760727.

Kongkaew, C., Jampachaisri, K., Chaturongkul, C.A. & Scholfield, C.N. (2014) Depression and adherence to treatment in diabetic children and adolescents: A systematic review and meta-analysis of observational studies. *European Journal of Pediatrics*, 173(2): 203–212. doi: 10.1007/s00431-013-2128-y.

Konstantis, G., Efstathiou, S., Pourzitaki, C., Kitsikidou, E., Germanidis, G. & Chourdakis, M. (2023) Efficacy and safety of probiotics in the treatment of irritable bowel syndrome: A systematic review and meta-analysis of randomised clinical trials using ROME IV criteria. *Clinical Nutrition*, 42(5): 800–809. doi:10.1016/j.clnu.2023.03.019.

Koops, T.U., Klein, V., Bei der Kellen, R., Hoyer, J., Löwe, B. & Briken, P. (2023) Association of sexual dysfunction according to *DSM-5* diagnostic criteria with avoidance of and discomfort during sex in a population-based sample. *Sexual Medicine*, 11(3): qfad037. doi:10.1093/sexmed/qfad037.

Kortsmit, K., Nguyen, A.T., Mandel, M.G., Hollier, L.M., Ramer, S., et al. (2023) Abortion surveillance: United States, 2021. *Morbidity and Mortality Weekly Report. Surveillance Summaries*, 72(9): 1–29. doi:10.15585/mmwr.ss7209a1.

Kovacs, W.J. & Ojeda, S.R. (2011) *Textbook of Endocrine Physiology* (6th edition). Oxford: Oxford University Press.

Kraiss, J.T., Ten Klooster, P.M., Moskowitz, J.T. & Bohlmeijer, E.T. (2020) The relationship between emotion regulation and well-being in patients with mental disorders: A meta-analysis. *Comprehensive Psychiatry*, 102: 152189. doi:10.1016/j.comppsych.2020.152189.

Krakower, D.S., Jain, S. & Mayer, K.H. (2015) Antiretrovirals for primary HIV prevention: The current status of pre- and post-exposure prophylaxis. *Current HIV/AIDS Reports*, 12(1): 127–138.

Kranzler, H.R. (2023) Overview of alcohol use disorder. *American Journal of Psychiatry*, 180: 565–572. doi:10.1176/appi.ajp.20230488.

Krauss, S., Dapp, L.C. & Orth, U. (2023) The link between low self-esteem and eating disorders: A meta-analysis of longitudinal studies. *Clinical Psychological Science*, 11: 1141–1158. doi:10.1177/21677026221144255.

Kreuter, M.W., Lukwago, S.N., Bucholtz, R.D., Clark, E.M. & Sanders-Thompson, V. (2003) Achieving cultural appropriateness in health promotion programs: Targeted and tailored approaches. *Health Education & Behavior*, 30(2): 133–146. doi:10.1177/1090198102251021.

Kriakous, S.A., Elliott, K.A., Lamers, C. & Owen, R. (2021) The effectiveness of mindfulness-based stress reduction on the psychological functioning of healthcare professionals: A systematic review. *Mindfulness*, 12(1): 1–28. doi: 10.1007/s12671-020-01500-9.

Kristeller, J. (2019) Cognitive behaviour therapy. In C.D. Llewellyn, S. Ayers, C. McManus, S. Newman, K.J. Petrie, T.A. Revenson & J. Weinman (eds), *The Cambridge Handbook of Psychology, Health and Medicine* (3rd edition). Cambridge: Cambridge University Press.

Kristensen, H.Ø., Thyø, A. & Christensen, P. (2019) Systematic review of the impact of demographic and socioeconomic factors on quality of life in ostomized colorectal cancer survivors. *Acta Oncologica*, 58(5): 566–572. doi: 10.1080/0284186X.2018.1557785.

Krittanawong, C., Maitra, N.S., Hassan Virk, H.U., Fogg, S., Wang, Z., et al. (2022) Association of optimism with cardiovascular events and all-cause mortality: Systematic review and meta-analysis. *American Journal of Medicine*, 135(7): 856–863.e2. doi:10.1016/j.amjmed.2021.12.023.

Kroenke, C.H. (2018) A conceptual model of social networks and mechanisms of cancer mortality, and potential strategies to improve survival. *Translational Behavioral Medicine*, 8(4): 629–642. doi: 10.1093/tbm/ibx061.

Krueger, R.F. & Eaton, N.R. (2015) Transdiagnostic factors of mental disorders. *World Psychiatry*, 14(1): 27–29.

Krzystanek, M., Surma, S., Stokrocka, M., Romańczyk, M., Przybyło, J., Krzystanek, N. & Borkowski, M. (2021) Tips for effective implementation of virtual reality exposure therapy in phobias – a systematic review. *Frontiers in Psychiatry*, 12: 737351. doi: 10.3389/fpsyt.2021.737351.

Kübler-Ross, E. (1969) *On Death and Dying*. New York: Macmillan.

Kunzler, L.S., Naves, L.A. & Casulari, L.A. (2018) Cognitive-behavioral therapy improves the quality of life of patients with acromegaly. *Pituitary*, 21: 323–333. doi:10.1007/s11102-018-0887-1.

Kurihara, H., Maeno, T. & Maeno, T. (2014) Importance of physicians' attire: Factors influencing the impression it makes on patients, a cross-sectional study. *Asia Pacific Family Medicine*, 13(1): 2.

Kurowski, M., Seys, S., Bonini, M., Del Giacco, S., Delgado, L., et al. (2022) Physical exercise, immune response, and susceptibility to infections-current knowledge and growing research areas. *Allergy*, 77(9): 2653–2664. do:10.1111/all.15328.

Kurz, M., Rosendahl, J., Rodeck, J., Muehleck, J. & Berger, U. (2022) School-based interventions improve body image and media literacy in youth: A systematic review and meta-analysis. *Journal of Prevention (2022)*, 43(1): 5–23. doi:10.1007/s10935-021-00660-1.

Kwekkeboom, K.L. & Gretarsdottir, E. (2006) Systematic review of relaxation interventions for pain. *Journal of Nursing Scholarship*, 38(3): 269–277.

Kyriakoulis, P. & Kyrios, M. (2023) Biological and cognitive theories explaining panic disorder: A narrative review. *Frontiers in Psychiatry*, 14: 957515. doi: 10.3389/fpsyt.2023.957515.

Labanski, A., Langhorst, J., Engler, H. & Elsenbruch, S. (2020) Stress and the brain-gut axis in functional and chronic-inflammatory gastrointestinal diseases: A transdisciplinary challenge. *Psychoneuroendocrinology*, 111, 104501. doi:10.1016/j.psyneuen.2019.104501.

Lacasse, K. & Jackson, T.E. (2020) Conformity to masculine norms predicts US men's decision-making regarding a new male contraceptive. *Culture, Health & Sexuality*, *22*(10): 1128–1144. doi:10.1080/13691058.2019.1658806.

Lackner, J.M. & Jaccard, J. (2021) Specific and common mediators of gastrointestinal symptom improvement in patients undergoing education/support vs. cognitive behavioral therapy for irritable bowel syndrome. *Journal of Consulting and Clinical Psychology, 89*(5): 435–453. doi:10.1037/ccp0000648.

Lacroix, E., Smith, A.J., Husain, I.A., Orth, U. & von Ranson, K.M. (2023) Normative body image development: A longitudinal meta-analysis of mean-level change. *Body Image, 45:* 238–264. doi:10.1016/j.bodyim.2023.03.003.

Lacy, B.E., Mearin, F., Chang, L., Chey, W.D., Lembo, A.J., Simren, M. & Spiller, R. (2016) Bowel disorders. *Gastroenterology, 150*(6): 1393–1407.

Ladwig, S., Zhou, Z., Xu, Y., Wang, X., Chow, C.K., Werheid, K. & Hackett, M.L. (2018) Comparison of treatment rates of depression after stroke versus myocardial infarction: A systematic review and meta-analysis of observational data. *Psychosomatic Medicine, 80*(8): 754–763. doi: 10.1097/PSY.0000000000000632.

Lahey, B.B. (2009) Public health significance of neuroticism. *The American Psychologist, 64*(4): 241–256. doi: 10.1037/a0015309.

Lam, C. & Chung, M.H. (2021) Dose–response effects of light therapy on sleepiness and circadian phase shift in shift workers: A meta-analysis and moderator analysis. *Science Reports, 11*(1): 11976. doi:10.1038/s41598-021-89321-1.

Lambez, B. & Vakil, E. (2021) The effectiveness of memory remediation strategies after traumatic brain injury: Systematic review and meta-analysis. *Annals of Physical and Rehabilitation Medicine, 64*(5): 101530. doi:10.1016/j.rehab.2021.101530.

Lameris, A.I., Hoenderop, J.G., Bindels, R.J. & Eijsvogels, T.M. (2015) The impact of formative testing on study behaviour and study performance of (bio)medical students: A smartphone application intervention study. *BMC Medical Education, 15:* 72.

Lamontagne, S.J., Pizzagalli, D.A. & Olmstead, M.C. (2021) Does inflammation link stress to poor COVID-19 outcome? *Stress and Health, 37*(3): 401–414. doi:10.1002/smi.3017.

Lamvu, G., Carrillo, J., Ouyang, C. & Rapkin, A. (2021) Chronic pelvic pain in women: A review. *JAMA, 325*(23): 2381–2391. doi:10.1001/jama.2021.2631.

Lanas, A. & Chan, F.K.L. (2017) Peptic ulcer disease. *Lancet, 390*(10094): 613–624. doi:10.1016/S0140-6736(16)32404-7.

Lanctôt, N. & Guay, S. (2014) The aftermath of workplace violence among healthcare workers: A systematic literature review of the consequences. *Aggression and Violent Behavior, 19*(5): 492–501. doi: 10.1016/j.avb.2014.07.010.

Lang, J., Kerr, D. M., Petri-Romão, P., McKee, T., Smith, H., et al. (2020) The hallmarks of childhood abuse and neglect: A systematic review. *PloS One, 15*(12): e0243639. doi:10.1371/journal.pone.0243639.

Laplante, D.P., Brunet, A. & King, S. (2016) The effects of maternal stress and illness during pregnancy on infant temperament: Project ice storm. *Pediatric Research, 79*(1–1): 107–113.

Laplante, D.P., Brunet, A., Schmitz, N., Ciampi, A. & King, S. (2008) Project ice storm: Prenatal maternal stress affects cognitive and linguistic functioning in 5½-year-old children. *Journal of the American Academy of Child and Adolescent Psychiatry, 47*(9): 1063–1072.

Lareyre, O., Gourlan, M., Stoebner-Delbarre, A. & Cousson-Gélie, F. (2021) Characteristics and impact of theory of planned behavior interventions on smoking behavior: A systematic review of the literature. *Preventive Medicine, 143:* 106327. doi:10.1016/j.ypmed.2020.106327.

Large, M.M., Ryan, C.J., Singh, S.P., Paton, M.B. & Nielssen, O.B. (2011) The predictive value of risk categorization in schizophrenia. *Harvard Review of Psychiatry*, *19*(1): 25–33.

Larkin, D., Birtle, A.J., Bradley, L., Dey, P., Martin, C.R., et al. (2022) A systematic review of disease related stigmatization in patients living with prostate cancer. *PloS One*, *17*(2): e0261557. doi:10.1371/journal.pone.0261557.

Larsson, S.C., Wallin, A., Wolk, A. & Markus, H.S. (2016) Differing association of alcohol consumption with different stroke types: A systematic review and meta-analysis. *BMC Medicine*, *14*(1): 178. doi: 10.1186/s12916-016-0721-4.

Lassen, R.H., Gonçalves, W., Gherman, B., Coutinho, E., Nardi, A.E., et al. (2024) Medication non-adherence in depression: A systematic review and metanalysis. *Trends in Psychiatry & Psychotherapy*, 9 Jan. doi: 10.47626/2237-6089-2023-0680. Epub ahead of print.

Latané, B. & Darley, J.M. (1970) *The Unresponsive Bystander*. New York: Appleton Century Crofts.

Laureati, M., Bergamaschi, V. & Pagliarini, E. (2014) School-based intervention with children: Peer-modeling, reward and repeated exposure reduce food neophobia and increase liking of fruits and vegetables. *Appetite*, *83*: 26–32.

Laursen, M., Johansen, C. & Hedegaard, M. (2009) Fear of childbirth and risk for birth complications in nulliparous women in the Danish National Birth Cohort. *British Journal of Obstetrics & Gynaecology*, *116*(10): 1350–1355.

Lautarescu, A., Craig, M.C. & Glover, V. (2020) Prenatal stress: Effects on fetal and child brain development. *International Review of Neurobiology*, *150*: 17–40. doi:10.1016/bs.irn.2019.11.002.

Lawrie, S.M., Martin, K., McNeill, G., Drife, J., Chrystie, P., et al. (1998) General practitioners' attitudes to psychiatric and medical illness. *Psychological Medicine*, *28*(6): 1463–1467.

Layard, R. (2006) *The Depression Report: A New Deal for Depression and Anxiety Disorders*. London: London School of Economics.

Lazarus, R.S. & Folkman, S. (1984) *Stress, Appraisal and Coping*. New York: Springer.

Leach, L.S., Poyser, C., Cooklin, A.R. & Giallo, R. (2016) Prevalence and course of anxiety disorders (and symptom levels) in men across the perinatal period: A systematic review. *Journal of Affective Disorders*, *190*: 675–686.

Leaviss, J., Davis, S., Ren, S., Hamilton, J., Scope, A., et al. (2020) Behavioural modification interventions for medically unexplained symptoms in primary care: Systematic reviews and economic evaluation. *Health Technology Assessment*, *24*(46): 1–490. doi:10.3310/hta24460.

Lee, J.H. (2016) The effects of music on pain: A meta-analysis. *Journal of Music Therapy*, *53*(4): 430–477.

Lee, R.T., Seo, B., Hladkyj, S., Lovell, B.L. & Schwartzmann, L. (2013) Correlates of physician burnout across regions and specialties: A meta-analysis. *Human Resouces for Health*, *11*: 48.

Lee, S., Holden, D., Webb, R. & Ayers, S. (2019) Pregnancy related risk perception in pregnant women, midwives & obstetricians: A cross-sectional survey. *BMC Pregnancy and Childbirth*, *19*: 335.

Lefler, L.L. & Bondy, K.N. (2004) Women's delay in seeking treatment with myocardial infarction: A meta-synthesis. *Journal of Cardiovascular Nursing*, *19*(4): 251–268.

Lefroy, J., Thomas, A., Harrison, C., Williams, S., O'Mahony, F., Gay, S., Kinston, R. & McKinley, R.K. (2014) Development and face validation of strategies for improving consultation skills. *Advances in Health Sciences Education: Theory & Practice*, *19*(5): 661–685.

Leichsenring, F., Abbass, A. & Heim, N. et al. (2023) The status of psychodynamic psychotherapy as an empirically supported treatment for common mental disorders – an umbrella review based on updated criteria. *World Psychiatry*, *22*: 286–304. doi:10.1002/wps.21104.

Leinberger-Jabari, A., Golob, M.M., Lindson, N. & Hartmann-Boyce, J. (2024) Effectiveness of culturally tailoring smoking cessation interventions for reducing or quitting combustible tobacco: A systematic review and meta-analyses. *Addiction*, *119*: 629–648. doi:10.1111/add.16400.

Leiter, M.P. & Maslach, C. (2000) Burnout and health. In A. Baum, T. Revenson & J. Singer (eds), *Handbook of Health Psychology*. Hillsdale, NJ: Lawrence Erlbaum. pp. 415–426.

Leiter, M.P. & Maslach, C. (2004) Areas of worklife: A structured approach to organizational predictors of job burnout. In P.L. Perrewe & D.C. Ganster (eds), *Research in Occupational Stress and Well-Being* (*Vol. 3*). Oxford: Elsevier (pp. 91–134).

Leonardi, M., Armour, M., Gibbons, T., Cave, A., As-Sanie, S., et al. (2021) Surgical interventions for the management of chronic pelvic pain in women. *Cochrane Database of Systematic Reviews*, *12*(12): CD008212. doi:10.1002/14651858. CD008212.pub2.

Leonhardt, C., Margraf-Stiksrud, J., Badners, L., Szerencsi, A. & Maier, R.F. (2014) Does the 'Teddy Bear Hospital' enhance preschool children's knowledge? A pilot study with a pre/post-case control design in Germany. *Journal of Health Psychology*, *19*(10): 1250–1260.

Leserman, J. (2008) Role of depression, stress, and trauma in HIV disease progression. *Psychosomatic Medicine*, *70*(5): 539–545.

Lett, H.S., Blumenthal, J.A., Babyak, M.A., Sherwood, A., Strauman, T., et al. (2004) Depression as a risk factor for coronary artery disease: Evidence, mechanisms, and treatment. *Psychosomatic Medicine*, *66*(3): 305–315.

Levenstein, S., Rosenstock, S., Jacobsen, R.K. & Jorgensen, T. (2015) Psychological stress increases risk for peptic ulcer, regardless of Helicobacter pylori infection or use of nonsteroidal anti-inflammatory drugs. *Clinical Gastroenterology and Hepatology*, *13*(3): 498–506.e1.

Leventhal, H., Nerenz, D.R. & Steele, D.J. (1984) Illness representations and coping with health threats. In A. Baum, S.E. Taylor & J.E. Singer (eds), *Handbook of Psychology and Health*. Hillsdale, NJ: Lawrence Erlbaum (pp. 219–252).

Leventhal, H., Phillips, L.A. & Burns, E. (2016) The common-sense model of self-regulation (CSM): A dynamic framework for understanding illness self-management. *Journal of Behavioral Medicine*, *39*(6): 935–936.

Levine, J.M. (2018) Socially-shared cognition and consensus in small groups. *Current Opinion in Psychology*, *23*: 52–56. doi: 10.1016/j.copsyc.2017.12.003.

Levinson, W., Hudak, P. & Tricco, A.C. (2013) A systematic review of surgeon–patient communication: Strengths and opportunities for improvement. *Patient Education and Counselling*, *93*(1): 3–17.

Lewin, B., Robertson, I.H., Cay, E.L., Irving, J.B. & Campbell, M. (1992) Effects of self-help post-myocardial-infarction rehabilitation on psychological adjustment and use of health services. *Lancet*, *339*(8800): 1036–1040.

Lewis, E. & Casement, P. (1986) The inhibition of mourning by pregnancy: A case study. *Psychoanalytic Psychotherapy*, *2*(1): 45–52.

Lexchin, J. (2006) Bigger and better: How Pfizer redefined erectile dysfunction. *PLoS Medicine*, *3*(4): e132.

Leyland, A.H. & Dundas, R. (2020) Declining cardiovascular mortality masks unpalatable inequalities. *Heart*, *106*: 6–7. doi:10.1136/ heartjnl-2019-315708.

Li, H., Boakye, D., Chen, X., Hoffeister, M. & Brenner, H. (2021) Association of Body Mass Index with risk of early-onset colorectal cancer: Systematic review and meta-analysis. *American Journal of Gastroenterology*, *116*(11): 2173–2183. doi:10.14309/ajg.0000000000001393.

Li, H., Cheng, B. & Zhu, X.P. (2018) Quantification of burnout in emergency nurses: A systematic review and meta-analysis. *International Emergency Nursing*, *39*: 46–54. doi: 10.1016/j.ienj.2017.12.005.

Li, J., Liu, F., Liu, Z., Li, M., Wang, Y., Shang, Y. & Li, Y. (2024) Prevalence and associated factors of depression in postmenopausal women: A systematic review and meta-analysis. *BMC Psychiatry*, *24*(1): 431. doi: 10.1186/s12888-024-05875-0.

Li, W.Y., Chiu, F.C., Zeng, J.K., Li, Y.W., Huang, S.-H., et al. (2020) Mobile health app with social media to support self-management for patients with chronic kidney disease: Prospective randomized controlled study. *Journal of Medical Internet Research*, *22*(12): e19452. doi:10.2196/19452.

Li, Z., Laginha, K.J., Boyle, F., Daly, M., Dinner, F., et al. (2024) Professionally led support groups for people living with advanced or metastatic cancer: A systematic scoping review of effectiveness and factors critical to implementation success within real-world healthcare and community settings. *Journal of Cancer Survivorship*, 8 January. doi: 10.1007/s11764-023-01515-w. Epub ahead of print.

Liang, W., Duan, Y., Li, F., Rhodes, R.E., Wang, X., et al. (2022) Psychosocial determinants of hand hygiene, facemask wearing, and physical distancing during the COVID-19 pandemic: A systematic review and meta-analysis. *Annals of Behavioral Medicine*, *56*(11): 1174–1187. doi:10.1093/abm/kaac049.

Lichtman, J.H., Froelicher, E.S., Blumenthal, J.A., Carney, R.M., Doering, L.V., et al. (2014) Depression as a risk factor for poor prognosis among patients with acute coronary syndrome: Systematic review and recommendations: A scientific statement from the American Heart Association. *Circulation*, *129*(12): 1350–1369. doi:10.1161/CIR.0000000000000019.

Liew, S.C. & Aung, T. (2021) Sleep deprivation and its association with diseases – a review. *Sleep Medicine*, *77*: 192–204. doi:10.1016/j.sleep.2020.07.048.

Lim, M.M. & Young, L.J. (2006) Neuropeptidergic regulation of affiliative behavior and social bonding in animals. *Hormones and Behavior*, *50*(4): 506–517. Review. Erratum in: *Hormones and Behaviour*, *51*(2): 292–293.

Lin, F.-L., Yeh, M.-L., Lai, Y.-H., Lin, K.-C., Yu, C.-J. & Chang, J.-S. (2019) Two-month breathing-based walking improves anxiety, depression, dyspnoea and quality of life in chronic obstructive pulmonary disease: A randomised controlled study. *Journal of Clinical Nursing*, *28*(19–20): 3632–3640. doi: 10.1111/jocn.14960.

Lin, L.-L., Gu, H.-Y., Yao, Y.-Y., Zhu, J., Niu, Y.-M., Luo, J. & Zhang, C. (2019) The association between watching football matches and the risk of cardiovascular events: A meta-analysis. *Journal of Sports Sciences*, *37*(24): 2826–2834. doi:10.1080/02640414.2019.1665246.

Linardon, J., Shatte, A., McClure, Z. & Fuller-Tyszkiewicz, M. (2023) A broad v. focused digital intervention for recurrent binge eating: A randomized controlled non-inferiority trial. *Psychological Medicine*, *53*(10): 4580–4591. doi:10.1017/S0033291722001477.

Lindegaard, T., Berg, M. & Andersson, G. (2020) Efficacy of internet-delivered psychodynamic therapy: Systematic review and meta-analysis. *Psychodynamic Psychiatry*, *48*(4): 437–454. doi: 10.1521/pdps.2020.48.4.437.

Lindsey, E.W. (2020) Relationship context and emotion regulation across the life span. *Emotion*, *20*: 59–62. doi:10.1037/emo0000666.

Lindson, N., Pritchard, G., Hong, B., Fanshawe, T.R., Pipe, A. & Papadakis, S. (2021) Strategies to improve smoking cessation rates in primary care. *Cochrane Database of Systematic Reviews*, *9*(9): CD011556. doi:10.1002/14651858.CD011556.pub2.

Lindstrom, K.N., Tucker, J.A. & McVay, M. (2023) Nudges and choice architecture to promote healthy food purchases in adults: A systematized review. *Psychology of Addictive Behaviors*, *37*(1): 87–103. doi:10.1037/adb0000892.

Linehan, M.M. (2014) *Skills Training Manual for Treating Borderline Personality Disorder* (2nd edition). New York: Guilford Press.

Ling, C., Bacos, K. & Rönn, T. (2022) Epigenetics of Type 2 diabetes mellitus and weight change – a tool for precision medicine? *Nature Reviews Endocrinology*, *18*(7): 433–448. doi:10.1038/s41574-022-00671-w.

Linhares, B.L., Miranda, E.P., Cintra, A.R., Reges, R. & Torres, L.O. (2022) Use, misuse and abuse of testosterone and other androgens. *Sexual Medicine Reviews*, *10*: 583–595. doi:10.1016/j.sxmr.2021.10.002.

Lipovac, K., ðerić, M., Tešić, M., Andrić, Z. & Marić, B. (2017) Mobile phone use while driving-literary review. *Transportation Research Part F: Traffic Psychology & Behaviour*, *47*: 132–142. doi: 10.1016/j.trf.2017.04.015.

Liu, J., Luo, C., Guo, Y., Cao, F. & Yan, J. (2023) Individual trigger factors for hemorrhagic stroke: Evidence from case-crossover and self-controlled case series studies. *European Stroke Journal*, *8*(3): 808–818. doi:10.1177/23969873231173285.

Liu, L., Xu, M., Marshall, I.J., Wolfe, C.D., Wang, Y. & O'Connell, M.D. (2023) Prevalence and natural history of depression after stroke: A systematic review and meta-analysis of observational studies. *PLoS Medicine*, *20*(3): e1004200. doi:10.1371/journal.pmed.1004200.

Liu, S.Y., Wrosch, C., Morin, A.J.S., Quesnel-Vallée, A. & Pruessner, J.C. (2019) Changes in self-esteem and chronic disease across adulthood: A 16-year longitudinal analysis. *Social Science & Medicine*, *242*: 112600. doi: 10.1016/j.socscimed.2019.112600.

Liu, X., Olsen, J., Agerbo, E., Yuan, W., Cnattingius, S., Gissler, M. & Li, J. (2013) Psychological stress and hospitalization for childhood asthma: A nationwide cohort study in two Nordic countries. *PLoS One*, *8*(10): e78816.

Liu, Y., Zhao, J. & Guo, W. (2018) Emotional roles of mono-aminergic neurotransmitters in major depressive disorder and anxiety disorders. *Frontiers in Psychology*, *9*: 2201. doi: 10.3389/fpsyg.2018.02201.

Liu, Y.-E., While, A.E., Norman, I.J. & Ye, W. (2012) Health professionals' attitudes toward older people and older patients: A systematic review. *Journal of Interprofessional Care*, *26*(5): 397–409. doi: 10.3109/13561820.2012.702146.

Lloyd-Williams, M., Shiels, C., Ellis, J., Abba, K., Gaynor, E., et al. (2018) Pilot randomised controlled trial of focused narrative intervention for moderate to severe depression in palliative care patients: DISCERN trial. *Palliative Medicine*, *32*(1): 206–215. doi: 10.1177/0269216317711322.

Lockhart, K.L. & Keil, F.C. (2018) Introduction: Understanding medicines and medical interventions. *Monographs of the Society for Research in Child Development*, *83*(2): 7–32. doi:10.1111/mono.12361.

Loijen, A., Vrijsen, J.N., Egger, J.I.M., Becker, E.S. & Rinck, M. (2020) Biased approach-avoidance tendencies in psychopathology: A systematic review of their assessment and modification. *Clinical Psychology Review*, *77*: 101825. doi:10.1016/j.cpr.2020.101825.

Loots, E., Goossens, E., Vanwesemael, T., et al. (2021) Interventions to improve medication adherence in patients with schizophrenia or bipolar disorders: A systematic review and meta-analysis. *International Journal of Environmental Research and Public Health*, *18*: 10213. doi:10.3390/ijerph181910213.

López, S.R., Grover, K.P., Holland, D., Johnson, M.J., Kain, C.D., et al. (1989) Development of culturally sensitive psychotherapists. *Professional Psychology: Research and Practice*, *20*(6): 369–376. doi:10.1037/0735-7028.20.6.369.

Lorber, W., Mazzoni, G. & Kirsch, I. (2007) Illness by suggestion: Expectancy, modeling, and gender in the production of psychosomatic symptoms. *Annals of Behavioral Medicine*, *33*(1): 112–116.

Lord, L., McKernon, D., Grzeskowiak, L., Kirsa, S. & Ilomaki, J. (2023) Depression and anxiety prevalence in people with cystic fibrosis and their caregivers: A systematic review and meta-analysis. *Social Psychiatry and Psychiatric Epidemiology*, *58*(2): 287–298. doi:10.1007/s00127-022-02307-w.

Lorig, K.R. & Holman, H. (2003) Self-management education: History, definition, outcomes, and mechanisms. *Annals of Behavioral Medicine, 26*(1): 1–7.

Lorig, K.R., Holman, H., Sobel, D., Laurent, D., Gonzalez, V. & Minor, M. (2007) *Self-Management of Long-Term Health Conditions: A Handbook for People with Chronic Disease*. London: UK Government/Expert Patients Programme Community Interest Company.

Lotfaliany, M., Agustini, B., Kowal, P., Berk, M., & Mohebbi, M. (2019) Co-occurrence of depression with chronic diseases among the older population living in low- and middle-income countries: A compound health challenge. *Annals of Clinical Psychiatry, 31*(2): 95–105.

Lotzin, A., Franc de Pommereau, A. & Laskowsky, I. (2023) Promoting recovery from disasters, pandemics, and trauma: A systematic review of brief psychological interventions to reduce distress in adults, children, and adolescents. *International Journal of Environmental Research and Public Health, 20*(7): 5339. doi: 10.3390/ijerph20075339.

Lourenço, O.M. (2016) Developmental stages, Piagetian stages in particular: A critical review. *New Ideas in Psychology, 40*: 123–137. doi: 10.1016/j.newideapsych.2015.08.002.

Lovallo, W.R. (2004) *Stress & Health: Biological and Psychological Interactions*. Thousand Oaks, CA: Sage.

Love, A.S. & Love, R. (2019) Anxiety disorders in primary care settings. *Nursing Clinics of North America, 54*(4): 473–493. doi:10.1016/j.cnur.2019.07.002.

Low, N.J.H., Leow, D.G.W. & Klainin-Yobas, P. (2024) Effectiveness of technology-based psychosocial interventions on psychological outcomes among adult cancer patients and caregivers: A systematic review and meta-analysis. *Seminars in Oncology Nursing, 40*(1): 151533. doi:10.1016/j.soncn.2023.151533.

Lowe, C.J., Safati, A. & Hall, P.A. (2017) The neurocognitive consequences of sleep restriction: A meta-analytic review. *Neuroscience & Biobehavioral Reviews, 80*: 586–604. doi: 10.1016/j.neubiorev.2017.07.010.

Lun, P., et al. (2022) A social ecological approach to identify the barriers and facilitators to COVID-19 vaccination acceptance: A scoping review. *PLoS One, 17*(10): e0272642. doi:10.1371/journal.pone.0272642.

Lundholm, L., Frisell, T., Lichtenstein, P. & Långström, N. (2015) Anabolic androgenic steroids and violent offending: Confounding by polysubstance abuse among 10,365 general population men. *Addiction, 110*(1): 100–108.

Luria, A.R. (1963 [1948]) *Restoration of Function after Brain Injury*. New York: Macmillan.

Luria, A.R. (1973) *The Working Brain: An Introduction to Neuropsychology*. New York: Basic Books.

Lustman, P.J., Anderson, R.J., Freedland, K.E., de Groot, M., Carney, R.M. & Clouse, R.E. (2000) Depression and poor glycemic control: A meta-analytic review of the literature. *Diabetes Care, 23*(7): 934–942.

Lynch, J.W., Kaplan, G.A., Cohen, R.D., Tuomilehto, J. & Solonen, J.T. (1996) Do cardiovascular risk factors explain the relation between socioeconomic status, risk of all-cause mortality, cardiovascular mortality, and acute myocardial infarction? *American Journal of Epidemiology, 144*(10): 934–942.

Ma, Y., Xie, T., Zhang, J. & Yang, H. (2023) The prevalence, related factors and interventions of oncology nurses' burnout in different continents: A systematic review and meta-analysis. *Journal of Clinical Nursing, 32*(19–20): 7050–7061. doi:10.1111/jocn.16838.

Maas, M.K. & Lefkowitz, E.S. (2015) Sexual esteem in emerging adulthood: Associations with sexual behavior, contraception use, and romantic relationships. *Journal of Sex Research, 52*(7): 795–806. doi: 10.1080/00224499.2014.945112.

Macêdo, T.M., Freitas, D.A., Chaves, G.S., Holloway, E.A. & Mendonça, K.M. (2016)

Breathing exercises for children with asthma. *Cochrane Database of Systematic Reviews, 4*: Art. CD011017. doi:10.1002/14651858. CD011017.pub2.

MacFarlane, A.E. (2020) Optimising individual and community involvement in health decision-making in general practice consultations and primary care settings: A way forward. *European Journal of General Practice, 26*(1): 196–201. doi: 10.1080/13814788.2020.1861245.

Machin, A.R., Babatunde, O., Haththotuwa, R., Scott, I., Blagojevic-Bucknall, M., et al. (2020) The association between anxiety and disease activity and quality of life in rheumatoid arthritis: A systematic review and meta-analysis. *Clinical Rheumatology, 39*(5): 1471–1482. doi:10.1007/s10067-019-04900-y.

Mackenbach, J.P., Valverde, J.R., Bopp, M. et al. (2019) Determinants of inequalities in life expectancy: An international comparative study of eight risk factors. *Lancet Public Health, 4*: e529–e537. doi:10.1016/S2468-2667(19)30147-1.

Maclachlan, L.R., Mills, K., Lawford, B.J., Egerton, T., Setchell, J., et al. (2020) Design, delivery, maintenance, and outcomes of peer-to-peer online support groups for people with chronic musculoskeletal disorders: Systematic review. *Journal of Medical Internet Research, 22*(4): e15822. doi:10.2196/15822.

MacLean, M.W., Hadid, V., Spreng, R.N., & Lepore, F. (2023) Revealing robust neural correlates of conscious and unconscious visual processing: Activation likelihood estimation meta-analyses. *NeuroImage, 273:* 120088. doi:0.1016/j.neuroimage. 2023.120088.

Madadin, M., Al Sahwan, H.S., Altarouti, K.K., Altarouti, S.A., Al Eswaikt, Z.S., & Menezes, R.G. (2020) The Islamic perspective on physician-assisted suicide and euthanasia. *Medicine, Science, and the Law, 60*(4): 278–286. doi:10.1177/0025802420934241.

Magill, M., Ray, L., Kiluk, B., Hoadley, A., Bernstein, M., Tonigan, J.S. & Carroll, K. (2019) A meta-analysis of cognitive-behavioral therapy for alcohol or other drug use disorders: Treatment efficacy by contrast condition. *Journal of Consulting and Clinical Psychology, 87*(12): 1093–1105. doi: 10.1037/ccp0000447.

Maglione, M.A., Maher, A.R., Ewing, B., Colaiaco, B., Newberry, S., et al. (2017) Efficacy of mindfulness meditation for smoking cessation: A systematic review and meta-analysis. *Addictive Behaviors, 69*: 27–34.

Magnolini, R., Falcato, L., Cremonesi, A., Schori, D. & Bruggmann, P. (2022) Fake anabolic androgenic steroids on the black market – a systematic review and meta-analysis on qualitative and quantitative analytical results found within the literature. *BMC Public Health, 22*(1): 1371. doi:10.1186/s12889-022-13734-4.

Mahendiran, M., Yeung, H., Rossi, S., Khosravani, H. & Perri, G.A. (2023) Evaluating the effectiveness of the SPIKES model to break bad news – a systematic review. *American Journal of Hospice and Palliative Medicine, 40*(11): 1231–1260. doi: 10.1177/10499091221146296.

Mahoney, L., Ayers, S. & Seddon, P. (2010) The association between parents' and healthcare professional's behavior and children's coping and distress during venipuncture. *Journal of Pediatric Psychology, 35*(9): 985–995.

Maier, A., Riedel-Heller, S.G., Pabst, A. & Luppa, M. (2021) Risk factors and protective factors of depression in older people 65+. A systematic review. *PloS One, 16*(5): e0251326. doi:10.1371/journal.pone.0251326.

Maier, K.J. & al'Absi, M. (2017) Toward a biopsychosocial ecology of the human microbiome, brain–gut axis, and health. *Psychosomatic Medicine, 79*(8): 947–957. doi: 10.1097/PSY.0000000000000515.

Maina, I.W., Belton, T.D., Ginzberg, S., Singh, A. & Johnson, T.J. (2018) A decade of studying implicit racial/ethnic bias in healthcare providers using the implicit association test. *Social Science & Medicine, 199*: 219–229. doi: 10.1016/j.socscimed. 2017.05.009.

Mainwaring, C., Gabbert, F. & Scott, A.J. (2023) A systematic review exploring variables related to bystander intervention in sexual violence contexts. *Trauma Violence Abuse*, *24*: 1727–1742. doi:10.1177/1524838 0221079660.

Makoul, G. (2001) The SEGUE Framework for teaching and assessing communication skills. *Patient Education and Counseling*, *45*(1): 23–34.

Makris, A.P., Karianaki, M., Tsamis, K. & Paschou, S.A. (2021) The role of the gut–brain axis in depression: Endocrine, neural, and immune pathways. *Hormones*, *20*(1): 1–12. doi:10.1007/s42000-020-00236-4.

Malik, A., Qureshi, H., Abdul-Razakq, H., et al. (2019) 'I decided not to go into surgery due to dress code': A cross-sectional study within the UK investigating experiences of female Muslim medical health professionals on bare below the elbows (BBE) policy and wearing headscarves (hijabs) in theatre. *BMJ Open*, *9*(3): e019954. doi:10.1136/bmjopen-2017-019954.

Mallery, L., MacLeod, T., Allen, M., McLean-Veysey, P. et al. (2019) Systematic review and meta-analysis of second-generation antidepressants for the treatment of older adults with depression: Questionable benefit and considerations for frailty. *BMC Geriatrics*, *19*(1): 306. doi:10.1186/s12877-019-1327-4.

Mamman, R., Grewal, J., Garrone, J.N. & Schmidt, J. (2024) Biopsychosocial factors of quality of life in individuals with moderate to severe traumatic brain injury: A scoping review. *Quality of Life Research*, *33*: 877–901. doi:10.1007/s11136-023-03511-0.

Mamukashvili-Delau, M., Koburger, N., Dietrich, S. & Rummel-Kluge, C. (2022) Efficacy of computer- and/or internet-based cognitive-behavioral guided self-management for depression in adults: A systematic review and meta-analysis of randomized controlled trials. *BMC Psychiatry*, *22*(1): 730. doi:10.1186/s12888-022-04325-z.

Mandal, M.K., Habel, U. & Gur, R.C. (2023) Facial expression-based indicators of schizophrenia: Evidence from recent research. *Schizophrenia Research*, *252*: 335–344. doi:10.1016/j.schres.2023.01.016.

Manninen, S.-M., Kero, K., Perkonoja, K., Vahlberg, T. & Polo-Kantola, P. (2021) General practitioners' self-reported competence in the management of sexual health issues – a web-based questionnaire study from Finland. *Scandinavian Journal of Primary Health Care*, *39*(3): 279–287. doi:10.1080/02813432.2021.1934983.

Marasigan, V., Perry, I., Bennett, K., Balanda, K., Capewell, S., O'Flaherty, M. & Kabir, Z. (2020) Explaining the fall in coronary heart disease mortality in the Republic of Ireland between 2000 and 2015 – IMPACT modelling study. *International Journal of Cardiology*, *310*: 159–161. doi:10.1016/j.ijcard.2020.03.067.

Marcano-Olivier, M.I., Horne, P.J., Viktor, S. & Erjavec, M. (2020) Using nudges to promote healthy food choices in the school dining room: A systematic review of previous investigations. *Journal of School Health*, *90*(2): 143–157. doi: 10.1111/josh.12861.

Marcano-Olivier, M., Sallaway-Costello, J., McWilliams, L., Horne, P.J., Viktor, S. & Erjavec, M. (2021) Changes in the nutritional content of children's lunches after the Food Dudes healthy eating programme. *Journal of Nutritional Science*, *10*: e40. doi:10.1017/jns.2021.31.

Marchetti, I. & Pössel, P. (2023) Cognitive triad and depressive symptoms in adolescence: Specificity and overlap. *Child Psychiatry & Human Development*, *54*(4): 1209–1217. doi:10.1007/s10578-022-01323-w.

Marcinkowska, U.M., Shirazi, T., Mijas, M. & Roney, J.R. (2023) Hormonal underpinnings of the variation in sexual desire, arousal and activity throughout the menstrual cycle – a multifaceted approach. *Journal of Sex Research*, *60*(9): 1297–1303. doi: 10.1080/00224499.2022.2110558.

Marmot, M. (2005) Social determinants of health inequalities. *Lancet*, *365*: 1099–1104.

Marmot, M. & Wilkinson, R. (2006) *Social Determinants of Health* (2nd edition). Oxford: Oxford University Press.

Marques A., Peralta, M., Gouveia, É.R., Chávez, F.G. & Valeiro, M.G. (2018) Physical activity buffers the negative relationship between multimorbidity, self-rated health and life satisfaction. *Journal of Public Health*, *40*(3): e328–e335. doi: 10.1093/pubmed/fdy012.

Marsh, A.A. & Blair, R.J. (2008) Deficits in facial affect recognition among antisocial populations: A meta-analysis. *Neuroscience and Biobehavioral Reviews*, *32*(3): 454–465.

Marshall, B.J. & Warren, J.R. (1984) Unidentified curved bacilli in the stomach of patients with gastritis and peptic ulceration. *Lancet*, *1*(8390): 1311–1315. doi:10.1016/s0140-6736(84)91816-6.

Marucha, P.T., Kiecolt-Glaser, J.K. & Favagehi, M. (1998) Mucosal wound healing is impaired by examination stress. *Psychosomatic Medicine*, *60*(3): 362–365.

Marziliano, A., Tuman, M. & Moyer, A. (2020) The relationship between post-traumatic stress and post-traumatic growth in cancer patients and survivors: A systematic review and meta-analysis. *Psycho-oncology*, *29*(4), 604–616. doi:10.1002/pon.5314.

Masedo, A., Grandón, P., Saldivia, S., et al. (2021) A multicentric study on stigma towards people with mental illness in health sciences students. *BMC Medical Education*, *21*(1): 324. doi:10.1186/s12909-021-02695-8.

Masood, B. & Moorthy, M. (2023) Causes of obesity: A review. *Clinical Medicine*, *23*: 284–91. doi:10.7861/clinmed.2023-0168.

Matcham, F., Davies, R., Hotopf, M., Hyrich, K.L., Norton, S., et al. (2018) The relationship between depression and biologic treatment Cresponse in rheumatoid arthritis: An analysis of the British society for rheumatology biologics register. *Rheumatology*, *57*(5): 835–843. doi: 10.1093/rheumatology/kex528.

Mathot, E., Liberman, K., Cao Dinh, H., Njemini, R. & Bautmans, I. (2021) Systematic review on the effects of physical exercise on cellular immunosenescence-related markers – An update. *Experimental Gerontology*, *149*, 111318. doi:10.1016/j.exger.2021.111318.

Matiz, A., Scaggiante, B., Conversano, C., Gemignani, A., Pascoletti, G., et al. (2024) The effect of mindfulness-based interventions on biomarkers in cancer patients and survivors: A systematic review. *Stress & Health*, *40*(4), e3375. doi: 10.1002/smi.3375. Epub ahead of print.

Mavis, S.C., Caruso, C.G., Dyess, N.F., Carr, C.B., Gerberi, D. & Dadiz, R. (2022) Implicit bias training in health professions education: A scoping review. *Medical Science Educator*, *32*(6): 1541–1552. doi:10.1007/s40670-022-01673-z.

Maxson, P.J., Edwards, S.E., Valentiner, E.M. & Miranda, M.L. (2016) A multidimensional approach to characterizing psychosocial health during pregnancy. *Maternal and Child Health Journal*, *20*(6): 1103–1113.

May, R.M. (1982) Vaccination programmes and herd immunity. *Nature*, *300*(5892): 481–483.

McAteer, G. & Gillanders, D. (2019) Investigating the role of psychological flexibility, masculine self-esteem and stoicism as predictors of psychological distress and quality of life in men living with prostate cancer. *European Journal of Cancer Care*, *28*(4): e13097. doi: 10.1111/ecc.13097.

McClure, C.C., Cataldi, J.R. & O'Leary, S.T. (2017) Vaccine hesitancy: Where we are and where we are going. *Clinical Therapeutics*, *39*(8): 1550–1562. doi: 10.1016/j.clinthera.2017.07.003.

McCombie, A., Gearry, R. & Mulder, R. (2014) Preferences of inflammatory bowel disease patients for computerised versus face-to-face psychological interventions. *Journal of Crohn's and Colitis*, *8*(6): 536–542.

McConville, J., McAleer, R. & Hahne, A. (2017) Mindfulness training for health profession students – The effect of mindfulness training on psychological well-being, learning and clinical performance of health professional students: A systematic review of randomized and non-randomized controlled trials. *Explore*, *13*(1): 26–45. doi:10.1016/j.explore.2016.10.002.

McCracken, L.M. & Morley, S. (2014) The psychological flexibility model: A basis for integration and progress in psychological approaches to chronic pain management. *Journal of Pain*, *15*(3): 221–234.

McCreary, D.R., Oliffe, J.L., Black, N., Flannigan, R., Rachert, J. & Goldenberg, S.L. (2020) Canadian men's health stigma, masculine role norms and lifestyle behaviors. *Health Promotion International*, *35*(3): 535–543. doi:10.1093/heapro/daz049.

McDermott, M.S., Oliver, M., Simnadis, T., Beck, E.J., Coltman, T., Iverson, D., Caputi, P. & Sharma, R. (2015) The theory of planned behaviour and dietary patterns: A systematic review and meta-analysis. *Preventive Medicine*, *81*: 150–156. doi: 10.1016/j.ypmed.2015.08.020.

McEwen, B.S. (1998) Stress, adaptation, and disease: Allostasis and allostatic load. *Annals of the New York Academy of Science*, *840*(1): 33–44.

McGettigan, M., Cardwell, C.R., Cantwell, M.M. & Tully, M.A. (2020) Physical activity interventions for disease-related physical and mental health during and following treatment in people with non-advanced colorectal cancer. *Cochrane Database of Systematic Reviews*, *5*(5): Art. CD012864. doi:10.1002/14651858. CD012864.pub2.

McGovern, C.M., Harrison, R. & Arcoleo, K. (2023) Integrative review of programs to improve outcomes for children with comorbid asthma and anxiety/depressive symptoms. *Journal of School Nursing*, *39*(1): 37–50. doi:10.1177/10598405211061508.

McGrady, M.E. & Pai, A.L.H. (2019) A systematic review of rates, outcomes, and predictors of medication non-adherence among adolescents and young adults with cancer. *Journal of Adolescent and Young Adult Oncolog*, *8*(5): 485–494. doi:10.1089/jayao.2018.0160.

McGraw, J., White, K.M. & Russell-Bennett, R. (2021) Masculinity and men's health service use across four social generations: Findings from Australia's *Ten to Men study*. *SSM – Population Health*, *15*: 100838. doi:10.1016/j.ssmph.2021.100838.

McGregor, G., Powell, R., Kimani, P. & Underwood, M. (2020) Does contemporary exercise-based cardiac rehabilitation improve quality of life for people with coronary artery disease? A systematic review and meta-analysis. *BMJ Open*, *10*(6): e036089. doi:10.1136/bmjopen-2019-036089.

McGowan, C. & Bland, R. (2023) The benefits of breastfeeding on child intelligence, behavior, and executive function: A review of recent evidence. *Breastfeeding Medicine*, *18*(3): 172–187. doi:10.1089/bfm.2022.0192.

McHugh, J., Saunders, E.J., Dadaev, T., McGrowder, E., Bancroft, E., et al. (2022) Prostate cancer risk in men of differing genetic ancestry and approaches to disease screening and management in these groups. *British Journal of Cancer*, *126*(10): 1366–1373. doi:10.1038/s41416-021-01669-3.

McHugh, P.R. (1989) The neuropsychiatry of basal ganglia disorders: A triadic syndrome and its explanation. *Neuropsychiatry, Neuropsychology & Behavioral Neurology*, *2*(4): 239–247.

McKnight, R., Price, J. & Geddes, J. (2019) *Psychiatry* (5th edition). Oxford: Oxford University Press.

Mclaren, S., Jhamb, M. & Unruh, M. (2021) Using patient-reported measures to improve outcomes in kidney disease. *Blood Purification*, *50*(4–5): 649–654. doi:10.1159/000515640

McManus, I.C., Keeling, A. & Paice, E. (2004) Stress, burnout and doctors' attitudes to work are determined by personality and learning style: A twelve-year longitudinal study of UK medical graduates. *BMC Medicine*, *2*(1): 1–12.

McMillan, D. & Lee, R. (2010) A systematic review of behavioral experiments vs. exposure alone in the treatment of anxiety disorders: A case of exposure while wearing the emperor's new clothes? *Clinical Psychology Review, 30*(5): 467–478. doi: 10.1016/j.cpr.2010.01.003.

McParlin, C., O'Donnell, A., Robson, S.C., Beyer, F., Moloney, E., et al. (2016) Treatments for hyperemesis gravidarum and nausea and vomiting in pregnancy: A systematic review. *JAMA, 316*(13): 1392–1401. doi: 10.1001/jama.2016.14337.

McPhee, G.M., Downey, L.A., Stough, C. (2019) Effects of sustained cognitive activity on white matter microstructure and cognitive outcomes in healthy middle-aged adults: A systematic review. *Ageing Research Reviews, 51*: 35–47. doi: 10.1016/j. arr.2019.02.004.

McWhinney, I. (1989) The need for a transformed clinical method. In M. Stewart & D. Roter (eds), *Communicating with Medical Patients*. Newbury Park, CA: Sage (pp. 25–40).

Meads, C. & Nouwen, A. (2005) Does emotional disclosure have any effects? A systematic review of the literature with meta-analyses. *International Journal of Technology Assessment in Health Care, 21*(2): 153–164.

Meechan, C.F., Laws, K.R., Young, A.H., McLoughlin, D.M. & Jauhar, S. (2022) A critique of narrative reviews of the evidence-base for ECT in depression. *Epidemiology and Psychiatric Sciences, 31*: e10. doi:10.1017/S2045796021000731.

Meeuwis, S.H., Wasylewski, M.T., Bajcar, E.A., Bieniek, H., Adamczyk, W.M., et al. (2023) Learning pain from others: A systematic review and meta-analysis of studies on placebo hypoalgesia and nocebo hyperalgesia induced by observational learning. *Pain, 164*(11): 2383–2396. doi:10.1097/j.pain.0000000000002943.

Mehrotra, R., Cukor, D., Unruh, M., Rue, T., Heagerty, P., et al. (2019) Comparative efficacy of therapies for treatment of depression for patients undergoing maintenance hemodialysis: A randomized clinical trial. *Annals of Internal Medicine, 170*(6): 369–379. doi: 10.7326/M18-2229.

Mehta, C.M., Arnett, J.J., Palmer, C.G. & Nelson, L.J. (2020) Established adulthood: A new conception of ages 30 to 45. *American Psychologist, 75*(4): 431–444. doi:10.1037/amp0000600.

Mehta, P.K., Sharma, A., Bremner, J.D. & Vaccarino, V. (2022) Mental stress-induced myocardial ischemia. *Current Cardiology Reports, 24*(12): 2109–2120. doi:10.1007/s11886-022-01821-2.

Meier, M., Wirz, L., Dickinson, P. & Pruessner, J.C. (2021) Laughter yoga reduces the cortisol response to acute stress in healthy individuals. *Stress, 24*(1): 44–52. doi:10.1080/10253890.2020.1766018.

Meissner, C.A. & Brigham, J.C. (2001) Thirty years of investigating the own-race bias in memory for faces: A meta-analytic review. *Psychology, Public Policy & Law, 7*(1): 3–35.

Meissner, K. (2009) Effects of placebo interventions on gastric motility and general autonomic activity. *Journal of Psychosomatic Research, 66*(5): 391–398.

Melby, M.K., Lock, M. & Kaufert, P. (2005) Culture and symptom reporting at menopause. *Human Reproduction Update, 11*(5): 495–512.

Melendez-Torres, G.J., Grant, S. & Bonell, C. (2015) A systematic review and critical appraisal of qualitative metasynthetic practice in public health to develop a taxonomy of operations of reciprocal translation. *Research Synthesis Methods, 6*(4): 357–371.

Melzack, R. (1999) From the gate to the neuromatrix. *Pain*, Suppl. *6*: S121–S126.

Melzack, R. & Wall, P.D. (1965) Pain mechanisms: A new theory. *Science, 150*(3699): 971–979.

Memon, A., Barber, J., Rumsby, E., et al. (2016) Opinions of women from deprived communities on the NHS stop smoking service in England. *European Journal of Person-Centered Healthcare, 4*: 346–351. doi:10.5750/EJPCH.V4I2.1101.

Memon, A., Taylor, K., Mohebati, L.M., Sundin, J., Cooper, M., Scanlon, T. & de Visser, R. (2016) Perceived barriers to accessing mental health services among Black and Minority Ethnic (BME) communities: A qualitative study in Southeast England. *BMJ Open*, *6*(11): e012337.

Mendell, L.M. (2014) Constructing and deconstructing the gate theory of pain. *Pain*, *155*(2): 210–216.

Menezes, P., Guraya, S.Y. & Guraya, S.S. (2021) A systematic review of educational interventions and their impact on empathy and compassion of undergraduate medical students. *Frontiers in Medicine*, *8*: 758377. doi: 10.3389/fmed.2021.758377.

Meng, J., Rains, S.A. & An, Z. (2021) How cancer patients benefit from support networks offline and online: Extending the model of structural-to-functional support. *Health Communication*, *36*: 198–206. doi:10.1080/10410236.2019.1673947.

Menz, F. & Al-Roubaie, A. (2008) Interruptions, status and gender in medical interviews: The harder you brake, the longer it takes. *Discourse & Society*, *19*(5): 645–666.

Mercer, D.A., Ditto, B., Lavoie, K.L., Campbell, T., Arsenault, A. & Bacon, S.L. (2018) Health locus of control is associated with physical activity and other health behaviors in cardiac patients. *Journal of Cardiopulmonary Rehabilitation & Prevention*, *38*(6): 394–399. doi: 10.1097/HCR.0000000000000350.

Mereish, E.H. & Bradford, J.B. (2014) Intersecting identities and substance use problems: Sexual orientation, gender, race, and lifetime substance use problems. *Journal of Studies on Alcohol and Drugs*, *75*(1): 179–188.

Merel, S.E., McKinney, C.M., Ufkes, P., Kwan, A.C. & White, A.A. (2016) Sitting at patients' bedsides may improve patients' perceptions of physician communication skills. *British Journal of Hospital Medicine*, *11*(12): 865–868.

Mesman, E., Vreeker, A. & Hillegers, M. (2021) Resilience and mental health in children and adolescents: An update of the recent literature and future directions. *Current Opinion in Psychiatry*, *34*(6): 586–592. doi:10.1097/YCO.0000000000000741.

Mesman, J., van Ijzendoom, M.H. & Bakermans-Kranenberg, M.J. (2009) The many faces of the Still-Face Paradigm: A review and meta-analysis. *Development Review*, *29*(2): 120–162.

Michie, S., van Stralen, M.M. & West, R. (2011) The behaviour change wheel: A new method for characterising and designing behaviour change interventions. *Implementation Science*, *6*: 42. doi: 10.1186/1748-5908-6-42.

Michie, S., Wood, C.E., Johnston, M., Abraham, C., Francis, J.J. & Hardeman, W. (2015) Behaviour change techniques: The development and evaluation of a taxonomic method for reporting and describing behaviour change interventions. *Health Technology Assessment*, *19*(99): 1–188.

Milad, E. & Bogg, T. (2020) Personality traits, coping, health-related behaviors, and cumulative physiological health in a national sample: 10 year prospective effects of conscientiousness via perceptions of activity on allostatic load. *Annals of Behavioral Medicine*, *54*: 880–892. doi:10.1093/abm/kaaa024.

Milgram, S. (1974) *Obedience to Authority*. New York: Harper & Row.

Millar, K., Purushotham, A.D., McLatchie, E., George, W.D. & Murray, G.D. (2005) A 1-year prospective study of individual variation in distress and illness perceptions, after treatment for breast cancer. *Journal of Psychosomatic Research*, *58*(4): 335–342.

Miller, G.A. (1956) The magical number seven, plus or minus two: Some limits on our capacity for processing information. *Psychological Review*, *63*(2): 81–97.

Miller, M., Mangano, C., Park, Y., Goel, R., Plotnick, G.D. & Vogel, R.A. (2006) Impact of cinematic viewing on endothelial function. *Heart*, *92*(2): 261–262.

Miller, W.R. & Rollnick, S. (2002) *Motivational Interviewing: Preparing People for Change*. New York: Guilford Press.

Miller, W.R. & Rollnick, S. (2013) *Motivational Interviewing: Helping People Change*. New York: Guilford Press.

Miller, W.R. & Rollnick, S. (2023) *Motivational Interviewing: Helping People to Change* (4th edition). New York: Guilford Press.

Mills, S.E.E., Nicolson, K.P. & Smith, B.H. (2019) Chronic pain: A review of its epidemiology and associated factors in population-based studies. *British Journal of Anaesthesia*, *123*(2): e273–e283. doi:10.1016/j.bja.2019.03.023.

Minano-Garrido, E.J., Catalan-Matamoros, D., & Gómez-Conesa, A. (2022) Physical therapy interventions in patients with anorexia nervosa: A systematic review. *International Journal of Environmental Research and Public Health*, *19*(21): 13921. doi:10.3390/ijerph192113921.

Mitchell, J.T., Zylowska, L. & Kollins, S.H. (2015) Mindfulness meditation training for Attention-Deficit/Hyperactivity Disorder in adulthood: Current empirical support, treatment overview, and future directions. *Cognitive and Behavioral Practice*, *22*(2): 172–191.

Mitchell, K.R., Brassil, K.J., Rodriguez, S.A., Tsai, E., Fujimoto, K., et al. (2020) Operationalizing patient-centered cancer care: A systematic review and synthesis of the qualitative literature on cancer patients' needs, values, and preferences. *Psychooncology*, *29*(11): 1723–1733. doi: 10.1002/pon.5500.

Mitchison, D. & Mond, J. (2015) Epidemiology of eating disorders, eating disordered behaviour, and body image disturbance in males: A narrative review. *Journal of Eating Disorders*, *3*: 20. doi: 10.1186/s40337-015-0058-y.

Mitte, K. (2005) Meta-analysis of cognitive-behavioral treatments for generalized anxiety disorder: A comparison with pharmacotherapy. *Psychological Bulletin*, *131*(5): 785–795.

Mjaaland, T.A. & Finset, A. (2009) Frequency of GP communication addressing the patient's resources and coping strategies in medical interviews: A video-based observational study. *BMC Family Practice*, *10*: 49.

Moberg, K.U., Handlin, L. & Petersson, M. (2020) Neuroendocrine mechanisms involved in the physiological effects caused by skin-to-skin contact – with a particular focus on the oxytocinergic system. *Infant Behavior and Development*, *61*: 101482. doi:10.1016/j.infbeh.2020.101482.

Modzelewski, S., Oracz, A., Żukow, X., Iłendo, K., Śledzikowka, Z. & Waszkiewicz, N. (2024) Premenstrual syndrome: New insights into etiology and review of treatment methods. *Frontiers in Psychiatry*, *15*: 1363875. doi: 10.3389/fpsyt.2024.1363875.

Mogk, C., Otte, S., Reinhold-Hurley, B. & Kroner-Herwig, B. (2006) Health effects of expressive writing on stressful or traumatic experiences: A meta-analysis. *Psycho-Social Medicine*, *16*(3): Doc06.

Mohamed, F.B.M., Cheng, L.J. Chia, W.E.R., Turunen, H. & He, H.G. (2024) Global prevalence and factors associated with workplace violence against nursing students: A systematic review, meta-analysis, and meta-regression. *Aggression and Violent Behavior*, *75*: 101907. doi:10.1016/j.avb.2023.101907.

Mohamud, M.A., Campbell, D.J.T., Wick, J., Leung, A.A., Fabreau, G.E., Tonelli, M. & Ronksley, P.E. (2023) 20-year trends in multimorbidity by race/ethnicity among hospitalized patient populations in the United States. *International Journal for Equity in Health*, *22*(1): 137. doi:10.1186/s12939-023-01950-2.

Mok, J.W., Oh, Y.H., Magge, D. & Padmanabhan, S. (2024) Racial disparities of gastric cancer in the USA: An overview of epidemiology, global screening guidelines, and targeted screening in a heterogeneous population. *Gastric Cancer*, *27*(3): 426–438. doi:10.1007/s10120-024-01475-9.

Mokdad, A.H., Forouzanfar, M.H., Daoud, F., Mokdad, A.A., El Bcheraoui, C., et al. (2016) Global burden of diseases, injuries, and risk factors for young people's health during 1990–2013: A systematic analysis for the global burden of disease study 2013. *Lancet*, *387*(10036): 2383–2401. doi: 10.1016/S0140-6736(16)00648-6.

Möller, S.P., Hayes, B., Wilding, H., Apputhurai, P., Tye-Din, J.A. & Knowles, S.R. (2021) Systematic review: Exploration of the impact of psychosocial factors on quality of life in adults living with coeliac disease. *Journal of Psychosomatic Research*, *147*: 110537. doi:10.1016/j.jpsychores.2021.110537.

Möller-Leimkuhler, A.M. (2002) Barriers to help-seeking by men: A review of sociocultural and clinical literature with particular reference to depression. *Journal of Affective Disorders, 71*(1–3): 1–9.

Molloy, G.J., Stamatakis, E., Randall, G. & Hamer, M. (2009) Marital status, gender and cardiovascular mortality: Behavioural, psychological distress and metabolic explanations. *Social Science & Medicine*, *69*(2): 223–228.

Monahan, J.L., Murphy, S.T. & Zajonc, R.B. (2000) Subliminal mere exposure: Specific, general and diffuse effects. *Psychological Science, 11*(6): 462–466.

Mondaini, N., Gontero, P., Giubilei, G., Lombardi, G., Cai, T., et al. (2007) Finasteride 5 mg and sexual side effects: how many of these are related to a nocebo phenomenon? *Journal of Sexual Medicine*, *4*(6): 1708–1712. doi:10.1111/j.1743-6109.2007.00563.x.

Moniruzzaman, M., Kadota, A., Akash, M.S., et al. (2021) Effects of physical activities on dementia-related biomarkers: A systematic review of randomized controlled trials. *Alzheimer's & Dementia, 6*(1): e12109. doi:10.1002/trc2.12109.

Mønsted, B. & Lehmann, S. (2022) Characterizing polarization in online vaccine discourse: A large-scale study. *PLoS One, 17*(2): e0263746. doi:10.1371/journal.pone.0263746.

Montgomery, A. & Maslach, C. (2019) Burnout in health professionals. In C.D. Llewellyn, S. Ayers, C. McManus, S. Newman, K.J. Petrie, T.A. Revenson & J. Weinman (eds), *The Cambridge Handbook of Psychology, Health and Medicine* (3rd edition). Cambridge: Cambridge University Press.

Montoya, R.M., Kershaw, C. & Prosser, J.L. (2018) A meta-analytic investigation of the relation between interpersonal attraction and enacted behavior. *Psychological Bulletin, 144*(7): 673–709. doi:10.1037/bul0000148.

Mooney, C.J., Elliot, A.J., Douthit, K.Z., Marquis, A. & Seplaki, C.L. (2016) Perceived control mediates effects of socioeconomic status and chronic stress on physical frailty: Findings from the health and retirement study. *Journal of Gerontology B: Psychological Sciences and Social Sciences, 73*(7): 1175–1184. doi: 10.1093/geronb/gbw096.

Moore, J.B., Rubin, K.C.R. & Heaney, C.A. (2023) Benefit finding and well-being over the course of the COVID-19 pandemic. *PLoS One, 18*(7): e0288332. doi:10.1371/journal.pone.0288332.

Moore R. (2022) Maximizing student clinical communication skills in dental education – a narrative review. *Dentistry Journal* (Basel), *10*(4): 57. doi: 10.3390/dj10040057.

Moos, R.H. & Schaefer, J.A. (1984) The crisis of physical illness: An overview and conceptual approach. In R.H. Moos (ed.), *Coping with Physical Illness*. Vol *2: New Perspectives*. New York: Plenum (pp. 3–25).

Moreau, C., Kågesten, A.E. & Blum, R.W. (2016) Sexual dysfunction among youth: An overlooked sexual health concern. *BMC Public Health, 16*(1): 1170.

Morgan, T., Bharmal, A., Duschinsky, R. & Barclay, S. (2020) Experiences of oldest-old caregivers whose partner is approaching end-of-life: A mixed-method systematic review and narrative synthesis. *PloS One, 15*(6): e0232401. doi:10.1371/journal.pone.0232401.

Morley, S. (2007) Pain management. In S. Ayers, A. Baum, C. McManus, S. Newman, K. Wallston, J. Weinman & R. West (eds), *Cambridge Handbook of Psychology, Health and Medicine* (2nd edition). Cambridge: Cambridge University Press (pp. 370–374).

Morris, J., Tattan-Birch, H., Albery, I.P., Heather, N. & Moss, A.C. (2024) Look away now! Defensive processing and unrealistic optimism by level of alcohol consumption. *Psychology & Health*, published online: 20 February. doi:10.1080/08870446.2024.2316681.

Morris, N., Moghaddam, N., Tickle, A. & Biswas, S. (2018) The relationship between coping style and psychological distress in people with head and neck cancer: A systematic review. *Psycho-oncology*, *27*(3): 734–747. doi:10.1002/pon.4509.

Morrison, A. (2023) Narrative and its discontents. *Medical Humanities*, *49*: 497–499. doi:10.1136/medhum-2022-012511.

Moseley, J.B., O'Malley, K., Petersen, N.J., Menke, T.J., Brody, B.A., Kuykendall, D.H., Hollingsworth, J.C., Ashton, C.M. & Wray, N.P. (2002) A controlled trial of arthroscopic surgery for osteoarthritis of the knee. *New England Journal of Medicine*, *347*(2): 81–88.

Mostafaei, H., Mori, K., Hajebrahimi, S., Abufaraj, M., Karakiewicz, P. I. & Shariat, S. F. (2021) Association of erectile dysfunction and cardiovascular disease: An umbrella review of systematic reviews and meta-analyses. *BJU International*, *128*(1): 3–11. doi:10.1111/bju.15313.

Motahari-Tabari, N.S., Nasiri-Amiri, F., Faramarzi, M., Shirvani, M.A., Bakhtiari, A. & Omidvar, S. (2023) The effectiveness of information–motivation–behavioral skills model on self-care practices in early pregnancy to prevent gestational diabetes mellitus in Iranian overweight and obese women: A randomized controlled trial. *Community Health Equity Research & Policy*, *43*(3): 257–264. doi:10.1177/0272684X211020300.

Mücke, M., Ludyga, S., Colledge, F. & Gerber, M. (2018) Influence of regular physical activity and fitness on stress reactivity as measured with the Trier social stress test protocol: A systematic review. *Sports Medicine*, *48*(11): 2607–2622. doi:10.1007/s40279-018-0979-0.

Mulligan, K. & Newman, S. (2019) Self-management interventions. In C.D. Llewellyn, S. Ayers, C. McManus, S. Newman, K.J. Petrie, T.A. Revenson & J. Weinman (eds), *The Cambridge Handbook of Psychology, Health and Medicine* (3rd edition). Cambridge: Cambridge University Press.

Mundle, R., Afenya, E. & Agarwal, N. (2021) The effectiveness of psychological intervention for depression, anxiety, and distress in prostate cancer: A systematic review of literature. *Prostate Cancer and Prostatic Diseases, 24*(3): 674–687. doi:10.1038/s41391-021-00342-3.

Munro, J., Angus, N. & Leslie, S.J. (2013) Patient focused internet-based approaches to cardiovascular rehabilitation – a systematic review. *Journal of Telemedicine and Telecare, 19*(6): 347–353. doi:10.1177/1357633X13501763.

Mura, G., Carta, M.G., Sancassiani, F., Machado, S. & Prosperini, L. (2018) Active exergames to improve cognitive functioning in neurological disabilities: A systematic review and meta-analysis. *European Journal of Physical and Rehabilitation Medicine, 54*(3): 450–462. doi:10.23736/S1973-9087.17.04680-9.

Murali, K.M., Mullan, J., Roodenrys, S., Hassan, H.C., Lambert, K. & Lonergan, M. (2019) Strategies to improve dietary, fluid, dialysis or medication adherence in patients with end stage kidney disease on dialysis: A systematic review and meta-analysis of randomized intervention trials. *PLoS One, 14*(1): e0211479. doi: 10.1371/journal.pone.0211479.

Muratore, A.F. & Attia, E. (2022) Psychopharmacologic management of eating disorders. *Current Psychiatry Reports, 24*: 345–351. doi:10.1007/s11920-022-01340-5.

Murphy, D.H., Hoover, K.M., Agadzhanyan, K., Kuehn, J.C. & Castel, A.D. (2022) Learning in double time: The effect of lecture video speed on immediate and delayed comprehension. *Applied Cognitive*

Psychology, 36(1): 69–82. doi:10.1002/acp.3899.

Murray, E. (2012) Web-based interventions for behavior change and self-management: Potential, pitfalls, and progress. *Medicine 2.0, 1*(2): e3.

Mustian, K.M., Alfano, C.M., Heckler, C., Kleckner, A.S., Kleckner, I.R., et al. (2017) Comparison of pharmaceutical, psychological, and exercise treatments for cancer-related fatigue: A meta-analysis. *JAMA Oncology, 3*(7): 961–968. doi: 10.1001/jamaoncol.2016.6914.

Myint, P.K., Luben, R.N., Wareham, N.J., Bingham, S.A. & Khaw, K.T. (2009) Combined effect of health behaviours and risk of first ever stroke in 20,040 men and women over 11 years' follow-up in Norfolk cohort of European Prospective Investigation of Cancer (EPIC Norfolk): Prospective population study. *British Medical Journal, 338*(2): b349. doi: 10.1136/bmj.b349.

Naeem, F., Phiri, P., Rathod, S. & Ayub, M. (2019) Cultural adaptation of cognitive–behavioural therapy. *BJPsych Advances. 25*(6): 387–395. doi:10.1192/bja.2019.15.

Naik, S.S., Nidhi, Y., Kumar, K. & Grover, S. (2023) Diagnostic validity of premenstrual dysphoric disorder: Revisited. *Frontiers in Global Women's Health, 4*: 1181583. doi: 10.3389/fgwh.2023.1181583.

Naji, L., Singh, B., Shah, A., Naji, F., Dennis, B., et al. (2021) Global prevalence of burnout among postgraduate medical trainees: A systematic review and meta-regression. *CMAJ Open, 9*(1): E189–E200. doi:10.9778/cmajo.20200068.

Naseralallah, L., Stewart, D., Azfar Ali, R., & Paudyal, V. (2022). An umbrella review of systematic reviews on contributory factors to medication errors in health-care settings. *Expert opinion on drug safety, 21*(11), 1379–1399. doi:10.1080/14740338.2022.2147921

Natale, P., Palmer, S.C., Ruospo, M., Saglimbene, V.M., Rabindranath, K.S. & Strippoli, G.F. (2019) Psychosocial interventions for preventing and treating depression in dialysis patients. *Cochrane Database of Systematic Reviews, 12*(12): Art. CD004542. doi: 10.1002/14651858.CD004542.pub3.

National Institute for Health and Care Excellence (2019) *Menopause: Diagnosis and Treatment.* NICE Guideline [NG23]. London: NICE. Available from www.nice.org.uk/guidance/ng23/chapter/Recommendations#managing-short-term-menopausal-symptoms (accessed 25 July 2024).

National Institute for Health and Care Excellence (2020) *Antenatal and Postnatal Mental Health: Clinical Management and Service Guidance.* Clinical Guideline [CG192]. London: NICE. Available from www.nice.org.uk/guidance/ng222 (accessed 25 July 2024).

National Institute for Health and Care Excellence (2022) *Depression in Adults: Treatment and Management.* Clinical Guideline [NG222]. London: NICE. Available from www.nice.org.uk/guidance/ng222 (accessed 30 July 2024).

Naylor, C., Parsonage, M., McDaid, D., Knapp, M., Fossey, M. & Galea, A. (2012) *Long-term Conditions and Mental Health: The Cost of Co-morbidities.* London: The Kings Fund and Centre for Mental Health.

Neimeyer, R.A., Wittkowski, J. & Moser, R.P. (2004) Psychological research on death attitudes: An overview and evaluation. *Death Studies, 28*(4): 309–340.

Nelson, J.E. (1999) Saving lives and saving deaths. *Annals of Internal Medicine, 130*(9): 776–777.

New Zealand Ministry of Social Development (2016) *The Social Report 2016 – Te pūrongo oranga tangata.* Wellington: NZMSD. Available from https://socialreport.msd.govt.nz/health/life-expectancy-at-birth.html (accessed 2 February 2024).

Newby, J.M., Twomey, C., YuanLi, S.S. & Andrews, G. (2016) Transdiagnostic computerised cognitive behavioural therapy for depression and anxiety: A systematic review and meta-analysis. *Journal of Affective Disorders, 199*: 30–41.

Newton, J.N. (2021) Trends in health expectancies across Europe: Countries that are achieving compression of morbidity and those that are not. *Lancet Regional Health Europe*, *3*: 100078. doi:10.1016/j.lanepe.2021.100078.

Nexø, M.A., Watt, T., Cleal, B., Hegedüs, L., Bonnema, S.J., Rasmussen, Å.K., Feldt-Rasmussen, U. & Bjorner, J.B. (2015) Exploring the experiences of people with hypo- and hyperthyroidism. *Qualitative Health Research*, *25*(7): 945–953.

Ng, Q.X., Soh, A., Loke, W., Venkatanarayanan, N., Lim, D.Y. & Yeo, W.S. (2019) Systematic review with meta-analysis: The association between post-traumatic stress disorder and irritable bowel syndrome. *Journal of Gastroenterology & Hepatology*, *34*: 68–73.

Nguyen, C.M., Koo, J. & Cordoro, K.M. (2016) Psycho-dermatologic effects of atopic dermatitis and acne: A review on self-esteem and identity. *Pediatric Dermatology*, *33*(2): 129–135. doi: 10.1111/pde.12802.

NHS Business Services Authority (2023) *Statistics and Data Science: Hormone Replacement Therapy – England – April 2015 to June 2023*. London: NHS Business Services Authority. Available from www.nhsbsa.nhs.uk/statistical-collections/hormone-replacement-therapy-england/hormone-replacement-therapy-england-april-2015-june-2023 (accessed 25 January 2025).

NHS Digital (2022) *Maternity Services Monthly Statistics*. June. Available from https://digital.nhs.uk/data-and-information/publications/statistical/maternity-services-monthly-statistics/june-2022-experimental-statistics (accessed 25 July 2024).

NHS England (2022) *NHS Workforce Race Equality Standard: 2021 Data Analysis Report for NHS Trusts*. March. London: NHS England. Available from www.england.nhs.uk/wp-content/uploads/2022/04/Workforce-Race-Equality-Standard-report-2021-.pdf (accessed 25 January 2025).

Ni, Y., Zhou, Y., Kivimäki, M., Cai, Y. et al. (2023) Socioeconomic inequalities in physical, psychological, and cognitive multimorbidity in middle-aged and older adults in 33 countries: A cross-sectional study. *Lancet Healthy Longevity*, *4*(11): e618–e628. doi:10.1016/S2666-7568(23)00195-2.

Niedenthal P.M. (2007) Embodying emotion. *Science*, *316*(5827), 1002–1005. https://doi.org/10.1126/science.1136930.

Nieuwlaat, R., Wilczynski, N., Navarro, T., Hobson, N., Jeffery, R., et al. (2014) Interventions for enhancing medication adherence. *Cochrane Database of Systematic Reviews*, *11*: Art. CD000011.

Nikolova, Y.S. & Hariri, A.R. (2015) Can we observe epigenetic effects on human brain function? *Trends in Cognitive Sciences*, *19*(7): 366–373. doi: 10.1016/j.tics.2015.05.003.

Nobile, S., Di Sipio Morgia, C. & Vento, G. (2022) Perinatal origins of adult disease and opportunities for health promotion: A narrative review. *Journal of Personalized Medicine*, *12*(2): 157. doi: 10.3390/jpm12020157.

Noble, L.M., Manalastas, G., Viney, R. & Griffin, A.E. (2022) Does the structure of the medical consultation align with an educational model of clinical communication? A study of physicians' consultations from a postgraduate examination. *Patient Education and Counseling*, *105*(6): 1449–1456. doi: 10.1016/j.pec.2021.10.001.

Nolsøe, A.B., Jensen, C.F.S, Østergren, P.B. & Fode, M. (2021) Neglected side effects to curative prostate cancer treatments. *International Journal of Impotence Research*, *33*(4): 428–438. doi:10.1038/s41443-020-00386-4.

Noone, J. & Najjar, R.H. (2021) Minimizing unconscious bias in nursing school admission. *Journal of Nursing Education*, *60*: 317–323. doi:10.3928/01484834-20210520-03.

Normansell, R., Kew, K.M. & Stovold, E. (2017) Interventions to improve adherence to inhaled steroids for asthma. *Cochrane Database of Systematic Reviews*, *4*(4): Art. CD012226. doi:10.1002/14651858.CD012226.pub2.

Nouwen, A., Adriaanse, M.C., van Dam, K., Iversen, M.M., Viechtbauer, W., et al. (2019) Longitudinal associations between depression and diabetes complications: A systematic review and meta-analysis. *Diabetic Medicine, 36*(12): 1562–1572. doi: 10.1111/dme.14054.

Nurius, P.S., Green, S., Logan-Greene, P. & Borja, S. (2015) Life course pathways of adverse childhood experiences toward adult psychological well-being: A stress process analysis. *Child Abuse & Neglect, 45*: 143–153. doi: 10.1016/j.chiabu.2015.03.008.

Nussbaumer-Streit, B., Mayr, V., Dobrescu, A.I., Chapman, A., Persad, E., et al. (2020) Quarantine alone or in combination with other public health measures to control COVID-19: A rapid review. *Cochrane Database of Systematic Reviews, 4*: Art. CD013574. doi: 10.1002/14651858.CD013574.

Nyssen, O.P., Taylor, S.J., Wong, G., Steed, E., Bourke, L., et al. (2016) Does therapeutic writing help people with long-term conditions? Systematic review, realist synthesis and economic considerations. *Health Technology Assessment, 20*(27): vii–367. doi: 10.3310/hta20270.

O'Brien, K.H., Putney, J.M., Hebert, N.W., Falk, A.M. & Aguinaldo, L.D. (2016) Sexual and gender minority youth suicide: Understanding subgroup differences to inform interventions. *LGBT Health, 3*(4): 248–251.

O'Connell, M.A., Leahy-Warren, P., Khashan, A.S., Kenny, L.C. & O'Neill, S.M. (2017) Worldwide prevalence of tocophobia in pregnant women: Systematic review and meta-analysis. *Acta Obstetricia et Gynecologica Scandinavica, 96*(8): 907–920. doi: 10.1111/aogs.13138.

O'Connor, M.F. & Seeley, S.H. (2022) Grieving as a form of learning: Insights from neuroscience applied to grief and loss. *Current Opinion in Psychology, 43*: 317–322. doi:10.1016/j.copsyc.2021.08.019.

O'Connor, S. & Andrews, T. (2018) Smartphones and mobile applications (apps) in clinical nursing education: A student perspective. *Nurse Education Today,* *69*: 172–178. doi:10.1016/j.nedt.2018.07.013.

O'Farrell, T.J. & Clements, K. (2012) Review of outcome research on marital and family therapy in treatment for alcoholism. *Journal of Marital and Familly Therapy, 38*(1): 122–144.

O'Sullivan, E.D. & Schofield, S.J. (2018) Cognitive bias in clinical medicine. *Journal of the Royal College of Physicians of Edinburgh, 48*(3): 225–232. doi: 10.4997/JRCPE.2018.306.

Ocañez, K.L., McHugh, R.K. & Otto, M.W. (2010) A meta-analytic review of the association between anxiety sensitivity and pain. *Depression and Anxiety, 27*(8): 760–767.

Ochsner, K.N. & Gross, J.J. (2005) The cognitive control of emotion. *Trends in Cognitive Science, 9*(5): 242–249.

Odor, P.M., Bampoe, S., Lucas, D.N., Moonesinghe, S.R., Andrade, J., et al. (2021) Incidence of accidental awareness during general anaesthesia in obstetrics: A multicentre, prospective cohort study. *Anaesthesia, 76*(6): 759–776. doi:10.1111/anae.15385.

Odgers, K., Kershaw, K.A., Li, S.H. & Graham, B.M. (2022) The relative efficacy and efficiency of single- and multi-session exposure therapies for specific phobia: A meta-analysis. *Behaviour Research and Therapy, 159*: 104203. doi:10.1016/j.brat.2022.104203.

Office for National Statistics (2020) *People with Long-term Health Conditions, UK: January to December 2019.* London: ONS. Available from www.ons.gov.uk/peoplepopulationand community/healthandsocialcare/conditions anddiseases/adhocs/11478peoplewithlong termhealthconditionsukjanuarytodecember 2019 (accessed 25 January 2025).

Office for National Statistics (2022) *Adult Smoking Habits in the UK: 2022.* London: ONS. Available from www.ons.gov.uk/peoplepopulationandcommunity/healthandsocialcare/healthandlifeexpectancies/bulletins/adultsmokinghabitsingreatbritain/2022 (accessed 25 January 2025).

Olander, E.K., Darwin, Z.J., Atkinson, L., Smith, D.M. & Gardner, B. (2016) Beyond the 'teachable moment': A conceptual analysis of women's perinatal behaviour change. *Women and Birth*, 29(3): e67–e71.

Olaniyan, F.V. & Hayes, G. (2022) Just ethnic matching? Racial and ethnic minority students and culturally appropriate mental health provision at British universities. *International Journal of Qualitative Studies on Health and Well-being*, 17(1): 2117444. doi:10.1080/17482631.2022.2117444.

Olsson, A., Mohammad, M.A., Rylance, R., Platonov, P.G., Sparv, D. & Erlinge, D. (2023) Sex differences in potential triggers of myocardial infarction. *European Heart Journal Open*, 3(2): oead011. doi:10.1093/ehjopen/oead011.

Olthuis, J.V., Watt, M.C., Bailey, K., Hayden, J.A. & Stewart, S.H. (2016) Therapist-supported internet cognitive behavioural therapy for anxiety disorders in adults. *Cochrane Database of Systematic Reviews*, 3: Art. CD011565.

Onakomaiya, M.M. & Henderson, L.P. (2016) Mad men, women and steroid cocktails: A review of the impact of sex and other factors on anabolic androgenic steroids effects on affective behaviors. *Psychopharmacology*, 233(4): 549–569.

Ong, D.S.M., Weibin, M.Z. & Vallabhajosyula, R. (2021) Serious games as rehabilitation tools in neurological conditions: A comprehensive review. *Technology and Health Care*, 29: 15–31. doi:10.3233/THC-202333.

Ong, J.J., Fu, H., Baggaley, R.C., Wi, T.E., Tucker, J.D., et al. (2021) Missed opportunities for sexually transmitted infections testing for HIV pre-exposure prophylaxis users: A systematic review. *Journal of the International AIDS Society*, 24(2): e25673. doi:10.1002/jia2.25673.

Onukwugha, F.I., Hayter, M. & Magadi, M.A. (2019) Views of service providers and adolescents on use of sexual and reproductive health services by adolescents: A systematic review. *African Journal of Reproductive Health*, 23(2): 134–147. doi:10.29063/ajrh2019/v23i2.13.

Orbell, S. & Phillips, L.A. (2019) Automatic processes and self-regulation of illness. *Health Psychology Review*, 13(4): 378–405. doi: 10.1080/17437199.2018.1503559.

Orenius, T., Säilä, H., Mikola, K. & Ristolainen, L. (2018) Fear of injections and needle phobia among children and adolescents: An overview of psychological, behavioral, and contextual factors. *SAGE Open Nursing*, 4. doi: 10.1177/2377960818759442.

Orth-Gomér, K., Schneiderman, N., Wang, H.X., Walldin, C., Blom, M. & Jernberg, T. (2009) Stress reduction prolongs life in women with coronary disease: The Stockholm Women's Intervention Trial for Coronary Heart Disease (SWITCHD). *Circulation: Cardiovascular Quality & Outcomes*, 2(1): 25–32.

Ortiz Worthington, R., Feld, L.D. & Volerman, A. (2019) Supporting new physicians and new parents: A call to create a standard parental leave policy for residents. *Academic Medicine: Journal of the Association of American Medical Colleges*, 94(11): 1654–1657. doi: 10.1097/ACM.0000000000002862.

Osborn, E., Brooks, J., O'Brien, P.M.S. & Wittkowski, A. (2021) Suicidality in women with Premenstrual Dysphoric Disorder: A systematic literature review. *Archives of Women's Mental Health*, 24(2): 173–184. doi: 10.1007/s00737-020-01054-8.

Osborne, M.T., Shin, L.M., Mehta, N.N., Pitman, R.K., Fayad, Z.A. & Tawakol, A. (2020) Disentangling the links between psychosocial stress and cardiovascular disease. *Circulation. Cardiovascular Imaging*, 13(8): e010931. doi:10.1161/CIRC IMAGING.120.010931.

Osmani, V., Hörner, L., Klug, S.J. & Tanaka, L. F. (2023) Prevalence and risk of psychological distress, anxiety and depression in adolescent and young adult (AYA) cancer survivors: A systematic review and meta-analysis. *Cancer medicine*, 12(17), 18354–18367. doi:10.1002/cam4.6435.

Öst, L.G. (2014) The efficacy of acceptance and commitment therapy: An updated systematic review and meta-analysis. *Behaviour Research and Therapy*, *61*: 105–121.

Öst, L.G., Enebrink, P., Finnes, A. et al. (2023) Cognitive behavior therapy for adult depressive disorders in routine clinical care: A systematic review and meta-analysis. *Journal of Affective Disorders*, *331*: 322–333. doi:10.1016/j.jad.2023.03.002.

Osterberg, L. & Blaschke, T. (2005) Adherence to medication. *New England Journal of Medicine*, *353*(5): 487–497.

Otis, M., Barber, S., Amet, M. & Nicholls, D. (2023) Models of integrated care for young people experiencing medical emergencies related to mental illness: A realist systematic review. *European Child & Adolescent Psychiatry*, *32*(12): 2439–2452. doi: 10.1007/s00787-022-02085-5.

Ougrin, D. (2011) Efficacy of exposure versus cognitive therapy in anxiety disorders: Systematic review and meta-analysis. *BMC Psychiatry*, *20*(11): 200.

Ozturk, F.O. & Tekkas-Kerman, K. (2022) The effect of online laughter therapy on depression, anxiety, stress, and loneliness among nursing students during the Covid-19 pandemic. *Archives of Psychiatric Nursing*, *41*: 271–276. doi:10.1016/j. apnu.2022.09.006.

Ozturk, F.O. & Tezel, A. (2021) Effect of laughter yoga on mental symptoms and salivary cortisol levels in first-year nursing students: A randomized controlled trial. *International Journal of Nursing Practice*, *27*: e12924. doi:10.1111/ijn.12924.

Pai, H.C., Li, C.C., Tsai, S.M. & Pai, Y.C. (2019) Association between illness representation and psychological distress in stroke patients: A systematic review and meta-analysis. *International Journal of Nursing Studies*, *94*: 42–50. doi: 10.1016/j. ijnurstu.2019.01.015.

Palagini, L., Bastien, C.H., Marazziti, D., Ellis, J.G. & Riemann, D. (2019) The key role of insomnia and sleep loss in the dysregulation of multiple systems involved in mood disorders: A proposed model.

Journal of Sleep Research, *28*(6): e12841. doi:10.1111/jsr.12841.

Palamenghi, L., Carlucci, M.M. & Graffigna, G. (2020) Measuring the quality of life in diabetic patients: A scoping review. *Journal of Diabetes Research*, 22 May: 5419298. doi:10.1155/2020/5419298.

Palmer, S., Vecchio, M., Craig, J.C., Tonelli, M., Johnson, D.W., et al. (2013) Prevalence of depression in chronic kidney disease: Systematic review and meta-analysis of observational studies. *Kidney International*, *84*(1): 179–191.

Pampati, S., Liddon, N., Dittus, P.J., Adkins, S.H. & Steiner, R.J. (2019) Confidentiality matters but how do we improve implementation in adolescent sexual and reproductive health care? *Journal of Adolescent Health*, *65*(3): 315–322. doi: 10.1016/j.jadohealth.2019.03.021.

Pan, A., Sun, Q., Okereke, O.I., Rexrode, K.M. & Hu, F.B. (2011) Depression and risk of stroke morbidity and mortality: A meta-analysis and systematic review. *JAMA*, *306*(11): 1241–1249.

Panagi, L., Poole, L., Hackett, R. A. & Steptoe, A. (2019) Happiness and inflammatory responses to acute stress in people with Type 2 diabetes. *Annals of Behavioral Medicine*, *53*(4): 309–320. doi:10.1093/abm/ kay039.

Panahi, F., Fakari, F.R., Nazarpour, S., Lotfi, R., Rahimizadeh, M., et al. (2022) Educating fathers to improve exclusive breastfeeding practices: A randomized controlled trial. *BMC Health Services Research*, *22*(1): 554. doi:10.1186/s12913-022-07966-8.

Paolacci, S., Kiani, A.K., Manara, E., Beccari, T., Ceccarini, M.R., et al. (2020) Genetic contributions to the etiology of anorexia nervosa: New perspectives in molecular diagnosis and treatment. *Molecular Genetics & Genomic Medicine*, *8*(7): e1244. doi: 10.1002/mgg3.1244.

Park, S.H., Cho, M.S., Kim, Y.S., Hong, J., Nam, E., et al. (2008) Self-reported health-related quality of life predicts survival for patients with advanced gastric cancer treated with first-line chemotherapy. *Quality of Life Research*, *17*(2): 207–214.

Park, Y., Sanscartier, S., Impett, E.A., Algoe, S. B., Leonhardt, N.D., et al. (2023) Meta-analytic evidence that attachment insecurity is associated with less frequent experiences of discrete positive emotions. *Journal of Personality*, *91*(5): 1223–1238. doi:10.1111/jopy.12796.

Parker, G. & Brotchie, H. (2017) Pancreatic cancer and depression: A narrative review. *Journal of Nervous and Mental Disease*, *205*(6): 487–490. doi: 10.1097/NMD.0000000000000593.

Parker, H.W., Abreu, A.M., Sullivan, M.C. & Vadiveloo, M.K. (2022) Allostatic load and mortality: A systematic review and meta-analysis. *American Journal of Preventive Medicine*, *63*(1): 131–140. doi:10.1016/j.amepre.2022.02.003.

Parry, C.H. (1825) *Collections from the Unpublished Writings of the Late C.H. Parry* (*Vol. 2*). London: Underwoods.

Parsons, T. (1975) The sick role and the role of the physician reconsidered. *Millbank Memorial Fund Quarterly*, *53*(3): 257–278.

Pascoe, L. & Edvardsson, D. (2013) Benefit finding in cancer: A review of influencing factors and health outcomes. *European Journal of Oncology Nursing*, *17*(6): 760–766.

Pascoe, M.C., Thompson, D.R., Jenkins, Z.M. & Ski, C.F. (2017) Mindfulness mediates the physiological markers of stress: Systematic review and meta-analysis. *Journal of Psychiatric Research*, *95*: 156–178. doi: 10.1016/j.jpsychires.2017.08.004.

Passchier, R.V., Abas, M.A., Ebuenyi, I.D. & Pariante, C.M. (2018) Effectiveness of depression interventions for people living with HIV in Sub-Saharan Africa: A systematic review & meta-analysis of psychological & immunological outcomes. *Brain, Behavior & Immunity*, *73*: 261–273. doi: 10.1016/j.bbi.2018.05.010.

Patel, T., Christy, K., Grierson, L., Shadd, J., Farag, A., et al. (2021) Clinician responses to legal requests for hastened death: A systematic review and meta-synthesis of qualitative research. *BMJ Supportive & Palliative Care*, *11*(1): 59–67. doi:10.1136/bmjspcare-2019-002018.

Patel, V., Burns, J.K., Dhingra, M., Tarver, L., Kohrt, B.A. & Lund, C. (2018) Income inequality and depression: A systematic review and meta-analysis of the association and a scoping review of mechanisms. *World Psychiatry*, *17*(1): 76–89. doi:10.1002/wps.20492.

Pateraki, E. & Morris, P.G. (2018) Effectiveness of cognitive behavioural therapy in reducing anxiety in adults and children with asthma: A systematic review. *Journal of Asthma*, *55*(5): 532–554. doi: 10.1080/02770903.2017.1350967.

Paterna, A., Alcaraz-Ibáñez, M., Fuller-Tyszkiewicz, M. & Sicilia, Á. (2021) Internalization of body shape ideals and body dissatisfaction: A systematic review and meta-analysis. *International Journal of Eating Disorders*, *54*(9): 1575–1600. doi:10.1002/eat.23568.

Patnode, C.D., Perdue, L.A., Rossom, R.C., Rushkin, M.C., Redmond, N., et al. (2020) *Screening for Cognitive Impairment in Older Adults: An Evidence Update for the U.S. Preventive Services Task Force*. Rockville, MD: Agency for Healthcare Research and Quality.

Patnode, C.D., Redmond, N., Iacocca, M.O. & Henninger, M. (2022) Behavioral counseling interventions to promote a healthy diet and physical activity for cardiovascular disease prevention in adults without known cardiovascular disease risk factors: Updated evidence report and systematic review for the US Preventive Services Task Force. *JAMA*, *328*(4): 375–388. doi:10.1001/jama.2022.7408.

Pauly, T., Michalowski, V.I., Nater, U.M., Gerstorf, D., Ashe, M.C., et al. (2019) Everyday associations between older adults' physical activity, negative affect, and cortisol. *Health Psychology*, *38*(6): 494–501. doi: 10.1037/hea0000743.

Payne, B.K. & Hannay, J.W. (2021) Implicit bias reflects systemic racism. *Trends in*

Cognitive Science, 25: 927–936. doi:10.1016/j.tics.2021.08.001.

Payne, H.E., Lister, C., West, J.H. & Bernhardt, J.M. (2015) Behavioral functionality of mobile apps in health interventions: A systematic review of the literature. *JMIR Mhealth Uhealth*, 3(1): e20.

Payne, S., Horn, S. & Relf, M. (1999) *Loss and Bereavement*. Buckingham: Open University Press.

Pearce, M., Garcia, L., Abbas, A., et al. (2022) Association between physical activity and risk of depression: A systematic review and meta-analysis. *JAMA Psychiatry*, 79(6): 550–559. doi:10.1001/jamapsychiatry. 2022.0609

Pearl, S.B. & Norton, P.J. (2017) Transdiagnostic versus diagnosis specific cognitive behavioural therapies for anxiety: A meta-analysis. *Journal of Anxiety Disorders*, 46: 11–24.

Pei, J., Amanvermez, Y., Vigo, D. et al. (2024) Sociodemographic correlates of mental health treatment seeking among college students: A systematic review and meta-analysis. *Psychiatric Services*, 31 January. Online first. doi:10.1176/appi. ps.20230414.

Peltzer, K. & Pengpid, S. (2015) Trying to lose weight among non-overweight university students from 22 low, middle and emerging economy countries. *Asia Pacific Journal of Clinical Nutrition*, 24(1): 177–183.

Pena-Polanco, J.E., Mor, M.K., Tohme, F.A., Fine, M.J., Palevsky, P.M. & Weisbord, S.D. (2017) Acceptance of antidepressant treatment by patients on hemodialysis and their renal providers. *Clinical Journal of the American Society of Nephrology*, 12(2): 298–303. doi: 10.2215/CJN.07720716.

Pennant, M.E., Loucas, C.E., Whittington, C., Creswell, C., Fonagy, P., et al. (2015) Computerised therapies for anxiety and depression in children and young people: A systematic review and meta-analysis. *Behaviour Research and Therapy*, 67: 1–18.

Pereira, L., Figueiredo-Braga, M. & Carvalho, I.P. (2016) Preoperative anxiety in

ambulatory surgery: The impact of an empathic patient-centered approach on psychological and clinical outcomes. *Patient Education & Counselling*, 99(5): 733–738. doi:10.1016/j.pec.2015.11.016.

Peres, D.S., Rodrigues, P., Viero, F.T., Frare, J. M., Kudsi, S.Q., Meira, G.M. & Trevisan, G., et al. (2022) Prevalence of depression and anxiety in the different clinical forms of multiple sclerosis and associations with disability: A systematic review and meta-analysis. *Brain, Behavior, & Immunity – Health*, 24, 100484. doi:10.1016/j. bbih.2022.100484.

Pérez-Aranda, A., Hofmann, J., Feliu-Soler, A., Ramírez-Maestre, C., Andrés-Rodríguez, L, et al. (2019) Laughing away the pain: A narrative review of humour, sense of humour and pain. *European Journal of Pain*, 23(2): 220–233. doi:10.1002/ejp.1309.

Perez-Bret, E., Altisent, R. & Rocafort, J. (2016) Definition of compassion in healthcare: A systematic literature review. *International Journal of Palliative Nursing*, 22(12): 599–606. doi: 10.12968/ijpn.2016.22. 12.599.

Perkins-Porras, L., Whitehead, D.L., Strike, P.C. & Steptoe, A. (2009) Pre-hospital delay in patients with acute coronary syndrome: Factors associated with patient decision time and home-to-hospital delay. *European Journal of Cardiovascular Nursing*, 8(1): 26–33.

Perrochon, A., Borel, B., Istrate, D., Compagnat, M. & Daviet, J.C. (2019) Exercise-based games interventions at home in individuals with a neurological disease: A systematic review and meta-analysis. *Annals of Physical Rehabilitation Medicine*, 62(5): 366–378. doi: 10.1016/j. rehab.2019.04.004.

Persson, B.N. & Kajonius, P.J. (2016) Empathy and universal values explicated by the empathy-altruism hypothesis. *Journal of Social Psychology*, 156: 610–619. doi:10.1080 /00224545.2016.1152212.

Persson, E., Asutay, E., Heilig, M., Löfberg, A., Pedersen, N., et al. (2019) Variation in the μ-Opioid Receptor Gene (OPRM1) does not moderate social-rejection sensitivity in humans. *Psychological Science*, *30*(7): 1050–1062. doi:10.1177/0956797619849894.

Pérusse, L., Jacob, R., Drapeau, V., Llewellyn, C., Arsenault, B.J., et al. (2022) Understanding gene-lifestyle interaction in obesity: The role of mediation versus moderation. *Lifestyle Genomics*, *15*(2): 67–76. doi:10.1159/000523813.

Peruzzolo, T.L., Pinto, J.V., Roza, T.H., Shintani, A.O., Anzolin, A.P., Gnielka, V., Kohmann, A.M., Marin, A.S., Lorenzon, V.R., Brunoni, A.R., Kapczinski, F. & Passos, I.C. (2022) Inflammatory and oxidative stress markers in post-traumatic stress disorder: A systematic review and metaanalysis. *Molecular Psychiatry*, 27(8): 3150–3163. https://doi.org/10.1038/s41380-022-01564-0.

Peters, M.D.J. (2022) Addressing vaccine hesitancy and resistance for COVID-19 vaccines. *International Journal of Nursing Studies*, *131*: 104241. doi:10.1016/j.ijnurstu.2022.104241.

Petersen, S., Taube, K., Lehmann, K., Van den Bergh, O. & von Leupoldt, A. (2012) Social comparison and anxious mood in pulmonary rehabilitation: The role of cognitive focus. *British Journal of Health Psychology*, *17*(3): 463–476.

Petrie, K.J. & Pennebaker, J.W. (2004) Health-related cognitions. In S. Sutton, A. Baum & M. Johnston (eds), *The SAGE Handbook of Health Psychology*. London: Sage (pp. 127–142).

Petrie, K.J., Faasse, K., Crichton, F. & Grey, A. (2014) How common are symptoms? Evidence from a New Zealand national telephone survey. *BMJ Open*, *4*(6): e005374.

Petrie, K.J., Moss-Morris, R., Grey, C. & Shaw, M. (2004) The relationship of negative affect and perceived sensitivity to symptom reporting following vaccination. *British Journal of Health Psychology*, *9*(1): 101–111.

Petrilli, C.M., Mack, M., Petrilli, J.J., Hickner, A., Saint, S. & Chopra, V. (2015) Understanding the role of physician attire on patient perceptions: A systematic review of the literature – targeting attire to improve likelihood of rapport (TAILOR) investigators. *BMJ Open*, *5*(1): e006578.

Petscher, E.S., Rey, C. & Bailey, J.S. (2009) A review of empirical support for differential reinforcement of alternative behavior. *Research in Developmental Disabilities*, *30*(3): 409–425.

Petticrew, M., Bell, R. & Hunter, D. (2002) Influence of psychological coping on survival and recurrence in people with cancer: Systematic review. *British Medical Journal*, *325*(7372): 1066.

Pfaeffli Dale, L., Whittaker, R., Dixon, R., Stewart, R., Jiang, Y., et al. (2015) Acceptability of a mobile health exercise-based cardiac rehabilitation intervention: A randomized trial. *Journal of Cardiopulmonary Rehabilitaion & Prevention*, *35*(5): 312–319. doi: 10.1097/HCR.0000000000000125.

Phan, D.Q., Zheng, C., Thai, T. et al. (2022) Cardiorespiratory fitness and mortality in patients aged 60 to 90 years. *American Journal of Cardiology*, *170*: 132–137. doi:10.1016/j.amjcard.2022.01.035.

Piaget, J. (1954) *The Construction of Reality in the Child*. New York: Basic Books.

Piasecka, M., Papakokkinou, E., Valassi, E., et al. (2020) Psychiatric and neurocognitive consequences of endogenous hypercortisolism. *Journal of Internal Medicine*, *288*: 168–182. doi:10.1111/joim.13056.

Pięta, M. & Rzeszutek, M. (2022) Posttraumatic growth and well-being among people living with HIV: A systematic review and meta-analysis in recognition of 40 years of HIV/AIDS. *Quality of Life Research*, *31*: 1269–1288. doi:10.1007/s11136-021-02990-3.

Piili, R.P., Hökkä, M., Vänskä, J., Tolvanen, E., Louhiala, P. & Lehto, J.T. (2024) Facing a request for assisted death: Views of Finnish physicians, a mixed method study. *BMC Medical Ethics*, *25*(1): 50. doi:10.1186/s12910-024-01051-x.

Piliavin, I.M., Rodin, J. & Piliavin, J.A. (1969) Good samaritanism: An underground phenomenon? *Journal of Personality and Social Psychology*, 13(4): 289–299.

Pilver, C.E., Kasl, S., Desai, R. & Levy, B.R. (2011) Exposure to American culture is associated with premenstrual dysphoric disorder among ethnic minority women. *Journal of Affective Disorders*, 130(1–2): 334–341.

Pincus, J.D. (2024) Theoretical and empirical foundations for a unified pyramid of human motivation. *Integrative Psychological and Behavioral Science*, 58: 731–756. doi:10.1007/s12124-022-09700-9.

Pinel, J.P.J. & Barnes, S. (2021) *Biopsychology* (11th edition). Boston, MA: Pearson.

Pinquart, M. & Duberstein, P.R. (2010) Associations of social networks with cancer mortality: A meta-analysis. *Critical Reviews in Oncology/Hematology*, 75(2): 122–137.

Pinquart, M. (2013) Self-esteem of children and adolescents with chronic illness: A meta-analysis. *Child: Care, Health & Development*, 39(2): 153–161. doi: 10.1111/j.1365-2214.2012.01397.x.

Pinto, P.R., McIntyre, T., Ferrero, R., Almeida, A. & Araújo-Soares, V. (2013) Predictors of acute postsurgical pain and anxiety following primary total hip and knee arthroplasty. *Journal of Pain*, 14(5): 502–515. doi:10.1016/j.jpain.2012.12.020.

Pitman, A., Marston, L., Lewis, G., Semlyen, J., McManus, S. & King, M. (2021) The mental health of lesbian, gay, and bisexual adults compared with heterosexual adults: Results of two nationally representative English household probability samples. *Psychological Medicine*, 52(15): 1–10. doi:10.1017/S0033291721000052.

Pivonello, R., Auriemma, R.S., Delli Veneri, A. et al. (2022) Global psychological assessment with the evaluation of life and sleep quality and sexual and cognitive function in a large number of patients with acromegaly: A cross-sectional study. *European Journal of Endocrinology*, 187: 823–845. doi:10.1530/EJE-22-0263.

Plasencia, G., Luedicke, J.M., Nazarloo, H.P., Carter, C.S. & Ebner, N.C. (2019) Plasma oxytocin and vasopressin levels in young and older men and women: Functional relationships with attachment and cognition. *Psychoneuroendocrinology*, 110: 104419. doi:10.1016/j.psyneuen.2019.104419

Plourde, A., Lavoie, K.L., Raddatz, C. & Bacon, S.L. (2017) Effects of acute psychological stress induced in laboratory on physiological responses in asthma populations: A systematic review. *Respiratory Medicine*, 127: 21–32. doi: 10.1016/j.rmed.2017.03.024.

Polakovská, L. & Řiháček, T. (2022) What is it like to live with medically unexplained physical symptoms? A qualitative meta-summary. *Psychology and Health*, 37(2): 580–596. doi:10.1080/08870446.2021.1901900.

Poletti, V., Pagnini, F., Banfi, P. & Volpato, E. (2022) The role of depression on treatment adherence in patients with heart failure: A systematic review of the literature. *Current Cardiology Reports*, 24(12): 1995–2008. doi: 10.1007/s11886-022-01815-0.

Polityńska, B., Pokorska, O., Wojtukiewicz, A. M., Sawicka, M., Myśliwiec, M., Honn, K. V., Tucker, S.C. & Wojtukiewicz, M.Z. (2022) Is depression the missing link between inflammatory mediators and cancer?. *Pharmacology & Therapeutics*, 240: 108293. https://doi.org/10.1016/j.pharmthera.2022.108293.

Pope, J.P., Pelletier, L. & Guertin, C. (2018) Starting off on the best foot: A review of message framing and message tailoring, and recommendations for the comprehensive messaging strategy for sustained behavior change. *Health Communication*, 33(9): 1068–1077. doi: 10.1080/10410236.2017.1331305.

Porter, A.C., Lash, J.P., Xie, D., Pan, Q., DeLuca, J., et al. (2016) Predictors and outcomes of health-related quality of life in adults with CKD. *Clinical Journal of the American Society of Nephrology*, 11(7): 1154–1162.

Potter, E.L., Hopper, I., Sen, J., Salim, A. & Marwick, T.H. (2019) Impact of socioeconomic status on incident heart failure and left ventricular dysfunction: Systematic review and meta-analysis. *European Heart Journal Quality of Care & Clinical Outcomes*, *5*(2): 169–179. doi: 10.1093/ehjqcco/qcy047.

Potthoff, S., Kwasnicka, D., Avery, L., Finch, T. et al. (2022) Changing healthcare professionals' non-reflective processes to improve the quality of care. *Social Science & Medicine*, *298*: 114840. doi:10.1016/j. socscimed.2022.114840.

Potthoff, S., Rasul, O., Sniehotta, F.F., Marques, M., Beyer, F., et al. (2019) The relationship between habit and healthcare professional behaviour in clinical practice: A systematic review and meta-analysis. *Health Psychology Review*, *13*(1): 73–90. doi: 10.1080/174 37199.2018.1547119.

Powell, R., Scott, N.W., Manyande, A., Bruce, J., Vögele, C., et al. (2016) Psychological preparation and postoperative outcomes for adults undergoing surgery under general anaesthesia. *Cochrane Database of Systematic Reviews*, *5*: Art. CD008646.

Pradas-Hernández, L., Ariza, T., Gómez-Urquiza, J.L., Albendín-García, L., De la Fuente, E.I. & Cañadas-De la Fuente, G.A. (2018) Prevalence of burnout in paediatric nurses: A systematic review and meta-analysis. *PLoS One*, *13*(4): e0195039. doi:10.1371/journal.pone.0195039.

Präg, P. (2020) Subjective socio-economic status predicts self-rated health irrespective of objective family socio-economic background. *Scandinavian Journal of Public Health*, *48*: 707–714. doi:10.1177/140349482 0926053.

Prather, A.A., Janicki-Deverts, D., Hall, M.H. & Cohen, S. (2015) Behaviorally assessed sleep and susceptibility to the common cold. *Sleep*, *38*(9): 1353–1359. doi: 10.5665/ sleep.4968.

Preis, H., Lobel, M. & Benyamini, Y. (2019) Between expectancy and experience: Testing a model of childbirth satisfaction.

Psychology of Women Quarterly, *43*(1): 105–117. doi: 10.1177/0361684318779537.

Presseau, J., Johnston, M., Heponiemi, T., Elovainio, M., Francis, J.J., et al. (2014) Reflective and automatic processes in health care professional behaviour: A dual process model tested across multiple behaviours. *Annals of Behavioral Medicine*, *48*(3): 347–358. doi: 10.1007/s12160-014-9609-8.

Pressman, S.D. & Cohen, S. (2005) Does positive affect influence health? *Psychological Bulletin*, *131*(6): 925–971.

Pressman, S.D., Jenkins, B.N. & Moskowitz, J. (2019) Positive affect and health: What do we know and where next should we go? *Annual Review of Psychology*, *70*: 627–650. doi:10.1146/annurev-psych-010418-102955.

Preti, E., Di Mattei, V., Perego, G., Ferrari, F., Mazzetti, M., et al. (2020) The psychological impact of epidemic and pandemic outbreaks on healthcare workers: Rapid review of the evidence. *Current Psychiatry Reports*, *22*(8): 43. doi: 10.1007/s11920-020-01166-z.

Price, D.D., Craggs, J., Verne, G.N., Perlstein, W.M. & Robinson, M.E. (2007) Placebo analgesia is accompanied by large reductions in pain-related brain activity in irritable bowel syndrome patients. *Pain*, *127*(1–2): 63–72.

Prigge, R., Wild, S.H. & Jackson, C.A. (2022) The individual and combined associations of depression and socioeconomic status with risk of major cardiovascular events: A prospective cohort study. *Journal of Psychosomatic Research*, *160*: 110978. doi:10.1016/j.jpsychores.2022.110978.

Prince, M., Wimo, A.G.M., Guerchet, M., Ali, G.C., Wu, Y.T. & Prina, M. (2015) *World Alzheimer Report 2015: The Global Impact of Dementia: An Analysis of Prevalence, Incidence, Cost and Trends*. London: Alzheimer's Disease International.

Pritchard, S.E., Garsed, K.C., Hoad, C.L., Lingaya, M., Banwait, R., et al. (2015) Effect of experimental stress on the small bowel and colon in healthy humans. *Neurogastroenterology & Motility*, *27*(4): 542–549.

Prochaska, J.O. & DiClemente, C.C. (1983) Stages and processes of self-change of smoking: Toward an integrative model of change. *Journal of Consulting and Clinical Psychology*, 51(3): 390–395.

Pyett, P., Rayner, J., Venn, A., Bruinsma, F., Werther, G. & Lumley, J. (2005) Using hormone treatment to reduce the adult height of tall girls: Are women satisfied with the decision in later years? *Social Science & Medicine*, 61(8): 1629–1639.

Pyle, D., Perry, A., Lamont-Mills, A., Tehan, G. & Chambers, S.K. (2021) A scoping review of the characteristics and benefits of online prostate cancer communities. *Psycho-oncology*, 30(5): 659–668. doi:10.1002/pon.5618.

Qiao, J., Lin, X., Wu, Y., Huang, X., Pan, X., et al. (2022) Global burden of non-communicable diseases attributable to dietary risks in 1990–2019. *Journal of Human Nutrition and Dietetics*, 35(1): 202–213. doi:10.1111/jhn.12904.

Qin, H.Y., Cheng, C.W., Tang, X.D. & Bian, Z.X. (2014) Impact of psychological stress on irritable bowel syndrome. *World Journal of Gastroenterology*, 20(39): 14126–14131. doi: 10.3748/wjg.v20.i39.14126.

Quenby, S., Gallos, I.D., Dhillon-Smith, R.K., Podesek, M., Stephenson, M.D., Fisher, J., et al. (2021) Miscarriage matters: The epidemiological, physical, psychological, and economic costs of early pregnancy loss. *Lancet*, 397(10285): 1658–1667. doi: 10.1016/S0140-6736(21)00682-6.

QuickStats (2021) Percentage of adults aged ≥18 years who received an influenza vaccination in the past 12 months, by sex and age group – National Health Interview Survey, United States, 2020. *Morbid and Mortality Weekly Report (MMWR)*, 70(45): 1586. Published 12 November 2021. doi:10.15585/mmwr.mm7045a5.

QuickStats (2022) Percentage of adults aged ≥18 years who always use sunscreen when outside for >1 hour on a sunny day, by sex and age group – National Health Interview Survey, United States, 2020. *Morbid and Mortality Weekly Report (MMWR)*, 71(22): 747. Published 3 June 2022. doi:10.15585/mmwr.mm7122a5.

Qureshi, A.A., Awosika, O., Baruffi, F., Rengifo-Pardo, M. & Ehrlich, A. (2019) Psychological therapies in management of psoriatic skin disease: A systematic review. *American Journal of Clinical Dermatology*, 20(5): 607–624. doi: 10.1007/s40257-019-00437-7.

Ragelienė, T. & Grønhøj, A. (2020) The influence of peers' and siblings' on children's and adolescents' healthy eating behavior: A systematic literature review. *Appetite*, 148: 104592. doi:10.1016/j.appet.2020.104592.

Ramos-Leví, A.M., Cañada, E. & Matias-Guiu, J.A. (2023) Cognitive dysfunction in patients with primary adrenal insufficiency: A systematic review. *Applied Neuropsychology: Adult*, 30: 802–813. doi:10.1080/23279095.2022.2090256.

Rank, S.G. & Jacobson, C.K. (1977) Hospital nurses' compliance with medication overdose orders: A failure to replicate. *Journal of Health & Social Behavior*, 18: 188–193.

Rasmussen, E.B. (2020) Making and managing medical anomalies: Exploring the classification of 'medically unexplained symptoms'. *Social Studies of Science*, 50: 901–931. doi:10.1177/0306312720940405.

Rasmussen, H.N., Scheier, M.F. & Greenhouse, J.B. (2009) Optimism and physical health: A meta-analytic review. *Annals of Behavioral Medicine*, 37(3): 239–256.

Rathod, S., Phiri, P., de Visser, R.O., et al. (2023) Applying the cultural adaption framework to the Early Youth Engagement (EYE-2) approach to early intervention in psychosis. *British Journal of Clinical Psychology*, 62(3): 537–555. doi:10.1111/bjc.12423.

Raven, B.H. (1965) Social influence and power. In I.D. Steiner & M. Fishbein (eds), *Current Studies in Social Psychology*. New York: Holt, Reinhart & Winston (pp. 399–444).

Ray, L.A., Meredith, L.R., Kiluk, B.D., Walthers, J., Carroll, K.M. & Magill, M. (2020) Combined pharmacotherapy and cognitive behavioral therapy for adults with alcohol or substance use disorders: A systematic review and meta-analysis. *JAMA Network Open*, *3*(6): e208279. doi: 10.1001/jamanetworkopen.2020.8279.

Rayan, A. & Ahmad, M. (2017) Mindfulness and parenting distress among parents of children with disabilities: A literature review. *Perspectives on Psychiatric Care*, March. doi: 10.1111/ppc.12217. Epub ahead of print.

Ream, E., Hughes, A.E., Cox, A., Skarparis, K. & Richardson, A. (2020) Telephone interventions for symptom management in adults with cancer. *Cochrane Database of Systematic Reviews*, *6*(6): Art. CD007568. doi:10.1002/14651858.CD007568.pub2.

Reas, D.L. & Grilo, C.M. (2021) Psychotherapy and medications for eating disorders: Better together? *Clinical Therapeutics*, *43*: 17–39. doi:10.1016/j.clinthera.2020.10.006.

Rehm, J., Gmel Sr, G.E., Gmel, G., Hasan, O.S.M., Imtiaz, S., Popova, S., Probst, C., Roerecke, M., Room, R., Samokhvalov, A.V., Shield, K.D. & Shuper, P.A. (2017) The relationship between different dimensions of alcohol use and the burden of disease – an update. *Addiction*, *112*(6): 968–1001. doi: 10.1111/add.13757.

Rehm, J., Rovira, P., Llamosas-Falcón, L. & Shield, K.D. (2021) Dose-response relationships between levels of alcohol use and risks of mortality or disease, for all people, by age, sex, and specific risk factors. *Nutrients*, *13*(8): 2652. doi:10.3390/nu13082652.

Reid, C., Seymour, J. & Jones, C. (2016) A thematic synthesis of the experiences of adults living with hemodialysis. *Clinical Journal of the American Society of Nephrology*, *11*(7): 1206–1218. doi: 10.2215/CJN.10561015.

Reilly, T.J., Patel, S., Unachukwu, I.C., Knox, C.L., Wilson, C.A., et al. (2024) The prevalence of premenstrual dysphoric disorder: Systematic review and meta-analysis. *Journal of Affective Disorders*, *349*: 534–540. doi: 10.1016/j.jad.2024.01.066.

Reith-Hall, E. & Montgomery, P. (2023) Communication skills training for improving the communicative abilities of student social workers. *Campbell Systematic Reviews*, *19*(1): e1309. doi: 10.1002/cl2.1309.

Ren, Y., Yang, H., Browning, C., Thomas, S. & Liu, M. (2015) Performance of screening tools in detecting major depressive disorder among patients with coronary heart disease: A systematic review. *Medical Science Monitor*, *21*: 646–653.

Renaud-Charest, O., Lui, L.M.W., Eskander, S., Ceban, F., Ho, R., et al. (2021) Onset and frequency of depression in post-COVID-19 syndrome: A systematic review. *Journal of Psychiatric Research*, *144*: 129–137. doi:10.1016/j.jpsychires.2021.09.054.

Rennung, M. & Göritz, A.S. (2016) Prosocial consequences of interpersonal synchrony: A meta-analysis. *Z Psychology*, *224*(3): 168–189.

Resnicow, K., Baranowski, T., Ahluwalia, J.S. & Braithwaite, R.L. (1999) Cultural sensitivity in public health: Defined and demystified. *Ethnicity & Disease*, *9*(1): 10–21.

Ribeiro, M., Benadjaoud, M.A., Moisy, L. et al. (2022) Symptoms of depression and anxiety in adults with high-grade glioma: A literature review and findings in a group of patients before chemoradiotherapy and one year later. *Cancers*, *14*: 5192. doi:10.3390/cancers14215192.

Richard, C., Glaser, E. & Lussier, M.T. (2017) Communication and patient participation influencing patient recall of treatment discussions. *Health Expectations*, *20*(4): 760–770. doi:10.1111/hex.12515.

Richardson, E.M., Schüz, N., Sanderson, K., Scott, J.L. & Schüz, B. (2017) Illness representations, coping, and illness outcomes in people with cancer: A systematic review and meta-analysis. *Psychooncology*, *26*(6): 724–737. doi: 10.1002/pon.4213.

Richardson, P. (2006) National Clinical Practice Guidelines (NICE Guidelines on Depression) – core interventions in the management of depression in primary & secondary care. *Association for Psychoanalytic Psychotherapy Newsletter, 34*: 2–5.

Richters, J., Altman, D., Badcock, P.B., Smith, A.M.A., de Visser, R.O., Grulich, A.E., et al. (2014) Sexual identity, sexual attraction and sexual experience: The second Australian study of health and relationships. *Sexual Health, 11*(5): 451–460. doi: 10.1071/SH14117.

Richters, J., Yeung, A., Rissel, C. & McGeechan, K. (2022) Sexual difficulties, problems, and help-seeking in a national representative sample: The second Australian Study of Health and Relationships. *Archives of Sexual Behavior, 51*(2): 1435–1446. doi:10.1007/s10508-021-02244-w.

Ricks, T.N., Abbyad, C. & Polinard, E. (2022) Undoing racism and mitigating bias among healthcare professionals: Lessons learned during a systematic review. *Journal of Racial and Ethnical Health Disparities, 9*: 1990–2000. doi:10.1007/s40615-021-01137-x.

Riddle, J.P., Smith, H.E. & Jones, C.J. (2016) Does written emotional disclosure improve the psychological and physical health of caregivers? A systematic review and meta-analysis. *Behaviour Research and Therapy, 80*: 23–32. doi:10.1016/j.brat.2016.03.004.

Riecke, J., Zerth, S.F., Schubert, A.K., Wiesmann, T., Dinges, H.C., et al. (2023) Risk factors and protective factors of acute postoperative pain: An observational study at a German university hospital with cross-sectional and longitudinal inpatient data. *BMJ Open, 13*(5): e069977. doi:10.1136/bmjopen-2022-069977.

Riegel, B., Jaarsma, T., Lee, C.S. & Strömberg, A. (2019) Integrating symptoms into the middle-range theory of self-care of chronic illness. *ANS: Advances in Nursing Science, 42*(3): 206–215. doi: 10.1097/ANS.0000000000000237.

Rissel, C.E., Richters, J., Grulich, A.E., de Visser, R.O. & Smith A.M.A. (2003) Attitudes toward sex in a representative sample of adults. *Australian & New Zealand Journal of Public Health, 27*(2): 118–123.

Ritchie, D., Van den Broucke, S. & Van Hal, G. (2021) The health belief model and theory of planned behavior applied to mammography screening: A systematic review and meta-analysis. *Public Health Nursing, 38*(3): 482–492. doi:10.1111/phn.12842.

Rivera, E., Corte, C., DeVon, H.A., Collins, E. G., & Steffen, A. (2020) A systematic review of illness representation clusters in chronic conditions. *Research in Nursing & Health, 43*(3): 241–254. doi:10.1002/nur.22013.

Roberts, N.P., Kitchiner, N. J., Kenardy, J., Robertson, L., Lewis, C. & Bisson, J.I. (2019) Multiple session early psychological interventions for the prevention of post-traumatic stress disorder. *Cochrane Database of Systematic Reviews, 8*(8): Art. CD006869. doi:10.1002/14651858.CD006869.pub3.

Robertson, L.M., Douglas, F., Ludbrook, A., Reid, G. & van Teijlingen, E. (2008) What works with men? A systematic review of health promoting interventions targeting men. *BMC Health Services Research, 8*: 141. doi:10.1186/1472-6963-8-141.

Robinaugh, D.J., Ward, M.J., Toner, E.R., Brown, M.L., Losiewicz, O.M., et al. (2019) Assessing vulnerability to panic: A systematic review of psychological and physiological responses to biological challenges as prospective predictors of panic attacks and panic disorder. *General Psychiatry, 32*(6): e100140. doi:10.1136/gpsych-2019-100140.

Robine, J.M., Michel, J.P. & Herrmann, F.R. (2007) Who will care for the oldest people in our ageing society? *British Medical Journal, 334*(7593): 570–571.

Robinson, C.H., Albury, C., McCartney, D., Fletcher, B., Roberts, N., et al. (2021) The relationship between duration and quality of sleep and upper respiratory tract infections: A systematic review. *Family Practice, 38*(6): 802–810. doi:10.1093/fampra/cmab033.

Rodondi, P.Y., Maillefer, J., Suardi, F., Rodondi, N., Cornuz, J. & Vannotti, M. (2009) Physician response to 'by-the-way' syndrome in primary care. *Journal of General Internal Medicine, 24*(6): 739–741. doi: 10.1007/s11606-009-0980-2.

Rodrigues, B., Carraça, E., Francisco, B.B. & Nobre, I. (2023) Theory-based physical activity and/or nutrition behavior change interventions for cancer survivors: A systematic review. *Journal of Cancer Survivorship, 18*(5): 1464–1480. doi:10.1007/s11764-023-01390-5.

Roessel, J., Schoel, C., Zimmermann, R. & Stahlberg, D. (2019) Shedding new light on the evaluation of accented speakers: Basic mechanisms behind non-native listeners' evaluations of non-native accented job candidates. *Journal of Language and Social Psychology, 38*(1): 3–32. doi: 10.1177/0261927X17747904.

Rogers, C. (1951) *Client-centered Therapy: Its Current Practice, Implications and Theory.* London: Constable.

Rogers, F., Rashidi, A. & Ewens, B. (2022) Education and support for erectile dysfunction and penile rehabilitation post prostatectomy: A qualitative systematic review. *International Journal of Nursing Studies, 130*: 104212. doi:10.1016/j.ijnurstu.2022.104212.

Rogerson, O., Wilding, S., Prudenzi, A. & O'Connor, D.B. (2024) Effectiveness of stress management interventions to change cortisol levels: A systematic review and meta-analysis. *Psychoneuroendocrinology, 159*: 106415. doi:10.1016/j.psyneuen.2023.106415.

Rogler, L.H., Malgady, R.G., Costantino, G. & Blumenthal, R. (1987) What do culturally sensitive mental health services mean? The case of Hispanics. *American Psychologist, 42*(6): 565–570. doi:10.1037//0003-066x.42.6.565.

Rohleder, N. (2019) Stress and inflammation – the need to address the gap in the transition between acute and chronic stress effects. *Psychoneuroendocrinology, 105*: 164–171. doi:10.1016/j.psyneuen.2019.02.021.

Rohling, M.L., Faust, M.E., Beverly, B. & Demakis, G. (2009) Effectiveness of cognitive rehabilitation following acquired brain injury: A meta-analytic re-examination of Cicerone et al.'s (2000, 2005) systematic reviews. *Neuropsychology, 23*(1): 20–39.

Rohrer, J.M., Egloff, B. & Schmukle, S.C. (2015) Examining the effects of birth order on personality. *Proceedings of the National Academy of Science USA, 112*(46): 14224–14229.

Roper, A., Pacas Fronza, G., Dobkin, R.D., Beaudreau, S.A., Mitchell, L.K., et al. (2024) A systematic review of psychotherapy approaches for anxiety in Parkinson's Disease. *Clinical Gerontologist, 47*(2): 188–214. doi:10.1080/07317115.2022.2074814.

Rosa Silva, J.P., Santiago Júnior, J.B., dos Santos, E.L. et al. (2020) Quality of life and functional independence in amyotrophic lateral sclerosis: A systematic review. *Neuroscience & Biobehavioral Reviews, 111*: 1–11. doi:10.1016/j.neubiorev.2019.12.032.

Rosendal, M., Olde Hartman, T.C., Aamland, A., van der Horst, H., Lucassen, P., et al. (2017) 'Medically unexplained' symptoms and symptom disorders in primary care: Prognosis-based recognition and classification. *BMC Family Practice, 18*(1): 18. doi: 10.1186/s12875-017-0592-6.

Rosenstock, I.M. (1974) Historical origins of the health belief model. *Health Education Monographs, 2*(4): 1–8.

Ross, L. (1977) The intuitive psychologist and his shortcomings. In L. Berkowitz (ed.), *Advances in Experimental Social Psychology* (*Vol. 10*). Orlando, FL: Academic Press (pp. 173–240).

Ross, M.C., Heilicher, M. & Cisler, J.M. (2021) Functional imaging correlates of childhood trauma: A qualitative review of past research and emerging trends. *Pharmacology, Biochemistry, and Behavior, 211*: 173297. doi:10.1016/j.pbb.2021.173297.

Rothman, A.J. & Salovey, P. (1997) Shaping perceptions to motivate healthy behavior: The role of message framing. *Psychological Bulletin, 121*(1): 3–19.

Rothman, I., Tennant, A., Mills, R.J. & Young, C.A. (2023) The association of health locus of control with clinical and psychosocial aspects of living with multiple sclerosis. *Journal of Clinical Psychology in Medical Settings*, *30*(4): 821–835. doi:10.1007/s10880-023-09938-4.

Rouhe, H., Salmela-Aro, K., Halmesmäki, E. & Saisto, T. (2009) Fear of childbirth according to parity, gestational age, and obstetric history. *British Journal of Obstetrics & Gynaecology*, *116*(1): 67–73.

Rovito, M.J., Cavayero, C., Leone, J.E. & Harlin, S. (2015) Interventions promoting testicular self-examination (TSE) performance: A systematic review. *American Journal of Men's Health*, *9*(6): 506–518.

Roy, D.N., Biswas, M., Islam, E. & Azam, M.S. (2022) Potential factors influencing COVID-19 vaccine acceptance and hesitancy: A systematic review. *PLoS One*, *17*(3): e0265496. doi:10.1371/journal.pone.0265496.

Rozin, P., Haidt, J. & McCauley, C. (2018) Disgust. In L. Feldman Barrett, M. Lewis & J.M. Haviland-Jones (eds), *Handbook of Emotions* (4th edition). New York: Guilford Press (pp. 815–834).

Rubinow, D.R., Johnson, S.L., Schmidt, P.J., Girdler, S. & Gaynes, B. (2015) Efficacy of estradiol in perimenopausal depression: So much promise and so few answers. *Depress Anxiety*, *32*(8): 539–549. doi: 10.1002/da.22391.

Ruffault, A., Czernichow, S., Hagger, M.S., Ferrand, M., Erichot, N., et al. (2017) The effects of mindfulness training on weight-loss and health-related behaviours in adults with overweight and obesity: A systematic review and meta-analysis. *Obesity Research & Clinical Practice*, *11*(5): 90–111. doi: 10.1016/j.orcp.2016.09.002.

Ruiter, R.A.C., Kessels, L.T.E., Peters, G.-J.Y. & Kok, G. (2014) Sixty years of fear appeal research: Current state of the evidence. *International Journal of Psychology*, *49*(2): 63–70.

Rush, K.L., Hickey, S., Epp, S. & Janke, R. (2017) Nurses' attitudes toward older people care: An integrative review. *Journal of Clinical Nursing*, *26*(23–24): 4105–4116. doi: 10.1111/jocn.13939.

Russell, S.L., Haynos, A.F., Crow, S.J. & Fruzzetti, A.E. (2017) An experimental analysis of the affect regulation model of binge eating. *Appetite*, *110*: 44–50. doi: 10.1016/j.appet.2016.12.007.

Ryback, R.S. & Lewis, O.F. (1971) Effects of prolonged bed rest on EEG sleep patterns in young, healthy volunteers. *Electroencephalography & Clinical Neurophysiology*, *31*(4): 395–399.

Saab, M.M., Landers, M. & Hegarty, J. (2016) Testicular cancer awareness and screening practices: A systematic review. *Oncology Nursing Forum*, *43*(1): E8–E23.

Sabini, J. & Silver, M. (2005) Ekman's basic emotions: Why not love and jealousy? *Cognition & Emotion*, *19*(5): 693–712.

Sadri, H., Oliaei, A., Sadri, S., Pezeshki, P., Chughtai, B. & Eltermand, D. (2024) Systematic review and meta-analysis of urinary incontinence prevalence and population estimates. *Neurourology Urodynamics*, *43*(1): 52–62. doi:10.1002/nau.25276.

Sætre, L.M.S., Raasthøj, I., Lauridsen, G.B., Balasubramaniam, K., Haastrup, P., et al. (2024) Revisiting the symptom iceberg based on the Danish symptom cohort: Symptom experiences and healthcare-seeking behaviour in the general Danish population in 2022. *Heliyon*, *10*(10): e31090. doi:10.1016/j.heliyon.2024.e31090.

Safer, J.D., Coleman, E., Feldman, J., Garofalo, R., et al. (2016) Barriers to healthcare for transgender individuals. *Current Opinion in Endocrinology, Diabetes and Obesity*, *23*(2): 168–171. doi:10.1097/MED.0000000000000227.

Sahani, V., Hurd, Y.L. & Bachi, K. (2022) Neural underpinnings of social stress in substance use disorders. *Current Topics in Behavioral Neurosciences*, *54*: 483–515. doi:10.1007/7854_2021_272.

Saharoy, R., Potdukhe, A., Wanjari, M. & Taksande, A.B. (2023) Postpartum depression and maternal care: Exploring the complex effects on mothers and infants. *Cureus*, *15*(7): e41381. doi: 10.7759/cureus.41381.

Sajadinejad, M.S., Asgari, K., Molavi, H., Kalantari, M. & Adibi, P. (2012) Psychological issues in inflammatory bowel disease: An overview. *Gastroenterology Research and Practice*, Art. 106502. doi: 10.1155/2012/106502.

Salomonsson, B., Gullberg, M.T., Alehagen, S. & Wijma, K. (2013) Self-efficacy beliefs and fear of childbirth in nulliparous women. *Journal of Psychosomatic Obstetrics and Gynaecology*, *34*(3): 116–121.

Salsberg, E., Richwine, C., Westergaard, S. et al. (2021) Estimation and comparison of current and future racial/ethnic representation in the US health care workforce. *JAMA Netw Open*, *4*(3): e213789. doi:10.1001/jamanetwork open.2021.3789.

Salvador, Á., Mansuklal, S.A., Moura, M., Crespo, C. & Barros, L. (2023) Facilitators and barriers to adherence to medical recommendations among adolescents with cancer: A systematic review. *Journal of Child Health Care*, 21 October: 13674935231208502. doi: 10.1177/13674935231208502. Epub ahead of print.

Salzmann, S., Euteneuer, F., Kampmann, S., Rienmüller, S. & Rüsch, D. (2023) Preoperative anxiety and need for support: A qualitative analysis in 1,000 patients. *Patient Education and Counseling*, *115*: 107864. doi:10.1016/j.pec.2023.107864.

Salzwedel, A., Koran, I., Langheim, E., Schlittt, A. et al. (2020) Patient-reported outcomes predict return to work and health-related quality of life six months after cardiac rehabilitation: Results from a German multi-centre registry (OutCaRe). *PLoS One*, *15*(5): e0232752. doi:10.1371/journal.pone.0232752.

Samuels, M.H. (2014) Psychiatric and cognitive manifestations of hypothyroidism. *Current Opinion in Endocrinology, Diabetes and Obesity*, *21*: 377–383. doi:10.1097/MED.0000000000000089.

Samulowitz, A., Gremyr, I., Eriksson, E. & Hensing, G. (2018) 'Brave men' and 'emotional women': A theory-guided literature review on gender bias in health care and gendered norms towards patients with chronic pain. *Pain Research & Management*, 25 February: 6358624. doi:10.1155/2018/6358624.

Sanaei Nasab, H., Yazdanian, M., Mokhayeri, Y., Latifi, M., Niksadat, N., Harooni, J. & Armoon, B. (2019) The role of psychological theories in oral health interventions: A systematic review and meta-analysis. *International Journal of Dental Hygiene*, *17*(2): 142–152. doi:10.1111/idh.12386.

Sanders, S. & Reinisch, J. (1999) Would you say you 'had sex' if …? *Journal of the American Medical Association*, *281*(3): 275–277.

Santiago, B.V.M., Oliveira, A.B.G., Silva, G.M.R.D., Silva, M.F.D., Bergamo, P.E., Parise, M. & Villela, N.R. (2023) Prevalence of chronic pain in Brazil: A systematic review and meta-analysis. *Clinics*, *78*: 100209. doi:10.1016/j.clinsp.2023.100209.

Santino, T.A., Chaves, G.S., Freitas, D.A., Fregonezi, G.A. & Mendonça, K.M. (2020) Breathing exercises for adults with asthma. *Cochrane Database of Systematic Reviews*, *3*(3): Art. CD001277. doi: 10.1002/146518 58.CD001277.pub4.

Santos, I., Sniehotta, F.F., Marques, M.M., Carraça, E.V. & Teixeira, P.J. (2017) Prevalence of personal weight control attempts in adults: A systematic review and meta-analysis. *Obesity Reviews*, *18*(1): 32–50. doi: 10.1111/obr.12466.

Sara, J.D., Prasad, M., Eleid, M.F., Zhang, M., Widmer, R.J. & Lerman, A. (2018) Association between work-related stress and coronary heart disease: A review of prospective studies through the job strain, effort-reward balance, and organizational justice models. *Journal of the American Heart Association*, *7*(9): e008073. doi: 10.1161/JAHA.117.008073.

Saracci, R. (1997) The World Health Organization needs to reconsider its definition of health. *British Medical Journal*, *314*(7091): 1409–1410.

Sarafino, E.P. (2002) *Health Psychology: Biopsychosocial Interactions* (5th edition). Hoboken, NJ: Wiley.

Sari Motlagh, R., Quhal, F., Mori, K., Miura, N., Aydh, A., Laukhtina, E., et al. (2021) The risk of new onset dementia and/or Alzheimer disease among patients with prostate cancer treated with androgen deprivation therapy: A systematic review and meta-analysis *Journal of Urology*, *205*(1): 60–67. doi:10.1097/JU.0000000000001341.

Sasson, A.N., Ananthakrishnan, A.N. & Raman, M. (2021) Diet in treatment of inflammatory bowel diseases. *Clinical Gastroenterology and Hepatology*, *19*(3): 425–435.e3. doi:10.1016/j.cgh.2019.11.054.

Savage, L.J. (1954) *The Foundations of Statistics*. New York: Wiley.

Savulescu, J., Roache, R., Davies, W. & Loebel, J.P. (eds) (2020) *Psychiatry Reborn: Biopsychosocial Psychiatry in Modern Medicine*. Oxford: Oxford University Press.

Sawyer, A., Ayers, S. & Field, A. (2010) Posttraumatic growth and adjustment among individuals with cancer or HIV/AIDS: A meta-analysis. *Clinical Psychology Review*, *30*(4): 436–447.

Saxby, D.E. (2017) Birth of a new perspective? A call for biopsychosocial research on childbirth. *Current Directions in Psychological Science*, *26*(1): 81–86.

Say, A., de la Piedad Garcia, X. & Mallan, K. M. (2023) The correlation between different operationalisations of parental restrictive feeding practices and children's eating behaviours: Systematic review and meta-analyss. *Appetite*, *180*: 106320. doi:10.1016/j.appet.2022.106320.

Sayette, M.A. (2007) Alcohol abuse. In S. Ayers, A. Baum, C. McManus, S. Newman, K. Wallston, J. Weinman & R. West (eds) *Cambridge Handbook of Psychology, Health and Medicine* (2nd edition). Cambridge: Cambridge University Press (pp. 534–537).

Schablon, A., Zeh, A., Wendeler, D., Peters, C., Wohlert, C., Harling, M. & Nienhaus, A. (2012) Frequency and consequences of violence and aggression toward employees in the German healthcare and welfare system: A cross-sectional study. *BMJ Open*, *2*(5): e001420.

Schaper, S.J. & Stengel, A. (2022) Emotional stress responsivity of patients with IBS – a systematic review. *Journal of Psychosomatic Research*, *153*: 110694. doi:10.1016/j.jpsychores.2021.110694.

Schaumberg, K. Anderson, D.A., Anderson, L.M., Reilly, E.E. & Gorrell, S. (2016) Dietary restraint: What's the harm? A review of the relationship between dietary restraint, weight trajectory and the development of eating pathology. *Clinical Obesity*, *6*(2): 89–100.

Schaumberg, K., Jangmo, A., Thornton, L.M., Birgegård, A., Almqvist, C., Norring, C., et al. (2019) Patterns of diagnostic transition in eating disorders: A longitudinal population study in Sweden. *Psychological Medicine*, *49*(5): 819–827. doi: 10.1017/S0033291718001472.

Schaumberg, K., Reilly, E. E., Gorrell, S., et al. (2021). Conceptualizing eating disorder psychopathology using an anxiety disorders framework: Evidence and implications for exposure-based clinical research. *Clinical Psychology Review*, *83*, 101952. doi:10.1016/j.cpr.2020.101952.

Schefft, C., Heinitz, C., Guhn, A., Brakemeier, E.L., Sterzer, P. & Köhler, S. (2023) Efficacy and acceptability of third-wave psychotherapies in the treatment of depression: A network meta-analysis of controlled trials. *Frontiers in Psychiatry*, *14*: 1189970. doi: 10.3389/fpsyt.2023.1189970.

Scheier, M.F. & Carver, C.S. (2018) Dispositional optimism and physical health: A long look back, a quick look forward. *American Psychology*, *73*: 1082–1094. doi:10.1037/amp0000384i

Scheier, M.F., Carver, C.S. & Bridges, M.W. (1994) Distinguishing optimism from neuroticism (and trait anxiety, self-mastery, and self-esteem): A re-evaluation of the Life Orientation Test. *Journal of Personality and Social Psychology, 67*(6): 1063–1078.

Scheier, M.F., Swanson, J.D., Barlow, M.A., Greenhouse, J.B., Wrosch, C. & Tindle, H.A. (2021) Optimism versus pessimism as predictors of physical health: A comprehensive reanalysis of dispositional optimism research. *American Psychology, 76*: 529–548. doi:10.1037/amp0000666.

Scheim, A.I., Rich, A.J., Zubizarreta, D., et al. (2024) Health status of transgender people globally: A systematic review of research on disease burden and correlates. *PLoS One, 19*(3): e0299373. doi:10.1371/journal. pone.0299373.

Schleifenbaum, L., Stern, J., Driebe, J.C., Wieczorek, L.L., Gerlach, T.M., Arslan, R.C. & Penke, L. (2024) Ovulatory cycle shifts in human motivational prioritisation of sex and food. *Hormones & Behavior, 162*: 105542. doi: 10.1016/j.yhbeh. 2024.105542.

Schmid Mast, M., Hall, J.A. & Roter, D.L. (2007) Disentangling physician sex and physician communication style: Their effects on patient satisfaction in a virtual medical visit. *Patient Education and Counseling, 68*(1): 16–22. doi:10.1016/j. pec.2007.03.020.

Scholliers, A., Cornelis, S., Tosi, M., Opsomer, T. et al. (2023) Impact of fatigue on anaesthesia providers: A scoping review. *British Journal of Anaesthesia, 130*(5): 622–635. doi:10.1016/j.bja.2022.12.011.

Schoot, T.S., Goto, N.A., van Marum, R.J., Hilbrands, L.B. & Kerckhoffs, A.P.M. (2022) Dialysis or kidney transplantation in older adults? A systematic review summarizing functional, psychological, and quality of life-related outcomes after start of kidney replacement therapy. *International Urology and Nephrology, 54*(11): 2891–2900. doi:10.1007/s11255-022-03208-2.

Schoretsanitis, G., Kutynia, A., Stegmayer, K., Strik, W. & Walther, S. (2016) Keep at bay! Abnormal personal space regulation as marker of paranoia in schizophrenia. *European Psychiatry, 31*: 1–7.

Schout, B.M.A., Hendrikx, A.J.M., Scheele, F., Bemelmans, B.M.H. & Scherpbier, A.J.J.A. (2010) Validation and implementation of surgical simulators: A critical review of present, past, and future. *Surgery & Endoscopy, 24*(3): 536–546.

Schouten, B.C. & Meeuwesen, L. (2006) Cultural differences in medical communication: A review of the literature. *Patient Education and Counselling, 64*(1–3): 21–34.

Schreiner, P.J. (2016) Emerging cardiovascular risk research: Impact of pets on cardiovascular risk prevention. *Current Cardiovascular Risk Reports, 10*(2): 8.

Schröder, D., Wrona, K.J., Müller, F., Heinemann, S., Fischer, F. & Dockweiler, C. (2023) Impact of virtual reality applications in the treatment of anxiety disorders: A systematic review and meta-analysis of randomized-controlled trials. *Journal of Behavior Therapy and Experimental Psychiatry, 81*: 101893. doi:10.1016/j.jbtep.2023.101893.

Schubbe, D., Scalia, P., Yen, R.W., Saunders, C.H., Cohen, S., Elwyn, G., et al. (2020) Using pictures to convey health information: A systematic review and meta-analysis of the effects on patient and consumer health behaviors and outcomes. *Patient Education and Counseling, 103*(10): 1935–1960. doi: 10.1016/j.pec.2020.04.010.

Schuster, R., Bornovalova, M. & Hunt, E. (2012) The influence of depression on the progression of HIV: Direct and indirect effects. *Behavior Modification, 36*(2): 123–45.

Schweizer, S., Satpute, A.B., Atzil, S., Field, A. P., Hitchcock, C., Black, M., et al. (2019) The impact of affective information on working memory: A pair of meta-analytic reviews of behavioral and neuroimaging evidence. *Psychological Bulletin, 145*(6), 566–609. doi:10.1037/bul0000193.

Schwenker, R., Dietrich, C. E., Hirpa, S., Nothacker, M., Smedslund, G., Frese, T. &

Unverzagt, S. (2023) Motivational interviewing for substance use reduction. *Cochrane Database of Systematic Reviews, 12*(12): CD008063. doi:10.1002/14651858. CD008063.pub3.

Scorza, P., Duarte, C.S., Hipwell, A.E., Posner, J., Ortin, A., Canino, G., et al. (2019) Research review: Intergenerational transmission of disadvantage: Epigenetics and parents' childhoods as the first exposure. *Journal of Child Psychology and Psychiatry, and Allied Disciplines, 60*(2): 119–132. doi: 10.1111/jcpp.12877.

Scott, A., Sudlow, M, Shaw, E. & Fisher, J. (2020) Medical education, simulation and uncertainty. *The Clinical Teacher, 17*(5): 497–502. doi:10.1111/tct.13119.

Scott, W. & McCracken, L.M. (2018) Chronic pain. In C.D. Llewellyn, S. Ayers, C. McManus, S. Newman, K. Petrie, T. Revenson & J. Weinman (eds), *The Cambridge Handbook of Psychology, Health and Medicine* (3rd edition). Cambridge: Cambridge University Press.

Scottish Intercollegiate Guidelines Network (SIGN) (2023) Perinatal Mental Health Conditions: A national clinical guideline. SIGN publication 169. Edinburgh: SIGN. Available from https:// www.sign.ac.uk/ media/2172/sign-169-perinatal.pdf (accessed 26 January 2025).

Scott-Sheldon, L.A.J., Balletto, B.L., Donahue, M.L., Feulner, M.M., Cruess, D.G., Salmoirago-Blotcher, E., et al. (2019) Mindfulness-based interventions for adults living with HIV/AIDS: A systematic review and meta-analysis. *AIDS & Behavior, 23*(1): 60–75. doi: 10.1007/s10461-018-2236-9.

Seale, C. (2008) *Constructing Death: The Sociology of Dying and Bereavement* (2nd edition). Cambridge: Cambridge University Press.

Sebastiani, G., Borrás-Novell, C., Casanova, M.A., Pascual Tutusaus, M., Ferrero Martínez, S., Gómez Roig, M.D. & García-Algar, O. (2018) The effects of alcohol and drugs of abuse on maternal nutritional profile during pregnancy. *Nutrients, 10*(8): 1008. doi:10.3390/nu10081008.

Sechrest, L. & Wallace, J. (1964) Figure drawings and naturally occurring events: Elimination of the expansive euphoria hypothesis. *Journal of Educational Psychology, 55*(1): 42–44.

Segal, Z.V., Williams, J.M.G. & Teasdale, J.D. (2002) *Mindfulness-Based Cognitive Therapy for Depression: A New Approach for Preventing Relapse.* New York: Guilford Press.

Segerstrom, S.C. & Miller, G.E. (2004) Psychological stress and the human immune system: A meta-analytic study of 30 years of inquiry. *Psychological Bulletin, 130*(4): 601–630. https://doi. org/10.1037/0033-2909.130.4.601.

Segerstrom, S.C., Taylor, S.E., Kemeny, M.E. & Fahey, J.L. (1998) Optimism is associated with mood, coping, and immune change in response to stress. *Journal of Personality and Social Psychology, 74*(6): 1646–1655.

Seidler, Z.E., Dawes, A.J., Rice, S.M., Oliffe, J.L. & Dhillon, H.M. (2016) The role of masculinity in men's help-seeking for depression: A systematic review. *Clinical Psychology Review, 49*: 106–118. doi: 10.1016/j.cpr.2016.09.002.

Selic, P., Svab, I., Repolusk, M. & Gucek, N.K. (2011) What factors affect patients' recall of general practitioners' advice? *BMC Family Practice, 12*: 141.

Seligman, M.E.P. (1975) *Helplessness: On Depression, Development, and Death.* San Francisco, CA: W.H. Freeman.

Semlyen, J., King, M., Varney, J. & Hagger-Johnson, G. (2016) Sexual orientation and symptoms of common mental disorder or low wellbeing: Combined meta-analysis of 12 UK population health surveys. *BMC Psychiatry, 16*, 67. doi:10.1186/s12888-016-0767-z.

Seng, J.J.B., Tan, J.Y., Yeam, C.T., Htay, H., & Foo, W.Y.M. (2020) Factors affecting medication adherence among pre-dialysis chronic kidney disease patients: A systematic review and meta-analysis of literature. *International Urology and Nephrology, 52*(5): 903–916. doi:10.1007/s11255-020-02452-8.

Senn, T.E., Scott-Sheldon, L.A. & Carey, M.P. (2014) Relationship-specific condom attitudes predict condom use among STD clinic patients with both primary and non-primary partners. *AIDS & Behavior*, *18*(8): 1420–1427. doi: 10.1007/s10461-014-0726-y.

Senra, H. & McPherson S. (2021) Depression in disabling medical conditions – current perspectives. *International Review of Psychiatry*, *33*: 312–325. doi:10.1080/09540261.2021.1887823.

Seoud, T., Syed, A., Carleton, N., Rossi, C., Kenner, B., Quershi, H., et al. (2020) Depression before and after a diagnosis of pancreatic cancer: Results from a national, population-based study. *Pancreas*, *49*(8): 1117–1122. doi:10.1097/MPA.0000000000001635.

Shafiee, A., Jafarabady, K., Rajai, S., Mohammadi, I. & Mozhgani, S.H. (2023) Sleep disturbance increases the risk of severity and acquisition of COVID-19: A systematic review and meta-analysis. *European Journal of Medical Research*, *28*(1): 442. doi:10.1186/s40001-023-01415-w.

Shahabi, N., Shahbazi, S., Kakhaki, H.E.S. & Mohseni, S. (2024) The effectiveness of a theory-based health education program on waterpipe smoking cessation in Iran: One year follow-up of a quasi-experimental research. *BMC Public Health*, *24*(1): 664. doi:10.1186/s12889-024-18169-7.

Shahid, S., Kelson, J. & Saliba, A. (2024) Effectiveness and user experience of virtual reality for social anxiety disorder: Systematic review. *JMIR Mental Health*, *11*: e48916. doi: 10.2196/48916.

Shangase, N., Kharsany, A.B.M, Ntombela, N. P., Pettifor, A. & McKinnon, L.R. (2021) A systematic review of randomized controlled trials of school based interventions on sexual risk behaviors and sexually transmitted infections among young adolescents in Sub-Saharan Africa. *AIDS and Behavior*, *25*(11): 3669–3686. doi:10.1007/s10461-021-03242-8.

Shapiro, D.E., Boggs, S.R, Melamed, B.G. & Graham-Pole, J. (1992) The effect of varied physician affect on recall, anxiety, and perceptions in women at risk for breast cancer: An analogue study. *Health Psychology*, *11*(1): 61–66.

Sharkiya, S.H. (2023) Quality communication can improve patient-centred health outcomes among older patients: A rapid review. *BMC Health Services Research*, *23*(1): 886. doi:10.1186/s12913-023-09869-8.

Sharko, M., Sharma, M.M., Benda, N.C., Chan, M., Wilsterman, E., Liu, L.G., Demetres, M., et al. (2022) Strategies to optimize comprehension of numerical medication instructions: A systematic review and concept map. *Patient Education and Counseling*, *105*(7): 1888–1903. doi:10.1016/j.pec.2022.01.018.

Sharma, S., Ferreira-Valente, A., de Williams, A.C., Abbott, J.H., Pais-Ribeiro, J. & Jensen, M.P. (2020) Group differences between countries and between languages in pain-related beliefs, coping, and catastrophizing in chronic pain: A systematic review. *Pain Medicine*, *21*(9): 1847–1862. doi:10.1093/pm/pnz373.

Sharpley, C.F., Halat, J., Rabinowicz, T., Weiland, B. & Stafford, J. (2001) Standard posture, postural mirroring, and client-perceived rapport. *Counselling Psychology Quarterly*, *14*(4): 267–280.

Shenefelt, P.D. (2011) Psychodermatological disorders: Recognition and treatment. *International Journal of Dermatology*, *50*(11): 1309–1322.

Shepperd, J.A., Pogge, G. & Howell, J.L. (2017) Assessing the consequences of unrealistic optimism: Challenges and recommendations. *Consciousness and Cognition*, *50*: 69–78. doi:10.1016/j.concog.2016.07.004.

Shepperd, J.A., Waters, E., Weinstein, N.D. & Klein, W.M. (2015) A primer on unrealistic optimism. *Current Directions in Psychological Science*, *24*(3): 232–237. doi: 10.1177/0963721414568341.

Shi, C., Taylor, S., Witthöft, M., Du, X., Zhang, T., Lu, S. & Ren, Z. (2022) Attentional bias toward health-threat in health anxiety: A systematic review and three-level meta-analysis. *Psychological Medicine*, *52*(4): 604–613. doi:10.1017/S0033291721005432.

Shi, W., Ghisi, G.L.M., Zhang, L., Hyun, K., Pakosh, M. & Gallagher, R. (2023) Systematic review, meta-analysis and meta-regression to determine the effects of patient education on health behaviour change in adults diagnosed with coronary heart disease. *Journal of Clinical Nursing*, 32(15–16): 5300–5327. doi:10.1111/jocn.16519.

Shields, M.C., Hollander, M.A.G., Busch, A.B., Kantawala, Z. & Rosenthal, M.B. (2023) Patient-centered inpatient psychiatry is associated with outcomes, ownership, and national quality measures. *Health Affairs Scholar*, *1*(1): qxad017. doi: 10.1093/haschl/qxad017.

Shiga, T. (2023) Depression and cardiovascular diseases. *Journal of Cardiology*, *81*: 485–490. doi:10.1016/j.jjcc.2022.11.010.

Shin, Y.H., Hwang, J., Kwon, R., Lee, S.W., Kim, M.S., GBD 2019 Allergic Disorders Collaborators, et al. (2023) Global, regional, and national burden of allergic disorders and their risk factors in 204 countries and territories, from 1990 to 2019: A systematic analysis for the Global Burden of Disease Study 2019. *Allergy*, *78*(8): 2232–2254. doi:10.1111/all.15807.

Shirazian, S., Grant, C.D., Aina, O., Mattana, J., Khorassani, F. & Ricardo, A.C. (2016) Depression in chronic kidney disease and end-stage renal disease: Similarities and differences in diagnosis, epidemiology, and management. *Kidney International Reports*, *2*(1): 94–107. doi: 10.1016/j.ekir.2016.09.005.

Shorey, S., Asurlekar, A.R., Chua, J.S. & Lim, L.H. (2023) Influence of oxytocin on parenting behaviors and parent–child bonding: A systematic review. *Developmental Psychobiology*, *65*(2): e22359. doi:10.1002/dev.22359.

Shraim, M., Mallen, C.D. & Dunn, K.M. (2013) GP consultations for medically unexplained physical symptoms in parents and their children: A systematic review. *British Journal of General Practice*, *63*(610): e318–e325.

Siegmann, E.M., Müller, H.H.O., Luecke, C., Philipsen, A., Kornhuber, J. & Grömer, T.W. (2018) Association of depression and anxiety disorders with autoimmune thyroiditis: A systematic review and meta-analysis. *JAMA Psychiatry*, *75*(6): 577–584. doi: 10.1001/jamapsychiatry.2018.0190.

Siewchaisakul, P., Luh, D.L., Chiu, S.Y.H., Yen, A.M.F., Chen, C.D., & Chen, H.H. (2020) Smoking cessation advice from healthcare professionals helps those in the contemplation and preparation stage: An application with transtheoretical model underpinning in a community-based program. *Tobacco Induced Diseases*, *18*: 57. doi:10.18332/tid/123427.

Silva, A.C., Dos Santos Ferreira, S., Alves, R.C., Follador, L. & Da Silva, S.G. (2016) Effect of music tempo on attentional focus and perceived exertion during self-selected paced walking. *International Journal of Exercise Science*, *9*(4): 536–544.

Silva, N.R.D.S., Rizardi, F.G., Fujita, R.A., Villalba, M.M., & Gomes, M.M. (2021) Preferred music genre benefits during strength tests: Increased maximal strength and strength-endurance and reduced perceived exertion. *Perceptual and Motor Skills*, *128*(1): 324–337. doi:10.1177/0031512520945084.

Silverman, J., Kurtz, S. & Draper, J. (2013) *Skills for Communicating with Patients* (3rd edition). Oxford: Radcliff Medical Press.

Simion, F., Di Giorgio, E., Leo, I. & Bardi, L. (2011) The processing of social stimuli in early infancy: From faces to biological motion perception. *Progress in Brain Research*, *189*: 173–193. doi: 10.1016/B978-0-444-53884-0.00024-5.

Simons, D.J., Boot, W.R., Charness, N., Gathercole, S.E., Chabris, C.F., Hambrick, D.Z. & Stine-Morrow, E.A. (2016) Do

'Brain-Training' programs work? *Psychological Science in the Public Interest*, *17*(3): 103–186. doi: 10.1177/1529100616661983.

Simons, G., Mallen, C.D., Kumar, K., Stack, R.J. & Raza, K. (2015) A qualitative investigation of the barriers to help-seeking among members of the public presented with symptoms of new-onset rheumatoid arthritis. *Journal of Rheumatology*, *42*(4): 585–592.

Simpson, R.J., Boßlau, T.K., Weyh, C., Niemiro, G.M., Batatinha, H., Smith, K.A., & Krüger, K. (2021) Exercise and adrenergic regulation of immunity. *Brain, Behavior, and Immunity*, *97*: 303–318. doi:10.1016/j.bbi.2021.07.010.

Skakoon-Sparling, S. & Cramer, K.M. (2021) Sexual risk taking intentions under the influence of relationship motivation, partner familiarity, and sexual arousal. *Journal of Sex Research*, *58*: 659–670. doi:10.1080/00224499.2020.1743227.

Skinner, B.F. (1957) *Verbal Behaviour*. Acton, MA: Copley.

Skyt, I., Lunde, S.J., Baastrup, C., Svensson, P., Jensen, T.S. & Vase, L. (2020) Neuro transmitter systems involved in placebo and nocebo effects in healthy participants and patients with chronic pain: A systematic review. *Pain*, *161*(1): 11–23. doi:10.1097/j.pain.0000000000001682.

Slee, A., Nazareth, I., Freemantle, N. & Horsfall, L. (2021) Trends in generalised anxiety disorders and symptoms in primary care: UK population-based cohort study. *British Journal of Psychiatry*, *218*(3): 158–164. doi:10.1192/bjp.2020.159.

Sletvold, H., Sagmo, L.A.B. & Torheim, E.A. (2020) Impact of pictograms on medication adherence: A systematic literature review. *Patient Education and Counseling*, *103*: 1095–1103. doi:10.1016/j.pec.2019.12.018.

Sliedrecht, W., Roozen, H.G., Witkiewitz, K., de Waart, R. & Dom, G. (2021) The association between impulsivity and relapse in patients with alcohol use disorder: A literature review. *Alcohol and Alcoholism*, *56*(6): 637–650. doi:10.1093/alcalc/agaa132.

Smaardijk, V.R., Maas, A.H.E.M., Lodder, P., Kop, W.J. & Mommersteeg, P.M.C. (2020) Sex and gender-stratified risks of psychological factors for adverse clinical outcomes in patients with ischemic heart disease: A systematic review and meta-analysis. *International Journal of Cardiology*, *302*: 21–29. doi: 10.1016/j.ijcard.2019.12.014.

Smeeth, D., Beck, S., Karam, E.G. & Pluess, M. (2021) The role of epigenetics in psychological resilience. *Lancet Psychiatry*, *8*(7): 620–629. doi:10.1016/S2215-0366(20)30515-0.

Smith, A.B., Rutherford, C., Butow, P., Olver, I. et al. (2018) A systematic review of quantitative observational studies investigating psychological distress in testicular cancer survivors. *Psychooncology*, *27*(4): 1129–1137. doi:10.1002/pon.4596.

Smith, J. (2007) From base evidence through to evidence base: A consideration of the NICE guidelines. *Psychoanalytic Psychotherapy*, *21*(1): 40–60.

Smith, M.M. & Hewitt, P.L. (2024) The equivalence of psychodynamic therapy and cognitive behavioral therapy for depressive disorders in adults: A meta-analytic review. *Journal of Clinical Psychology*, *80*(5): 945–967. doi: 10.1002/jclp.23649.

Smith, R.C. (2020) It's time to view severe medically unexplained symptoms as red-flag symptoms of depression and anxiety. *JAMA Network Open*, *3*(7): e2011520. doi:10.1001/jamanetworkopen.2020.11520.

Smith, T.W. (2022) Intimate relationships and coronary heart disease: Implications for risk, prevention, and patient management. *Current Cardiology Reports*, *24*: 761–774. doi:10.1007/s11886-022-01695-4.

Smyth, A., O'Donnell, M., Hankey, G.J., Rangarajan, S. et al. (2022) Anger or emotional upset and heavy physical exertion as triggers of stroke: The INTERSTROKE study. *European Heart Journal*, *43*(3): 202–209. doi:10.1093/eurheartj/ehab738.

Smyth, J.M. & Arigo, D. (2009) Recent evidence supports emotion-regulation interventions for improving health in at-risk and clinical populations. *Current Opinion in Psychiatry*, 22(2): 205–210. doi: 10.1097/YCO.0b013e3283252d6d.

Sneddon, H., Gojkovic Grimshaw, D., Livingstone, N. & Macdonald, G. (2020) Cognitive-behavioural therapy (CBT) interventions for young people aged 10 to 18 with harmful sexual behaviour. *Cochrane Database of Systematic Reviews*, 6(6): Art. CD009829. doi: 10.1002/14651858. CD009829.pub2.

Soenens, B. & Vansteenkiste, M. (2020) Taking adolescents' agency in socialization seriously: The role of appraisals and cognitive-behavioral responses in autonomy-relevant parenting. *New Directions for Child and Adolescent Development*, 173: 7–26. doi:10.1002/cad.20370.

Soh, Y., Kawachi, I., Kubzansky, L.D., Berkman, L.F. & Tiemeier, H. (2024) Chronic loneliness and the risk of incident stroke in middle and late adulthood: A longitudinal cohort study of U.S. older adults. *eClinicalMedicine*, 73: 102639. doi:10.1016/j.eclinm.2024.102639.

Solaro, C., Gamberini, G. & Masuccio, F.G. (2018) Depression in multiple sclerosis: Epidemiology, aetiology, diagnosis and treatment. *CNS Drugs*, 32(2): 117–133. doi: 10.1007/s40263-018-0489-5.

Solazzo, A., Gorman, B. & Denney, J. (2020) Does sexual orientation complicate the relationship between marital status and gender with self-rated health and cardiovascular disease? *Demography*, 57(2): 599–626. doi:10.1007/s13524-020-00857-9.

Soler, J.K., Yaman, H., Esteva, M., Dobbs, F., Asenova, R.S., Katic, M., Ozvacic, Z., Desgranges, J.P., Moreau, A., Lionis, C., Kotányi, P., Carelli, F., Nowak, P.R., de Aguiar Sá Azeredo, Z., Marklund, E., Churchill, D. & Ungan, M. (2008) European General Practice Research Network Burnout Study Group. Burnout in European family doctors: The EGPRN study. *Journal of Family Practice*, 25(4): 245–265.

Solmi, M., Wade, T.D., Byrne, S., Del Giovane, C. et al. (2021) Comparative efficacy and acceptability of psychological interventions for the treatment of adult outpatients with anorexia nervosa: A systematic review and network meta-analysis. *Lancet Psychiatry*, 8(3): 215–224. doi:10.1016/S2215-0366(20)30566-6.

Sonino, N. & Fava, G.A. (2012) Improving the concept of recovery in endocrine disease by consideration of psychosocial issues. *Journal of Clinical Endocrinology and Metabolism*, 97(8): 2614–2616.

Sonnenberg, P., Clifton, S., Beddows, S., Field, N., Soldan, K., Tanton, C., Mercer, C.H., da Silva, F.C., Alexander, S., Copas, A.J., Phelps, A., Erens, B., Prah, P., Macdowall, W., Wellings, K., Ison, C.A. & Johnson, A.M. (2013) Prevalence, risk factors, and uptake of interventions for sexually transmitted infections in Britain: Findings from the National Surveys of Sexual Attitudes and Lifestyles (Natsal). *Lancet*, 382(9907): 1795–1806.

Soo, C.A., Tate, R.L., Catroppa, C. et al. (2024) A randomized controlled trial of cognitive behavioural therapy for managing anxiety in adolescents with acquired brain injury. *Neuropsychological Rehabilitation*, 34(1): 74–102. doi:10.1080/09602011.2022.2154811.

Soorenian, A. & Olsen, J. (2024) *Exploring the Everyday Lives of Disabled People*. Available from www.gov.uk/government/publications/exploring-the-everyday-lives-of-disabled-people/exploring-the-everyday-lives-of-disabled-people (accessed 14 June 2024).

Sørensen, N.V., Frandsen, B.H., Orlovska-Waast, S., Buus, T.B. et al. (2023) Immune cell composition in unipolar depression: A comprehensive systematic review and meta-analysis. *Molecular Psychiatry*, 28(1): 391–401. doi:10.1038/s41380-022-01905-z.

Soundararajan, K., Prem, V. & Kishen, T.J. (2022) The effectiveness of mindfulness-based stress reduction intervention on physical function in individuals with chronic low back pain: Systematic review and meta-analysis of randomized controlled trials. *Complementary Therapies in Clinical Practice, 49*: 101623. doi: 10.1016/j. ctcp.2022.101623.

Sousa, H., Ribeiro, O., Paúl, C., Costa, E., Miranda, V., Ribeiro, F. & Figueiredo, D. (2019) Social support and treatment adherence in patients with end-stage renal disease: A systematic review. *Seminars in Dialysis, 32*(6): 562–574. doi: 10.1111/ sdi.12831.

Southwick, S.M., Bonanno, G.A., Masten, A.S., Panter-Brick, C. & Yehuda, R. (2014) Resilience definitions, theory, and challenges: Interdisciplinary perspectives. *European Journal of Psychotraumatology, 5*(1): 25338. doi: 10.3402/ejpt.v5.25338.

Spătaru, B., Podină, I.R., Tulbure, B.T. & Maricuţoiu, L.P. (2024) A longitudinal examination of appraisal, coping, stress, and mental health in students: A cross-lagged panel network analysis. *Stress and Health, 40*(5): e3450. doi:10.1002/ smi.3450.

Spector, A., Li, Z., He, L., Badawy, Y. & Desai, R. (2024) The effectiveness of psychosocial interventions on non-physiological symptoms of menopause: A systematic review and meta-analysis. *Journal of Affective Disorders, 352*: 460–472. doi: 10.1016/j. jad.2024.02.048.

Spelten, E., Thomas, B., O'Meara, P.F., Maguire, B.J., FitzGerald, D. & Begg, S.J. (2020) Organisational interventions for preventing and minimising aggression directed towards healthcare workers by patients and patient advocates. *Cochrane Database of Systematic Reviews, 4*(4): Art. CD012662. doi:10.1002/14651858.CD012662.pub2.

Spencer, C., Reed, R.G., Votruba-Drzal, E. & Gianaros, P.J. (2024) Psychological stress and the longitudinal progression of subclinical atherosclerosis. *Health Psychology, 43*(1): 58–66. doi:10.1037/ hea0001333.

Spiegel, B., Schoenfeld, P. & Naliboff, B. (2007) Systematic review: The prevalence of suicidal behaviour in patients with chronic abdominal pain and irritable bowel syndrome. *Alimentary Pharmacology & Therapeutics, 26*(2): 183–193.

Spiegel, D., Bloom, J.R., Kraemer, H.C. & Gottheil, E. (1989) Effect of psychosocial treatment on survival of patients with metastatic breast cancer. *Lancet, 2*(8668): 888–891.

Squier, R.W. (1990) A model of empathic understanding and adherence to treatment regimens in practitioner-patient relationships. *Social Science & Medicine, 30*(3): 325–339.

St Clair, D. & Lang, B. (2021) Schizophrenia: A classic battle ground of nature versus nurture debate. *Science Bulletin, 66*: 1037–1046. doi:10.1016/j.scib.2021.01.032.

Stamps, A.E. III (2012) How distance mitigates perceived threat at 30–90 m. *Perceptual and Motor Skills, 114*(3): 709–716. doi: 10.2466/24.20.27.

Stamu-O'Brien, C., Jafferany, M., Carniciu, S. & Abdelmaksoud, A. (2021) Psychodermatology of acne: Psychological aspects and effects of acne vulgaris. *Journal of Cosmetic Dermatology, 20*(4): 1080–1083. doi:10.1111/jocd.13765.

Stanford, F.C. (2020) The importance of diversity and inclusion in the healthcare workforce. *Journal of the National Medical Association, 112*(3): 247–249. doi:10.1016/j. jnma.2020.03.014.

Stanton, R., Rosenbaum, S., Rebar, A. & Happell, B. (2019) Prevalence of chronic health conditions in Australian adults with depression and/or anxiety. *Issues in Mental Health Nursing, 40*(10): 902–907. https:// doi.org/10.1080/01612840.2019. 1613701.

Starfelt Sutton, L.C. & White, K.M. (2016) Predicting sun-protective intentions and behaviours using the theory of planned behaviour: A systematic review and meta-analysis. *Psychology & Health, 31*: 1272–1292. doi: 10.1080/08870446. 2016.1204449.

Stavely, R., Abalo, R. & Nurgali, K. (2020) Targeting enteric neurons and plexitis for the management of inflammatory bowel disease. *Current Drug Targets*, 21(14) 1428–1439. doi:10.2174/138945012166620 0516173242.

Stavropoulou, I., Sakellari, E., Barbouni, A. & Notara, V. (2024) Community-based virtual reality interventions in older adults with dementia and/or cognitive impairment: A systematic review. *Experimental Aging Research*, 7 July. doi: 10.1080/036107 3X.2024.2377438. Epub ahead of print.

Stead, L.F., Buitrago, D., Preciado, N., Sanchez, G., Hartmann-Boyce, J. & Lancaster, T. (2013) Physician advice for smoking cessation. *Cochrane Database of Systematic Reviews*, 5 (Art. CD000165).

Steinfeldt, J.A., Clay, S.L. & Priester, P.E. (2020) Prevalence and perceived importance of racial matching in the psychotherapeutic dyad: A national survey of addictions treatment clinical practices. *Substance Abuse Treatment, Prevention, and Policy*, 15: 76. doi:10.1186/s13011-020-00318-x.

Stellern, J., Xiao, K.B., Grennell, E., Sanches, M., Gowin, J.L. & Sloan, M.E. (2023) Emotion regulation in substance use disorders: A systematic review and meta-analysis. *Addiction, 118*(1), 30–47. https://doi.org/10.1111/add.16001.

Steptoe, A. & Brydon, L. (2009) Emotional triggering of cardiac events. *Neuroscience and Biobehavioral Reviews*, 33(2): 63–70.

Stevenson, F.A., Barry, C.A., Britten, N., Barber, N. & Bradley, C.P. (2000) Doctor–patient communication about drugs: The evidence for shared decision making. *Social Science & Medicine*, 50(6): 829–840. doi: 10.1016/s0277-9536(99)00376-7.

Stewart, T.L., Chipperfield, J.G., Perry, R.P. & Hamm, J.M. (2016) Attributing heart attack and stroke to 'Old Age': Implications for subsequent health outcomes among older adults. *Journal of Health Psychology*, 21(1): 40–49. doi: 10.1177/1359105314521477.

Stewart, T.M., Martin, C.K. & Williamson, D.A. (2022) The complicated relationship between dieting, dietary restraint, caloric restriction, and eating disorders: Is a shift in public health messaging warranted? *International Journal of Environmental Research and Public Health*, 19(1): 491. doi:10.3390/ijerph19010491.

Stice, E., Onipede, Z.A. & Marti, C.N. (2021) A meta-analytic review of trials that tested whether eating disorder prevention programs prevent eating disorder onset. *Clinical Psychology Review*, 87: 102046. doi:10.1016/j.cpr.2021.102046.

Still, L. & Dolen, W.K. (2016) The perception of asthma severity in children. *Current Allergy and Asthma Reports*, 16(7): 50. doi:10.1007/s11882-016-0629-2.

Stinson, J., Connelly, M., Kamper, S.J., Herlin, T. & Toupin April, K. (2016) Models of care for addressing chronic musculoskeletal pain and health in children and adolescents. *Best Practice & Research: Clinical Rheumatology*, 30(3): 468–482.

Stockhorst, U., Wiener, J.A., Klosterhalfen, S., Klosterhalfen, W., Aul, C. & Steingrüber, H.J. (1998) Effects of overshadowing on conditioned nausea in cancer patients: An experimental study. *Physiology & Behaviour*, 64(5): 743–753.

Stoffers-Winterling, J.M., Storebø, O.J., Pereira Ribeiro, J. et al. (2022) Pharmacological interventions for people with borderline personality disorder. *Cochrane Database of Systematic Review*, 11(11): Art. CD012956. doi:10.1002/14651858.CD012956.pub2.

Stone, E.M., Chen, L.N., Daumit, G.L., Linden, S. & McGinty, E.E. (2019) General medical clinicians' attitudes toward people with serious mental illness: A scoping review. *Journal of Behavioral Health Services & Research*, 46(4): 656–679. doi: 10.1007/s11414-019-09652-w.

Storebø, O.J., Stoffers-Winterling, J.M., Völlm, B.A., Kongerslev, M.T., Mattivi, J.T., Jørgensen, M.S., Faltinsen, E., Todorovac, A., Sales, C.P., Callesen, H.E., Lieb, K. & Simonsen, E. (2020) Psychological therapies for people with borderline personality disorder. *Cochrane Database of Systematic*

Reviews, 5(5): Art. CD012955. doi:10.1002/14651858.CD012955.pub2.

Størksen, H.T., Garthus-Niegel, S., Vangen, S. & Eberhard-Gran, M. (2013) The impact of previous birth experiences on maternal fear of childbirth. *Acta Obstetricia et Gynecologica Scandinavica*, 92(3): 318–324.

Stott, N., Fox, J.R.E. & Williams, M.O. (2021) Attentional bias in eating disorders: A meta-review. *International Journal of Eating Disorders*, 54: 1377–1399. doi:10.1002/eat.23560.

Strack, F. & Deutsch, R. (2004) Reflective and impulsive determinants of social behavior. *Personality & Social Psychology Review*, 8(3): 220–247. doi: 10.1207/s15327957pspr0803_1.

Straus, S.E., Richardson, W.S., Glasziou, P. & Haynes, R.B. (2018) *Evidence-Based Medicine: How to Practice and Teach EBM* (5th edition). London: Elsevier.

Street, R.L., Makoul, G., Arora, N.K. & Epstein, R.M. (2009) How does communication heal? Pathways linking clinician–patient communication to health outcomes. *Patient Education and Counseling*, 74(3): 295–301.

Stroebe, M., Schut, H. & Stroebe, W. (2007) Coping with bereavement. In S. Ayers, A. Baum, C. McManus, S. Newman, K. Wallston, J. Weinman & R. West (eds), *Cambridge Handbook of Psychology, Health and Medicine* (2nd edition). Cambridge: Cambridge University Press (pp. 41–46).

Stuijfzand, S., Deforges, C., Sandoz, V., Sajin, C.T., Jaques, C., Elmers, J. & Horsch, A. (2020) Psychological impact of an epidemic/pandemic on the mental health of healthcare professionals: A rapid review. PREPRINT (Version 1), *BMC Public Health* 20(1): 1230. doi: 10.21203/rs.3.rs-30156/v1.

Sturgeon, J.A. & Zautra, A.J. (2016) Social pain and physical pain: shared paths to resilience. *Pain Management*, 6: 63–74. doi:10.2217/pmt.15.56.

Subar, A.R. & Rozenman, M. (2021) Like parent, like child: Is parent interpretation bias associated with their child's interpretation bias and anxiety? A systematic review and meta-analysis. *Journal of Affective Disorders*, 291: 307–314. doi:10.1016/j.jad.2021.05.020.

Subramanian, S.W., Elwert, F. & Christakis, N. (2008) Widowhood and mortality among the elderly: The modifying role of neighborhood concentration of widowed individuals. *Social Science & Medicine*, 66(4): 873–884.

Suls, J., Green, P.A. & Boyd, C.M. (2019) Multimorbidity: Implications and directions for health psychology and behavioral medicine. *Health Psychology*, 38(9): 772–782. doi: 10.1037/hea0000762.

Suls, J., Martin, R. & Wheeler, L. (2002) Social comparison: Why, with whom and with what effect? *Current Directions in Psychological Science*, 11(5): 159–163.

Suls, J. & Rothman, A. (2004) Evolution of the biopsychosocial model: Prospects and challenges for health psychology. *Health Psychology*, 23(2): 119–125.

Sun, S., Qian, J., Wang, F., Tian, Y., Sun, Y., Zheng, Q. & Yu, X. (2023) Impact of contact with the baby following stillbirth on parental mental health and well-being: A systematic review and meta-analysis. *International Journal of Nursing Practice*, 29(6): e13146. doi: 10.1111/ijn.13146.

Sung, H., Ferlay, J., Siegel, R.L., Laversanne, M., Soerjomataram, I., Jemal, A. & Bray, F. (2021) Global cancer statistics 2020: GLOBOCAN estimates of incidence and mortality worldwide for 36 cancers in 185 countries. *CA: A Cancer Journal for Clinicians*, 71(3): 209–249. https://doi.org/10.3322/caac.21660.

Surall, V. & Steppacher, I. (2020) How to deal with death: An empirical path analysis of a simplified model of death anxiety. *Omega*, 82(2): 261–277. doi:10.1177/0030222818808145.

Suskind, A.M., Berry, S.H., Ewing, B.A., Elliott, M.N., Suttorp, M.J. & Clemens, J.Q. (2013) The prevalence and overlap of interstitial cystitis/bladder pain syndrome and chronic prostatitis/chronic pelvic pain syndrome in men: Results of the RAND Interstitial Cystitis Epidemiology male study. *Journal of Urology*, 189(1): 141–145.

Süss, H., & Ehlert, U. (2020) Psychological resilience during the perimenopause. *Maturitas, 131*, 48–56. https://doi.org/10.1016/j.maturitas.2019.10.015.

Sustainable Development Solutions Network (2012) *Indicators and a Monitoring Framework: Launching a Data Revolution for the Sustainable Development Goals. Target 3.4.* New York: Sustainable Development Solutions Network. Available from https://indicators.report/targets/3-4/ (accessed 8 April 2024).

Sverre, K.T., Nissen, E.R., Farver-Vestergaard, I., Johannsen, M. & Zachariae, R. (2023) Comparing the efficacy of mindfulness-based therapy and cognitive-behavioral therapy for depression in head-to-head randomized controlled trials: A systematic review and meta-analysis of equivalence. *Clinical Psychology Review, 100*: 102234. doi:10.1016/j.cpr.2022.102234.

Taddio, A., McMurtry, C.M., Logeman, C., Gudzak, V. et al. (2022) Prevalence of pain and fear as barriers to vaccination in children – systematic review and meta-analysis. *Vaccine, 40*(52): 7526–7537. doi:10.1016/j.vaccine.2022.10.026.

Tajfel, H. & Turner, J. (1986) An integrative theory of intergroup conflict. In S. Worchel & W. Austin (eds), *Psychology of Intergroup Relations*. Chicago, IL: Nelson-Hall (pp. 2–24).

Tak, H., Ruhnke, G.W. & Shih, Y.-C.T. (2015) The association between patient-centered attributes of care and patient satisfaction. *Patient, 8*(2): 187–197.

Talaulikar, V. (2022) Menopause transition: Physiology and symptoms. *Best Practice & Research Clinical Obstetrics & Gynaecology, 81*: 3–7. doi: 10.1016/j.bpobgyn.2022.03.003.

Talevski, J., Shee, A.W., Rasmussen, B., Kemp, G. & Beachamp, A. (2020) Teach-back: A systematic review of implementation and impacts. *PLoS One, 15*(4): e0231350. doi:10.1371/journal.pone.0231350.

Talsma, D., Senkowski, D., Soto-Faraco, S. & Woldorff, M.G. (2010) The multifaceted interplay between attention and multisensory integration. *Trends in Cognitive Science, 14*(9): 400–410.

Tamminga, S.J., Emal, L.M., Boschman, J.S., Levasseur, A., Thota, A., Ruotsalainen, J.H., et al. (2023) Individual-level interventions for reducing occupational stress in healthcare workers. *Cochrane Database of Systematic Reviews, 5*(5): CD002892. doi:10.1002/14651858.CD002892.pub6.

Tan, C.C., Cheng, K.K. & Wang, W. (2015) Self-care management programme for older adults with diabetes: An integrative literature review. *International Journal of Nursing Practice, 21*(Suppl. 2): 115–124.

Tanaka, Y., Ikeda, K., Kaneko, Y., Ishiguro, N., & Takeuchi, T. (2024) Why does malaise/fatigue occur? Underlying mechanisms and potential relevance to treatments in rheumatoid arthritis. *Expert Review of Clinical Immunology, 20*(5): 485–499. doi:10.1080/1744666X.2024.2306220.

Tang, J.A., Oh, T., Scheer, J.K. & Parsa, A.T. (2014) The current trend of administering a patient-generated index in the oncological setting: A systematic review. *Oncology Reviews, 8*(1): 245. doi:10.4081/oncol.2014.245.

Tang, M., Liu, X., Wu, Q. & Shi, Y. (2020) The effects of cognitive-behavioral stress management for breast cancer patients. *Cancer Nursing, 43*(3), 222–237. doi:10.1097/NCC.0000000000000804.

Tanofsky-Kraff, M., Haynos, A., Kotler, L., Yanovski, S. & Yanovski, J. (2007) Laboratory-based studies of eating among children and adolescents. *Current Nutrition & Food Science, 3*(1): 55–74.

Tasbihgou, S.R., Vogels, M.F. & Absalom, A.R. (2018) Accidental awareness during general anaesthesia – a narrative review. *Anaesthesia, 73*: 112–122. doi:10.1111/anae.14124.

Tavakoli, P., Vollmer-Conna, U., Hadzi-Pavlovic, D. & Grimm, M.C. (2021) A review of inflammatory bowel disease: A model of microbial, immune and neuropsychological integration. *Public Health Reviews, 42*: 1603990. doi:10.3389/phrs.2021.1603990.

Taylor, C.B., Miller, N.H., Smith, P.M. & DeBusk, R.F. (1997) The effect of a home-based, case-managed, multifactorial risk-reduction program on reducing psychological distress in patients with cardiovascular disease. *Journal of Cardiopulmonary Rehabilitation, 17*(3): 157–162.

Taylor, S., Pinnock, H., Epiphanou, E., Pearce, G., Parke, H., Schwappach, A., Purushotham, N., Jacob, S., Griffiths, C., Greenhalgh, T. & Sheikh, A. (2014) A rapid synthesis of the evidence on interventions supporting self-management for people with long-term conditions: PRISMS – Practical systematic Review of Self-Management Support for long-term conditions. *Health Services and Delivery Research, 4/2*(53): 1–580.

Taylor, S.E. (2006) Tend and befriend: Biobehavioral bases of affiliation under stress. *Current Directions in Psychological Science, 15*(6): 273–277.

Taylor, S.E. (2012) Tend and befriend theory. In P.A.M. van Lange, A.W. Kruglanski & E.T. Higgins (eds), *Handbook of Theories of Social Psychology (Vol. 1)*. London: Sage (pp. 32–94).

Taylor, S.E. (2020) How are social ties protective? *Spanish Journal of Psychology, 23*: e41. doi:10.1017/SJP.2020.35.

Taylor, S.E., Saphire-Bernstein, S. & Seeman, T. E. (2009) Plasma oxytocin in women and plasma vasopressin in men are markers of distress in primary relationships. *Psychological Science, 21*(1): 3–7.

Teasdale, E.J., Leydon, G., Fraser, S., Roderick, P., Taal, M.W. & Tonkin-Crine, S. (2017) Patients' experiences after CKD diagnosis: A meta-ethnographic study and systematic review. *American Journal of Kidney Diseases, 70*(5): 656–665. doi: 10.1053/j.ajkd.2017.05.019.

Tedeshi, R.G. & Calhoun, L.G. (2004) *Posttraumatic Growth: Conceptual Foundation and Empirical Evidence*. Philadelphia, PA: Lawrence Erlbaum Associates.

Tedstone, J.E. & Tarrier, N. (2003) Posttraumatic stress disorder following medical illness and treatment. *Clinical Psychology Review, 23*(3): 409–448.

Tekampe, J., van Middendorp, H., Meeuwis, S.H., van Leusden J.W.R., Pacheco-López, G., Hermus, A.R.M.M. & Evers, A.W.M. (2017) Conditioning immune and endocrine parameters in humans: A systematic review. *Psychotherapy and Psychosomatics, 86*(2): 99–107.

Teshale, A.B., Htun, H.L., Owen, A., Gasevic, D. et al. (2023) The role of social determinants of health in cardiovascular diseases: An umbrella review. *Journal of the American Heart Association, 12*(13): e029765. doi:10.1161/JAHA.123.029765.

Tetui, M., Grindrod, K., Waite, N., VanderDoes, J. & Taddio, A. (2022) Integrating the CARD (Comfort Ask Relax Distract) system in a mass vaccination clinic to improve the experience of individuals during COVID-19 vaccination: A pre-post implementation study. *Human Vaccines & Immunotherapeutics, 18*(5): 2089500. doi:10.1080/21645515.2022.2089500.

Teye-Kwadjo, E., Kagee, A. & Swart, H. (2017) Predicting the intention to use condoms and actual condom use behaviour: A three-wave longitudinal study in Ghana. *Applied Psychology: Health and Well-being, 9*(1): 81–105. doi: 10.1111/aphw.12082.

Thacher, J.D., Gehring, U., Gruzieva, O., Standl, M., Pershagen, G., Bauer, C.-P., et al. (2018) Maternal smoking during pregnancy and early childhood and development of asthma and rhinoconjunctivitis: A MeDALL project. *Environmental Health Perspectives, 126*(4): 047005. doi: 10.1289/EHP2738.

Thier, S.L., Yu-Isenberg, K.S., Leas, B.F., Cantrell, C.R., DeBussey, S., Goldfarb, N.I. & Nash, D.B. (2008) In chronic disease, nationwide data show poor adherence by patients to medication and by physicians to guidelines. *American Journal of Managed Care, 17*: 48–57.

Thomsen, E.L., Boisen, K.A., Andersen, A., Jørgensen, S.E., Teilman, G. & Michelsen, S.I. (2023) Low level of well-being in young people with physical-mental multimorbidity: A population-based study.

Journal of Adolescent Health, 73(4): 707–714 doi:10.1016/j.jadohealth.2023.05.014.

Thomson, G. & Garrett, C. (2019) Afterbirth support provision for women following a traumatic/distressing birth: Survey of NHS hospital trusts in England. *Midwifery, 71*: 63–70. doi: 10.1016/j.midw.2019.01.004.

Thorn, B.E., Ward, L.C., Sullivan, M.J. & Boothby, J.L. (2003) Communal coping model of catastrophizing: Conceptual model building. *Pain, 107*(3): 280.

Thornton, C.P., Ruble, K. & Kozachik, S. (2020) Psychosocial interventions for adolescents and young adults with cancer: An integrative review. *Journal of Pediatric Hematology/Oncology Nursing, 37*(6): 408–422. doi:10.1177/1043454220919713.

Thumfart, K.M., Jawaid, A., Bright, K., Flachsmann, M. & Mansuy, I.M. (2022) Epigenetics of childhood trauma: Long term sequelae and potential for treatment. *Neuroscience & Biobehavioral Reviews, 132*: 1049–1066. doi:10.1016/j.neubiorev.2021.10.042.

Tian, X., Tang, R.Y., Xu, L.L., Xie, W., Chen, H., Pi, Y.P. & Chen, W.Q. (2020) Progressive muscle relaxation is effective in preventing and alleviating of chemotherapy-induced nausea and vomiting among cancer patients: A systematic review of six randomized controlled trials. *Supportive Care in Cancer, 28*(9): 4051–4058. doi:10.1007/s00520-020-05481-2.

Timmermans, I., Denollet, J., Pedersen, S.S., Meine, M. & Versteeg, H. (2018) Patient-reported causes of heart failure in a large European sample. *International Journal of Cardiology, 258*: 179–184. doi:10.1016/j.ijcard.2018.01.113.

Timmers, T., Janssen, L., Kool, R.B., & Kremer, J.A. (2020) Educating patients by providing timely information using smartphone and tablet apps: Systematic review. *Journal of Medical Internet Research, 22*(4): e17342. doi:10.2196/17342.

Tindle, H.A., Stevenson Duncan, M., Greevy, R.A., Vasan, R.S., Kundu, S., Massion, P.P. & Freiberg, M.S. (2018) Lifetime smoking history and risk of lung cancer: Results from the Framingham Heart Study. *Journal of the National Cancer Institute, 110*(11): 1201–1207. doi: 10.1093/jnci/djy041.

Tjepkema, M., Bushnik, T. & Bougie, E. (2019) Life expectancy of First Nations, Métis and Inuit household populations in Canada. *Health Reports, 30*: 3–10. doi:10.25318/82-003-x201901200001-eng.

Toates, F. (2009) An integrative theoretical framework for understanding sexual motivation, arousal, and behavior. *Journal of Sex Research, 46*(2–3): 168–193. doi:10.1080/00224490902747768.

Tobin, E.T., Kane, H.S., Saleh, D.J., Naar-King, S., Poowuttikul, P., Secord, E., Pierantoni, W., Simon, V.A. & Slatcher, R.B. (2015) Naturalistically observed conflict and youth asthma symptoms. *Health Psychology, 34*(6): 622–631.

Todd, J., Coutts-Bain, D., Wilson, E. & Clarke, P. (2023) Is attentional bias variability causally implicated in emotional vulnerability? A systematic review and meta-analysis. *Neuroscience and Biobehavioral Reviews, 146*: 105069. doi:10.1016/j.neubiorev.2023.105069.

Tolomeo, S., Chiao, B., Lei, Z., Chew, S.H. & Ebstein, R.P. (2020) A novel role of CD38 and oxytocin as tandem molecular moderators of human social behavior. *Neuroscience and Biobehavioral Reviews, 115*: 251–272. doi:10.1016/j.neubiorev.2020.04.013.

Tomori, C., Hernández-Cordero, S., Busath, N., Menon, P. & Pérez-Escamilla, R. (2022) What works to protect, promote and support breastfeeding on a large scale: A review of reviews. *Maternal & Child Nutrition, 18 Suppl 3*(Suppl 3): e13344. doi:10.1111/mcn.13344.

Torbahn, G., Brauchmann, J., Axon, E., Clare, K., Metzendorf, M.I., Wiegand, S., et al. (2022) Surgery for the treatment of obesity in children and adolescents. *Cochrane Database of Systematic Reviews, 9*(9): CD011740. doi:10.1002/14651858.CD011740.pub2.

Tortella-Feliu, M., Fullana, M.A., Pérez-Vigil, A. et al. (2019) Risk factors for posttraumatic stress disorder: An umbrella review. *Neuroscience & Biobehaioral Reviews, 107*: 154–165. doi:10.1016/j.neubiorev. 2019.09.013.

Toselli, S., Grigoletto, A., Zaccagni, L., Rinaldo, N., Badicu, G., Grosz, W.R. & Campa, F. (2021) Body image perception and body composition in early adolescents: A longitudinal study of an Italian cohort. *BMC Public Health, 21*(1): 1381. doi:10.1186/s12889-021-11458-5.

Toyama, N. (2016) Adults' explanations and children's understanding of contagious illnesses, non-contagious illnesses, and injuries. *Early Child Development & Care, 186*(4): 526–543. doi: 10.1080/0300 4430.2015. 1040785.

Trajkova, S., d'Errico, A., Soffietti, R., Sacerdote, C. & Ricceri, F. (2019) Use of antidepressants and risk of incident stroke: A systematic review and meta-analysis. *Neuroepidemiology, 53*(3–4): 142–151. doi: 10.1159/000500686.

Trauer, J.M., Qian, M.Y., Doyle, J.S., Rajaratnam, S.M. & Cunnington, D. (2015) Cognitive behavioral therapy for chronic insomnia: A systematic review and meta-analysis. *Annals of Internal Medicine, 163*(3): 191–204. doi:10.7326/M14-2841.

Travagin, G., Margola, D. & Revenson, T.A. (2015) How effective are expressive writing interventions for adolescents? A meta-analytic review. *Clinical Psychology Review, 36*: 42–55. doi:10.1016/j. cpr.2015.01.003.

Triolo, F., Harber-Aschan, L., Belvederi Murri, M., Calderón-Larrañaga, A., Vetrano, D.L., Sjöberg, L., et al. (2020) The complex interplay between depression and multimorbidity in late life: Risks and pathways. *Mechanisms of Ageing and Development, 192*: 111383. doi:10.1016/j. mad.2020.111383.

Tronieri, J.S., Wadden, T.A., Chao, A.M. & Tsai, A.G. (2019) Primary care interventions for obesity: Review of the evidence. *Current Obesity Reports, 8*: 128–136. doi: 10.1007/ s13679-019-00341-5.

Trueba, A.F. & Ritz, T. (2013) Stress, asthma, and respiratory infections: Pathways involving airway immunology and microbial endocrinology. *Brain, Behavior, and Immunity, 29*: 11–27. doi:10.1016/j. bbi.2012.09.012.

Trzepacz, P.T. & Baker, R.W. (1993) *The Psychiatric Mental Status Examination.* Oxford: Oxford University Press.

Tsao, C.W., Aday, A.W., Almarzooq, Z.I., Anderson, C.A.M., Arora, P., Avery, C.L., et al. (2023) Heart disease and stroke statistics-2023 update: A report from the American Heart Association. *Circulation, 147*(8): e93–e621. doi:10.1161/ CIR.0000000000001123.

Tsodikov, A., Gulati, R., Heijnsdijk, E.A.M., Pinsky, P.F., Moss, S.M., Qiu, S., et al. (2017) Reconciling the effects of screening on prostate cancer mortality in the ERSPC and PLCO trials. *Annals of Internal Medicine, 167*(7): 449–455. doi: 10.7326/ M16-2586.

Tsunematsu, T. (2023) What are the neural mechanisms and physiological functions of dreams? *Neuroscience Research, 189*: 54–59. doi:10.1016/j.neures.2022.12.017.

Turiano, N.A., Chapman, B.P., Agrigoroaei, S., Infurna, F.J. & Lachman, M. (2014) Perceived control reduces mortality risk at low, not high, education levels. *Health Psychology, 33*(8): 883–890.

Turiano, N.A., Chapman, B.P., Gruenewald, T.L. & Mroczek, D. K. (2015) Personality and the leading behavioral contributors of mortality. *Health Psychology, 34*(1): 51–60.

Turk Charles, S., Gatz, M., Kato, K. & Pedersen, N.L. (2008) Physical health 25 years later: The predictive ability of neuroticism. *Health Psychology, 27*(3): 369–378.

Turnbull, A., Seitz, A., Tadin, D. & Lin, F.V. (2022) Unifying framework for cognitive training interventions in brain aging. *Ageing Research Reviews, 81*: 101724. doi:10.1016/j.arr.2022.101724.

Turner, G., Green, R., Alae-Carew, C. & Dangour, A.D. (2021) The association of dimensions of fruit and vegetable access in the retail food environment with consumption; a systematic review. *Global Food Security*, 29: 100528. doi:10.1016/j.gfs.2021.100528.

Turner, J.S., Pettit, K.E., Buente, B.B., Humbert, A.J., Perkins, A.J. & Kline, J.A. (2016) Medical student use of communication elements and association with patient satisfaction: A prospective observational pilot study. *BMC Medical Education, 21*(16): 150.

Turner-Cobb, J.M. & Katsampouris, E. (2019) Stress. In C.D. Llewellyn, S. Ayers, C. McManus, S. Newman, K.J. Petrie, T.A. Revenson & J. Weinman (eds), *The Cambridge Handbook of Psychology, Health and Medicine* (3rd edition). Cambridge: Cambridge University Press.

Tversky, A. & Kahneman, D. (1974) Judgment under uncertainty: Heuristics and biases. *Science, 185*(4157): 1124–1130.

Tzelepis, F., Rose, S.K., Sanson-Fisher, R.W., Clinton-McHarg, T., Carey, M.L. & Paul, C.L. (2014) Are we missing the Institute of Medicine's mark? A systematic review of patient-reported outcome measures assessing quality of patient-centred cancer care. *BMC Cancer, 14*(1): 41.

Uchino, B.N., Kent de Grey, R.G., Cronan, S. & Trettevik, R. (2019) Social relationships. In C.D. Llewellyn, S. Ayers, C. McManus, S. Newman, K.J. Petrie, T.A. Revenson & J. Weinman (eds), *The Cambridge Handbook of Psychology, Health and Medicine* (3rd edition). Cambridge: Cambridge University Press.

Uchino, B.N., Trettevik, R., Kent de Grey, R.G., Cronan, S., Hogan, J. & Baucom, B.R.W. (2018) Social support, social integration, and inflammatory cytokines: A meta-analysis. *Health Psychology, 37*(5): 462–471. doi: 10.1037/hea0000594.

Uddenberg, E.R., Safwan, N., Saadedine, M., Hurtado, M.D., Faubion, S.S. & Shufelt, C.L. (2024) Menopause transition and cardiovascular disease risk. *Maturitas, 185*: 107974. doi:10.1016/j.maturitas.2024.107974.

UK Parliament Women and Equalities Committee (2022) *Menopause and the Workplace*. First Report of Session 2022–23, 28 July. London: UK Parliament. Available from https://publications.parliament.uk/pa/cm5803/cmselect/cmwomeq/91/report.html (accessed 25 July 2024).

Ukai, T., Tabuchi, T. & Iso, H. (2022) The impact of spousal behavior changes on smoking, drinking and physical activity: The longitudinal survey of middle-aged and elderly persons in Japan. *Preventive Medicine, 164*: 107293. doi:10.1016/j.ypmed.2022.107293.

UN Office on Drugs and Crime (2023) *Global Study on Homicide 2023*. New York: UN Office on Drugs and Crime.

UNAIDS (2024) *UNAIDS Data 2023*. Geneva: UNAIDS.

Ünal, B., Critchley, J.A., Fidan, D. & Capewell, S. (2005) Life-years gained from modern cardiological treatments and population risk factor changes in England and Wales, 1981–2000. *American Journal of Public Health, 95*(1): 103–108.

Ungar, M. & Theron, L. (2020) Resilience and mental health: How multisystemic processes contribute to positive outcomes. *Lancet Psychiatry, 7*: 441–448. doi:10.1016/S2215-0366(19)30434-1.

Ungar, N., Sieverding, M., Weidner, G., Ulrich, C.M. & Wiskemann, J. (2016) A self-regulation-based intervention to increase physical activity in cancer patients. *Psychology, Health & Medicine, 21*(2): 163–175. doi:10.1080/13548506.2015.1081255.

United Nations Department of Economic and Social Affairs, Population Division (2020) *Fertility among Young Adolescents Aged 10 to 14 Years*. New York: UNDESA.

Urech, C., Grossert, A., Alder, J., Scherer, S., Handschin, B., Kasenda, B., et al. (2018) Web-based stress management for newly diagnosed patients with cancer (STREAM): A randomized, wait-list controlled intervention study. *Journal of Clinical Oncology, 36*: 780–788.

Uribe, F.A.R., de Oliveira, S.B., Junior, A.G. & da Silva Pedroso, J. (2021) Association between the dispositional optimism and depression in young people: A systematic review and meta-analysis. *Psicologia, Reflexao e Critica*, *34*(1): 37. doi:10.1186/s41155-021-00202-y

Ussher, J.M. (2010) Are we medicalizing women's misery? A critical review of women's higher rates of reported depression. *Feminism & Psychology*, *20*(1): 9–35.

Ussher, J.M. (2019) Premenstrual syndrome. In C.D. Llewellyn, S. Ayers, C. McManus, S. Newman, K.J. Petrie, T.A. Revenson & J. Weinman (eds), *The Cambridge Handbook of Psychology, Health and Medicine* (3rd edition). Cambridge: Cambridge University Press.

Ussher, J.M., Hunter, M. & Cariss, M. (2002) A woman-centred psychological intervention for premenstrual symptoms, drawing on cognitive-behavioural and narrative therapy. *Clinical Psychology and Psychotherapy*, *9*(5): 319–331.

Vaghela, R., Santoro, C. & Braham, L. (2023) The psychological adjustment needs of individuals following an acquired brain injury: A systematic review. *Applied Neuropsychology: Adult*, *30*(5): 469–482. doi:10.1080/23279095.2021.1956927.

Valadez, E.A., Pine, D.S., Fox, N.A. & Bar-Haim, Y. (2022) Attentional biases in human anxiety. *Neuroscience & Biobehavioral Reviews*, *142*: 104917. doi:10.1016/j.neubiorev.2022.104917.

Valtorta, N.K., Kanaan, M., Gilbody, S. & Hanratty, B. (2018) Loneliness, social isolation and risk of cardiovascular disease in the English Longitudinal Study of Ageing. *European Journal of Preventive Cardiology*, *25*(13): 1387–1396. doi:10.1177/2047487318792696.

Vambheim, S.M., Kyllo, T.M., Hegland, S. & Bystad, M. (2021) Relaxation techniques as an intervention for chronic pain: A systematic review of randomized controlled trials. *Heliyon*, *7*(8): e07837. doi:10.1016/j.heliyon.2021.e07837.

van Bunderen, C.C. & Olsson, D.S. (2023) Meta-analysis of mortality in adults with growth hormone deficiency: Does growth hormone replacement therapy really improve mortality rates? *Best Practice & Research Clinical Endocrinology & Metabolism*, *37*(6): 101835. doi:10.1016/j.beem.2023.101835.

van den Dries, L., Juffer, F., van Ijzendoorn, M.H. & Bakermans-Kranenburg, M.J. (2009) Fostering security? A meta-analysis of attachment in adopted children. *Children and Youth Services Review*, *31*(3): 410–421.

van der Bruggen, C.O., Stams, G.J. & Bogels, S.M. (2008) Research review: The relation between child and parent anxiety and parental control. *Journal of Child Psychology and Psychiatry, and Allied Disciplines*, *49*(12): 1257–1269.

van der Feltz-Cornelis, C., Allen, S.F., Holt, R.I.G., Roberts, R., Nouwen, A. & Sartorius, N. (2021) Treatment for comorbid depressive disorder or subthreshold depression in diabetes mellitus: Systematic review and meta-analysis. *Brain and Behavior*, *11*(2): e01981. doi:10.1002/brb3.1981.

van Dessel, N., den Boeft, M., van der Wouden, J.C., Kleinstäuber, M., Leone, S.S., Terluin, B., et al. (2014) Non-pharmacological interventions for somatoform disorders and medically unexplained physical symptoms (MUPS) in adults. *Cochrane Database of Systematic Reviews*, *11*: Art. CD011142.

van Dis, E.A.M., van Veen, S.C., Hagenaars, M.A., Batelaan, N.M., Bockting, C.L.H., van den Heuvel, R.M., et al. (2020) Long-term outcomes of cognitive behavioral therapy for anxiety-related disorders: A systematic review and meta-analysis. *JAMA Psychiatry*, *77*(3): 265–273. doi: 10.1001/jamapsychiatry.2019.3986.

van Dixhoorn, J. & White, A. (2005) Relaxation therapy for rehabilitation and prevention in ischaemic heart disease: A systematic review and meta-analysis. *European Journal of Cardiovascular Prevention and Rehabilitation*, *12*(3): 193–202.

van Duinkerken, E., Snoek, F.J. & de Wit, M. (2020) The cognitive and psychological effects of living with Type 1 diabetes: A narrative review. *Diabetic Medicine*, *37*(4): 555–563. doi:10.1111/dme.14216.

van Eeden, A.E., van Hoeken, D. & Hoek, H.W. (2021) Incidence, prevalence and mortality of anorexia nervosa and bulimia nervosa. *Current Opinion in Psychiatry*, *34*(6): 515–524. doi:10.1097/YCO.0000000000000739.

van Gils, A., Schoevers, R.A., Bonvanie, I.J., Gelauff, J.M., Roest, A.M. & Rosmalen, J.G. (2016) Self-help for medically unexplained symptoms: A systematic review and meta-analysis. *Psychosomatic Medicine*, *78*(6): 728–739.

Van Heertum, K. & Rossi, B. (2017) Alcohol and fertility: How much is too much? *Fertility Research and Practice*, *3*(1): 10. First published 10 July. doi: 10.1186/s40738-017-0037-x.

van Hoorn, J., Shablack, H., Lindquist, K.A. & Telzer, E.H. (2019) Incorporating the social context into neurocognitive models of adolescent decision-making: A neuroimaging meta-analysis. *Neuroscience and Biobehavioral Reviews*, *101*: 129–142. doi:10.1016/j.neubiorev.2018.12.024.

van Ijzendoorn, M.H. & Kroonenberg, P.M. (1988) Cross-cultural patterns of attachment: A meta-analysis of the Strange Situation. *Child Development*, *59*(1): 147–156.

van Loon, A.W.G., Creemers, H.E., Okorn, A. et al. (2022) The effects of school-based interventions on physiological stress in adolescents: A meta-analysis. *Stress Health*, *38*: 187–209. doi:10.1002/smi.3081.

van Mulukom, V., Pummerer, L.J., Alper, S., Bai, H., Čavojová, V., Farias, J., et al. (2022) Antecedents and consequences of COVID-19 conspiracy beliefs: A systematic review. *Social Science & Medicine*, *301*: 114912. doi:10.1016/j.socscimed.2022.114912.

van Oosterhout, R.E.M., de Boer, A.R., Maas, A.H.E.M., Rutten, F.H., Bots, M.L. & Peters, S.A.E. (2020) Sex differences in symptom presentation in acute coronary syndromes: A systematic review and meta-analysis. *Journal of the American Heart Association*, *9*(9): e014733. doi:10.1161/JAHA.119.014733.

van Tuijl, L.A., Basten, M., Pan, K.Y., Vermeulen, R., Portengen, L., de Graeff, A., et al. (2023) Depression, anxiety, and the risk of cancer: An individual participant data meta-analysis. *Cancer*, *129*(20): 3287–3299. doi:10.1002/cncr.34853.

Van Wilder, L., Pype, P., Mertens, F. & Rammant, E. et al. (2021) Living with a chronic disease: Insights from patients with a low socioeconomic status. *BMC Family Practice*, *22*(1): 233. doi:10.1186/s12875-021-01578-7.

Vancampfort, D., Vanderlinden, J., De Hert, M., Soundy, A., Adámkova, M., Skjaerven, L.H., Catalán-Matamoros, D., Gyllensten, A.L., Gómez-Conesa, A. & Probst, M. (2014) A systematic review of physical therapy interventions for patients with anorexia and bulimia nervosa. *Disability and Rehabilitation*, *36*(8): 628–634.

Vargas-Román, K., Díaz-Rodríguez, C.L., Cañadas-De la Fuente, G.A., Gómez-Urquiza, J.L., Ariza, T. & De la Fuente-Solana, E. I. (2020) Anxiety prevalence in lymphoma: A systematic review and meta-analysis. *Health Psychology*, *39*(7): 580–588. doi:10.1037/hea0000869.

Vaz, J.S., Maia, M.F.S., Neves, P.A.R., Santos, T.M., Vidaletti, L.P. & Victora, C. (2021) Monitoring breastfeeding indicators in high-income countries: Levels, trends and challenges. *Maternal & Child Nutrition*, *17*(3): e13137. doi:10.1111/mcn.13137.

Veehof, M.M., Trompetter, H.R., Bohlmeijer, E.T. & Schreurs, K.M. (2016) Acceptance- and mindfulness-based interventions for the treatment of chronic pain: A meta-analytic review. *Cognitive Behaviour Therapy*, *5*(1): 5–31.

Veettil, S.K., Wong, T.Y., Loo, Y.S., Playdon, M.C., Lai, N.M., Giovannucci, E.L. & Chaiyakunapruk, N. (2021) Role of diet in colorectal cancer incidence: Umbrella review of meta-analyses of prospective observational studies. *JAMA Network Open*, *4*(2): e2037341. doi:10.1001/jamanetworkopen.2020.37341.

Vela, M.B., Erondu, A.I., Smith, N.A., Peek, M.E., Woodruff, J.N. & Chin, M.H. (2022) Eliminating explicit and implicit biases in health care: Evidence and research needs. *Annual Review of Public Health, 43*: 477–501. doi:10.1146/annurev-publhealth-052620-103528.

Velloza, J., Roche, S., Concepcion, T. & Ortblad, K.F. (2023) Advancing considerations of context in the evaluation and implementation of evidence-based biomedical HIV prevention interventions: A review of recent research. *Current Opinion in HIV and AIDS, 18*(1): 1–11. doi:10.1097/COH.0000000000000768.

Venktaramana, V., Loh, E.K.Y., Wong, C.J.W., Yeo, J.W., Teo, A.Y.T., Chiam, C.S.Y., et al. (2022) A systematic scoping review of communication skills training in medical schools between 2000 and 2020. *Medical Teacher, 44*(9): 997–1006. doi: 10.1080/0142159X.2022.2054693.

Venn, A., Bruinsma, F., Werther, G., Pyett, P., Baird, D., Jones, P., et al. (2004) The use of oestrogen to reduce the adult height of tall girls: Long-term effects on fertility. *Lancet, 364*(9444): 1513–1518.

Vernooij, R.W.M., Lancee, M., Cleves, A., Dahm, P., Bangma, C.H. & Aben, K.K.H. (2020) Radical prostatectomy versus deferred treatment for localised prostate cancer. *Cochrane Database of Systematic Reviews, 6*(6): Art. CD006590. doi: 10.1002/14651858.CD006590.pub3.

Victora, C.G., Bahl, R., Barros, A.J.D., França, G.V.A., Horton, S., Krasevec, J., et al. (2016) Breastfeeding in the 21st century: Epidemiology, mechanisms, and lifelong effect. *Lancet, 387*(10017): 475–490. doi: 10.1016/S0140-6736(15)01024-7.

Vilchinsky, N., Ginzburg, K., Fait, K. & Foa, E.B. (2017) Cardiac-disease-induced PTSD: A systematic review. *Clinical Psychology Review, 55*: 92–106. doi: 10.1016/j.cpr.2017.04.009.

Villanacci, V., Bassotti, G., Nascimbeni, R., Antonelli, E., Cadei, M., Fisogni, S., et al. (2008) Enteric nervous system abnormalities in inflammatory bowel diseases. *Neurogastroenterology & Motility, 20*(9): 1009–1016.

Visser, L.N.C, Tollenaar, M.S., de Haes, H.C.J.M. & Smets, E.M.A. (2017) The value of physicians' affect-oriented communication for patients' recall of information. *Patient Education and Counseling, 100*(11): 2116–2120. doi: 10.1016/j.pec.2017.06.005.

Vogeley, K. & Bente, G. (2010) 'Artificial humans': Psychology and neuroscience perspectives on embodiment and nonverbal communication. *Neural Networks, 23*(8–9): 1077–1090.

von Blanckenburg, P. & Leppin, N. (2018) Psychological interventions in palliative care. *Current Opinion in Psychiatry, 31*: 389–395. doi:10.1097/YCO.0000000000000441.

Vos, M.S. & de Haes, J.C.J.M. (2007) Denial in cancer patients: An explorative review. *Psycho-Oncology, 16*(1): 12–25. doi: 10.1002/pon.1051.

Voth, J. & Sirois, F.M. (2009) The role of self-blame and responsibility in adjustment to inflammatory bowel disease. *Rehabilitation Psychology, 54*(1): 99–108.

Vuilleumier, P. & Huang, Y.M. (2009) Emotional attention: Uncovering the mechanisms of affective biases in perception. *Current Directions in Psychological Science, 18*(3): 148–152.

Wadden, T.A., Tronieri, J.S., & Butryn, M.L. (2020) Lifestyle modification approaches for the treatment of obesity in adults. *American Psychology, 75*: 235–251. doi:10.1037/amp0000517

Walburn, J., Vedhara, K., Hankins, M., Rixon, L. & Weinman, J. (2009) Psychological stress and wound healing in humans: A systematic review and meta-analysis. *Journal of Psychosomatic Research, 67*(3): 253–271.

Walker, D.C., White, E.K. & Srinivasan, V.J. (2018) A meta-analysis of the relationships between body checking, body image avoidance, body image dissatisfaction, mood, and disordered eating. *International Journal of Eating Disorders, 51*(8): 745–770. doi: 10.1002/eat.22867.

Walker, E.R. & Druss, B.G. (2017) Cumulative burden of comorbid mental disorders, substance use disorders, chronic medical conditions, and poverty on health among adults in the USA. *Psychology, Health & Medicine*, *22*(6): 727–735. doi: 10.1080/13548506.2016.1227855.

Walker, J. (2001) *Control and the Psychology of Health*. Buckingham: Open University Press.

Walker, Z.J., Xue, S., Jones, M.P. & Ravindran, A.V. (2021) Depression, anxiety, and other mental disorders in patients with cancer in low- and lower-middle-income countries: A systematic review and meta-analysis. *JCO Global Oncology*, *7*: 1233–1250. doi:10.1200/GO.21.00056.

Wallis, C.J.D., Glaser, A., Hu, J.C., Huland, H., Lawrentschuk, N., Moon, D., et al.. (2018) Survival and complications following surgery and radiation for localized prostate cancer: An international collaborative review. *European Urology*, *73*(1): 11–20. doi: 10.1016/j.eururo.2017.05.055.

Wallston, K.A., Wallson, B.S. & DeVellis, R. (1978) Development of the multidimensional health locus of control (MHLC) scales. *Health Education Monographs*, *6*(2): 160–170.

Walsh, A.L., Lehmann, S., Zabinski, J., Truskey, M., Purvis, T., Gould, N.F., et al. (2019) Interventions to prevent and reduce burnout among undergraduate and graduate medical education trainees: A systematic review. *Academic Psychiatry*, *43*(4): 386–395. doi:10.1007/s40596-019-01023-z.

Walsh, J.C., Lynch, M., Murphy, A.W. & Daly, K. (2004) Factors influencing the decision to seek treatment for symptoms of acute myocardial infarction: An evaluation of the self-regulatory model of illness behaviour. *Journal of Psychosomatic Research*, *56*(1): 67–73.

Wampold, B.E., Minami, T., Tierney, S.C., Baskin, T.W. & Bhati, K.S. (2005) The placebo is powerful: Estimating placebo effects in medicine and psychotherapy from randomised clinical trials. *Journal of Clinical Psychology*, *61*(7): 835–854.

Wan, S.W., Chng, Y.J.D., Lim, S.H., Chong, C.S., Pikkarainen, M. & He, H.G. (2022) A systematic review and meta-analysis on the effectiveness of web-based psychosocial interventions among patients with colorectal cancer. *Journal of Advanced Nursing*, *78*(7): 1883–1896. doi:10.1111/jan.15258.

Wang, A.W., Hsu, W.Y. & Chang, C.S. (2023) Curvilinear prediction of posttraumatic growth on quality of life: A five-wave longitudinal investigation of breast cancer survivors. *Quality of Life Research*, *32*(11): 3185–3193. doi:10.1007/s11136-023-03464-4.

Wang, L., Liang, C., Chen, P., Cao, Y. & Zhang, Y. (2023) Effect of antidepressants on psychological comorbidities, disease activity, and quality of life in inflammatory bowel disease: A systematic review and meta-analysis. *Therapeutic Advances in Gastroenterology*, *16*: 17562848231155022. doi:10.1177/17562848231155022.

Wang, N., Pei, L., Zhang, M., Wang, G., Zheng, S., Kou, X. & Chen, H. (2024) The impact of psychological interventions on surgical site wound healing post-surgery in psoriasis patients: A meta-analysis. *International wound journal*, *21*(4), *Wound Journal*, *21*(4): e14509. doi:10.1111/iwj.14509.

Wang, Q., Sun, W. & Wu, H. (2022) Associations between academic burnout, resilience and life satisfaction among medical students: A three-wave longitudinal study. *BMC Medical Education, 22*(1): 248. doi:10.1186/s12909-022-03326-6.

Wang, S., Zhai, H., Wei, L., Shen, B. & Wang, J. (2020) Socioeconomic status predicts the risk of stroke death: A systematic review and meta-analysis. *Preventive Medicine Reports*, *19*: 101124. doi: 10.1016/j.pmedr.2020.101124.

Wang, T., Li, Y. & Zheng, X. (2024) Association of socioeconomic status with cardiovascular disease and cardiovascular risk factors: A systematic review and meta-analysis. *Journal of Public Health*, *32*: 385–399. doi:10.1007/s10389-023-01825-4.

Wang, T., Xu, M., Bi, Y. & Ning, G. (2018) Interplay between diet and genetic susceptibility in obesity and related traits. *Frontiers of Medicine*, *12*(6): 601–607. doi 10.1007/s11684-018-0648-6.

Wang, X., Dai, Z., Zhu, X., Li, Y., Ma, L., Cui, X. & Zhan, T. (2024) Effects of mindfulness-based stress reduction on quality of life of breast cancer patient: A systematic review and meta-analysis. *PLoS One*, *19*(7): e0306643. doi: 10.1371/journal.pone.0306643.

Wang, Y., Jiao, Y., Nie, J., O'Neil, A., Huang, W., Zhang, L., et al. (2020). Sex differences in the association between marital status and the risk of cardiovascular, cancer, and all-cause mortality: A systematic review and meta-analysis of 7,881,040 individuals. *Global Health Research and Policy*, *5*: 4. doi:10.1186/s41256-020-00133-8.

Wang, Z., Chen, X., Zhou, J., Loke, A.Y. & Li, Q. (2023) Posttraumatic growth in colorectal cancer survivors: A systematic review. *Clinical Psychology & Psychotherapy*, *30*(4): 740–753. doi:10.1002/cpp.2838.

Wankhar, D., Kumar, A.P., Vijayakumar, V., Balakrishnan, V.A.A., Ravi, P., Rudra, B. & K, M. (2024) Effect of meditation, mindfulness-based stress reduction, and relaxation techniques as mind–body medicine practices to reduce blood pressure in cardiac patients: A systematic review and meta-analysis. *Cureus*, *16*(4): e58434. doi: 10.7759/cureus.58434.

Warriach, Z.I., Patel, S., Khan, F. & Ferrer, G.F. (2022) Association of depression with cardiovascular diseases. *Cureus*, *14*(6): e26296. doi:10.7759/cureus.26296.

Watkins, E.R. (2016) *Rumination-Focused Cognitive-Behavioural Therapy for Depression.* New York: Guilford Press.

Watson, D. & Tellegen, A. (1985) Toward a consensual structure of mood. *Psychological Bulletin*, *98*(2): 219–223.

Watson, P.W.B. & McKinstry, B. (2009) A systematic review of interventions to improve recall of medical advice in healthcare consultations. *Journal of the Royal Society of Medicine*, *102*(6): 235–243.

Waxmonsky, J.G., Baweja, R., Bansal, P.S. & Waschbusch, D.A. (2021) A review of the evidence base for psychosocial interventions for the treatment of emotion dysregulation in children and adolescents. *Child and Adolescent Psychiatry Clinics of North America*, *30*(3): 573–594. doi:10.1016/j.chc.2021.04.008

Webb, R. & Ayers, S. (2015) Cognitive biases in processing infant emotion by women with depression, anxiety and post-traumatic stress disorder in pregnancy or after birth: A systematic review. *Cognition & Emotion*, *29*(7): 1278–1294.

Webb, R., Bond, R., Romero-Gonzalez, B., Mycroft, R. & Ayers, S. (2021) Interventions to treat fear of childbirth in pregnancy: A systematic review and meta-analysis. *Psychological Medicine*, *51*(12): 1964–1977. doi: 10.1017/S0033291721002324.

Webb, R., Ford, E., Easter, A., Shakespeare, J., Holly, J., Hogg, S., et al. (2023a) MATRIx Study Team. Conceptual frameworks of barriers and facilitators to perinatal mental healthcare: The MATRIx models. *BJPsych Open*, *9*(4): e127. doi: 10.1192/bjo.2023.510.

Webb, R., Uddin, N., Constantinou, G., Ford, E., Easter, A., Shakespeare, J., et al. (2023b) MATRIx Study Team. Meta-review of the barriers and facilitators to women accessing perinatal mental healthcare. *BMJ Open*, *13*(7): e066703. doi: 10.1136/bmjopen-2022-066703.

Wegwarth, O. & Gigerenzer, G. (2018) The barrier to informed choice in cancer screening: Statistical illiteracy in physicians and patients. *Recent Results Cancer Research*, *210*: 207–221. doi: 10.1007/978-3-319-64310-6_13.

Weight, C.J., Sellon, J.L., Lessard-Anderson, C.R., Shanafelt, T.D., Olsen, K.D. & Laskowski, E.R. (2013) Physical activity, quality of life, and burnout among physician trainees: The effect of a team-based, incentivized exercise program. *Mayo*

Clinic Proceedings, *88*(12): 1435–1442. doi:10.1016/j.mayocp.2013.09.010.

Weintraub, D., Aarsland, D., Chaudhuri, K.R., et al. (2022) The neuropsychiatry of Parkinson's disease: Advances and challenges. *Lancet Neurology*, *21*: 89–102. doi:10.1016/S1474-4422(21)00330-6.

Weisz, G. & Knaapen, L. (2009) Diagnosing and treating premenstrual syndrome in five western nations. *Social Science & Medicine*, *68*(8): 1498–1505.

Weiten, W. (2004) *Psychology Themes and Variations* (6th edition). Belmont, CA: Wadsworth/Thomson Learning.

Wells, A. (2010) Metacognitive theory and therapy for worry and generalized anxiety disorder: Review and status. *Journal of Experimental Psychopathology*, *1*(1): 133–145.

Welsh, J., Bishop, K., Booth, H., et al. (2021) Inequalities in life expectancy in Australia according to education level: A whole-of-population record linkage study. *International Journal for Equity in Health*, *20*(1): 178. doi:10.1186/s12939-021-01513-3.

Wen, Y., Yang, Y., Shen, J. & Luo, S. (2021) Anxiety and prognosis of patients with myocardial infarction: A meta-analysis. *Clinical Cardiology*, *44*(6): 761–770. doi:10.1002/clc.23605.

West, C. & Zimmerman, D.H. (1987) Doing gender. *Gender & Society*, *1*(2): 125–151.

Wettergren, L., Kettis-Lindblad, A., Sprangers, M. & Ring, L. (2009) The use, feasibility and psychometric properties of an individualised quality-of-life instrument: A systematic review of the SEIQoL-DW. *Quality of Life Research*, *18*(6): 737–746.

Wettstein, M., Wahl, H.W. & Siebert, J.S. (2020) 20-year trajectories of health in midlife and old age: Contrasting the impact of personality and attitudes toward own aging. *Psychology and Aging*, *35*(6): 910–924. doi:10.1037/pag0000464.

Whalley, B., Rees, K., Davies, P., Bennett, P., Ebrahim, S., Liu, Z., West, R., Moxham, T., Thompson, D.R. & Taylor, R.S. (2011) Psychological interventions for coronary heart disease. *Cochrane Database of Systematic Reviews*, *8*: Art. CD002902.

Whiteley, L.B., Olsen, E.M., Haubrick, K.K., Odoom, E., Tarantino, N. & Brown, L.K. (2021) A review of interventions to enhance HIV medication adherence. *Current HIV/AIDS Reports*, *18*(5): 443–457. doi:10.1007/s11904-021-00568-9.

Whittaker, A.C., Ginty, A., Hughes, B.M., Steptoe, A. & Lovallo, W.R. (2021) Cardiovascular stress reactivity and health: Recent questions and future directions. *Psychosomatic Medicine*, *83*(7): 756–766. doi:10.1097/PSY.0000000000000973.

Whitten, C.E., Donovan, M. & Cristobal, K. (2005) Treating chronic pain: New knowledge, more choices. *The Permanente Journal*, *9*(4): 9–18.

Widmer, R.J., Prasad, M., Gomaa, M., Sara, J.D.S., Reriani, M.K., Lerman, L.O., Suwaidi, J.A. & Lerman A. (2020) Vascular reactivity to mental stress is associated with poor cardiovascular disease outcomes in females following acute coronary syndrome. *Coronary Artery Disease*, *31*(3): 300–305. doi:10.1097/MCA.0000000000000831.

Wieser, M.J., Pauli, P., Alpers, G.W. & Mühlberger, A. (2009) Is eye to eye contact really threatening and avoided in social anxiety? An eye-tracking and psychophysiology study. *Journal of Anxiety Disorders*, *23*(1): 93–103. doi: 10.1016/j.janxdis.2008.04.004.

Wilkinson, H., Whittington, R., Perry, L. & Eames, C. (2017) Examining the relationship between burnout and empathy in healthcare professionals: A systematic review. *Burnout Research*, *6*: 18–29. doi: 10.1016/j.burn.2017.06.003.

Wilkinson, N., Paikan, A., Gredebäck, G., Rea, F. & Metta, G. (2014) Staring us in the face? An embodied theory of innate face preference. *Developmental Science*, *17*(6): 809–825. doi:10.1111/desc.12159.

Wilkinson, T.A., Jenkins, K., Hawryluk, B.A., Moore, C.M., Wiehe, S.E. & Kottke, M.J. (2022) Dual protection messaging for adolescents and young adults in the setting of over-the-counter hormonal contraception: A human-centered design approach. *Journal of Pediatric and Adolescent Gynecology, 35*(6): 669–675. doi:10.1016/j.jpag.2022.08.009.

Williams, A.C. & Craig, K.D. (2016) Updating the definition of pain. *Pain, 157*(11): 2420–2423.

Williams, A.C.C., Fisher, E., Hearn, L. & Eccleston, C. (2020) Psychological therapies for the management of chronic pain (excluding headache) in adults. *Cochrane Database of Systematic Review, 8*(8): Art. CD007407. doi: 10.1002/14651858.CD007407.pub4.

Willroth, E.C., Luo, J., Atherton, O.E., Weston, S.J., Drewelies, J., Batterham, P.J., et al. (2023) Personality traits and health care use: A coordinated analysis of 15 international samples. *Journal of Personality and Social Psychology, 125*(3): 629–648. doi:10.1037/pspp0000465.

Wilson, L.F., Doust, J., Mishra, G.D. & Dobson, A.J. (2023) Symptom patterns and health service use of women in early adulthood: A latent class analysis from the Australian Longitudinal Study on Women's Health. *BMC Public Health, 23*(1): 147. doi:10.1186/s12889-023-15070-7.

Wilson, T.E., Gousse, Y., Joseph, M.A. et al. (2019) HIV prevention for Black heterosexual men: The Barbershop Talk with Brothers cluster randomized trial. *American Journal of Public Health, 109*(8): 1131–1137. doi:10.2105/AJPH.2019.305121.

Wilson, T.E., Weedon, J., Cohen, M.H., Golub, E.T. et al. (2017) Positive affect and its association with viral control among women with HIV infection. *Health Psychology, 36*(1): 91–100. doi:10.1037/hea0000382.

Windover, A.K., Boissy, A., Rice, T.W., Gilligan, T., Velez, V.J. & Merlino, J. (2014) The REDE model of healthcare communication: Optimizing relationship as a therapeutic agent. *Journal of Patient Experience, 1*(1): 8–13. doi: 10.1177/237437431400100103.

Witkop, M., Morgan, G., O'Hara, J., et al. (2021). Patient preferences and priorities for haemophilia gene therapy in the US: A discrete choice experiment. *Haemophilia, 27*(5): 769–782. doi:10.1111/hae.14383.

Wolchik, S.A., Schenck, C.E. & Sandler, I.N. (2009) Promoting resilience in youth from divorced families: Lessons learned from experimental trials of the new beginnings program. *Journal of Personality, 77*(6): 1833–1868. doi: 10.1111/j.1467-6494.2009.00602.x.

Wolff, A., Schumacher, N.U. & Pürner, D. et al. (2023) Parkinson's disease therapy: What lies ahead? *Journal of Neural Transmission, 130*: 793–820. doi:10.1007/s00702-023-02641-6.

Worden, J.W. (2018) *Grief Counselling and Grief Therapy: A Handbook for the Mental Health Practitioner* (5th edition). New York: Springer.

World Health Organization (1992) *Basic Documents* (39th edition). Geneva: WHO.

World Health Organization (1996) *Diagnostic and Management Guidelines for Mental Disorders in Primary Care. ICD-10 Chapter V Primary Care Version.* Geneva: WHO.

World Health Organization (2006) *Report of a Technical Consultation on Sexual Health, 28–31 January 2002.* Geneva: WHO.

World Health Organization (2008) *Closing the Gap in a Generation: Health Equity through Action on the Social Determinants of Health.* Geneva: WHO, Commission on Social Determinants of Health.

World Health Organization (2009) *Surgical Safety Checklist.* Geneva: WHO.

World Health Organization (2013) *Long-term Effects of Breastfeeding: A Systematic Review.* Geneva: WHO.

World Health Organization (2015) Caesarean sections should be performed only when necessary. *News Release.* Geneva: WHO.

World Health Organization (2018) *Global Status Report on Alcohol and Health*, 2018. Geneva: WHO.

World Health Organization (2019a) *International Classification of Diseases for*

Mortality and Morbidity Statistics (ICD-11 MMS), 2018 version. Geneva: WHO.

World Health Organization (2019b) Global and regional STI estimates. *The Global Health Observatory.* Available from www.who.int/data/gho/data/themes/topics/global-and-regional-sti-estimates (accessed 11 May 2024).

World Health Organization (2020a) *World Health Statistics 2020: Monitoring Health for the SDGs, Sustainable Development Goals.* Geneva: WHO.

World Health Organization (2020a) The top 10 causes of death. *Newsroom: Fact Sheets.* Geneva: WHO. Available from www.who.int/news-room/fact-sheets/detail/the-top-10-causes-of-death (accessed 26 July 2024).

World Health Organization (2020b) Palliative care. *Health Topics.* Geneva: WHO. Available from www.who.int/cancer/palliative/definition/en/ (accessed 14 July 2020).

World Health Organization (2020c) Healthy diet. *Newsroom: Fact Sheets.* Geneva: WHO. Available from www.who.int/news-room/fact-sheets/detail/healthy-diet (accessed 25 May 2024).

World Health Organization (2021) Caesarean section rates continue to rise, amid growing inequalities in access. *News*, 16 June. Available from www.who.int/news/item/16-06-2021-caesarean-section-rates-continue-to-rise-amid-growing-inequalities-in-access (accessed 30 July 2024).

World Health Organization (2022) Mental disorders. *Newsroom: Fact Sheets.* Geneva: WHO. Available from www.who.int/news-room/fact-sheets/detail/mental-disorders (accessed 30 July 2024).

World Health Organization (2023a) *Advancing the Global Agenda on Prevention and Control of Communicable Diseases 2000 to 2020: Looking Forwards to 2030.* Geneva: WHO.

World Health Organization (2023b) *World Health Statistics 2023: Monitoring Health for the SDGs, Sustainable Development Goals.* Geneva: WHO.

World Health Organization (2024a) Tobacco. *Newsroom: Fact Sheets.* Geneva: WHO. Available from www.who.int/news-room/fact-sheets/detail/tobacco (accessed 25 June 2024).

World Health Organization (2024b) *World Mental Health Report: Transforming Mental Health for All.* Geneva: WHO. Available from www.who.int/publications/i/item/9789240049338 (accessed 19 July 2024).

World Health Organization (2024c) Cause-specific mortality, 2000–2019. *The Global Health Observatory.* Available from www.who.int/data/gho/data/themes/mortality-and-global-health-estimates/ghe-leading-causes-of-death (accessed 6 May 2024).

World Health Organization (2024d) Life expectancy at birth (years). *The Global Health Observatory.* Available from www.who.int/data/gho/data/indicators/indicator-details/GHO/life-expectancy-at-birth-(years) (accessed 7 May 2024).

World Health Organization (2024e) Social determinants of health. *Health Topics.* Available from www.who.int/health-topics/social-determinants-of-health#tab=tab_1 (accessed 17 January 2024).

World Health Organization (2024f) Disability. *Health Topics.* Available from www.who.int/health-topics/disability (accessed 14 June 2024).

World Health Organization (2024g) *International Statistical Classification of Diseases and Related Health Problems* (ICD-11). Geneva: WHO.

World Health Organizaton Human Reproduction Programme (2019) *Adolescent Pregnancy.* Geneva: WHO

Wright, B. & Bragge, P. (2018) Interventions to promote healthy eating choices when dining out: A systematic review of reviews. *British Journal of Health Psychology*, 23(2): 278–295. doi: 10.1111/bjhp.12285.

Wright, D.B. & Loftus, E.F. (2008) Eyewitness memory. In G. Cohen & M. Conway (eds), *Memory in the Real World* (3rd edition). New York: Psychology (pp. 91–105).

Wu, A.D., Lindson, N., Hartmann-Boyce, J., Wahedi, A., Hajizadeh, A., Theodoulou, A., et al. (2022) Smoking cessation for secondary prevention of cardiovascular disease. *Cochrane Database of Systematic Reviews, 8*(8): CD014936. doi:10.1002/14651858.CD014936.pub2.

Wu, Y., Strating, M., Ahaus, C.T.B. & Buljac-Samardzic, M. (2024) Prevalence, risk factors, consequences, and prevention and management of patient aggression and violence against physicians in hospitals: A systematic review. *Aggression and Violent Behavior, 74*: 101892. doi:10.1016/j.avb.2023.10189.

Wutz, M., Hermes, M., Winter, V. & Köberlein-Neu, J. (2023). Factors influencing the acceptability, acceptance, and adoption of conversational agents in health care: Integrative review. *Journal of Medical Internet Research, 25*: e46548. doi:10.2196/46548.

Wynn, M. & Holloway, S. (2019) The impact of psychological stress on wound healing: A theoretical and clinical perspective. *Wounds UK, 15*(3): 20–27.

Xavier, M.J., Roman, S.D., Aitken, R.J. & Nixon, B. (2019) Transgenerational inheritance: How impacts to the epigenetic and genetic information of parents affect offspring health. *Human Reproduction Update, 25*(5): 518–540. doi:10.1093/humupd/dmz017.

Xia, W., Ding, J., Yan, Y., Chen, F., Yan, M. & Xu, X. (2024) Effectiveness of virtual reality technology in symptom management of patients at the end of life: A systematic review and meta-analysis. *Journal of the American Medical Directors Association*, 13 June: 105086. doi: 10.1016/j.jamda.2024.105086. Epub ahead of print.

Xu, M., Luo, Y., Zhang, Y., Xia, R., Qian, H. & Zou, X. (2023) Game-based learning in medical education. *Frontiers in Public Health, 11*: 1113682. doi: 10.3389/fpubh.2023.1113682.

Yaegashi, H., Kirino, S., Remington, G., Misawa, F. & Takeuchi, H. (2020) Adherence to oral antipsychotics measured by electronic adherence monitoring in schizophrenia: A systematic review and meta-analysis. *CNS Drugs, 34*(6): 579–598. doi: 10.1007/s40263-020-00713-9.

Yaghmour, S.M. (2022) Impact of settings and culture on nurses' knowledge of and attitudes and perceptions towards people with dementia: An integrative literature review. *Nursing Open, 9*: 66–93. doi:10.1002/nop2.1106.

Yamamoto, T., Shimoyama, T. & Kuriyama, M. (2017) Dietary and enteral interventions for Crohn's disease. *Current Opinion in Biotechnology, 44*: 69–73. doi: 10.1016/j.copbio.2016.11.011.

Yan, T., Chan, C.W.H., Chow, K.M., Zheng, W. & Sun, M. (2020) A systematic review of the effects of character strengths-based intervention on the psychological well-being of patients suffering from chronic illnesses. *Journal of Advanced Nursing, 76*(7): 1567–1580. doi: 10.1111/jan.14356.

Yang, J.J. & Jiang, W. (2020) Immune biomarkers alterations in post-traumatic stress disorder: A systematic review and meta-analysis. *Journal of Affective Disorders, 268*: 39–46. doi: 10.1016/j.jad.2020.02.044.

Yang, L., Cambou, M.C. & Nielsen-Saines, K. (2023) The end is in sight: Current strategies for the elimination of HIV vertical transmission. *Current HIV/AIDS Reports, 20*(3): 121–130. doi:10.1007/s11904-023-00655-z.

Yau, K.W., Tang, T.S., Görges, M., Pinkney, S., Kim, A.D., Kalia, A. & Amed, S. (2022) Effectiveness of mobile apps in promoting healthy behavior changes and preventing obesity in children: Systematic review. *JMIR Pediatrics and Parenting, 5*(1): e34967. doi: 10.2196/34967.

Yayan, J. & Rasche, K. (2023) Risk factors for depression in patients with chronic obstructive pulmonary disease. *Respiratory Physiology & Neurobiology, 315*: 104110. doi:10.1016/j.resp.2023.104110.

Ye, G., Baldwin, D.S. & Hou, R. (2021) Anxiety in asthma: A systematic review and meta-analysis. *Psychological Medicine, 51*(1): 11–20. doi:10.1017/S0033291720005097.

Yedidia, M.J., Gillespie, C.C., Kachur, E., Schwartz, M.D., Ockene, J., Chepaitis, A.E., Snyder, C.W., Lazare, A. & Lipkin Jr., M. (2003) Effect of communications training on medical student performance. *Journal of the American Medical Association, 290*(9): 1157–1165.

Yi, S., Kanetkar, V. & Brauer, P. (2022) Nudging food service users to choose fruit- and vegetable-rich items: Five field studies. *Appetite, 173*: 105978. doi:10.1016/j.appet.2022.105978.

Yih, J., Uusberg, A., Taxer, J.L. & Gross, J.J. (2019) Better together: A unified perspective on appraisal and emotion regulation. *Cognition and Emotion, 33*(1): 41–47. doi:10.1080/02699931.2018.1504749.

Yildiz, P.D., Ayers, S. & Phillips, L. (2017) The prevalence of posttraumatic stress disorder in pregnancy and after birth: A systematic review and meta-analysis. *Journal of Affective Disorders, 208*: 634–645. doi: 10.1016/j.jad.2016.10.009.

Ying, M., Shao, X., Qin, H., Yin, P., Lin, Y., Wu, J., et al. (2024) Disease burden and epidemiological trends of chronic kidney disease at the global, regional, national levels from 1990 to 2019. *Nephron, 148*(2): 113–123. doi:10.1159/000534071.

Yorke, J., Fleming, S., Shuldham, C., Rao, H. & Smith, H.E. (2015) Nonpharmacological interventions aimed at modifying health and behavioural outcomes for adults with asthma: A critical review. *Clinical & Experimental Allergy, 45*(12): 1750–1764. doi: 10.1111/cea.12511.

Young, H.N., Len-Rios, M.E., Brown, R., Moreno, M.M. & Cox, E. (2016) How does patient-provider communication influence adherence to asthma medications? *Patient Education and Counseling, 100*(4): 696–702.

Young, Q.R., Ignaszewski, A., Fofonoff, D. & Kaan, A. (2007) Brief screen to identify five of the most common forms of psychosocial distress in cardiac patients: Validation of the screening tool for psychological distress (STOP-D). *Journal of Cardiovascular Nursing, 22*(6): 525–534.

Yousef, M., Rundle-Thiele, S. & Dietrich, T. (2023) Advertising appeals effectiveness: A systematic literature review. *Health Promotion Internationals, 38*(4): daab204. doi: 10.1093/heapro/daab204.

Youssef, N.A., McCall, W.V. & Andrad, C. (2017) The role of ECT in posttraumatic stress disorder: A systematic review. *Annals of Clinical Psychiatry, 29*(1): 62–70.

Yussof, I., Tahir, N.A.M., Hatah, E. & Shah, N.M. (2022) Factors influencing five-year adherence to adjuvant endocrine therapy in breast cancer patients: A systematic review. *Breast, 62*: 22–35. doi:10.1016/j.breast.2022.01.012

Zagaria, A., Vacca, M., Cerolini, S., Ballesio, A., & Lombardo, C. (2022) Associations between orthorexia, disordered eating, and obsessive-compulsive symptoms: A systematic review and meta-analysis. *The International Journal of Eating Disorders, 55*(3), 295–312. doi:10.1002/eat.23654.

Zaharias, G. (2018) What is narrative-based medicine? Narrative-based medicine 1. *Canadian Family Physician, 64*(3): 176–180.

Zaki, J. & Williams, W.C. (2013) Interpersonal emotion regulation. *Emotion, 13*(5): 803–810.

Zamani, M. & Alizadeh-Tabari, S. (2023) Anxiety and depression prevalence in digestive cancers: A systematic review and meta-analysis. *BMJ Supportive & Palliative Care, 13*(e2): e235–e243. doi:10.1136/bmjspcare-2021-003275.

Zamani, M., Alizadeh-Tabari, S. & Zamani, V. (2019) Systematic review with meta-analysis: The prevalence of anxiety and depression in patients with irritable bowel syndrome. *Alimentary Pharmacology & Therapeutics, 50*(2): 132–143. doi: 10.1111/apt.15325.

Zanatta, F., Tabernero, C., Steca, P., Castillo-Mayén, R., Cuadrado, E. & Luque, B. (2024) Predicting physical activity and quality of life in coronary heart disease patients: An 18-month path analysis of motivational and emotional factors. *Health Psychology, 43*(5): 352–364. doi:10.1037/hea0001348.

Zanella, E. & Lee, E. (2022) Integrative review on psychological and social risk and prevention factors of eating disorders including anorexia nervosa and bulimia nervosa: Seven major theories. *Heliyon*, 8(11): e11422. doi:10.1016/j.heliyon.2022. e11422.

Zautra, A.J. & Reich, J.W. (2010) Resilience: The meanings, methods, and measures of a fundamental characteristic of human adaptation. In S. Folkman (ed.), *The Oxford Handbook of Stress, Health, and Coping*. Oxford: Oxford University Press.

Zeng, Y., Wang, J., Cai, X., Zhang, X., Zhang, J., Peng, M., et al. (2023) Effects of physical activity interventions on executive function in older adults with dementia: A meta-analysis of randomized controlled trials. *Geriatric Nursing*, 51: 369–377. doi:10.1016/j.gerinurse.2023.04.012.

Zhang, A., Borhneimer, L.A., Weaver, A., Franklin, C., Hai, A.H., Guz, S. & Shen, L. (2019) Cognitive behavioral therapy for primary care depression and anxiety: A secondary meta-analytic review using robust variance estimation in meta-regression. *Journal of Behavioral Medicine*, 42(6): 1117–1141. doi: 10.1007/s10865-019-00046-z.

Zhang, C., Xu, S., Wen, X. & Liu, M. (2023) The effect of expressive writing on Chinese cancer patients: A systematic review and meta-analysis of randomized control trails. *Clinical Psychology & Psychotherapy, 30*(6): 1357–1368. doi:10.1002/cpp.2878.

Zhang, J., Wu, M., Li, J., Song, W., Lin, X. & Zhu, L. (2024) Effects of virtual reality-based rehabilitation on cognitive function and mood in multiple sclerosis: A systematic review and meta-analysis of randomized controlled trials. *Multiple Sclerosis and Related Disorders*, 87: 105643. doi: 10.1016/j.msard.2024.105643.

Zhang, L., Ni, Z., Liu, Y. & Chen, H. (2023) The effectiveness of e-health on reducing stigma, improving social support and quality of life among people living with HIV: A systematic review and meta-analysis of randomized controlled trials. *International Journal of Nursing Studies, 148*: 104606. doi:10.1016/j. ijnurstu.2023.104606.

Zhang, S., Xu, M., Liu, Z.J., Feng, J. & Ma, Y. (2020) Neuropsychiatric issues after stroke: Clinical significance and therapeutic implications. *World Journal of Psychiatry*, 10: 125–138. doi:10.5498/wjp. v10.i6.125.

Zhang, X., Li, L., Zhang, Q., Le, L.H. & Wu, Y. (2024) Physician empathy in doctor–patient communication: A systematic review. *Health Communication*, 39(5): 1027–1037. doi: 10.1080/10410236.2023.2201735.

Zhang, Y. & Han, B. (2016) Positive affect and mortality risk in older adults: A meta-analysis. *PsyCh Journal*, 5: 125–138. doi:10.1002/pchj.129.

Zhang, Y., Joshy, G., Glass, K. & Banks, E. (2020) Physical functional limitations and psychological distress in people with and without colorectal cancer: Findings from a large Australian study. *Journal of Cancer Survivorship*, 14(6): 894–905. doi:10.1007/s11764-020-00901-y.

Zhang, Y., Ren, R., Yang, L., Zhang, H., Shi, Y., Shi, J., Sanford, L.D., Lu, L., Vitiello, M.V. & Tang, X. (2022) Comparative efficacy and acceptability of psychotherapies, pharmacotherapies, and their combination for the treatment of adult insomnia: A systematic review and network meta-analysis. *Sleep Medicine Reviews*, 65: 101687. doi: 10.1016/j.smrv.2022.101687.

Zhang, Y. & Zhao, X. (2021) Effects of the Health Belief Model-Based intervention on anxiety, depression, and quality of life in chronic obstructive pulmonary disease. *Neuroimmunomodulation*, 28: 129–136. doi:10.1159/000512993.

Zhang, Y.B., Chen, C., Pan, X.F., Guo, J., Li, Y., Franco, O.H., et al. (2021) Associations of healthy lifestyle and socioeconomic status with mortality and incident cardiovascular disease: two prospective cohort studies. *BMJ (Clinical Research Ed.), 373*: n604. doi:10.1136/ bmj.n604.

Zhao, X. (2023) Challenges and barriers in intercultural communication between patients with immigration backgrounds and health professionals: A systematic literature review. *Health Communication*, 8: 24–33. doi:10.1080/10410236.2021.1980188.

Zheng, R., Wang, S., Zhang, S., Zeng, H., Chen, R., Sun, K., et al. (2023) Global, regional, and national lifetime probabilities of developing cancer in 2020. *Science Bulletin*, 68(21): 2620–2628. doi:10.1016/j.scib.2023.09.041.

Zhou, Y., Graham, L. & West, C. (2016) The relationship between study strategies and academic performance. *International Journal of Medical Education*, 7: 324–332. doi: 10.5116/ijme.57dc.fe0f.

Zhu, J., Fang, F., Sjölander, A., Fall, K., Adami, H.O. & Valdimarsdóttir, U. (2017) First-onset mental disorders after cancer diagnosis and cancer-specific mortality: A nationwide cohort study. *Annals of Oncology*, 28(8): 1964–1969. doi: 10.1093/annonc/mdx265s.

Zhu, J., Hay, P.J., Yang, Y., Le Grange, D., Lacey, J.H., Lujic, S., Smith, C. & Touyz, S. (2023) Specific psychological therapies versus other therapies or no treatment for severe and enduring anorexia nervosa. *Cochrane Database of Systematic Reviews*. 8. Art. No.: CD011570. DOI: 10.1002/14651858.CD011570.pub2.

Zipkin, D.A., Umscheid, C.A., Keating, N.L., Allen, E., Aung, K., Beyth, R., Kaatz, S., Mann, D.M., Sussman, J.B., Korenstein, D.,

Schardt, C., Nagi, A., Sloane, R. & Feldstein, D.A. (2014) Evidence-based risk communication: A systematic review. *Annals of Internal Medicine*, 161(4): 270–280. doi: 10.7326/M14-0295.

Zivkovic, S., Koh, C.H., Kaza, N. & Jackson, C.A. (2019) Antipsychotic drug use and risk of stroke and myocardial infarction: A systematic review and meta-analysis. *BMC Psychiatry*, 19(1): 189. doi: 10.1186/s12888-019-2177-5.

Zorbas, C., Reeve, E., Naughton, S., Batis, C., Whelan, J., Waqa, G. & Bell, C. (2020) The relationship between feasting periods and weight gain: A systematic scoping review. *Current Obesity Reports*, 9(1): 39–62. doi:10.1007/s13679-020-00370-5.

Zou, H., Cao, X. & Chair, S.Y. (2021) A systematic review and meta-analysis of mindfulness-based interventions for patients with coronary heart disease. *Journal of Advanced Nursing*, 77(5): 2197–2213. doi:10.1111/jan.14738.

Zuelke, A.E., Luppa, M., Löbner, M., Pabst, A., Schlapke, C., Stein, J. & Riedel-Heller, S.G. (2021) Effectiveness and feasibility of internet-based interventions for grief after bereavement: Systematic review and meta-analysis. *JMIR Mental Health*, 8(12): e29661. doi:10.2196/29661.

Zvolensky, M.J. & Eifert, G.H. (2001) A review of psychological factors/processes affecting anxious responding during voluntary hyperventilation and inhalations of carbon dioxide-enriched air. *Clinical Psychology Review*, 21(3): 375–400.

INDEX

Page numbers followed by "f" indicate figures; those followed by "t" indicate tables.